Handbook of Behavioral Health Disability Management

Pamela A. Warren
Editor

Handbook of Behavioral Health Disability Management

Springer

Editor
Pamela A. Warren
Carle Physician Group
and University of Illinois Medical School
Department of Psychiatry
Monticello, IL, USA

ISBN 978-3-030-07879-9 ISBN 978-3-319-89860-5 (eBook)
https://doi.org/10.1007/978-3-319-89860-5

Printed on acid-free paper

This Springer imprint is published by the registered company Springer International Publishing AG part of Springer Nature.
The registered company address is: Gewerbestrasse 11, 6330 Cham, Switzerland

Contents

Chapter 1
A Critique of the Behavioral Health Disability System

Pamela A. Warren

1.1 Overview of the Explosion of Behavioral Health Concerns

There is an increased recognition of behavioral health (BH) concerns occurring with increasing frequency both with treating professionals and within disability systems. However, there is also confusion about what this term encompasses. The behavioral health spectrum is comprised of mental health disorders, such as Major Depressive Disorder (MDD) and also psychosocial issues, such as job dissatisfaction, workplace conflict, and a lack of balance between personal life and work. BH concerns are a huge cost to society as well as to the individual. A review of the empirical literature (Agency for Healthcare Research and Quality, 2009; American Psychiatric Foundation, 2005; Talmage & Melhorn, 2005; Warren, 2013a, 2013b) and the actuarial data from federal disability programs, such as the Social Security Administration (SSA, 2015) and insurers (Warren & Hubbard, 2008), have demonstrated 300% + increases in behavioral disability claims over the past two decades. Based on direct medical costs, such as medical, medication, absenteeism, and short- and long-term disability, the annual costs of mental health disorders total $253 billion (Warren, 2005). However, when indirect costs, such as presenteeism and psychosocial issues are considered, the total costs rise to a staggering $1.265 trillion. In the USA alone, workplace behavioral health disorders cost employers $114 billion per year (DMEC, 2009). These concerns are not isolated to the USA alone. The World Health Organization (WHO) has predicted that by the year 2020, MDD will be the leading cause of disability, globally. Currently, MDD is the second leading cause of disability (WHO, 2004).

P. A. Warren (✉)
Carle Physician Group and University of Illinois Medical School, Department of Psychiatry, Monticello, IL, USA

P. A. Warren (ed.), *Handbook of Behavioral Health Disability Management*,
https://doi.org/10.1007/978-3-319-89860-5_1

1.2 Problematic Factors that Complicate Behavioral Healthcare

1.2.1 Comorbid Physical and Psychological Concerns

BH issues have been identified as occurring both as individual concerns and as a comorbidity issue with physical injuries and illnesses (American Medical Association, 2008; American Psychiatric Association and American Psychiatric Foundation, 2006, 2005). The term "behavioral health" currently is used by professionals to encompass true psychiatric disorders, such as those that meet the *Diagnostic Statistical Manual of Mental Disorders, 5th Edition* (American Psychiatric Association, *DSM-5*, 2013), as well as psychosocial issues, such as workplace difficulties or personal life matters (American Medical Association, 2008). Moreover, the review of empirical research has revealed that the majority of physical concerns also have a concurrent psychiatric component (Buist-Bouwman, de Graaf, Vollebergh, & Ormel, 2005; Chellappa & Ramaraj, 2009; Dersh, Gatchel, Polatin, & Mayer, 2002; Dewa & Lin, 2000; de Waal et al., 2009; DiMatteo, Lepper, & Croghan, 2000; Evans et al., 2005; Fava et al., 2006; Gatchel, 2004; ;Gatchel, Peng, Peters, Fuchs, & Turk, 2007; Gros, Antony, McCabe, & Swinson, 2009; Hutter, Scheidt-Nave, & Baumeister, 2009; McGlynn et al., 2003; Merikangas et al., 2007; Kessler, Ormel, Dernier, & Stang, 2003; Kessler et al., 2005, 2006; Kroenke, 2003; Kroenke, et al., 1994; Ormel et al., 2008; Roy-Byrne et al., 2008; Scott et al., 2007, 2009; Simon, Grothaus, Durham, Von Korff & Rabiniak, 1996; Suls & Bunde, 2005). Thus, it is essential for all professionals involved in the treatment and disability management processes to acknowledge the broader scope of BH concerns, as well as incorporating a biopsychosocial approach across professions (Bruns et al., 2010). The term *biopsychosocial* addresses the biological, psychological, and psychosocial factors in a combined manner that better account for the complexity of impairment issues, particularly with comorbid concerns (Bruns & Disorbio, 2005).

The scope of this book will examine the occurrence of BH concerns and how to begin to move past the Cartesian duality model that had artificially separated the mind from the physical (Campbell, Clauw, & Keefe, 2003; Wade, 2006). Further, this exploration will also investigate how the occurrence of BH concerns typically occurs across multiple professions and what are the current problems that occur as well as strategies for the enhancement of treatment outcomes. However, there are multiple present barriers that occur within the treatment and management processes that currently impede the implementation of the synthesis of a more comprehensive approach. One of the primary barriers, despite this knowledge, is the current trend in the medical, mental, rehabilitation health, assessment, treatment, and disability fields to still artificially separate behavioral and physical health concerns. Consequently, this leads to the lack of identification and treatment of BH concerns, an underestimate of the actual prevalence of BH in the professional and disability fields, as well as the potential for unwarranted workplace absence and inappropriate labeling of an individual as being permanently disabled and unfit to function in everyday life activities indefinitely (Bagenstos, 2000; DMEC, 2009). The current BH treatment and disability systems have been noted to have major contributing factors in the explosion of BH concerns that is presently occurring (Centers for Disease Control and Prevention; National Center for Injury Prevention and Control 2006; Center for Disease Control & Prevention (CDC), 2015a, 2015b).

1.3 The Systemic Problems in the Treatment and Management of BH Concerns

1.3.1 The De Facto Behavioral Healthcare System in the USA

In this time of managed healthcare, most BH concerns are not addressed from a coordinated and standardized approach. Instead, in the current system, most individuals with BH concerns are initially evaluated by a primary care physician (PCP) (Koike, Unutzer, & Wells, 2002; National Committee for Quality Assurance 2009). Thus, the de facto BH care system is occurring within the general medical system and does not typically involve the inclusion of BH professionals, at the outset of treatment (Norquist & Regier, 1996). In the typical treatment process, the PCP is likely to prescribe medication only and request that the individual returns for further evaluation at some time in the future, usually around 6 weeks. The individual may or may not be referred to a mental healthcare professional. Thus, there is little to no follow-up of the individual in terms of the appropriateness of the selected treatment, side effects, and compliance with treatment. Consequently, any type of treatment provided is typically confined to what the PCP can accomplish within a short time span due to time-limited appointments. Empirical research has demonstrated that the amount of time that a physician is able to spend with a patient is very brief. This limited amount of time must address the evaluation of the presenting problem, the development of the treatment plan, and the dictation that summarizes the key points of the appointment and current actions taken by the physician. Not surprisingly, while PCPs can diagnosis and treat BH disorders, such as Major Depressive Disorder, a high percentage frequently will miss recognizing or assessing symptoms and not make the diagnosis altogether (Seelig & Katon, 2008). Thus, the de facto BH healthcare system significantly contributes to iatrogenic disability.

Despite the availability of effective treatments for Major Depressive Disorder, rates of appropriate treatment for MDD remain low nationally, particularly in primary care, where only about one-fourth of depressed patients receive appropriate care, including receiving either any diagnosis of a mental health concern or even the correct psychological diagnosis (Kroenke, 2003, 2006). In most instances, the person's diagnosis is made based solely on the symptoms noted. Thus, this complicates the professional treatment. Moreover, unlike physical concerns which are diagnosed based on a standardized evaluation and treatment process, the same is not true of behavioral healthcare (Gask, 2005).

Additional issues include the societal stigma of being diagnosed with a BH concern, and obtaining appropriate professional treatment due to the individual's reluctance to receive care outside of the medical setting. Consequently, a BH professional may or may not be involved in the care of the individual with a BH issue. Moreover, after the referral is made to the BH, the PCP's diagnosis is likely to be assumed accurate and, thus, influencing the professional treatment that the person receives from the BH professional (Seelig & Katon, 2008).

Although the focus was on the PCP, it is important to realize that these concerns are not unique to the medical primary care profession alone. Unfortunately, due to the lack of professional training, the majority of professionals currently involved in both the treatment and disability management fields have little to no training in appropriate evidence-based evaluation, treatment, and management of BH concerns and how to appropriately synthesize this in an effective manner. This is particularly troubling since this leaves the individual with a BH issue left to navigate the BH system without strong assistance.

1.3.2 The Contributory Factors of the Behavioral Health Treatment System and Insurers

The Surgeon General's 1999 report specifically focused on BH issues and the overall mental health system. It was initially reported that although the USA spent over $69 billion on mental health services, there was substantial disparity in the quality of treatment provided. This resulted in abysmal treatment outcomes. Consequently, there was a recommendation for a complete overhaul of the BH treatment system. Moreover, the ability to receive treatment was directly impacted by whether an individual had insurance coverage to provide professional treatment as well as the ability to navigate of obtaining approval from the insurer for care.

After some changes in the BH treatment, systems were put into place; BH expenditures were reviewed. The total medical expenditure spent in 2011 was $48.2 billion. Forty-five percent ($21.7 billion) of this was spent on BH medications. The 27.1% of BH expenditures ($13.1 billion) were spent on outpatient treatment. Inpatient expenditures total 16.5% or $7.95 billion (Zibman, 2014). This demonstrates that there has been a substantial decrease from monetary amounts previously spent on: 1) the treatment of mental health concerns; 2) the issues of obtaining approval from the insurer(s); and 3) how the amount paid for specific services differed from the payor and the treating professional. However, these figures do not include State or federal disability systems. This is of concern since it demonstrates that simply decreasing payment for BH treatment does not necessarily result in improved treatment quality or treatment outcomes. Instead, there are multifactorial issues that contribute to the current fragmented treatment and management processes. Thus, the improvement of increased recognition of BH concerns and subsequent treatment must also address current barriers that lead to poorly defined and open-ended care and sustained poor treatment outcomes as well as an astronomical increase in BH disability claims (Anssea et al., 2004; Kessler et al., 2003; National Business Group on Health, 2007; National Institute of Mental Health, 2008).

Finally, these data do not include those individuals with BH conditions who do not receive BH treatment. In 2014, it was estimated that 27.5% of insured adults in the U.S. with a mental health condition, did not receive BH treatment. To put this in perspective, this represents 8.3 million adults in the USA who have a serious mental health condition. There were 1.6 million uninsured adults in the U.S. with a mental health condition did not receive BH treatment. This illustrates that the estimates of both US adults with a mental health condition as well as expenditures in the USA are suppressed and do not adequately reflect the extent of mental health issues within the USA. In addition, these data do not reflect those individuals with physical conditions or substance abuse disorders that are known to have high comorbidity with mental health issues (Substance Abuse and Mental Health Administration (SAMHA, 2015). When put into this context, it is clear that the BH conditions are still not fully recognized in annualized data and that many are not receiving treatment.

1.3.3 Federal Agencies and the Incidence of Behavioral Health Disability

The SSA's (2015) actuarial data provide ample evidence of the considerable increase in BH concerns over the past two decades. In 2015, disabled workers accounted for 87% of SSA disability beneficiaries. The average age for disability benefits as called in the SSA's Social Security Disability Insurance (SSDI) program is 54. The majority of beneficiaries are male (52%). Slightly over 14% applied and also received SSI benefits as well. When the Supplemental Security Income (SSI) program disability benefits are considered, the percentage of disabled workers increased to 90% of all disability benefits. BH concerns represented 34.8% of all of the SSA's disability beneficiaries group. Thus, BH disorders represented the SSA's largest disability beneficiary group.

Musculoskeletal concerns represented 28.6% of all disability benefits. It is the second largest group which receives SSA disability benefits.

However, randomized controlled research has consistently demonstrated a high comorbidity prevalence (64% and higher) with BH concerns. Because a significant number of chronic physical concerns also have been found to have a concurrent BH concern, it becomes evident the potential impact of BH concerns within the largest public disability program in the USA. (SSA, 2015).

The Veterans Affairs (VA) has its own stand-alone disability program. Typically, a veteran can only apply for disability pertaining to limited mental health conditions: Post Traumatic Stress Disorder (PTSD) an eating disorder, and a few mental health conditions (other than PTSD).

As of March 31, 2017, there are 918,591 veterans who have received disability compensation benefits for PTSD. When this PTSD figure is compared to the 4.44 million veterans receiving disability compensation, it is clear that mental health disability accounts for just a small portion of the total VA disability expenditure. Moreover, a veteran is rated for the percentage of disability that corresponds to varying amounts of VA disability payment. For perspective, the 4.4 million veterans received disability compensation within the VA system in 2016, yet only 569,673 were rated to 100% disabled (United States Department of Veteran Affairs, 2017).

Thus, these figures demonstrate that that primarily PTSD or eating disorders are currently viewed by the VA systems as causing impairment in functioning sufficient to be disabled. In contrast, the VA provides mental health treatment for Major Depressive Disorder, anxiety disorders, PTSD, bipolar disorder, schizophrenia, suicide prevention, military sexual trauma, and substance abuse. Yet, there is no breakdown for medical expenditures per non-PTSD mental disorders (DVA Information Technology Center, 2017). Consequently, the VA data demonstrate an undercounting in both treatment expenditures and veterans who are treated with a mental health condition.

There are other disability systems such as the Railroad Retirement Board (RRB) (2017), the States and federal Workers' Compensation Systems (Federal Employees' Compensation Act (FECA), 1916) that have unique mental health disability data that are not included in the overall US mental health disability treatment expenditure or disability compensation totals. When all of each of these systems are considered together, it demonstrates that the current estimation of mental health disability and treatment data is grossly under-counted. The reason is that each State and federal disability system has unique laws and rules that apply to that system alone. Therefore, the analyzed data are not included in any other mental health disability figures.

A more in-depth discussion of each of these systems will take place in Chap. 7.

1.4 The Need for Improvement in Communications Among Professionals Involved in the BH Fields to Reduce BH Disability

This brief overview discussed in this chapter notes some of the primary systemic problems that must be addressed to set a different course of action needed to both treat and manage BH concerns and disorders. One of the primary ways in which the system can immediately improve is with enhanced communication among professionals in the treatment fields with those professionals in the disability management fields (DMEC, 2009; Talmage, 2007; Talmage & Melhorn, 2005). The other chapters of this book will explore these problems in a more in-depth manner. Further, the scope of BH concerns will be examined across multiple disciplinary perspectives to provide a unique synthesis of addressing BH concerns in a comprehensive manner and across the entire behavioral health spectrum. Typically, in addition to the PCP, the other professionals involved in this process are occupational medicine physician; psychologist; psychiatrist; rehabilitation professionals, such as a physical therapist and rehabilitation vocational counselor; attorney; nurse case manager; and insurer. Each of these different perspectives will address: 1) factors specific to each professional discipline; 2) the determination of psychological and behavioral health functioning related to the identified concern; 3) gaps in determining functioning; and 4) fostering collaborative communications with other professionals (Talmage, 2007). This type of cross-communication is essential in developing much-needed improvements to bridge the current problems rampant within the BH disability field (Warren, 2009).

References

Agency for Healthcare Research and Quality. (2009). *National Healthcare Quality Report, 2008* (pp. 09–0001). Rockville, MD: Agency for Healthcare Research and Quality (Publication No.

American Medical Association. (2008). *Guides to the evaluation of permanent impairment* (6th ed.). Chicago: American Medical Association.

American Psychiatric Association. (2013). *Diagnostic and statistical manual on mental disorders* (5th ed.). Washington, DC: American Psychiatric Association. (DSM-5).

American Psychiatric Foundation, Partnership for Workplace Mental Health. (2005). *Assessing and treating psychiatric occupational disability, executive report.* Washington, DC: American Psychiatric Association.

American Psychiatric Association. (2006). *Practice guidelines for the treatment of psychiatric disorders: Compendium.* Arlington, VA: American Psychiatric Association Press.

Anssea, M., Dierick, M., Buntink, F., et al. (2004). High prevalence of mental disorders in primary care. *Journal of Affective Disorders, 78*(1), 49–55.

Bagenstos, S. R. (2000). Subordination, stigma, and "disability". *Virginia Law Review, 86*, 397–534.

Bruns, D., & Disorbio, J. M. (2005). Chronic pain and biopsychosocial disorders. *Practical Pain Management, 5*(7), 2–9.

Bruns, D., Mueller, K., & Warren, P. A. (2010). A review of evidence-based biopsychosocial laws governing the treatment of pain and injury. *Psychological Injury and Law, 3*, 169–181.

Buist-Bouwman, M. A., de Graaf, R., Vollebergh, W. A. M., & Ormel, J. (2005). Comorbidity of physical and mental disorders and the effect on work-loss days. *Acta Psychiatrica Scandinavica, 111*(6), 436–443.

Campbell, L. C., Clauw, D. J., & Keefe, F. J. (2003). Persistent pain and depression: A biopsychosocial perspective. *Biological Psychiatry, 54*, 399–409.

Centers for Disease Control and Prevention. (2015a). *Behavioral risk factor surveillance system prevalence data.* Atlanta, GA: CDC.

Center for Disease Control and Prevention. (2015b). Health, United States-Mental Health. https://www.cdc.gov/nchs/hus/mentalhealth.htm#access

Centers for Disease Control and Prevention; National Center for Injury Prevention and Control. (2006). Web-based injury statistics query and reporting system (WISQARS). Retrieved from http://www.cdc.gov/ncipc/wisqars/default.htm

Chellappa, P., & Ramaraj, R. (2009). Depression, homocysteine concentration, and cardiovascular events. *Journal of the American Medical Association, 301*(15), 1542.

de Waal, M. W. M., Arnold, I. A., Spinhoven, P., et al. (2009). The role of comorbidity in the detection of psychiatric disorders with checklists for mental and physical symptoms in primary care. *Social Psychiatry and Psychiatric Epidemiology, 44*(1), 78–85.

Dersh, J., Gatchel, R. J., Polatin, P., & Mayer, T. (2002). Prevalence of psychiatric disorders in patients with chronic, work-related musculoskeletal pain disability. *Journal of Occupational and Environmental Medicine, 44*, 459–469.

Dewa, C., & Lin, E. (2000). Chronic physical illness, psychiatric disorder and disability in the workplace. *Social Science & Medicine, 51*, 41–50.

DiMatteo, M. R., Lepper, H. S., & Croghan, T. W. (2000). Depression is a risk factor for noncompliance with medical treatment: Meta-analysis of the effects of anxiety and depression on patient adherence. *Archives of Internal Medicine, 160*, 2101–2107.

Disability Management Employer Coalition (DMEC). (2009). *Tools of the trade: A compilation of programs and processes for the absence, disability, health and productivity professional*. San Diego, CA: Disability Management Employer Coalition.

DVA Information Technology Center; Health Services Training Report; VBA Education Service; VBA Office of Performance Analysis & Integrity; 1 VHA OABI and VSSC (10E2A); 2 DoD. Produced by the National Center for Veterans Analysis and Statistics. http://www.va.gov/vetdata/pocketcard/index.asp

Evans, D. L., Charney, D. S., Lewis, L., et al. (2005). Mood disorders in the medically ill: Scientific review and recommendations. *Biological Psychiatry, 58*, 175–189.

Federal Employees' Compensation Act (FECA), Department of Labor, Federal Employees' CompensationAct (1916), Sept. 7, 1916, ch. 458, 39 Stat. 742, 39 Stat. 742, ch. 458.

Fava, M., Rush, A. J., Alpert, J. E., et al. (2006). What clinical and symptom features and comorbid disorders characterize outpatients with anxious major depressive disorder: A replication and extension. *Canadian Journal of Psychiatry, 51*(13), 823–835.

Gask, L. (2005). Overt and covert barriers to the integration of primary and specialist mental health care. *Social Science & Medicine, 61*(8), 1785–1794.

Gatchel, R. J. (2004). Comorbidity of chronic mental and physical health conditions: The biopsychosocial perspective. *American Psychologist, 59*, 792–805.

Gatchel, R. J., Peng, Y. B., Peters, M. L., Fuchs, P. N., & Turk, D. C. (2007). The biopsychosocial approach to chronic pain: Scientific advances and future directions. *Psychological Bulletin, 133*(4), 581–624.

Gros, D. F., Antony, M. M., McCabe, R. E., & Swinson, R. P. (2009). Frequency and severity of the symptoms of irritable bowel syndrome across the anxiety disorders and depression. *Journal of Anxiety Disorders, 23*(2), 290–296.

Hutter, N., Scheidt-Nave, C., & Baumeister, H. (2009). Health care utilisation and quality of life in individuals with diabetes and comorbid mental disorders. *General Hospital Psychiatry, 31*(1), 33–35.

Kessler, R. C., Akiskal, H. S., Ames, M., et al. (2006). Prevalence and effects of mood disorders on work performance in a nationally representative sample of U.S. workers. *American Journal of Psychiatry, 163*(9), 1561–1568.

Kessler, R. C., Demler, O., Frank, R. G., et al. (2005). Prevalence and treatment of mental disorders, 1990 to 2003. *The New England Journal of Medicine, 352*(24), 2515–2523.

Kessler, R. C., Ormel, J., Dernier, O., & Stang, P. E. (2003). Co-morbid mental disorders account for the role impairment of commonly occurring chronic physical disorders: Results from the National Comorbidity Survey. *Journal of Occupational and Environmental Medicine, 45*, 1257–1266.

Koike, A. K., Unutzer, J., & Wells, K. B. (2002). Improving the care for depression in patients with comorbid medical illness. *American Journal of Psychiatry, 159*(10), 1738–1745.

Kroenke, K. (2003). Patients presenting with somatic complaints: Epidemiology, psychiatric comorbidity and management. *International Journal of Methods in Psychiatric Research, 12*, 34–43.

Kroenke, K. (2006). Review of biopsychosocial medicine: An integrated approach to understanding illness. *Journal of Psychosomatic Research, 60*(4), 433.

Kroenke, K., Spitzer, R. L., Williams, J. B., et al. (1994). Physical symptoms in primary care: Predictors of psychiatric disorders and functional impairment. *Archives of Family Medicine, 3*, 774–779.

McGlynn, E. A., Asch, S. M., Adams, J., et al. (2003). The quality of health care delivered to adults in the United States. *The New England Journal of Medicine, 348*, 2635–2645.

Merikangas, K. R., Ames, M., Cui, L., et al. (2007). The impact of comorbidity of mental and physical conditions on role disability in the US adult household population. *Archives of General Psychiatry, 64*, 1180–1188.

National Business Group on Health. (2007). *An employer's guide to behavioral health services* (p. 100). Washington, DC: National Business Group on Health.

National Committee for Quality Assurance. (2009). *Healthcare effectiveness data and information set (HEDIS)*. Washington, DC: National Committee for Quality Assurance.

National Institute of Mental Health. (2008). *The numbers count: Mental disorders in America*. Washington, DC: National Institute of Mental Health.

Norquist, G. S., & Regier, D. A. (1996). The epidemiology of psychiatric disorders and the de facto mental health care system. *Annual Review of Medicine, 47*, 473–479.

Ormel, J., Petukhova, M., Chatterji, S., et al. (2008). Disability and treatment of specific mental and physical disorders across the world. *British Journal of Psychiatry, 192*, 368–375.

Railroad Retirement Board (RRB). https://www.rrb.gov/mep/ee/forms_ret_surv_dis.asp, retrieved May 10, 2017.

Roy-Byrne, P. P., Davidson, K., Kessler, R. C., et al. (2008). Anxiety disorders and comorbid medical illness. *General Hospital Psychiatry, 30*(3), 208–225.

Scott, K. M., Bruffaerts, R., Tsang, A., et al. (2007). Depression–anxiety relationships with chronic physical conditions: Results from the world mental health surveys. *Journal of Affective Disorders, 103*, 113–120.

Scott, K. M., Von Korff, M., Alonso, J., et al. (2009). Mental–physical co-morbidity and its relationship with disability: Results from the world mental health surveys. *Psychological Medicine, 39*(1), 33–43.

Seelig, M. D., & Katon, W. (2008). Gaps in depression care: Why primary care physicians should hone their depression screening, diagnosis, and management skills. *Journal of Occupational and Environmental Medicine, 50*(4), 451–458.

Simon, G. E., Grothaus, L., Durham, M. L., Von Korff, M., & Rabiniak, C. (1996). Impact of visit copayments on outpatient mental health utilization by members of a health maintenance organization. *American Journal of Psychiatry, 153*(3), 331–338.

Social Security Administration. (2015). *Annual statistical report on the social security disability insurance program, 2015*. Baltimore, MD: Social Security Administration.

Substance Abuse and Mental Health Services Administration. (2015). *Behavioral health barometer: United States, 2015. HHS Publication No. SMA–16–Baro–2015*. Substance Abuse and Mental Health Services Administration: Rockville, MD.

Suls, J., & Bunde, J. (2005). Anger, anxiety, and depression as risk factors for cardiovascular disease: The problems and implications of overlapping affective dispositions. *Psychological Bulletin, 131*, 260–300.

Talmage, J. B. (2007). Failure to communicate: How terminology and forms confuse the work ability/disability evaluation process. *Journal of Insurance Medicine, 39*, 192–198.

Talmage, J. B., & Melhorn, J. M. (Eds.). (2005). *A physician's guide to return to work*. Chicago, IL: American Medical Association Press.

United States Department of Veteran Affairs., http://benefits.va.gov/compensation/. Retrieved May 1, 2017.

Wade, D. (2006). Why physical medicine, physical disability and physical rehabilitation? We should abandon Cartesian dualism. *Clinical Rehabilitation, 20*, 185–190.

Warren, P. A. (2005). *The management of workplace mental health issues and appropriate disability prevention strategies*. San Diego, CA: Work Loss Data Institute.

Warren, P. A. (2009). Behavioral health as a causation issue in workers' compensation and disability claims. *IAIABC Journal, 46*(2), 17–56.
Warren, P. A. (2013a). Those who hesitate are lost: The case for setting behavioral health treatment and disability standards, part I. *Psychological Injury and Law, 6*(3), 183–195.
Warren, P. A. (2013b). Those who hesitate are lost: The case for setting behavioral health treatment and disability standards, part II. *Psychological Injury and Law, 6*(3), 196–207.
Warren, P. A., & Hubbard, J. D. (2008). Psychosocial issues related to behavioral health disability claims. Dearborn National Life Insurance Company.
WHO. (2004). *The world health report 2004: Changing history*. Geneva, Switzerland: The World Health Organization.
Zibman, C. (2014, October). Expenditures for Mental Health among Adults, Ages 18–64, 2009–2011: Estimates for the U.S. Civilian Noninstitutionalized Population. Statistical brief #454. Agency for Healthcare Research and QualityRockville, MD. http://meps.ahrq.gov/mepsweb/data_files/publications/st454/stat454.shtml

Chapter 2
Prevalence of Behavioral Health Concerns

Pamela A. Warren

2.1 Prevalence of Behavioral Health Concerns

In the fields of disability and disease management, the term "behavioral health" (BH) has been coined to encompass both psychological diagnoses, such as major depressive disorder (MDD) as well as psychosocial concerns, such as job dissatisfaction or fear of reinjury. In the most recent two decades, there has been an explosion of BH disability claims despite the development of new, empirically based BH treatments that have been demonstrated to quickly and effectively treat psychological disorders to return an individual to one's previous level of functioning. However, to understand this phenomenon, it is essential to examine the prevalence of BH concerns to better understand some of the current problematic issues that occur in both the treatment and disability management fields (Wainberg et al., 2017). In general, the prevalence of psychological disorders has been found to vary across each type of Diagnostic and Statistical Manual, 5th edition diagnostic categories (ApA, 2013). The current body of empirical research (Bogner, de Vries, Maulik, & Unützer, 2009; Fichter, Narrow, Roper, et al., 1996; U.S. Department of Health and Human Services, 1999) has revealed that there is a general prevalence rate of approximately 20% across all objectively determined mental health (MH) concerns in the US general population. One of the primary Psychological Disorders that occur is Major Depressive Disorder, which has been found to have a prevalence rate of 10–20% in the general population (American Psychiatric Association (ApA), 2013; Kessler et al., 1994). The Substance Abuse and Mental Health Services Administration (SAMHSA, 2007a, 2007b, 2015) placed the prevalence rate of a behavioral health disorder much higher, with 30% of the population experiencing

P. A. Warren (✉)
Carle Physician Group and University of Illinois Medical School, Department of Psychiatry, Monticello, IL, USA

P. A. Warren (ed.), *Handbook of Behavioral Health Disability Management*,
https://doi.org/10.1007/978-3-319-89860-5_2

a BH disorder in any given year (age group 15–54). Moreover, over the lifetime course, approximately 48% of the population has had at least one BH disorder, while 27% have had two or more BH disorders. SAMHSA (2015) reported that the most common BH disorders were depressive disorders (Major Depressive Disorder and Dysthymic Disorder), the anxiety disorder spectrum (e.g., Generalized Anxiety Disorder, Social Phobia, Panic Disorder, etc.), and substance abuse. In those individuals who typically apply for disability benefits, the prevalence rate is estimated to range from a conservative 30% up to a greater estimate of 60–70% when including comorbid physical and psychological concerns (Aronoff, Mandel, Genovese, et al., 2007; Binder & Rohling, 1996; Buist-Bouwman, de Graaf, Vollebergh, & Ormel, 2005; Campbell, Clauw, & Keefe, 2003; CDC, 2006; Dersh, Gatchel, Polatin, & Mayer, 2002; Dersh, Polatin, Leeman, & Gatchel, 2005; DMEC, 2008; Evans, Charney, Lewis, et al., 2005; Gatchel, 2004; Kessler, Anthony, Blazer, et al., 1997; Kessler, Ormel, Dernier, & Stang, 2003; Kouzis & Eaton, 1997; MacDonald-Wilson, Rogers, & Anthony, 2001; Whiteford, Ferrari, Degenhardt, Feigin, & Vos, 2015; Whiteford et al., 2013).

The National Institute of Mental Health (NIMH) (2008) examined the disability associated with specific conditions. The amount of disability is broken into units called disability-adjusted life years (DALYs). In 2013, the NIMH reported that the leading cause of disability in the United States for the age group of 15–44 is Major Depressive Disorder. This observation is supported by other empirical data which noted the same leading cause of disability (CDC, 2013; CDC, 2017; SAMHSA, 2015). Consequently, it quickly becomes clear that those individuals who are diagnosed with a BH concern are the very people who have a substantial impact on the initiation of current BH disability claims and attendant costs associated with the claims, particularly those that do not resolve in the anticipated timeframe. It is the astronomic expanse of BH concerns, poor treatment outcomes, and open-ended disability leaves that are of noteworthy interest since these aspects dramatically increase the costs of BH disability (American Psychiatric Foundation (APF), 2005; DMEC, 2008). Therefore, it is imperative for all professionals to both recognize and understand the importance of appropriate management of BH concerns (DMEC, 2009). Moreover, with the anticipated increase of MDD as a leading cause of disability worldwide, it makes clear that BH issues are not merely minor concerns when it comes to professional treatment and assisting the individual in the stay-at-work (SAW) and return-to-work (RTW) processes, but are critical components to be addressed (ACOEM, 2006; Bruns & Disorbio, 2005; Gask, 2005; GBD 2013 DALYs & HALE Collaborators, 2015; Greenberg & Shuman, 1997; Greene, 2007; Kessler & Wang, 2008; Kessler et al., 2008; Ormel, Petukhova, Chatterji, et al., 2008; Patel, Chisholm, Dua, et al., 2016; Reggers & Ansseau, 1999; Roy-Byrne, Davidson, Kessler, et al., 2006; Seedat, Scott, Angermeyer, et al., 2009; U.S. Burden of Disease Collaborators, 2013; Wang, Berglund, & Kessler, 2000; Zechmeister, Kilian, & McDaid, 2008; WHO, 2004).

Currently, there is a great deal of misperception among all professionals regarding all aspects of BH disability. Many of these issues, such as the lack of the following, are:

- Appropriate training to complete a thorough and competent BH evaluation required to evaluate an individual in a comprehensive manner regarding functioning
- Objective data to support a lengthy BH disability leave
- The medicalization of psychosocial concerns
- Providing treatment that is in line with current empirical research and best practice standards
- A RTW goal in treatment planning and long-term workplace absences which will be discussed to provide a more thorough understanding of the underlying issues with the current BH evaluation and treatment process (Warren, 2009, 2013a, b; Warren & Hubbard, 2006, 2008)

2.2 BH Professionals Involved in the BH Disability Process and Problematic Issues

There are several different types of BH professionals currently providing professional treatment. A cursory comparison of each professional will be provided. However, it is essential to keep in mind that it is not possible to provide comprehensive information in the scope of a single chapter regarding each profession. Instead, this comparison is provided to understand the basic differences among each profession to be seen at a glance in Table 2.1.

2.2.1 Problematic Inconsistencies in Professional BH Training

When looking at Table 2.1, it becomes evident that there are limitations across each profession in what constitutes usual care as well as the clinical focus with each type of profession. It becomes clear too that there are substantial differences in the breadth of professional training that may result in specific clinical competency in the BH evaluation process, particularly in regard to the types of objective standardized psychological testing that can be conducted to adequately assess an individual's current functioning. Consequently, an immediate observation regarding this potential lack of additional training specific to the evaluation of objectively determined BH disability is essential for any consumer of such services to be aware. This may necessarily limit what types of clinical services and treatment the professional may offer in regard to BH and the evaluation of permanent impairment (Warren, 2005, 2013a, b).

In addition to training differences for each profession, there are also limitations in what each type of professional is taught as regarding the pertinent diagnosis, evaluation, selection, and determination of appropriate clinical treatment. The evaluation process becomes more complex when the assessment of the individual from

Table 2.1 Demonstration of differences in professional training experiences and professional services provided by each type of behavioral health professional

Type of professional	Counselors (LCPC, LPC)	Social workers (LCSW, MSW)	Nurse practitioners/ physician assistants (NP, PA)	Counseling psychologists	Clinical psychologists (Ph.D., Psy.D., and occasionally, Ed.D.)	Physicians (FP, GP, psychiatrists	Physicians (OEM)
Educational degree	Masters' degree + internship	Masters' degree + internship	Bachelor's degree + additional advanced training to become a licensed NP or PA or specific specialty	Doctoral degree + practicum + internship	Doctoral degree + practicum + internship	Medical degree (M.D. or D.O.) + residency + additional training for any specialty	Medical degree (M.D. or D.O.) + residency + additional training for OM specialty
Number of years to earn degree beyond bachelor's degree	2–3	2–3	4+, if obtaining specialty training	8–9	8–9	4–8	4–8
Can practice without supervision	Maybe. In a few states, a master's level professional can be licensed as a psychologist.	Yes	Maybe. Most states require a physician to oversee the NP treatment, particularly in psychiatric treatment	Yes	Yes	Yes	Yes

Type of professional	Counselors (LCPC, LPC)	Social workers (LCSW, MSW)	Nurse practitioners/ physician assistants (NP, PA)	Counseling psychologists	Clinical psychologists (Ph.D., Psy.D., and occasionally, Ed.D.)	Physicians (FP, GP, psychiatrists	Physicians (OEM)
Can make a professional diagnosis	Yes, but many states require this is reviewed by a licensed, supervising BH professional	Yes	Maybe. Most states require a physician to oversee the NP's or PA's treatment, particularly in psychiatric treatment	Yes	Yes	Yes	Yes
Can provide professional treatment	Yes, with supervision by a licensed BH professional	Yes	Yes, but with supervision in most states	Yes	Yes	Yes	Yes

(continued)

Table 2.1 (continued)

Type of professional	Counselors (LCPC, LPC)	Social workers (LCSW, MSW)	Nurse practitioners/ physician assistants (NP, PA)	Counseling psychologists	Clinical psychologists (Ph.D., Psy.D., and occasionally, Ed.D.)	Physicians (FP, GP, psychiatrists	Physicians (OEM)
Can administer standardized psychological testing and interpret the results for the evaluation of impairment in functioning	No, except in those states that allow the professional to become licensed as a psychologist. However, many of the tests are restricted to doctoral or MD practitioners only	No, except in those states that allow the professional to become licensed as a psychologist. However, many of the tests are restricted to doctoral or MD practitioners only	No	Yes, provided the professional has had graduate level training in psychological assessment and has had supervised practical experience	Yes, particularly clinical and neuropsychologists. Both types of these professionals can typically complete the testing required to determine objective impairment in functioning	Yes, but only if the physician has had appropriate graduate level psychological assessment training and has had supervised practical experience	Yes, but only if the physician has had appropriate graduate level psychological assessment training and has had supervised practical experience

Type of professional	Counselors (LCPC, LPC)	Social workers (LCSW, MSW)	Nurse practitioners/physician assistants (NP, PA)	Counseling psychologists	Clinical psychologists (Ph.D., Psy.D., and occasionally, Ed.D.)	Physicians (FP, GP, psychiatrists	Physicians (OEM)
Can prescribe psychotropic medication	No	No	Yes, but most states require a physician to review, particularly in a psychiatric setting	No	Generally, no. however, following states do, Idaho, Illinois, Iowa, Louisiana, and New Mexico. The US territories of Guam and Puerto Rico allow clinical psychologists with additional professional training to prescribe. This is also true in the US armed forces. Other states are considering allowing psychologists' prescription rights. Thus, this may change in the future (Bethune, 2017; Warren, 2005, 2013a, b)	Yes	Yes

(continued)

Table 2.1 (continued)

Type of professional	Counselors (LCPC, LPC)	Social workers (LCSW, MSW)	Nurse practitioners/ physician assistants (NP, PA)	Counseling psychologists	Clinical psychologists (Ph.D., Psy.D., and occasionally, Ed.D.)	Physicians (FP, GP, psychiatrists	Physicians (OEM)
Has professional experience related to prevention and disability management as well as occupational health	No	No	Perhaps if the NP or PA has specialty training in occupational health. However, the complexities of disability management are not typically taught with professional training	No	Perhaps, with the integration of BH + primary care, there is more overlap. However, most graduate schools do not provide disability management or occupational health training. Clinical health psychologists as well as neuropsychologists are likely to have more training	Maybe	Yes

multiple domains occurs. Moreover, when the biopsychosocial model that is utilized in current practice is considered, the evaluating professional must take a thoughtful and thorough assessment of the physical, psychological, emotional, developmental, and social aspects of the person's life. While talking with the individual is one way to obtain this information, it is insufficient to only consider what the person has to say since reality can be clouded by an individual's perceptions of it (e.g., cognitive biases). Consequently, the evaluating professional must strive to corroborate subjective information (e.g., the person's perceptions) with more objective information in BH evaluations.

Two types of professionals who tend to have better training in the assessment of individual are clinical psychologists and psychiatrists pertaining to psychological assessment and treatment. A brief discussion of the type of training highlights the differences in training.

2.2.2 *Clinical Psychologists*

Most clinical psychology doctoral programs, particularly those that are APA-approved, have a standardized sequence of 4 years of coursework training, including clinical practica, the completion of a scientific study (dissertation, usually 1–2-year process) for which the student has primary control of designing and conducting, and a required 2-year supervised internship before the professional may sit for a state licensure examination. The American Psychological Association (APA, 2009) is the primary professional organization that governs the ethical standards and the determination of appropriate professional training and clinical practice. Clinical psychologists traditionally receive professional training to evaluate, diagnose, and treat a broad variety of psychological disorders and in addressing common problems experienced by most individuals in the course of everyday life. While some counseling psychologists may receive this type of coursework and training, the majority does not, as can be ascertained from examining the typical graduate programs in counseling psychology.

Of note, even if a psychologist is not a member of the APA, the clinician is bound to follow what is considered to be appropriate clinical practice standards, in particular with regard to appropriate psychological testing. Any professional who utilizes standardized psychological testing is bound to follow the Standards for Educational and Psychological Testing (APA, 2014). While the breadth of this professional training is essential to practice as a competent clinician, there may be gaps in professional training and real-life application of clinical skills, particularly in regard to professional training regarding the prevention and management of psychological disorders that are primary catalysts for BH disability (APA, 2001, 2002, 2007a, 2007b, 2009).

2.2.3 Physicians

While all physicians receive basic training regarding BH concerns and treatment of them, not all physicians have completed rigorous professional training to treat the complexity of most BH disorders. As noted in Chap. 1, the primary care medicine system is viewed as being the de facto behavioral health system in the United States. While this type of model has improved medical care access, it has not necessarily improved the quality of care. A typical comprehensive BH evaluation takes approximately 45–90 min to complete. The average time spent in face-to-face patient visits with most primary care doctors is between 15.7–20 min (Mauksch, Dugdale, Dodson, & Epstein, 2008; Ming, Thomas, & Weimin, 2007). Thus, it is not surprising that other studies found the substantial variance among PCPs in terms of assessing for a BH diagnosis and the level of accuracy of diagnosis made (Baumeister & Hutter, 2012; Epstein et al., 2008; Goodrich et al., 2013; Hooper et al., 2012). It is important to note that significant improvements have been made in diagnosing and treating BH disorders in the primary care setting. But, unless further improvements are made in both the diagnosis and the implementation of current best practice standards as well as close collaboration with BH professionals, then a poor treatment outcome remains a distinct potential outcome.

Those physicians who have trained as psychiatrists have completed medical training and then have undergone intensive supervised training pertaining to the diagnosis of psychiatric illnesses and the medical treatment of such conditions. In Chap. 7, a deeper discussion of some of the issues that impact on psychiatrists providing care is provided. However, it is important to note that because a psychiatrist specializes in the treatment of BH disorders, there is specific training that occurs with an emphasis on the treatment of mental health disorders as a medical condition and the usage of medications to treat them (ACOEM, 2006). Moreover, any consumer in the utilization of BH services and in the disability management spectrum must carefully screen whether the psychiatrist has sufficient training in the evaluation of BH functional impairment.

2.2.4 Lack of Objective Assessment in the BH Evaluation Process

There is frequent confusion among professionals as to why objective assessment must occur as well as what constitutes objective information. The reason for this approach is that it provides a more accurate picture about the person's actual level of functioning and allows the professional to discuss functioning from an objective standpoint versus a perceptual/subjective one. A professional must attempt to provide as accurate data and facts as possible report regarding functioning. If a professional does not follow this approach, then serious questions regarding the objectivity and accuracy of the professional's clinical report can be made. Objective documentation pertaining to an individual's psychological functioning considers physical data (e.g., blood work, X-rays, and MRIs) and psychological and psychosocial data which are determined through comprehensive standardized testing. Moreover, any psychological testing must be specific to the reported concern and not simply administered without a particular reason. Otherwise, testing in this manner does not follow current appropriate psychological testing standards set forth by the APA (2014). While a professional may note that one is not a member of the American Psychological Association (APA), all psychological tests, in particular, standardized psychological testing and the administration of such tests, are under the APA's jurisdiction. Thus, all professionals who utilize psychological tests must comply with the rules set forth by the APA, even if not a professional member.

The testing data provide data and information that are synthesized and then examined in a more comprehensive manner to allow the professional to assess the individual from the physical, psychological, cognitive, emotional, development, and psychosocial aspects that may be impacting on the person (Turner et al., 2001). This synthesis is considered objective data because the standardized tests are administered in a specific manner each time the test is administered from individual to individual (Marchetti et al., 2016). Moreover, the test user must follow the interpretation protocol set forth in the standardization process in order for the testing results to be considered valid. Unfortunately, many professionals do not follow this step and end up reporting psychological test data that were either nonstandardized or invalid due to the manner in which it was administered and/or interpreted.

Many master's level clinicians as well as other BH professionals tend to overutilize subjective tools, such as surveys, questionnaires, and fill-in-the-blank devices (AMA, 2008; Bruns, Mueller, & Warren, 2010). There are three primary issues with these types of tools:

1. Usually, these tools have been validated for research settings, but not clinical settings. This is important because both the AMA (2008) and APA (2001, 2002, 2014) require appropriate psychological test usage in which the test administrator must employ the test in the setting for which it was designed as well as follow appropriate testing administration protocol.
2. These tools have been found to be excellent screening devices to identify potential BH concerns, but that they are inappropriate to use in the actual assessment of psychological functioning because of limitations in their validity (accurately measuring what the test purports to measure) and reliability (consistently measuring the same clinical issue or domain each time the test is employed) and thus do not provide meaningful data about the individual's current level of functioning.
3. Users of screening tools frequently make changes to address a different clinical issue, but without going through the standardization process (ACOEM, 2008; Bruns et al., 2010; Warren, 2009). Thus, this arbitrary process deviates from mandated psychological testing protocol as noted by the APA (2001, 2002, 2014). When a change in a tool takes place, it is uncertain if the tool still screens for the issues for which it originally designed to assess and because the changes were made without completing the required stringent validation process. (APA, 2014).

2.2.5 Problematic Selection of BH Treatment

The type of treatment that is provided by the clinician is likely based on the course-work and professional supervised experience in graduate or medical training. It is important to note that there are different types of treatment associated with different psychological theories, and thus, the selection of treatment is likely to be substantially influenced by the clinician's theoretical orientation. These treatments may or may not align with empirical research and best practice standards. Consequently, there is the potential that a professional may provide treatment that was learned in clinical training, but is no longer deemed appropriate or effective. Types of professional services are generally determined by two governing bodies: (1) the profession itself sets standards regarding what constitutes thorough training and (2) each state has laws that legally limit as to what services a professional is able to provide. Any consumer of BH services should take steps to familiarize oneself with these standards and laws. It is beyond the scope of this chapter to address them here. (Heilburn, Grisso, & Goldstein, 2009; Lerner & Henke, 2008; Merikangas et al., 2007).

Unfortunately, not all behavioral health treatments are effective for the treatment of all BH concerns (Warren, 2009, 2013a, b). It is critical to know that there are current scientifically based treatments for true individual BH disorders (e.g., major depressive disorder) that are the most likely to result in efficient care and the facilitation of the individual's return to previous level of functioning. Thus, the limitation in professional training that was discussed earlier can have negative implications throughout the diagnostic process, assessment process, and the type of treatment provided (Kane, 2008; Koocher & Keith-Speigel, 2016; Koocher et al., 2013).

It is important for non-BH professionals to understand the differences in training among BH professionals. Furthermore, it is essential that non-BH professionals become better acquainted with current scientifically based treatments for true psychological disorders in order to both understand typical treatment of the disorder and in order to ask the treating professional (TP) about different aspects of the treatment provided, treatment goals, medications, and transition plans for the RTW process (ACOEM, 2008, 2006; Melhorn & Ackerman, 2008; Warren, 2009). While some BH TPs may balk at a non-clinician asking these type of clarifying questions, in reality, there is nothing inherently wrong with a non-BH professional asking questions pertaining to professional care received. In the age of the Internet, it is common for a person to informally research different topics of interest, including professional care. Thus, BH TPs must recognize this and use asked questions as an opportunity to discuss the current state-of-the-art treatment and be prepared to discuss any deviations in the care they have provided. Moreover, the TP must also explain how the RTW goal and process are being addressed and will be accomplished as well as the expected timeline for treatment. Any deviations from the above must be grounded in scientifically based standards versus subjective clinical opinion (Warren, 2013a, b).

In addition, there is wide variation in the quality of BH health treatment provided currently (American Psychiatric Foundation (APF), 2005; NBGH, 2007; Warren, 2005, 2013a, b; Warren & Hubbard, 2008). This has resulted in poor and unpredictable treatment outcomes in the BH treatment process. These poor outcomes have caused some non-BH professionals to become skeptical as to the veracity of the BH impairment in functioning claim, particularly if there is poor documentation provided to support such a claim. Consequently, non-clinicians involved in the BH disability process have come to ask questions of the BH TP regarding treatment for a variety of reasons, including BH disability claim determination. With the advent of HIPAA (Health Insurance Portability and Accountability Act of 1996), new changes were mandated regarding what types of health information could be released and imposed new requirements to protect health information. However, HIPAA also allowed that certain protected health information (PHI) could be disclosed without a signed release by the individual receiving treatment, in some cases, such as the application for disability. Frequently, BH TPs inappropriately use HIPAA as a shield to avoid disclosing essential information, often to the detriment of the person being treated, such as in the case of obtaining disability benefits. It is important to note that HIPAA specifically allows both TPs and non-clinicians to exchange information in regard to workers' compensation (WC) and other disability issues, such as with short-term (STD), long-term (LTD), Social Security Administration Disability Insurance (SSDI), and other disability systems. Moreover, if there is sustained concern about the release of potentially protected health information, any professional may alleviate this by simply asking the person receiving treatment to sign a release of information. This effectively reduces the potential concern of the person not assenting to the release of pertinent information. Although this is not always necessary with these types of disability disclosures as noted in HIPAA, it provides additional protection to all involved parties (ARRA, 2009; HIPAA, 1996; Warren, 2009).

2.2.6 Problematic Utilization of Inappropriate or Nonevidence-Based Treatment

It is also essential to note that the empirical research is clear that there are evidence-based treatments for the majority of BH diagnoses and that recovery is the norm, not the exception (APF, 2005; Barlow, 2005; Bush & Heilbronner, 2012; Bush & Martin, 2008; Bush & Martin, 2010a, b; Bush et al., 2017; DMEC, 2008, 2009; Melhorn & Ackerman, 2008; Messer, 2004; Nathan & Gorman, 1998; NBGH, 2007; Reed, Kihlstrom, & Messer, 2006; Rush, Warden, Wisniewski, et al., 2009; Sing, Hill, & Puffer, 2001; Warren, 2005, 2013a, b). Thus, this is an essential issue for professionals to address throughout the BH evaluation and treatment process. Unfortunately, as the American Psychiatric Foundation's Partnership for Workplace Mental Health (2005) has noted, there seems to be professional disconnect between the empirical literature and its application by BH professionals in current common clinical practice. This problem is of great concern since two of the primary reasons empirical research takes place are to develop and identify new or more efficacious ways in which to provide treatment in clinical practice and to improve treatment outcomes. Thus, there are several questions that can be raised about the type of professional treatment provided by a BH TP:

1. Has the implementation of best practice standards into current clinical treatment occurred?
2. Has a RTW goal been set as a part of the treatment plan?
3. What are the ethical and professional implications of not providing such treatment to individuals?
4. What are the inherent problems with providing less-than-excellent care and the likelihood of poor treatment outcomes? (Warren, 2009).

There are several professional treatment guidelines and best practice standards for physical concerns, such as the American College of Occupational Medicine (ACOEM, 2008), the American Medical Association's *Guides to the Evaluation of Permanent Impairment* (AMA, 2008), the Colorado State Division of Workers' Compensation Chronic Pain guidelines (2007), the Colorado Division of Workers' Compensation (2009), as well as commercially available guidelines such as the Official Disability Guidelines (ODGs, 2016) and the Reed Group Medical Disability Guidelines (MDG, 2017). However, there are relatively few guidelines explicitly for BH concerns: the *American Psychiatric Association's Practice Guidelines for the Treatment of Psychiatric Disorders (2006)*, the Work Loss Data Institute's ODG (2015), and the book *The Management of Workplace Mental Health Issues and Appropriate Disability Prevention Strategies* (Warren, 2005). The ACOEM and the AMA guidelines both have chapters on mental and behavioral health issues. However, at the time of this chapter, the ACOEM guidelines are being updated for the inclusion of current empirical research. The AMA guidelines focus more on the assessment of permanent impairment, not the specifics of professional BH treatment. Another considerable concern, at present, is that the importance of providing current evidence-based treatments is not regularly taught in professional training of BH clinicians nor mandated by professional organizations such as the American Psychological Association or the American Psychiatric Association (APA) (Warren, 2013a, b). While it can be appreciated that there are different theoretical bases for treatment, the importance of providing the most efficient treatment to alleviate an individual's suffering and to greatly facilitate the person's return to previous functioning is of tantamount concern. This is a professional deficit that must be remediated in order to provide quality BH assessment and treatment processes.

While there are limitations in the professional training of BH professionals that contribute to uneven treatment and poor treatment outcomes, there are also several misperceptions arise with that all professionals, both BH and non-BH, that will be explored further (Pope & Vasquez, 2016).

2.3 Common Misperceptions that Occur with by all Professionals Involved in the BH Disability Process

There are multiple misperceptions that occur across the BH disability spectrum that contribute to adversarial interactions, arbitrary decision-making, treatment, disability claim, and legal outcomes.

2.3.1 Determination of Functional Impairment Versus Disability

There is a common misunderstanding among professionals regarding the terms of "disability" and "impairment in functioning." Frequently, many professionals appear to believe that the terms of impairment and disability are synonymous and use them interchangeably. The term "disability" is a socioeconomic and legal term which varies with each state statute, federal statute, insurance carrier, governmental agency, or organization (Warren, 2009). Because of the variability of the definition of disability across organizations and laws, there is little to no standardization of language and criteria regarding disability. Thus, currently, there is no single set of criteria recognized as to define disability in a standardized manner. Consequently, there is a great deal of confusion about among professionals in using the term "disability" and the belief that using one organization or law's specific criteria will be sufficient to constitute disability and more specifically, whether an individual has true physical or psychological impairment (Schultz & Gatchel, 2005). However, frequently, the primary issue at stake for clinicians is in the professional determination process of whether the individual can actually work. Thus, this relates directly to ability to function in the workplace (and other settings) versus simply noting that a person is "disabled." Unfortunately, by using an organization's disability definition and criteria, such as, for example, the Social Security Administration (SSA, 2017), there is a tendency to refocus the treating professional to solely address whether the individual's current concerns meet the organization's disability criteria. A significant problem with this approach is that the organization's disability criteria may or may not utilize current clinical practice standards to objectively determine what the individual is and is not objectively capable of doing. Consequently, the question regarding objective impairment in functioning remains unanswered.

SSA (2017) revised their mental disorders criteria and medical evidence rules.

SSA now requires psychological testing to be completed before any SSA disability claim is considered. However, this is still an over-reliance on subjective information (e.g., the claimant's and medical professionals' opinions) versus more objective data to ascertain whether any valid impairment in functioning exists. This creates a dilemma for both the TP and the individual who is reported to be disabled since both have moved away from an active treatment model and recovery as an outcome goal and more to declaring the individual is disabled and incapable of recovery, including work. Moreover, once a person obtains disability status through an organization, such as SSA, then there is little to no incentive to help the individual continue professional treatment or to recover and return to one's previous lifestyle, including work (Warren & Hubbard, 2006, 2008). Thus, this is essential for professionals in the BH disability field to be aware and to ask the following general questions:

- What is the current *DSM* diagnosis for this individual?
- Do the reported symptoms and impairment in functioning fit the *DSM* diagnostic criteria?

- If no, does any *DSM* diagnosis exist?
- What is the current best practice standard for this diagnosis?
- Is this the actual treatment being provided?
- If yes, is the person making appreciable progress in treatment?
- If no, what are the barriers to the person making progress that need to be addressed?
- Has a RTW goal been set as an integral part of BH treatment?
- If yes, how will be this addressed? For example, a good place to start is by contacting the individual's human resources department.
- If no, how is this supported in the current empirical research?

Generally, it is not supported to provide an "off-label" or nonevidence-based treatment for any psychological condition. Without the benefit of empirical research to support the selection of a particular treatment, the clinician is simply making a subjective choice that frequently leads to lengthy workplace absences and no change in the person's functioning.

These questions will quickly help any professional to quickly focus on the pertinent issues at hand and avoid tangential concerns that may be interesting but have little impact on the clinical issue of functioning. As noted earlier, when the issue of BH disability is examined, it quickly becomes apparent that there are even fewer definitive criteria than can be found with the physical disability criteria. Again, many of the difficulties are related to the nonstandardization of criteria in the initial defining of disability. Thus, "disability" is a term that is used among professionals to convey a wide variety of psychological diagnoses and BH concerns, but without a sufficient standardized mode in which to note occurrence of objective impairment (Warren, 2005, 2013a, b).

While disability is primarily a nonstandardized term that has little to no meaning, the same is not true for impairment of functioning. Impairment relates to the actual objectively determined functioning of the individual across many different physical systems, such as, for example, cardiac, respiratory, emotional, neurological, and cognitive functioning. Importantly, there are specific means to measure functioning in each of these systems that is both standardized and utilized across different professions and will be discussed more fully in the later chapters. However, in summarization, this objectively determined process provides a means for professionals to discuss if specific deficits exist and how these deficits relate to the individual's ability to complete daily activities of everyday living as well as in performing a variety of workplace duties (AMA, 2013; ACOEM, 2008; Warren, 2005, 2009).

2.3.2 A BH Diagnosis Is Automatically Equal to Impairment in Functioning

A common, problematic issue in the field of behavioral health evaluation process is the apparent belief among most professionals involved in the BH evaluation, treatment, and disability process that a mental health diagnosis is equal to a disability (Talmage, 2007; Talmage & Melhorn, 2005). While there is no question that some psychological diagnoses have considerable impact on an individual's life, there is not a substantial body of empirical research to date, which demonstrates that the majority of the psychiatric diagnoses necessarily result in a permanent inability to function in multiple settings, including work (Alpert, Biggs, Davis, et al., 2006; AMA, 2008; APF, 2005; Centers for Disease Control (CDC), 2013, 2017; Kahn & Langlieb, 2005; Warren, 2005, 2013a, b). Yet, this perception permeates across all professional fields involved in the prevention and management of BH disability. Typically, with both treating and case management professionals, the current standard has been to utilize a psychological diagnosis as the means to justify an application of a disability claim. However, starting from this point, it clearly illustrates how strongly it is presumed that a psychological diagnosis is synonymous with impairment. Thus, using this line of reasoning and to continue to its logical conclusion, it would stand to reason that once a psychological diagnosis is made, then all persons with a psychological diagnosis would be both permanently disabled and impaired. Yet, it is clear from casual observation – such as having a family member with a diagnosed psychological condition, empirical research, as well as in clinical practice – that even though some individuals do receive a psychological diagnosis, there are variations in the severity of that clinical concern (Warren, 2009).

Moreover, many continue to function in all aspects of life, despite receiving a psychological diagnosis. For example, the *DSM-5* (American Psychiatric Association (ApA, 2013) has a clear system of rating for the severity of MDD. This rating system is to be used to denote milder symptoms of MDD to more severe symptoms that are highly likely to impact on the person's ability to functioning effectively in life. Thus, while an individual may receive a diagnosis of MDD, it may not currently be impacting on the person's ability to function. Therefore, despite the diagnosis, the person is likely to be able to participate in everyday life activities. Once an exception to an assumption can be found, such as in this case, then it clearly brings into the question the soundness of utilizing over-generalities in clinical practice as well as in nonclinical settings regarding BH disability.

It is incumbent for the TP to evaluate actual functioning beyond a diagnosis. One way to do this is to employ the *DSM* coding system for the specific psychological condition to denote severity of the current status. This coding system can also be used to reflect the positive changes in the individual's recovery and return to functioning. An example of this is when a person is diagnosed with major depressive disorder and noted to be consistent moderate impairment. Yet, over time with appropriate treatment, the person will still have the diagnosis of MDD, but it will be noted to be in full remission once treatment ends. Consequently, *DSM* diagnostic system is not a unilateral system, but a bidirectional one.

Furthermore, in the review of several thousand psychological disability claims, the change in severity of the *DSM* diagnosis is rarely seen in follow-up after a disability claim has been approved and even with professional treatment (Warren, 2005, 2009; Warren & Hubbard, 2008). This does not necessarily accurately represent that the person is still severely impaired, but begs the questions regarding whether:

1. Has the TP made the correct diagnosis initially?
2. Has the diagnosis been confirmed with objective, standardized psychological testing?
3. Has the TP reevaluated the individual since the treatment began?
4. Does the professional treatment provided meet the current best practice standards?
5. What are the barriers to further improvement?
6. Is the person being treated fully complying with treatment? (Warren, 2009). Evidence-based treatment and best practice standards will be discussed in more depth in Chap. 4, and the usage of objective standardized psychological testing will be examined in Chap. 4.

2.3.3 Behavioral Health Impairment in Functioning Is Permanent

Frequently, both BH and disability professionals as well as individuals with true, objectively determined BH impairment tend to believe that this impairment is permanent and recovery requires the individual to avoid those situations that exacerbate one's symptoms, as well as withdraw from everyday activities, including work. However, this viewpoint is a deviation from the recognition of necessary and appropriate rehabilitation required with most chronic physical injuries and illnesses in the medical and rehabilitation fields. When one is physically ill or injured, the medical standard is to facilitate an increasing activity level in order to keep the person as physically active as possible to preserve and strengthen physical health. Even after cardiac or orthopedic surgery, it is common practice for the individual to be gotten up and moving as soon as it is deemed medically safe to facilitate the healing process and to prevent complications, such as DVTs, bedsores, and muscle atrophy (AMA, 2008). However, unfortunately, there is not an analogous standard in the current BH treatment practice (Warren, 2013a, b). Instead, BH TPs frequently tend to confuse empathy with actual professional treatment, and the person is encouraged to recover by withdrawing from life. This is not to say that empathy is not important in the treatment of BH concerns, because it is essential to have professional empathy to the condition of human suffering (Koocher, Norcross, & Hill, 2005). But, empathy alone is not noted anywhere in the empirical research, as a current stand-alone professional treatment nor does it help the person to maintain a more active lifestyle, make appropriate changes, focus on developing sound coping skills, as well as regroup and re-engage fully in all activities of living, including work.

This observation should not be taken to mean that no person should ever be placed on permanent disability, since there are some BH diagnoses, such as traumatic brain injury, Schizophrenia, or dementia (Lee, Lyketsos, & Rao, 2003; Rao & Lyketsos, 2003; Schretlen et al., 2007; Schretlen, Munro, Anthony, & Pearlson, 2003) that may potentially result in permanent impairment in functioning. However, it is essential to note there are serious issues with professionally opining that an individual is completely and totally impaired in all spheres of life, even with the completion of objective determination of impairment in functioning (Gold & Shuman, 2009; Gold & Davidson, 2007; Gold et al., 2008; Weber, 2008; Weiner & Hess, 2005). If this was actually the case, then this represents profound impairment in which the person cannot take even basic needs and is totally reliant on others. Yet, the review of BH disability claims typically demonstrates that the person is often able to take part in complete activities of daily living, taking medication, and even driving a car. It is important to note that the act of driving utilizes every cognitive domain (e.g., memory, spatial recognition, sense of direction, short-term and long-term memory to name a few). Thus, if clinician opines that an individual is completely unable of any functioning and yet is cleared to drive a car, this does not make sense from a neuropsychological professional point of view.

Empirical research has demonstrated that the quality of one's life dramatically decreases when one is unemployed or once placed on disability. Gerdtham and Johannesson (2003) found that one's social relationships and financial and physical status substantially decreased, so much so, that after 10–17 years the individual became unemployed and that there was a 50% increased probability of committing suicide. This effectively illustrates that being declared disabled is not a panacea for BH concerns and may actually cause or worsen a BH condition. In the field of psychology, this is called *learned helplessness* (Seligman & Maier, 1967).

2.3.4 Inappropriate Usage of Subjective Information Versus Objective Data for Behavioral Health Concerns

Because of the inherent nonstandardized definition of BH disability, many professionals across the disability spectrum tend to over-rely on subjective information (from either the person being evaluated or the professional) as "evidence" of disability versus utilizing objective data of impairment in functioning in the BH disability determination process. Examples of subjective information are the individual's self-report of distressing symptoms, family members' report of symptoms, the clinician's professional opinion without the inclusion of objective, standardized psychological testing to offset any underlying professional bias, and the usage of screening tools, such as a Beck Depression Inventory (BDI) (which is appropriate for research settings and basic screening, but inappropriate for the comprehensive assessment of individual's perceived BH impairment), questionnaires, surveys, and the like. This listing is not meant to be all-inclusive, but rather to illustrate common problematic issues that arise across the BH field. This is not to say that this type of information should not be gathered and noted in the assessment and treatment process, but it must be cross-checked with more objective means of confirming or ruling out impairment in functioning. The importance of objective assessment is a critical component of the BH evaluation and assessment process. Some examples of objective evidence are standardized objective psychological testing, blood work, as well as PET scans and MRIs (Melhorn & Ackerman, 2008; Warren, 2009). The process of objective psychological testing will be discussed later in Chaps. 3 and 4.

2.3.5 Over-Reliance on Subjective Information in the Diagnostic Process

Frequently, professionals involved in the BH field use psychological symptoms and their clinical opinions as shortcuts or heuristics to render a clinical diagnosis. Although this certainly is a component of assessment in which professionals are trained, using this approach alone leaves the professional vulnerable to over-relying on one's opinion and an underlying apparent assumption of infallibility in one's professional decision-making.

Using the physical treatment model, when a person consults with a physician, symptoms are noted and discussed but then further explored through a variety of more objective measures, such as cultures, blood assays, X-rays, CT, MRIs, and the like. Consequently, the physician is able to quickly narrow the clinical focus and use clinical tools available to confirm or rule out specific diagnoses and to delineate an appropriate treatment for the issue. While BH professionals have similar objective, clinical tools available, they are not regularly utilized so that the person's subjective report is often viewed as completely accurate and without bias. This is further compounded by the BH professional employing one's clinical opinion alone as the final arbiter in the ruling out or confirmation of a psychological condition and/or diagnosis. Thus, if the BH diagnosis is based solely on subjective information versus objectively determined data, and the diagnosis is incorrect, then conceivably, the person could receive the inappropriate professional treatment for reported concern. Unfortunately, this can result in lengthy and expensive professional treatment with little to no progress made in facilitating the person's return to one's previous level of functioning. The potential ethical and legal implications that could arise with this approach should give pause to all professionals (Hadjistavropoulos & Bieling, 2001; Hamm, Reiss, Paul, & Bursztajn, 2007; Harding, 2004; Warren, 2005, 2013a, b; Warren & Hubbard, 2008).

This more subjective type of approach taken by professionals is frequently observed in the BH disability claims process. Unfortunately, the majority of applications for BH disability have important missing documentation that impedes the claim management decision-making process. For example in the review of a large, national insurer, frequent missing information found in BH claims were:

1. A missing *DSM-5* (or current version) diagnosis.
2. A clinical evaluation is missing or is of poor quality.
3. A person's symptoms are provided as "proof" of impairment.
4. There are no objective data, such as valid, standardized psychological testing provided to support the reported diagnosis.
5. Treating professionals have not collaborated.
6. A treating professional has noted that the workplace must be changed before the person can return to work.
7. Open-ended workplace leave is reported as being required.
8. The person is reported to have sustained symptoms, even after lengthy treatment.

9. Evidence of poor quality of treatment provided by the BH professional (Warren & Hubbard, 2008).

This type of missing documentation results in a cycle that causes the need for additional documentation, delays in decision-making, mistrust, and frustration for all involved parties. Moreover, this increases the costs to the claimant and the insurer alike since it is necessary to have the claimant request additional information and perhaps reevaluation and for the insurer to have the file materials reviewed by a psychologist or psychiatrist trained in disability management. Because of lengthy delays, arbitrary decisions may be made and result in an adversarial stance between the BH professional, claimant, and insurer (Hadjistavropoulos & Bieling, 2001; Hamm et al., 2007; Warren, 2005, 2013a, b; Warren & Hubbard, 2006, 2008).

2.3.6 Physical Disability Concerns Represent the Majority of the Disability Claims

As noted earlier, there is a great deal of physical and BH comorbidity occurring in the disability management field. While various organizations may have databases specific to limited populations, by examining the SSA (2015) actuarial data, it can provide clear data to illustrate overall disability patterns. In 2015, there were 10, 237,204 SSA beneficiaries. These beneficiaries are broken into diagnostic groups. BH concerns represent the largest group (34.8% or 3,563,074 people) receiving disability benefits. However, most of the mental health group is comprised of intellectual disability or psychotic disorders, such as schizophrenia. The largest subgroup within the SSA mental health group is the mood disorders group. It's comprised of 1,394,271 SSA beneficiaries. There is another subgroup called "other mental disorders." This subgroup had 391,350 SSA beneficiaries in 2015. Typically, "other" is used to denote that a person has some type of mental disorder that does not cleanly fit into one of the other sub-diagnostic categories. This is an important factor to consider since most insurers will no longer accept indistinct diagnoses. Instead, a definitive *DSM* diagnosis is required. Yet, SSA does not consider this and lumps several hundred thousand into an "other" category in its actuarial data.

Instead, SSA's rules indicate that for the person to be eligible for SSA benefits, the person must have a mental health condition that will last at least 2 years and negatively impacts on the person's ability to work. Most psychological conditions are determined through the psychological evaluation process and are further assessed with standardized psychological testing. It is also important to note that the majority of psychological conditions which are treated with empirically supported treatment resolve in less than a year. The usual time frame that most psychological conditions resolve is typically within weeks to several months. Consequently, this is an important clue regarding the SSA disability determination claims process since SSA requires that a psychological condition must be present for at least 2 years into order to quality for SSA disability benefits. Moreover, SSA includes an "other" subgroup for those SSA psychological disability claims that do not have clear *DSM* diagnoses. Instead, both the person who is filing for SSA benefits and the professional(s) providing documentation "believe" that the person has a substantial mental health condition, but cannot say what it is. This necessarily means that there is no standardized psychological testing that confirms any *DSM* diagnosis since that is one of the primary purposes of psychological testing. That is, psychological testing confirms or rules out a psychological condition. Moreover, this also means that there is no clear diagnosis for the "other" subgroup, but treatment is being given anyhow. In the medical field, it is viewed as unethical and potentially fraudulent to provide treatment where no condition exists. Yet, this consideration of this problematic stance does not appear to be an issue within the SSA disability claim determination process. Based on the concerning issues just discussed, it is clear that SSA rules for the mental health disability claims filing are not aligned with current professional standards of care and allow subjective opinion as "documentation."

Moreover, when the mood disorder subgroup and "other" group are added, they account for 50% of the total MH diagnostic group receiving SSA benefits. To put this into greater perspective, the SSA beneficiaries in these two subgroups account for 17% of the total SSA disability benefits that are paid annually.

The second largest SSA beneficiary group is the musculoskeletal concerns (28.6%, 2,932,328). Of note, empirical research has consistently demonstrated that approximately 64% of individuals with musculoskeletal concerns (1,876,724 beneficiaries) have a comorbid BH diagnosis as well. Typical comorbid psychological conditions are MDD and several different anxiety disorders. By employing this information with the SSA data, this results in an additional 18.3% of individuals diagnosed with a musculoskeletal concern who have a concurrent BH diagnosis. This pushes both the totals of the overall mental health diagnostic group and the mood disorder subgroup to 5,439,798 and 3,327,099, respectively. This demonstrates that BH concerns account to 53% of the SSA disability benefits budget.

Moreover, as noted earlier, empirical research has demonstrated that there is approximately 50–60% prevalence rate of behavioral health comorbidity with other physical concerns, such as, for example, cardiac, stroke, diabetes, cancer, and morbid obesity (Buist-Bouwman et al., 2005; Campbell et al., 2003; CDC, 2006; Chellappa & Ramaraj, 2009; de Waal, Arnold, Spinhoven, et al., 2009; Dersh et al., 2002, 2005; Evans et al., 2005; Fava, Rush, Alpert, et al., 2006; Gros, Antony, McCabe, & Swinson, 2009; Hutter, Scheidt-Nave, & Baumeister, 2009; Kessler, Akiskal, Ames, et al., 2006; Kessler et al., 1997; Kessler et al., 2003; Kessler, McGonagle, Zhao, et al., 1994). Using this assumption, of the remaining 40.2% of individuals receiving SSDI benefits, approximately another 20.1–24.12% has a comorbid BH diagnosis. Thus, in taking SSA's data, and incorporating the empirical research demonstrating a high prevalence of physical and BH comorbidity, there are approximately 70.3–74.32% of individuals with a comorbid BH diagnosis within the SSA disability system. Even with the subtraction for intellectual and psychotic disorders which are permanent in nature, there are still 65.5–69.52% of individuals with a BH diagnosis. While these data illustrate the SSA BH comorbidity issue, it is essential to note that the same issue occurs within the private insurance industry which pays STD and LTD disability benefits. This is known because those individuals receiving STD and LTD disability benefits and who do not experience resolution of their concern typically go on to apply for SSA disability benefits. Consequently, this quickly demonstrates the true scope of the BH disability issue. Therefore, BH disability concerns represent the largest portion of disability recipients across the board of STD, LTD, and SSA (SSA, 2015).

Further illustration of the expanse of BH disability issues can be seen by examining the SSA for those 30 States and US territories with higher BH prevalence rates than the overall SSA average in Table 2.2.

Of note, the higher the BH disability percentage of SSA beneficiaries, the lower the second highest category of musculoskeletal concerns, except for three States. This can be observed in Table 2.3.

Table 2.4 demonstrates the overall BH prevalence rates with the SSA actuarial data when the BH and the musculoskeletal concerns only are included. Thus, this provides a clear picture of the extent of BH disability within one federal disability system.

There is not only a higher rate of BH disability in each of these States, but also the inclusion of the 64% of the musculoskeletal concerns that have a comorbid psychological disorder pushes the BH disability percentage even higher in all states (Dersh et al., 2002, 2005). Thus, it becomes clear the extent that BH disorders impact on federal disability. Because short-term disability (STD) and long-term disability (LTD) are the stepping stones for SSA disability benefits, it is clear that a similar pattern in the private insurance industry as well (Agency for Healthcare Research & Quality, 2015; National Committee for Quality Assurance, 2009).

Unfortunately, there is not a similar breakdown of data available for the WC system since statutes vary from State to State regarding the allowance of a BH concern as being compensable. For example, the State of Montana does not allow a BH concern under its WC laws. In other instances, some States such as IL may allow a BH claim under its WC law, but if a BH concern is not identified as a part of a physical claim. There is likely to result in an under-reporting of BH issues in the State's reported WC data (Kroenke & Unutzer, 2017; Kroenke et al., 2015). In addition, when a BH concern has been identified, but not confirmed with objective psychological assessment, it is likely that there will be an inaccurate over-counting of BH concerns within the data (Warren, 2005). Further discussion of the States and federal WC systems will take place in Chap. 6.

2.3.7 *Disability Concerns Can Only Be Physical or Behavioral in Nature, But Not Both*

By looking at the empirical research, it is abundantly clear that while an impairment issue can be either a physical or behavioral disorder, it is equally probable that an impairment concern can also be a comorbid concern. Thus, it is essential to move from an "either–or" approach and more to the integration of the biopsychosocial issues that have been to occur with all types of disorders and is the current model employed in empirical research. The biopsychosocial model was discussed in Chap. 1.

Table 2.2 States and territories with BH disability percentages higher than SSA BH disability percentage of 34.8%

Alabama: 37.7 Alaska: 37.8	**Hawaii: 44.7**	**Maine: 42.8**	**New Hampshire: 51.4**	Utah: 39.3
Arizona: 36.2	Idaho: 36.5	**Massachusetts: 49.6**	New Mexico: 36.0	**Vermont: 46.3**
California: 36.7	Illinois: 37.4	Michigan: 36.3	**North Dakota: 40.0**	Washington: 39.6 **Wisconsin: 40.0**
Connecticut: 43.8	Indiana: 36.9		Ohio: 39.0	Wyoming: 35.06
		Minnesota: 46.0	Oregon: 336.0	**Puerto Rico: 48.4**
District of Columbia: 42.9	Kansas: 37.0	Montana: 34.9 Nebraska: 37.1	**Rhode Island: 47.0** South Dakota: 38.1	**Foreign countries: 41.0**

The bold-print states represent over 40% of SSA BH disability in the State or territory

Table 2.3 States and territories with musculoskeletal disability percentages lower than SSA musculoskeletal percentage of 28.6%

Arizona: 27.3 California: 28.0	**Illinois 24.3** Indiana: 27.06 **Iowa: 24.3**	Maryland: 25.4 **Massachusetts: 21.8** Mississippi: 27.1 Nebraska: 25.4	New Jersey: 28.1 **North Dakota: 24.2** Ohio: 25.8 Rhode Island: 24.5	Utah: 24.8 Washington: 28.0 Wisconsin: 27.1
Connecticut: 22.6	Kansas: 27.2	**New Hampshire: 21.5**	Texas: 27.3	**Foreign countries: 19.5**
District of Columbia: 18.1 **Hawaii: 19.3**	Maine: 27.0		Utah: 24.8	

This demonstrates an overall inverse relationship between the States with higher BH disability and the lower disability beneficiaries with musculoskeletal concerns

2.3.8 BH Issues Must Be Treated Differently from Physical Issues

Most physical concerns have clear treatment standards that have been developed to quickly and effectively treat the underlying issue. Thus, a physician does not have to struggle to identify the assessment or treatment process. Instead, the majority of medical treatments are strongly based on the melding of clinical practice with scientifically based research. This type of information is typically taught during medical training as well as with continuing education throughout the professional career. This allows for a standardization of medical assessment and treatment from physician to physician. Consequently, a physical ailment, such as a broken bone, is treated in similar fashion by each professional (Warren, 2013a, b).

While there are similar standards in the graduate and medical training for the evaluation and assessment in the BH field, the same is not true when it comes to the

Table 2.4 The SSA BH disability group and the 64% of psychological comorbidity demonstrated in the empirical research and taken from the SSA musculoskeletal disability group

Hawaii: **56.3** Idaho: **54.2** Illinois: **52.5**	Iowa: **53.1** Kansas: **50.8** Kentucky: **53.5**	Minnesota: **53.5** Montana: **50.7** Nebraska: **51.3**	New Jersey: **50.1** New Mexico: **53.6** North Dakota: **53.5**	Oregon: **52.5** Pennsylvania: **50.2** Rhode Island: **55.0**
Indiana: **50.1**	Massachusetts: **60.9**	New Hampshire: **60.5**	Ohio: **55.0**	Puerto Rico: **63.6**

These percentages are added together for a cumulative totals

actual provision of professional BH treatment. Instead, it is common for a mélange of BH treatments provided without regard to empirical research and its synthesis into clinical practice. The problem with this approach is that appropriate treatment that is specific to the BH diagnosis may or may not be conducted. Instead, each BH professional is left to determine a type of treatment based on the professional's theoretic orientation, such as, for example, psychoanalysis, humanistic, or behavioral. While many BH professionals profess to provide eclectic psychotherapy, this is particularly problematic in regard to providing a cohesive treatment from start to finish. Many times, this type of treatment can result in poorly focused treatment that is both lengthy and open-ended. Thus, this type of approach can substantially reduce the likelihood of good treatment outcome, including facilitating the person's return to the previous level of functioning, if it is not strongly supported by scientific research. Furthermore, the treatment process issue is compounded by the tendency for many BH professionals to believe that BH issues should not be standardized because this is somehow uncaring and that behavioral health care must be treated differently from physical concerns. The problem with this approach is that it ignores/bypasses the biopsychosocial aspect of disability as well as overlooking the current scientifically based treatments available. Thus, this type of approach may result in the unintentional continuation of the individual's suffering. Most importantly, because many individuals with physical concerns also experience a concurrent psychological disorder, it is imperative to evaluate and treat BH issues in tandem with physical concerns (ACOEM, 2006, 2008; AMA, 2008; APA, 2009).

2.3.9 Treating Professionals Are the Most Appropriate to Evaluate BH Impairment in Functioning Issues

There is a tendency among all professionals in the disability field to believe that TPs are the best professionals to evaluate BH disability issues, particularly in regard to those individuals receiving treatment. However, there are several problems with this belief. First, when a TP is in the treating role, most professional organizations, such as the APA's ethical guidelines (2013), do not permit the professional to have a dual professional relationship with an individual receiving treatment. For example, a TP can be a TP, but cannot later switch roles to that of an objective evaluator, such as a forensic evaluator of the same person and who then purports to reexamine the individual and look current level of functioning. Other organizations, such as ACOEM (2008) and the AMA (2008), have noted similar restrictions for professionals as well. Thus, a professional may be a TP or an objective evaluator in more of a forensic role, but not both simultaneously. The primary reason is that there are conflicting professional responsibilities associated with each professional role (Table 2.5).

Another important issue is that most BH professionals are trained in assessment and treatment, but do not receive professional training in regard to disability prevention and management strategies since these professional skills are not typically taught at the present in most BH graduate programs or medical schools. Thus, while it is true that the TP may have spent more time with the person who is reporting impairment, clinical observation and opinion alone are insufficient to note whether the individual actually is impaired. Instead, this must be determined through more objective means, such as with standardized psychological testing (Bruns et al., 2010).

The argument of deference being expressly given to the TP's professional opinion over an independent evaluating professional has not been supported by the US Supreme Court. It held the following:

> ERISA does not require plan administrators to accord special deference to the opinions of treating physicians. The "treating physician rule" imposed by the Ninth Circuit was originally developed by Courts of Appeals as a means to control disability determinations by administrative law judges under the Social Security Act. In 1991, the Commissioner of Social Security adopted regulations approving and formalizing use of the rule in the Social Security disability program. Nothing in ERISA or the Secretary of Labor's ERISA regulations, however, suggests that plan administrators must accord special deference to the opinions of treating physicians, or imposes a heightened burden of explanation on administrators when they reject a treating physician's opinion…
>
> Finally, and of prime importance, courts have no warrant to require administrators automatically to accord special weight to the opinions of a claimant's physician; nor may courts impose on administrators a discrete burden of explanation when they credit reliable evidence that conflicts with a treating physician's evaluation. (U.S. Supreme Court, Black & Decker Disability Plan v. Nord, 538 U.S., No. 02-469, 2003, pp. 5–11).

In summary, while TP opinions can be provided as some documentation in the disability determination process, the inclusion of an independent evaluating professional's opinion and evaluation carries the same weight as that of the TP. While there will still be questions raised by professionals regarding whether the TP is the best professional to evaluate the individual regarding impairment in functioning, the specific limitations noted here dispose of those questions.

2.3.10 Ten BH Concerns Can Only Be Work- or Nonoccupationally Related

Because of the arbitrary ordinal (work-related, not work-related; event caused impairment, the event did not cause impairment) system that many legal systems, particularly the WC system, utilize, a BH professional is likely to be asked to give

Table 2.5 The differences in professional responsibilities between the treating and forensic roles in psychology

Treating psychologist role	Independent or forensic psychologist role
An individual selects the psychologist for psychological treatment	A third party selects the psychologist for an independent evaluation of the individual
The individual is considered the patient or the client	The third party is considered the client, not the individual being evaluated
The individual's treatment information is considered PHI	The data collected in the evaluation are not considered PHI. However, the APA restrictions of releasing raw test data only to qualified professionals must still be followed
HIPAA applies to all information, data, and health-care information	HIPAA is not likely to apply to some information or data gathered due to exceptions related to separate disability and workers' compensation laws and need to have specific information to make decisions. However, the information is limited in scope to what can be provided to a third party
No information may be released without written consent by the patient	Information gathered may be released to a third party without consent by the individual, such as with disability evaluations
A court order or subpoena is required for release of information in a lawsuit	In the case of some legal and disability procedures, clinical information can be released without consent of the individual
The state mental health laws apply where the psychologist practices	The state mental health law is less likely to apply due to HIPAA exceptions for the management of disability claims and workers' compensations laws
A summarization of diagnosis, treatment, and outcome to date can occur with appropriate signed release	Typically, no release is needed to release only information pertinent to the disability procedures and where the professional is serving as an expert in a legal proceeding
Test data are considered PHI. Summarizations of testing may occur only with signed release	Raw test data are considered PHI, but a summarization of test results are not. The summarization may be released without signed consent
The goal of treatment is to alleviate symptoms and teach appropriate coping strategies. Treatment usually occurs for 6+ sessions	The goal of the evaluation is to objectively evaluate the individual's current cognitive, psychological, and emotional functioning related to (1) job fitness and ability to complete current job responsibilities, (2) disability claim resolution, and (3) legal proceeding
The patient may be seen in the future, if the need arises	The individual is not typically seen after the evaluation
The patient may request a copy of the evaluation and treatment records	The individual may not request a copy of the evaluation records or report directly from the evaluating psychologist evaluee's. However, records may be obtained by an attorney[a]

[a]All professionals are strongly encouraged to become trained in their individual State laws and in regard to federal laws related to the different disability processes. Moreover, professionals should consult with an attorney regarding the specifics of each law

opinion regarding whether the BH concern is work- or nonoccupationally related. However, because of the complexity of biopsychosocial issues inherent in the BH model of evaluation, this question cannot be easily answered. Instead, it is essential to first examine the issues related to legal causality and the current BH model of evaluation (Warren, 2009, 2013a, b, 2016).

2.4 Causality and Behavioral Health Concerns

Causality is a legal issue related specifically to tort law and the WC system. The legal standard for professional opinions of cause in civil legal settings is based upon "a more probable than not basis" (Kahn & Langlieb, 2005). Specifically, the issue of causality is one that behavioral health professionals are asked to address frequently both the workers' compensation and tort legal systems. However, the issue of causality, particularly within the WC system, is at odds with the multidimensional behavioral health (e.g., psychological and psychiatric competent evaluation and treatment approach) which is currently followed in the behavioral health field. The primary reason for the problematic opposition is that the WC standard follows an approach in which all injuries, illnesses, and impairments are considered work-related when they are "caused or worsened by work-related injury, even if the employee is predisposed to the impairment" (Kahn & Langlieb; Melhorn & Ackerman, 2008). Therefore, the WC system follows an ordinal means of measurement delineating between only two categories of work-related or not work-related. There are no gradations between the two categories. Moreover, the system does not consider the reported psychological disorder in terms of predisposition toward impairment, past development issues, or biological causes. Consequently, there are many problems with this WC definition and its inability to translate directly to the highly complex assessment models employed by psychologists and psychiatrists.

In a greatly simplified overview of the BH assessment model, BH professionals must evaluate the person from multiple aspects of the person's life, health, psychological, cognitive, emotional, and psychosocial factors to determine the appropriate diagnosis and then, treatment. In addition, BH impairment in functioning is multifactorial in nature. It is this lack of translation of legal terminology and an arbitrary categorization of work- or nonwork-related causation to the application of the BH treatment system that leads to a great deal of frustration and misconceptions. In order for a BH professional to attempt to answer the issue of causality, it is incumbent upon the other individuals involved in the disability process: employee/claimant, employer, families, coworkers, treating professionals, insurers, and attorneys to recognize:

1. The difference between impairment and disability.
2. What constitutes appropriate roles for the treating and evaluating professionals.
3. The essential criteria of an accurate diagnosis, appropriate best practice standard-based treatment.

4. The expectation of setting RTW as a required treatment goal.
5. The high probability in remission of the majority of psychological disorders and reduction in objectively determined impairment.
6. The ultimate goal of the BH treatment process is to restore the person to one's previous level of functioning (Warren, 2009).

This last aspect is of particular importance because if the person is to improve to one's previous level of functioning, then it may potentially reduce the monetary award or benefits paid to the individual. In addition, because the actual cause of a true objectively determined psychological disorder is multifactorial in nature, the majority of BH disorders cannot always be readily connected with a single interaction, setting, event, or person. Moreover, many true objective psychological disorders do not occur/begin directly after a specific event which is often identified as a trigger for a disorder. Instead, the development of true objective psychological impairment in functioning is a complex process comprised of genetic, social, psychosocial, and biological (biopsychosocial) factors that gradually converge across an indeterminate time period before a psychological disorder becomes apparent. Thus, absolute determination from a behavioral health standpoint is not usually possible (Caine, 2003; Heilburn, 2001; Heilburn et al., 2003; Heilburn, Marczyk, & DeMatteo, 2002; Heilburn, Marczyk, DeMatteo, & Mack-Allen, 2007; Heilburn, Warren, & Picarello, 2003).

Another issue that arises within legal causality is that all individuals involved in the disability determination process tend to use their own perceptions (accurate or inaccurate) to link a specific event as being the cause of the person's psychological disorder. This is particularly true in the legal system. The inherent problem with this approach is that it does not always incorporate clear and objective data to support the perception or in some instances, the professional opinion. Consequently, when subjective information is utilized as "proof," it further muddies the water regarding the causation issue (Melhorn & Ackerman, 2008; Warren, 2009).

In order for a BH professional to attempt to answer the legal issue of causality, the clinician must possess a thorough and competent understanding of the diagnostic process, how the correct diagnosis drives the selection of the appropriate treatment, and the emotional meaning that the individual has attached to the subjective symptoms s/he is experiencing. It is important to note that all parties, patients/employees/claimants, treating professionals, and attorneys frequently inappropriately subscribe cause to events and situations without the consideration of the necessary components of development, personality, and biological issues. Thus, this line of reasoning is often overly simplistic, circular in nature, and inaccurate. Most importantly, this ignores the significant complexity of the true development of a psychological disorder and that the majority of individuals with a psychological disorder still continue to function in life, including work (Grove, Zald, Lebow, Smitz, & Nelson, 2000; Melhorn & Ackerman, 2008; Warren, 2009; Young, Kane, & Nicholson, 2007).

There are several factors that must be examined and evaluated by the BH professional in order to complete a more thorough evaluation and to rule out potential treatment issues that are not psychological disorders and/or misperceptions, but may negatively impact on treatment outcome. These issues are:

- *Primary gain.* The person experiences relief with the symptom that helps to avoid an unconscious and internal conflict. It provides an acceptable excuse to avoid a situation. For example, a person with a severe headache is excused from going to work. The person has been having some dissatisfaction at work. Thus, the headache allows the person to avoid work. Thus, primary gain is an internalized motivation (Melhorn & Ackerman, 2008; Warren, 2009).
- *Secondary gain.* Any type of disorder may have a secondary gain component. In general, the motivation is externally based and is linked to obtaining or avoiding something. Examples of secondary gains can be increased attention from one's spouse, avoiding a household chore or a jail sentence, or monetary awards. The key element is that the person is consciously aware of the motivation (Melhorn & Ackerman, 2008; Warren, 2009).
- *Lack of training and/or misperception.* Frequently, a person or professional will inappropriately associate an event as a cause of a BH disorder, but without full knowledge of the complex evaluative process. This is not done maliciously or with intent. It is simply due to a lack of knowledge or in the case of the professional, either lack of training or a bias in clinical opinion that is not supported by objective data (Melhorn & Ackerman, 2008; Warren, 2009).
- *Malingering* versus *symptom exaggeration.* Malingering occurs when a person knowingly and willingly fakes one's symptomology for financial gain, such as in a lawsuit. It is not a psychological disorder. Instead, it is fraudulent behavior and one that may be criminal (Aronoff et al., 2007; Barsky, 2002; Iverson, 2007; McCracken & Gatchel, 2000; Mittenberg, Patton, Canyock, & Condit, 2002; Rogers, 1988, 1997; Rogers & Bender, 2003; Rohling, Binder, & Langhinrichsen-Rohling, 1995; Scott, Bruffaerts, Tsang, et al., 2007; Scott, Von Korff, Alonso, et al., 2009; Thompson, LeBourgeois, & Black, 2004; Warren, 2009; Wiley, 1998).
- *Symptom exaggeration is a conscious act.* Although symptom exaggeration can be a component of malingering, it does not automatically equate to malingering. For example, a person may exaggerate one's symptoms because of wanting assistance with a problem and fearing the concern will not be taken seriously without consciously increasing one's symptoms. Instead, the individual may exaggerate one's symptoms as a means to ensure help is obtained for the concern. If the concern is objectively determined to exist, then, the professional will need to explore whether the exaggeration is simply an exaggeration or if it is a willful intent to purposely mislead the professional and the concern does not exist. The latter is an example of malingering. Malingering is a conscious act of knowing that a disorder or symptoms do not exist and yet fabricates the disorder or symptoms. Malingering is fraud (Aronoff et al., 2007; Barsky, 2002; Iverson, 2007; McCracken & Gatchel, 2000; Mittenberg et al., 2002; Rogers, 1988, 1997; Rogers & Bender, 2003; Thompson et al., 2004; Warren, 2009; Wiley, 1998).
- Because empirical research has revealed that there is a higher rate (30–40%) of symptom exaggeration and malingering with disability concerns due to motiva-

tion for a favorable outcome, it is imperative that all BH professionals evaluate for these types of issues (Aronoff et al., 2007; Iverson, 2007; Mittenberg et al., 2002; Rogers, 1988, 1997; Rogers & Bender, 2003). Moreover, the AMA's *Guides to the Evaluation of Permanent Impairment* (AMA, 2008) requires this as a part of the BH evaluation.

- *Denial of a BH disorder*. In our society, there is still a stigma of having a psychological disorder. Thus, it is frequently difficult for some individuals to openly acknowledge the possibility of a psychological disorder. Instead, the person is likely to attribute the symptoms to another, more personally acceptable situation. This is a face-saving mechanism on the part of the involved person (Bagenstos, 2000).

It is essential to note that many BH symptoms are actually defenses used by the person for protection from one's emotional distress. Because of this, the individual cannot typically provide objective and accurate descriptions and a factually based explanation of the psychological concern. Thus, the person's description is more likely to be subjective in nature and must be corroborated against other types of more objective data (Warren, 2009).

2.4.1 Professional Barriers to Objective BH Causality Determination

There are several additional issues that arise with professionals that further compromise one's ability to infer with the BH causality determination process. These are:

- *Incomplete or cursory evaluation and assessment of the individual*. This occurs with the professional that does not follow all of the required components necessary to evaluate the person in a competent and comprehensive manner. Thus, the professional bases one's professional opinion on incomplete professional data (Warren, 2009).
- *Lack of clinical objectivity*. In this instance, the professional is influenced by conscious or unconscious feelings. The professional then moves away from professional objectivity (Grove et al., 2000; Harding, 2004).
- *Utilization of clinical heuristics*. Heuristics represent clinical generalizations or shortcuts that a professional may use in either the evaluation or treatment process that is based upon incorrect assumptions (Harding, 2004).
- *Differences in clinical opinion*. This commonly occurs when professionals focus on select clinical information or data, while ignoring data that do not support one's professional opinion or based on the lack of comprehensive synthesis of developmental, social, and biological factors (Warren, 2013a, b, 2016).
- *Potential loss of insurance*. Because some systems such as the WC system only pay for work-related concerns, this may leave a person without health insurance to pay for treatment (Pransky et al., 2004). Thus, the individual may be inclined to claim that the condition is work-related. At the same time, the professional

may feel a quandary either in not treating the person or in opining that the concern is related to the workplace (Warren, 2013a, b, 2016).

- *A professional desire to not upset patients and referral sources*. Most professionals want their patients as well as referral sources to be happy with them. Therefore, the professional may experience a wish to avoid conflict. In this circumstance, the professional may avoid issues and comprehensive evaluation as well as not stating the objective data findings clearly as a means to "keep everyone happy." However, this greatly decreases the professional's integrity as well as substantially degrades the credibility of the professional's opinion (Warren, 2009).
- *Lack of routine assessment of symptom exaggeration and malingering*. In the evaluation of symptom exaggeration and malingering, many professionals are quick to avoid a comprehensive assessment of these issues because of the distasteful nature of having to note that a person is purposefully misrepresenting the severity of symptoms. It is important to note that the current American Medical Association's *Guides to the Evaluation of Permanent Impairment* (AMA, 2008) requires the professional to evaluate for symptom exaggeration and malingering as part of the evaluation for any reported BH impairment in functioning. It must be noted that neither symptom exaggeration nor malingering is something that a professional can simply opine based on clinical opinion alone. Instead, it takes careful, comprehensive evaluation and includes looking at overall patterns across objective, standardized psychological tests (Aronoff et al., 2007; Iverson, 2007; Warren, 2009).
- *Medicalization*. This occurs when a professional identifies everyday situations, events, and occurrences and inappropriately mislabels them as medical or psychological disorders. Medicalization is at the heart of separating psychosocial issues from true objectively determined psychological disorders. Examples of psychosocial concerns are "stress," job dissatisfaction, workplace conflict, and relationship discord, which may aggravate a psychological disorder, but are not actual psychological disorders themselves. The *DSM-5* does not have diagnostic criteria for psychosocial concerns. Instead, the multiaxial system that existed in previous *DSM* versions no longer exists in *DSM-5*. When the *DSM-5* was being revised, the *DSM-5* Task Force selected a few of the *International Classification of Diseases* (*ICD-9-CM*) V codes and the *ICD-10-CM* Z codes to take the place of *DSM* Axis IV (psychosocial issues). In addition, the Global Assessment of Functioning (GAF) scale was removed from the *DSM-5* due to its lack of clinical reliability. Now, users of the *DSM-5* are to use the World Health Organization (WHO) Disability Assessment Schedule (WHODAS 2.0) as a clinician measure of the individual's functioning (ApA, 2013). However, many of the same problems exist with the *WHODAS* as existed with the GAF due to the lack of validity and reliability measures. While psychosocial issues may cause situational distress, they are not currently accepted as being a recognized psychological diagnosis. Moreover, if a professional artificially separates a psychosocial concern from the biopsychosocial model but ignores the contribution of these other complex aspects, then this should be viewed as a deviation from current practice standards (Barsky & Borus, 1995; Warren, 2003, 2009).

2.5 Conclusion

It is clear that BH health issues are a critical component in the multiple US disability processes. BH concerns cannot be simply assumed based on opinion or exposure to certain events. Instead, there are multiple individual and professional factors that negatively contribute across the current BH disability spectrum. In Chap. 5, strong, scientifically based strategies will be discussed in order to positively improve the BH treatment and disability process and, most importantly, to accurately assess the potential underlying BH concerns in order to facilitate the individual's return to health.

References

Agency for Healthcare Research and Quality. (2015). National Healthcare Quality and Disparities Report and 5th Anniversary update on the national quality strategy. Content last reviewed June, 2017. Agency for Healthcare Research and Quality. Rockville, MD. http://www.ahrq.gov/research/findings/nhqrdr/nhqdr15/index.html

Alpert, J. E., Biggs, M. M., Davis, L., et al. (2006). Enrolling research subjects from clinical practice: Ethical and procedural issues in the sequenced-treatment alternatives to relieve depression (STAR*D) trial. *Psychiatry Research, 141*(2), 193–200.

American College of Occupational and Environmental Medicine (ACOEM). (2008). *Occupational medicine practice guidelines: Evaluation and management of common health problems and functional recovery in workers* (3rd ed.). Beverly Farms, MA: OEM Health Information Press.

American College of Occupational and Environmental Medicine's Stay-at-Work and Return-to-Work Process Improvement Committee, Christian, J., Martin, D., Brown, D., Colledge, A., Gean, C., et al. (2006). Introduction to ACOEM's new work disability prevention guideline: "Preventing needless work disability by helping people stay employed". *Journal of Occupational and Environmental Medicine, 48*(9), 972–987.

American Educational Research Association, the American Psychological Association, and the National Council on Measurement in Education. (2014). *Standards for educational and psychological testing* (3rd ed.). Washington, DC: American Educational Research Association, the American Psychological Association, and the National Council on Measurement in Education.

American Medical Association (AMA). (2008). *Guides to the evaluation of permanent impairment* (6th ed.). Chicago, IL: American Medical Association.

American Medical Association (AMA). (2013). *Guides to the evaluation of disease and injury causation* (2nd ed.). Chicago: American Medical Association.

American Psychiatric Association (ApA). (2006). *Practice guidelines for the treatment of psychiatric disorders: Compendium, 2006*. Arlington, VA: American Psychiatric Association.

American Psychiatric Association (ApA). (2013). *Diagnostic and statistical manual of mental disorders: DSM-5*. Washington, DC: American Psychiatric Association.

American Psychiatric Foundation's Partnership for Workplace Mental Health. (2005). *Assessing and treating psychiatric occupational disability, executive report*. Washington, DC: American Psychiatric Association.

American Psychological Association (APA). (2001). APA's guidelines for test user qualifications: An executive summary. *American Psychologist, 56*(12), 1099–1113.

American Psychological Association (APA). (2002). Ethical principles of psychologists and code of conduct. *American Psychologist, 57*, 1060–1073.

American Psychological Association (APA). (2013). Specialty guidelines for forensic psychology. *The American Psychologist, 68*, 7–19. https://doi.org/10.1037/a0029889.

American Psychological Association (APA). (2007a). *Recent developments affecting the disclosure of test data and materials: Comments regarding the 1996 statement on the disclosure of test data* (pp. 1–7). Washington, DC: American Psychological Association.

American Psychological Association (APA). (2007b). Record keeping guidelines. *American Psychologist, 62*, 993–1004.

American Psychological Association (APA). (2009). *Guidelines and principles for accreditation of programs in professional psychology* (pp. 1–38). Washington, DC: American Psychological Association.

American Recovery and Reinvestment Act of 2009 (ARRA), Pubic Law No. 111–5.

Aronoff, G. M., Mandel, S., Genovese, E., et al. (2007). Evaluating malingering in contested injury or illness. *Pain Practice, 7*(2), 178–204.

Bagenstos, S. R. (2000). Subordination, stigma, and "disability". *Virginia Law Review, 86*, 397–534.

Barlow, D. H. (2005). What's new about evidenced-based assessment? *Psychological Assessment, 17*, 308–311.

Barsky, A. J. (2002). Forgetting, fabricating, and telescoping: The instability of medical history. *Archives of Internal Medicine, 162*, 981–984.

Barsky, A. J., & Borus, J. F. (1995). Somatization and medicalization in the era of managed care. *Journal of the American Medical Association, 274*, 1931–1934.

Baumeister, H., & Hutter, N. (2012). Collaborative care for depression in medical ill patients. *Current Opinion in Psychiatry, 25*(5), 405–414. https://doi.org/10.1097/YCO.0b013e3283556c63.

Bethune, S. (2017). And idaho makes five. American Psychological Association. *The Monitor, 48*(6), 18.

Binder, L. M., & Rohling, M. L. (1996). Money matters: A meta-analytic review of the effects of financial incentives on recovery after closed head injury. *American Journal of Psychiatry, 153*, 7–10.

Bogner, H. R., de Vries, H. F., Maulik, P. K., & Unützer, J. (2009). Mental health services use: Baltimore epidemiologic catchment area follow-up. *The American Journal of Geriatric Psychiatry, 17*(8), 706–715.

Bruns, D., & Disorbio, J. M. (2005). Chronic pain and biopsychosocial disorders. *Practical Pain Management, 5*(7), 2–9.

Bruns, D., Mueller, K., & Warren, P. (2010). The development of biopsychosocial laws governing treatment of pain and injury. *Psychological Injury and Law, 3*, 169–181.

Buist-Bouwman, M. A., de Graaf, R., Vollebergh, W. A. M., & Ormel, J. (2005). Comorbidity of physical and mental disorders and the effect on work-loss days. *Acta Psychiatrica Scandinavica, 111*(6), 436–443.

Bush, S. S., Demarkis, G. J., & Rohling, M. L. (2017). *APA handbook of forensic neuropsychology*. Washington, D.C.: American Psychological Association.

Bush, S. S., & Heilbronner, R. L. (2012). The neuropsychological IME. In S. S. Bush & G. L. Iverson (Eds.), *Neuropsychological assessment of work-related injuries* (pp. 280–302). New York: Guilford Press.

Bush, S. S., & Martin, T. A. (2008). Confidentiality in neuropsychological practice. In J. A. M. Horton & D. Wedding (Eds.), *The neuropsychology handbook* (3rd ed., pp. 515–530). New York: Springer.

Bush, S. S., & Martin, T. A. (2010a). The ethical and clinical practice of disclosing raw test data: Addressing the ongoing debate. *Applied Neuropsychology : Adult, 13*, 115–124. https://doi.org/10.1207/s15324826an1302_6.

Bush, S. S., & Martin, T. A. (2010b). Privacy, confidentiality, and privilege in forensic neuropsychology. In A. M. Horton Jr. & L. C. Hartlage (Eds.), *The handbook of forensic neuropsychology* (2nd ed., pp. 235–244). New York: Springer.

Caine, E. D. (2003). Determining causation in psychiatry. In K. A. Phillips, M. B. First, & H. A. Pincus (Eds.), *Advancing DSM: Dilemmas in psychiatric diagnosis*. Washington, DC: American Psychiatric Association.

Campbell, L. C., Clauw, D. J., & Keefe, F. J. (2003). Persistent pain and depression: A biopsychosocial perspective. *Biological Psychiatry, 54*, 399–409.

Centers for Disease Control and Prevention (CDC). (2013). Behavioral risk factor surveillance system prevalence data, 2010. In *62(ss01);1–247.Atlanta*. CDC: GA.

Centers for Disease Control and Prevention (CDC); National Center for Injury Prevention and Control. (2006). Web-based injury statistics query and reporting system (WISQARS). *Journal*. In *Retrieved from*. http://www.cdc.gov/ncipc/wisqars/default.htm.

Centers for Disease Control and Prevention (CDC): Mental health basics. https://www.cdc.gov/mentalhealth/basics.htm, accessed June 4, 2017.

Chellappa, P., & Ramaraj, R. (2009). Depression, homocysteine concentration, and cardiovascular events. *Journal of the American Medical Association, 301*(15), 1542.

Colorado Division of Workers' Compensation. (2007). Rule 17, exhibit 9: chronic pain disorder medical treatment guidelines. In *Retrieved from*. http://www.coworkforce.com/dwc/Rules/Rules%202007/New%20MTG/EX_9_Chronic_Pain.pdf.

Colorado Division of Workers' Compensation. (2009). Rule 17: Medical treatment guidelines. Retrieved June 9, 2009. In *From*. http://www.colorado.gov/cs/Satellite/CDLE-WorkComp/CDLE/1248095316866.

de Waal, M. W. M., Arnold, I. A., Spinhoven, P., et al. (2009). The role of comorbidity in the detection of psychiatric disorders with checklists for mental and physical symptoms in primary care. *Social Psychiatry and Psychiatric Epidemiology, 44*(1), 78–85.

Dersh, J., Gatchel, R. J., Polatin, P., & Mayer, T. (2002). Prevalence of psychiatric disorders in patients with chronic work-related musculoskeletal pain disability. *Journal of Occupational and Environmental Medicine, 44*, 459–469.

Dersh, J., Polatin, P., Leeman, G., & Gatchel, R. J. (2005). Secondary gains and losses in the medicolegal setting. In I. Z. Schultz & R. Gatchel (Eds.), *Handbook of complex occupational disability claims: Early risk identification, intervention, and prevention*. New York: Springer Science + Business Media. 566 pp.

Disability Management Employer Coalition (DMEC). (2008). *DMEC 2008 employer behavioral risk survey*. San Diego, CA: Disability Management Employer Coalition.

Disability Management Employer Coalition (DMEC). (2009). Tools of the trade: A compilation of programs and processes for the absence, disability. In *Health and productivity professional*. San Diego, CA: Disability Management Employer Coalition.

Epstein, S. A., Hooper, L. M., Weinfurt, K. P., DePuy, V., Cooper, L. A., Harless, W. G., & Tracy, C. M. (2008). Primary care physicians' evaluation and treatment of depression: Results of an experimental study using video vignettes. *Medical Care Research and Review : MCRR, 65*(6), 674–695. https://doi.org/10.1177/1077558708320987.

Evans, D. L., Charney, D. S., Lewis, L., et al. (2005). Mood disorders in the medically ill: Scientific review and recommendations. *Biological Psychiatry, 58*, 175–189.

Fava, M., Rush, A. J., Alpert, J. E., et al. (2006). What clinical and symptom features and comorbid disorders characterize outpatients with anxious major depressive disorder: A replication and extension. *Canadian Journal of Psychiatry, 51*(13), 823–835.

Fichter, M. M., Narrow, W. E., Roper, M. T., et al. (1996). Prevalence of mental illness in Germany and the United States: Comparison of the upper Bavarian study and the epidemiologic catchment area program. *Journal of Nervous and Mental Disease, 184*(10), 598–606.

Gask, L. (2005). Overt and covert barriers to the integration of primary and specialist mental health care. *Social Science & Medicine, 61*(8), 1785–1794.

Gatchel, R. J. (2004). Comorbidity of chronic mental and physical health conditions: The biopsychosocial perspective. *American Psychologist, 59*, 792–805.

GBD 2013 DALYs and HALE Collaborators. (2015). Global, regional, and national disability-adjusted life years (DALYs) for 306 diseases and injuries and healthy life expectancy (HALE) for 188 countries, 1990–2013: Quantifying the epidemiological transition. Lancet (London, England), 386(10009), 2145–2191. https://doi.org/10.1016/S0140-6736(15)61340-X.

Gerdtham, U. G., & Johannesson, M. (2003). A note on the effect of unemployment on mortality. *Journal of Health Economics, 22*, 505–518.

Gold, L. H., Anfang, S. A., Drukteinis, A. M., et al. (2008). AAPL practice guideline for the forensic evaluation of psychiatric disability. *Journal of the American Academy of Psychiatry and the Law, 36*(Suppl. 4), S3–S50.

Gold, L. H., & Davidson, J. E. (2007). Do you understand your risk? Liability and third-party evaluations in civil litigation. *The Journal of the American Academy of Psychiatry and the Law, 35*, 200–210. Retrieved from http://bit.ly/1mlf3vT.

Gold, L. H., & Shuman, D. W. (2009). Employment evaluations and the law. In *Evaluating mental health disability in the workplace* (pp. 25–42). New York: Springer.

Goodrich, D. E., Kilbourne, A. M., Nord, K. M., & Bauer, M. S. (2013). Mental health collaborative care and its role in primary care settings. *Current Psychiatry Reports, 15*(8), 383. https://doi.org/10.1007/s11920-013-0383-2.

Greenberg, S. A., & Shuman, D. W. (1997). Irreconcilable conflict between therapeutic and forensic roles. *Professional Psychology: Research and Practice, 28*, 50–57.

Greenberg, S. A., & Shuman, D. W. (2007). When worlds collide: Therapeutic and forensic roles. *Professional Psychology:Research and Practice, 38*(2), 129–132. https://doi.org/10.1037/0735-7028.38.2.129.

Greene, R. L. (2007). Forensic applications of the Minnesota multiphasic personality Inventory-2. In A. M. Goldstein (Ed.), *Forensic psychology: Emerging topics and expanding roles* (pp. 73–96). Hoboken, NJ: John Wiley & Sons.

Gros, D. F., Antony, M. M., McCabe, R. E., & Swinson, R. P. (2009). Frequency and severity of the symptoms of irritable bowel syndrome across the anxiety disorders and depression. *Journal of Anxiety Disorders, 23*(2), 290–296.

Grove, W. M., Zald, D. H., Lebow, B. S., Smitz, B. E., & Nelson, C. (2000). Clinical versus mechanical prediction: A meta-analysis. *Psychological Assessment, 12*(1), 19–30.

Hadjistavropoulos, T., & Bieling, P. (2001). File review consultation in the adjudication of mental health and chronic pain disability claims. *Consulting Psychology Journal: Practice and Research, 53*(1), 52–63.

Hamm, R. M., Reiss, D. M., Paul, R. K., & Bursztajn, H. J. (2007). Knocking at the wrong door: Insured workers' inadequate psychiatric care and workers' compensation claims. *International Journal of Law and Psychiatry, 30*, 416–426.

Harding, T. P. (2004). Psychiatric disability and clinical decision making: The impact of judgment error and bias. *Clinical Psychology Review, 24*, 707–729.

Health Insurance Portability and Accountability Act of 1996 (HIPAA), Pubic Law No. 104–191.

Heilburn, K. (2001). *Principles of forensic mental health assessment.* New York: Kluwer Academic/Plenum Publishers.

Heilburn, K., Grisso, T., & Goldstein, A. M. (2009). *Foundations of forensic mental health assessment.* New York: Oxford University Press. 180 pp.

Heilburn, K., Marczyk, G., & DeMatteo, D. (2002). *Forensic mental health assessment: A casebook.* New York: Oxford University Press.

Heilburn, K., Marczyk, G., DeMatteo, D., & Mack-Allen, J. (2007). A principles-based approach to forensic mental health assessment: Utility and update. In A. M. Goldstein (Ed.), *Forensic psychology: Emerging topics and expanding roles* (pp. 45–72). Hoboken, NJ: John Wiley & Sons.

Heilburn, K., Marczyk, G., DeMatteo, D., Zillmer, E., Harris, J., & Jennings, T. (2003). Principles of forensic mental health assessment: Implications for neuropsychological assessment in forensic contexts. *Assessment, 10*, 329–343.

Heilburn, K., Warren, J., & Picarello, K. (2003). Third party information in forensic assessment. In A. M. Goldstein (Ed.), *Forensic psychology: Vol. 11 of handbook of psychology* (pp. 69–86). Hoboken, NJ: John Wiley & Sons.

Hooper, L. M., Epstein, S. A., Weinfurt, K. P., DeCoster, J., Qu, L., & Hannah, N. J. (2012). Predictors of primary care physicians' self-reported intention to conduct suicide risk assessments. *The Journal of Behavioral Health Services & Research, 39*(2), 103–115. https://doi.org/10.1007/s11414-011-9268-5.

Hutter, N., Scheidt-Nave, C., & Baumeister, H. (2009). Health care utilisation and quality of life in individuals with diabetes and comorbid mental disorders. *General Hospital Psychiatry, 31*(1), 33–35.

Iverson, G. L. (2007). Identifying exaggeration and malingering. *Pain Practice, 7*(2), 94–102.

Kahn, J. P., & Langlieb, A. M. (Eds.). (2005). *Mental health and productivity in the workplace: A handbook for organizations and clinicians*. San Francisco, CA: Jossey-Bass.

Kane, A. W. (2008). Forensic psychology, psychological injuries, and the law. *Psychological Injury and Law, 1*(1), 36–58. https://doi.org/10.1007/s12207-007-9000-1.

Kessler, R. C., Akiskal, H. S., Ames, M., et al. (2006). Prevalence and effects of mood disorders on work performance in a nationally representative sample of U.S. workers. *American Journal of Psychiatry, 163*(9), 1561–1568.

Kessler, R. C., Anthony, J. C., Blazer, D. G., et al. (1997). The US comorbidity National Survey: Overview and future directions. *Epidemiologia e Psichiatria Sociale, 6*(1), 4–16.

Kessler, R. C., McGonagle, K., Zhao, S., et al. (1994). Lifetime and 12-month prevalence of DSM-III-R psychiatric disorders in the United States: Results from the National Comorbidity Survey. *Archives of General Psychiatry, 51*, 8–19.

Kessler, R. C., Ormel, J., Dernier, O., & Stang, P. E. (2003). Co-morbid mental disorders account for the role impairment of commonly occurring chronic physical disorders: Results from the National Comorbidity Survey. *Journal of Occupational and Environmental Medicine, 45*, 1257–1266.

Kessler, R. C., & Wang, P. S. (2008). The descriptive epidemiology of commonly occurring mental disorders in the United States. *Annual Review of Public Health, 29*, 115–129.

Koocher, G. P., & Keith-Spiegel, P. (2016). *Ethics in psychology and the mental health professions* (4th ed.). Oxford: NY. Oxford University Press.

Koocher, G. P., Norcross, J. C., & Greene, B. A. (2013). *Psychologist' desk reference* (3rd ed.). Oxford, NY: Oxford University Press.

Koocher, G. P., Norcross, J. C., & Hill, S. S. (2005). *Psychologists' desk reference* (2nd ed.). Oxford, NY: Oxford University Press.

Kouzis, A. C., & Eaton, W. W. (1997). Psychopathology and the development of disability. *Social Psychiatry and Psychiatric Epidemiology, 32*(7), 379–386.

Kroenke, K., Monahan, P. O., & Kean, J. (2015). Pragmatic characteristics of patient-reported outcome measures are important for use in clinical practice. *Journal of Clinical Epidemiology, 68*(9), 1085–1092. https://doi.org/10.1016/j.jclinepi.2015.03.023.

Kroenke, K., & Unutzer, J. (2017). Closing the false divide: Sustainable approaches to integrating mental health services into primary care. *Journal of General Internal Medicine, 32*(4), 404–410. https://doi.org/10.1007/s11606-016-3967-9.

Lee, H. C., Lyketsos, C. G., & Rao, V. (2003). Pharmacological management of the psychiatric aspects of traumatic brain injury. *International Review of Psychiatry, 15*(4), 359–370.

Lerner, D., & Henke, R. M. (2008). What does research tell us about depression, job performance, and work productivity? *Journal of Occupational and Environmental Medicine, 50*(4), 401–410.

MacDonald-Wilson, K., Rogers, E. S., & Anthony, W. A. (2001). Unique issues in assessing work function among individuals with psychiatric disabilities. *Journal of Occupational Rehabilitation, 11*(3), 217–232.

Marchetti, I., Loeys, T., Alloy, L. B., & Koster, E. H. W. (2016). Unveiling the structure of cognitive vulnerability for depression: Specificity and overlap. *PLoS One, 11*(12), e0168612. https://doi.org/10.1371/journal.pone.0168612.

Mauksch, L. B., Dugdale, D. C., Dodson, S., & Epstein, R. (2008). Relationship, communication, and efficiency in the medical encounter: Creating a clinical model from a literature review. *Archives of Internal Medicine, 168*(13), 1387–1395.

McCracken, L. M., & Gatchel, R. J. (2000). The magnification of psychopathology sequelae associated with multiple chronic medical conditions. *Journal of Applied Biobehavioral Research, 5*(1), 92–99.

Melhorn, J. M., & Ackerman, W. E. (Eds.). (2008). *Guides to the evaluation of disease and injury causation*. Chicago, IL: American Medical Association.

Merikangas, K. R., Ames, M., Cui, L., Stang, P. D., Ustun, B., Von Korff, M., et al. (2007). The impact of comorbidity of mental and physical conditions on role disability in the US adult household population. *Archives of General Psychiatry, 64*, 1180–1188.

Messer, S. B. (2004). Evidence-based practice: Beyond empirically supported treatments. *Professional Psychology: Research and Practice, 35*, 580–588.

Ming, T.-S., Thomas, G. M., & Weimin, Z. (2007). Physician and patient behaviour, time allocation in primary care office visits. *Health Services Research, 42*(5), 1871–1894.

Mittenberg, W., Patton, C., Canyock, E. M., & Condit, D. C. (2002). Base rates of malingering and symptom exaggeration. *Journal of Clinical and Experimental Neuropsychology, 24*(8), 1094–1102.

Nathan, P. E., & Gorman, J. M. (Eds.). (1998). *A guide to treatments that work*. New York: Oxford University Press.

National Business Group on Health (NBGH). (2007). *An employer's guide to behavioral health services* (p. 100). Washington, DC: National Business Group on Health.

National Committee for Quality Assurance. (2009). *Healthcare effectiveness data and information set (HEDIS)* (p. 2009). Washington, DC: National Committee for Quality Assurance.

National Institute of Mental Health. (2008). *The numbers count: Mental disorders in America*. Bethesda, MD: National Institute of Mental Health.

Ormel, J., Petukhova, M., Chatterji, S., et al. (2008). Disability and treatment of specific mental and physical disorders across the world. *The British Journal of Psychiatry: the Journal of Mental Science, 192*(5), 368–375.

Patel, V., Chisholm, D., Dua, T., et al. (2016). *Mental, neurological, and substance use disorders: Disease control priorities* (Vol. Volume 4, 3rd ed.). Washington (DC): The International Bank for Reconstruction and Development/The World Bank. https://doi.org/10.1596/9781464804267_ch1.

Pope, K. S., & Vasquez, M. J. T. (2016). *Ethics in psychotherapy and counseling* (5th ed.). Hoboken, NJ: Wiley & Sons.

Pransky, G. S., Shaw, W. S., Franche, R. L., & Clarke, A. (2004). Disability prevention and communication among workers, physicians, employers, and insurers: Current models and opportunities for improvement. *Disability & Rehabilitation, 26*(11), 625–634.

Rao, V., & Lyketsos, C. G. (2003). Psychiatric aspects of traumatic brain injury: New solutions to an old problem. *International Review of Psychiatry, 15*(4), 299–301.

Reed, G. M., Kihlstrom, J. F., & Messer, S. B. (2006). What qualifies as evidence of effective practice? In J. C. Norcross, L. E. Beutler, & R. F. Levant (Eds.), *Evidence-based practice in mental health: Debate and dialogue on fundamental questions* (pp. 13–55). Washington, DC: American Psychological Association.

Reed Group. (2017). Medical disability advisor. 6th Ed. Retrieved June, 10, 2017, from http://www.medicaldisabilityadvisor.com/

Reggers, J., & Ansseau, M. (1999). Specific phobias in women. *Revue Médicale de Liège, 54*(4), 329–334.

Rogers, R. (Ed.). (1988). *Clinical assessment of malingering and deception*. New York: Guilford Press.

Rogers, R. (Ed.). (1997). *Clinical assessment of malingering and deception* (2nd ed.). New York: Guilford Press.

Rogers, R., & Bender, S. D. (2003). Evaluation of malingering and deception. In A. M. Goldstein (Ed.), *Forensic psychology: Vol. 11 of handbook of psychology* (pp. 109–132). Hoboken, NJ: John Wiley & Sons.

Rohling, M. L., Binder, L. M., & Langhinrichsen-Rohling, J. (1995). Money matters: A meta-analytic review of the association between financial compensation and the experience and treatment of chronic pain. *Health Psychology, 14*, 537–547.

Roy-Byrne, P. P., Davidson, K. W., Kessler, R. C., et al. (2008). Anxiety disorders and comorbid medical illness. *General Hospital Psychiatry, 30*(3), 208–225.

Rush, A. J., Warden, D., Wisniewski, S. R., et al. (2009). STAR*D: Revising conventional wisdom. *CNS Drugs, 23*(8), 627–647.

SAMHSA. (2007a). *CMHS uniform reporting system output tables*. Rockville, MD: Substance Abuse and Mental Health Services Administration (Publication No. SMA 06–4195).

SAMHSA. (2007b). *Results from the 2006 National Survey on drug use and health: National findings*. Rockville, MD: Substance Abuse and Mental Health Services Administration, Office of Applied Studies (Publication No. SMA 07–4293, NSDUH Series H-32).

SAMHSA. (2015). *Substance Abuse and Mental Health Services Administration. Behavioral health barometer: United States, 2015. HHS publication no. SMA–16–Baro–2015*. Substance Abuse and Mental Health Services Administration: Rockville, MD.

Schretlen, D. J., Cascella, N. G., Meyer, S. M., Kingery, L. R., Testa, S. M., Munro, C. A., et al. (2007). Neuropsychological functioning in bipolar disorder vs. schizophrenia. *Biological Psychiatry, 62*(2), 179–186.

Schretlen, D. J., Munro, C. A., Anthony, J. C., & Pearlson, G. D. (2003). Examining the range of normal intra-individual variability in neuropsychological test performance. *Journal of the International Neuropsychological Society, 9*, 864–870.

Schultz, I. Z., & Gatchel, R. J. (Eds.). (2005). *Handbook of complex occupational disability claims*. New York: Springer.

Scott, K. M., Bruffaerts, R., Tsang, A., et al. (2007). Depression–anxiety relationships with chronic physical conditions: Results from the world mental health surveys. *Journal of Affective Disorders, 103*, 113–120.

Scott, K. M., Von Korff, M., Alonso, J., et al. (2009). Mental–physical co-morbidity and its relationship with disability: Results from the world mental health surveys. *Psychological Medicine, 39*(1), 33–43.

Seedat, S., Scott, K. M., Angermeyer, M. C., et al. (2009). Cross-national associations between gender and mental disorders in the World Health Organization world mental health surveys. *Archives of General Psychiatry, 66*(7), 785–795.

Seligman, M. E. P., & Maier, S. F. (1967). Failure to escape traumatic shock. *Journal of Experimental Psychology, 74*, 1–9.

Sing, M., Hill, S., & Puffer, L. (2001). *Improving mental health insurance benefits without increasing costs*. Rockville, MD: Center for Mental Health Services, Substance Abuse and Mental Health Services Administration (DHHS Publication No. SMA 01–3542).

Social Security Administration (SSA). (2015). *Research, statistics, & policy analysis. Annual statistical report on the social security disability insurance program, 2015*. Baltimore, MD: Social Security Administration.

Social Security Administration (SSA). (2017). Revisions to rules regarding the evaluation of medical evidence. 82 FR 5844. https://www.federalregister.gov/documents/2017/01/18/2017-00455/revisions-to-rules-regarding-the-evaluation-of-medical-evidence. Accessed on June 5, 2017.

Talmage, J. B. (2007). Failure to communicate: How terminology and forms confuse the work ability/disability evaluation process. *Journal of Insurance Medicine, 39*, 192–198.

Talmage, J. B., & Melhorn, J. M. (Eds.). (2005). *A physician's guide to return to work*. Chicago, IL: American Medical Association.

Thompson, J., LeBourgeois, H., & Black, R. (2004). Malingering. In R. Simon & L. Gold (Eds.), *Textbook of forensic psychiatry* (pp. 427–448). Washington, DC: American Psychiatric Publishing.

Turner, S. M., DeMers, S. T., Fox, H., Roberts, H., & Reed, G. (2001). APA's guidelines for test user qualifications: An executive summary. *American Psychologist, 56*(12), 1099–1113.

U. S. Supreme Court. (2003). Black & Decker Plan V. Nord. 538 U. S., No. 02-469, pp. 5–11.

U. S. Department of Health and Human Services. (1999). *Mental health: A report of the surgeon general – Executive summary*. Rockville, MD: U.S. Department of Health and Human Services, Substance Abuse and Mental Health Services Administration, Center for Mental Health Services, National Institutes of Health, National Institute of Mental Health. Available online at. http://www.surgeongeneral.gov/library/mentalhealth/home.html.

US Burden of Disease Collaborators. (2013). The state of US health, 1990-2010: Burden of diseases, injuries, and risk factors. *JAMA, 310*(6), 591–608. https://doi.org/10.1001/jama.2013.13805.

Wainberg, M. L., Scorza, P., Shultz, J. M., Helpman, L., Mootz, J. J., Johnson, K. A., et al. (2017). Challenges and opportunities in global mental health: A research-to-practice perspective. *Current Psychiatry Reports, 19*(5), 28. https://doi.org/10.1007/s11920-017-0780-z.

Wang, P. S., Berglund, P., & Kessler, R. C. (2000). Recent care of common mental disorders in the United States: Prevalence and conformance with evidence-based recommendations. *Journal of General Internal Medicine, 15*(5), 284–292.

Warren, P. A. (2003). The evaluation of stress concerns in the workplace. *Duke University Return to Work Newsletter*. Duke University, Durham North Carolina.

Warren, P. A. (2005). *The management of workplace mental health issues and appropriate disability prevention strategies*. San Diego, CA: Work Loss Data Institute.

Warren, P. A. (2009). Behavioral health as a causation issue in workers' compensation and disability claims. *IAIABC Journal, 46*(2), 17–56.

Warren, P. A. (2013a). Those who hesitate are lost: The case for setting behavioral health treatment and disability standards, part I. *Psychological Injury and Law, 6*(3), 183–195.

Warren, P. A. (2013b). Those who hesitate are lost: The case for setting behavioral health treatment and disability standards, part II. Psychological Injury and Law, 6(3), 196–207.

Warren, P.A. (2016). Imprecision in the evalulation of workers' compensation psychological injury claims. American Medical Association Guides Newsletter, May/June, 5-16. Chicago, IL

Warren, P. A., & Hubbard, J. D. (2006). The disability claims process and determining mental health diagnoses versus workplace dissatisfaction. *American Academy of Disability Evaluating Physicians, 5*(2), 13–24.

Warren, P. A., & Hubbard, J.D. (2008). Psychosocial issues related to behavioral health disability claims. Fort Dearborn National Insurance Company.

Weber, M. C. (2008). AAPL guideline for forensic evaluation of psychiatric disabilities: A disability law perspective. *Journal of the American Academy of Psychiatry and the Law, 36*(4), 558–562.

Weiner, I., & Hess, A. (Eds.). (2005). *The handbook of forensic psychology* (3rd ed.). New York: John Wiley & Sons.

Whiteford, H. A., Degenhardt, L., Rehm, J., Baxter, A. J., Ferrari, A. J., Erskine, H. E., et al. (2013 Nov 9). Global burden of disease attributable to mental and substance use disorders: Findings from the global burden of disease study 2010. *Lancet, 382*(9904), 1575–1586. https://doi.org/10.1016/S0140-6736(13)61611-6.

Whiteford, H. A., Ferrari, A. J., Degenhardt, L., Feigin, V., & Vos, T. (2015). The global burden of mental, neurological and substance use disorders: An analysis from the global burden of disease study 2010. *PLoS One, 10*(2), e0116820. https://doi.org/10.1371/journal.pone.0116820.

WHO. (2004). *The world health report 2004: Changing history*. Geneva, Switzerland: The World Health Organization.

Wiley, S. D. (1998). Deception and detection in psychiatric diagnosis. *Psychiatric Clinics of North America, 21*(4), 869–894.

Work Loss Data Institute. (2008). *Official disability guidelines*. Encinitas, CA: Work Loss Data Institute.

Young, G., Kane, A. W., & Nicholson, K. (2007). *Causality of psychological injury: Presenting evidence in court*. New York: Springer.

Zechmeister, I., Kilian, R., & McDaid, D. (2008). Is it worth investing in mental health promotion and prevention of mental illness? A systematic review of the evidence from economic evaluations. *BMC Public Health, 8*, 20.

Chapter 3
Contributory Factors Leading Behavioral Health Disability

Pamela A. Warren

3.1 Personal Factors That May Contribute to Behavioral Health Disability

A professional can contribute to one's perception of being disabled a number of ways. First, a person may have had past experience with a family member or friend who was diagnosed and treated for a BH concern. In talking with the other individual, one's perception may be shaped by what the individual has noted was experienced and what the TP said. A different way for this to occur is through simply observing other people with the reported concern. By researching a BH concern on the Internet, there is considerable variance in the quality of the information that can be found. While there are many reputable websites that provide a true service with accurate information, there are many others that provide unsubstantiated information that may misdirect the individual in understanding what constitutes appropriate care and in terms of expected recovery. This type of misinformation may contribute to treatment compliance issues and poor treatment outcomes. Thus, the person who seeks treatment is frequently in need of careful assessment of misperceptions and education about the normal course of the condition in order to prepare the individual for treatment and for improved treatment outcomes (Warren, 2009, 2013a, 2013b; Warren & Hubbard, 2006, 2008).

P. A. Warren (✉)
Carle Physician Group and University of Illinois Medical School, Department of Psychiatry, Monticello, IL, USA

P. A. Warren (ed.), *Handbook of Behavioral Health Disability Management*,
https://doi.org/10.1007/978-3-319-89860-5_3

3.2 Treating Professional Causes of Iatrogenic Disability

Treating professional iatrogenic disability is caused by one of three ways: (1) injury occurs through overt action by the professional, such as prescribing the wrong medication and a negative reaction is experienced; (2) the TP provides information that conveys the message that the person is disabled or that the workplace is the source of the individual's concerns; or (3) the TP makes an inaccurate diagnosis based on Professional opinion alone without objective methods of evaluation, such as blood tests, X-rays, standardized psychological testing etc (American College of Occupational and Environmental Medicine (ACOEM), 2008; American College of Occupational and Environmental Medicine (ACOEM), 2006; American Psychiatric Association (ApA), 2013; Aronoff, Mandel, & Genovese, 2007; Norquist & Regier, 1996; Robinson, Gatchel, & Whitfill, 2005; Schultz & Gatchel, 2005; Talmage & Melhorn, 2005).

It is essential that comprehensive mental health professional care encompasses a deeper understanding of how the label of disability generally introduces a clinical bias on the part of the professional that may interfere without considering other types of data that do not support a clinical conclusion of permanent impairment in functioning (Harding, 2004). Moreover, when a professional conveys to the individual that a diagnosis equates functioning impairment, it is quite possible for this to become a self-fulfilling prophesy, leading the person to strongly identify with the disability role and believing that one is unable to function actively in life (American Medical Association (AMA), 2008; Warren, 2003). This can lead to iatrogenic disability caused by incorrect information and assumptions. The importance of the professional taking a broad view approach to facilitate understanding in the individual being evaluated and treated as to what choices the individual can make, how a diagnosis may or may not impact on one's life, how treatment will be structured to help ameliorate any current impairment, the inclusion of a RTW goal as a required part of the treatment process, and most importantly, how to resume living an active life – despite a psychological diagnosis – are critical components in the treatment of BH health concerns (ACOEM, 2008; ACOEM, 2006; Aronoff et al., 2007; Norquist & Regier, 1996; Robinson et al., 2005; Schultz & Gatchel, 2005; Talmage & Melhorn, 2005; Warren, 2009).

3.3 Employer Contributory Factors to Iatrogenic Behavioral Health Disability

The employers also play a role in the creation of iatrogenic disability. Employers need to be aware that without appropriate training, employees, supervisors, and administrators alike are likely to flounder. This can create a workplace where expectations and standards are not conveyed or that there is inconsistency in how employees are treated. Moreover, this stance causes confusion and frustration to occur and without an adequate means in which to address BH workplace concerns appropriately. Thus, job dissatisfaction can quickly occur and impact on work quality and productivity. Moreover, this can be compounded by supervisory evaluation of poor workplace performance (Disability Management Employer Coalition [DMEC], 2009, 2016; Kahn & Langlieb, 2005; Warren, 2009).

It is essential for employers to have workplace policy for both physical and BH concerns. It is still common for employers to have a workplace policy for physical concerns only. However, this leaves both the employee and employer in a poor position to address BH issues when they arise (DMEC, 2009, 2016; Kahn & Langlieb, 2005; Warren, 2013a, 2013b). For example, presenteeism may occur slowly before a person has a fully developed psychological disorder. Presenteeism occurs when the individual continues to work, but not up to one's full responsibilities or potential. Over time, the employee's workplace performance decreases substantially. Initially, this can be difficult to distinguish from job dissatisfaction. Having a workplace BH policy in place and ensuring that employees are aware of the policy encourages employees to obtain professional assistance. In addition, it opens the door for employers and employees to discuss a health concern from a work perspective and to address a temporary workplace accommodation, if necessary. It should be noted that not all BH disorders require a workplace accommodation. As pointed out earlier, there are variations with a psychological diagnosis, with some people experiencing little change in everyday functioning, to some people experiencing moderate impairment, to the most extreme situations where a person is severely impaired. However, as the APF (2005) noted, this constitutes a crisis in which intensive care is required. In worse cases, an individual may need to be hospitalized in order to be stabilized quickly. If an accommodation is needed, it should be linked objectively to determined impairment in functioning as well as linked to specific job duties. Because the normal outcome of BH is recovery, it stands to reason that any accommodation will be temporary only. By having a BH policy within the workplace, both the employer and employee have a means to address a BH concern with consistency, so that all employees are treated in a similar fashion.

There is increased workplace stress occurring in the workplace due to many factors, such as layoffs and increased workplace productivity expectations, to name a few (Wang, Demler, & Kessler, 2002). This stress as well as interpersonal differences can lead to workplace conflict. While many employers have workplace policy regarding appropriate workplace behavior and the lack of tolerance for any workplace violence, this does not always address issues, such as communication difficulties with a supervisor or a specific coworker or if the person is attempting to transfer to a different position or department because of these ongoing concerns. It is not always enough to simply have the people involved to sit down and discuss an issue. There are times when, despite taking this action, there are still interpersonal difficulties. A more winning strategy is to take a commonsense approach in allowing an employee to transfer (if possible) to another department. Moreover, if there are several employees from the same department who transfer in a relatively short amount of time, an employer should address whether there is an issue with the supervisor. It is better for an employer to keep an employee, particularly an employee who has performed well in the past, than to simply ignore the workplace interpersonal conflict (Kahn & Langlieb, 2005; Warren, 2009).

It is important for an employer to address workplace motivation issues and to recognize that not all negative motivation concerns, such as marital distress, lack of autonomy, work burnout, job dissatisfaction, job security, and disregard for workplace policies, are necessarily representative of psychological disorders. Instead, these can be representative of psychosocial issues. Psychosocial issues usually are feelings, events, or situations that are typical in everyday life. They are not objective psychological disorders. Warren and Hubbard (2006, 2008) found that job dissatisfaction is a primary cause of negative workplace motivation.

It should be noted that inappropriate employee behavior tends to share the trait of workplace conflict. However, there are also instances where some inappropriate employee behavior is frank criminal behavior, such as with a serious threat to do harm to another person, theft, vandalism, or sexual harassment. In most instances, this type of behavior is not related to a psychological disorder and is under voluntary control. Thus, it should be recognized by the employer, and the workplace policy dealing with each of these situations must be followed (Warren, 2009, 2013a, 2013b).

3.4 Attorney Contributory Factors to Iatrogenic Behavioral Health Disability

The discussion of how attorneys can promote iatrogenic disability will be brief since there is an entire chapter devoted to attorneys and BH disability. Defense attorneys can promote disability by denying that the plaintiff has any concerns at all and indicating that the person is faking or greatly exaggerating. This is inherently upsetting to the person reporting problematic symptomology and may cause the person to become more entrenched. Conversely, plaintiff attorneys represent individuals who have been injured. Some plaintiff attorneys in legal proceedings may directly or indirectly note that the monetary value of the case is directly related to the severity of the injury. Thus, the person is encouraged to seek multiple professional opinions to buttress the individual's claim of serious injury. While both types of attorneys have roles in the disability process, both defense and plaintiff attorneys must take care to practice in an ethical manner, not just to win the case. Long after the case is settled, the person with the reported injury will have to live with both the positive and negative outcomes (Gold et al., 2008; Goldstein, 2003a, 2003b; Heilburn, 2001; Heilburn, Marczyk, & DeMatteo, 2002; Heilburn et al., 2003; Heilburn, Marczyk, DeMatteo, & Mack-Allen, 2007; Heilburn, Warren, & Picarello, 2003; Melton, Petrila, Poythress, & Slobogin, 2007; Schultz & Gatchel, 2005; Simon & Gold, 2004; Van Gorp, 2007).

3.5 Insurer Contributory Factors to Behavioral Health Disability

The discussion of insurers will be equally brief since a later chapter will examine issues related to BH disability. However, insurers play a role in the iatrogenic BH disability process. There are a number of common issues that occur that serve to increase the probability of an adversarial interaction between the insurer and the claimant (Kemper, Tu, Reschovsky, & Schaefer, 2002; Hamm, Reiss, Paul, & Bursztajn, 2007). These issues are:

- *Lack of appropriate training for the case management of BH disability.* By not providing appropriate training to case management employees and by not becoming educated in appropriate evidence-based treatment, this can directly cause arbitrary decision-making. This and other factors will be discussed in Chap. 15 regarding the insurance industry and behavioral health disability.
- *A systemic lack of standardization in the types of objective data required to make a decision regarding the BH disability claim.* Each insurer has its own internalized system regarding the types of documentation required for the claim adjudication process. Currently, some insurers request objective data, while others simply request the evaluation and treatment notes and make a determination based on the insurer's internal criteria. Moreover, many insurers do not require the usage of *DSM-5* diagnoses and objective standardized psychological testing in the claim adjudication process (Binder & Rohling, 1996; Brodsky, 1996; Gold & Davidson, 2007; Gold & Shuman, 2009; Greene, 2007; Kane, 2008; Mittenberg et al., 2002; Thompson et al., 2004; Wiley, 1998; Young, et al., 2007). Because of this, frequently arbitrary decisions are made regarding the outcome of the claim, such as paying a claim that is unsubstantiated, but importantly, not paying a claim that may be substantiated with appropriate objective documentation (Hadjistavropoulos & Bieling, 2001; Hamm et al., 2007; Heilburn, 2001; Heilburn, Grisso & Goldstein, 2009; Heilburn et al., 2002, 2003, 2007; Warren, 2009; Warren & Hubbard, 2008; Weber, 2008; Weiner & Hess, 2005).
- *Differences in how BH disability issues are handled* versus *physical disability claims as well as not recognizing comorbid health concerns.* Frequently, despite changes in laws requiring the elimination of limiting BH treatment to ensure adequacy of care, some insurers still are limiting BH treatment. This is done by indicating that the insurer will only pay for an evaluation and then the TP must send the notes, so that the insurer's utilization review professional deems whether any further treatment is necessary from the insurer's perspective. This process is repeated when psychological testing services are requested by the TP. This is a slippery slope for the insurer because while an insurer cannot, by law, make treatment decisions, since this can be perceived as practicing without a license, this may result in this outcome unintentionally (Hadjistavropoulos & Bieling, 2001; Hamm et al., 2007; Warren, 2009, 2013a, 2013b; Warren & Hubbard, 2008).

Moreover, many insurers do not regularly assess for BH disorders with a physical disability claim. This is because many insurers still do not recognize the high prevalence of comorbid health concerns.

- *Lengthy review process for both treatment and the claim itself.* Some insurers also note that all BH treatment must be precertified. (Again, this is typically by a utilization review professional.) However, only after the TP has sent records and the precertification process has been completed can any further treatment be given without the person having to self-pay for services. In one instance, this author had called an insurer who then directed the query to a BH claim triage professional (who worked exclusively for the insurer to approve clinicians' requests for treatment). The BH professional approving treatment requests indicated that it was at least a 2-week process before any decision about beginning professional treatment would be made. It was also noted that the process could take even longer than the 2 weeks. This is an unfortunate process that certainly does not allow for expedient professional care (Hadjistavropoulos & Bieling, 2001; Hamm et al., 2007; Warren, 2009, 2013a, 2013b Warren & Hubbard, 2008).
- *Lack of direct interaction with the TP.* Many insurers require the TP to send records, but do not allow the TP to discuss the pertinent issues with either a case manager (CM) or the medical director to quickly address issues. An example of this occurred when this author was requested to send all documentation to an insurer pertaining to an individual with rapidly progressing Huntington's disease. The author contacted the insurer directly and asked to speak with the medical director to expedite the process. This request was denied the ability to talk by the CM with the medical director to discuss the pressing issues; later the medical director called the author directly. At that point, the disability claim was quickly approved (Melhorn & Ackerman, 2008; National Business Group on Health [NBGH], 2007; Otto, Slobogin, & Greenberg, 2007; Pransky, Shaw, Franche, & Clarke, 2004; Schultz & Gatchel, 2005; Talmage, 2007; Talmage & Melhorn, 2005).
- *Lack of incorporation of scientifically based practice guidelines into the treatment and claim review processes.* Currently, most insurers have not brought scientifically based practice guidelines into the precertification and claim review processes. This is curious since the insurer is making decisions as part of its internalized system. It would be quite easy to incorporate these types of evidence-based standards as a means both to streamline the precertification and claim review processes and to ensure decision made within the insurance company that were in line with the scientifically based standards (ACOEM et al., 2006; Melhorn & Ackerman, 2008; Warren, 2009, 2013a, 2013b).
- *The insurer employs psychologists or psychiatrists, but does not assess whether the professional has received appropriate training in disability assessment, evaluation, treatment, and prevention.* Therefore, those professionals may make the same mistakes as other non-BH professionals. A primary issue with this for the insurer is that it makes the organization vulnerable to potential legal challenges,

as has successfully occurred in the past several years (Robinson et al., 2005; Rogers, 1997, 1988; Rogers & Bender, 2003; Rohling, Binder & Langhinrichsen-Rohling, 1995; Schultz & Gatchel, 2005; Simon & Gold, 2004; Warren & Hubbard, 2008).

3.6 Conclusion

There are multiple stakeholders involved in the BH disability process. Frequently, those stakeholders inadvertently contribute BH disability through the actions that they take. It is the actions that treating professionals, employers, and insurers take that contribute to iatrogenic BH disability. In the next chapter, the contribution of laws and differing diagnostic systems related to BH disability are explored further.

References

American College of Occupational and Environmental Medicine (ACOEM). (2008). *Occupational medicine practice guidelines: Evaluation and management of common health problems and functional recovery in workers* (3rd ed.). Beverly Farms, MA: OEM Health Information Press.

American College of Occupational and Environmental Medicine's Stay-at-Work and Return-to-Work Process Improvement Committee, Christian, J., Martin, D., Brown, D., Colledge, A., Gean, C., et al. (2006). Introduction to ACOEM's new work disability prevention guideline: "Preventing needless work disability by helping people stay employed". *Journal of Occupational and Environmental Medicine, 48*(9), 972–987.

American Medical Association (AMA). (2008). *Guides to the evaluation of permanent impairment* (6th ed.). Chicago: American Medical Association.

American Psychiatric Association (ApA). (2013). *Diagnostic and statistical manual of mental disorders: DSM-5*. Washington, DC: American Psychiatric Association.

American Psychiatric Foundation's Partnership for Workplace Mental Health. (2005). *Assessing and treating psychiatric occupational disability, executive report*. Washington, DC: American Psychiatric Association.

Aronoff, G. M., Mandel, S., Genovese, E., et al. (2007). Evaluating malingering in contested injury or illness. *Pain Practice, 7*(2), 178–204.

Binder, L. M., & Rohling, M. L. (1996). Money matters: A meta-analytic review of the effects of financial incentives on recovery after closed head injury. *American Journal of Psychiatry, 153*, 7–10.

Brodsky, C. M. (1996). Psychiatric aspects of fitness for duty. *Occupational Medicine, 11*(4), 719–726. 443.

Disability Management Employer Coalition (DMEC). (2009). *Tools of the trade: A compilation of programs and processes for the absence, disability, health and productivity professional*. San Diego, CA: Disability Management Employer Coalition.

Disability Management Employer Coalition (DMEC). (2016). *DMEC 2016 employer behavioral risk survey*. San Diego, CA: Disability Management Employer Coalition.

Gold, L. H., Anfang, S. A., Drukteinis, A. M., et al. (2008). AAPL practice guideline for the forensic evaluation of psychiatric disability. *Journal of the American Academy of Psychiatry and the Law, 36*(Suppl. 4), S3–S50.

Gold, L. H., & Davidson, J. E. (2007). Do you understand your risk? Liability and third-party evaluations in civil litigation. *The Journal of the American Academy of Psychiatry and the Law, 35*, 200–210. Retrieved from http://bit.ly/1mlf3vT

Gold, L. H., & Shuman, D. W. (2009). Employment evaluations and the law. In *Evaluating mental health disability in the workplace* (pp. 25–42). New York: Springer.

Goldstein, A. M. (Ed.). (2003a). *Forensic psychology: Vol. 11 of handbook of psychology*. Hoboken, NJ: Wiley.

Goldstein, A. M. (2003b). Overview of forensic psychology. In A. M. Goldstein (Ed.), *Forensic psychology: Vol. 11 of handbook of psychology* (pp. 3–20). Hoboken, NJ: Wiley.

Greenberg, S. A., & Shuman, D. W. (1997). Irreconcilable conflict between therapeutic and forensic roles. *Professional Psychology: Research and Practice, 28*, 50–57.

Greene, R. L. (2007). Forensic applications of the Minnesota multiphasic personality inventory-2. In A. M. Goldstein (Ed.), *Forensic psychology: Emerging topics and expanding roles* (pp. 73–96). Hoboken, NJ: Wiley.

Hadjistavropoulos, T., & Bieling, P. (2001). File review consultation in the adjudication of mental health and chronic pain disability claims. *Consulting Psychology Journal: Practice and Research, 53*(1), 52–63.

Hamm, R. M., Reiss, D. M., Paul, R. K., & Bursztajn, H. J. (2007). Knocking at the wrong door: Insured workers' inadequate psychiatric care and workers' compensation claims. *International Journal of Law and Psychiatry, 30*, 416–426.

Harding, T. P. (2004). Psychiatric disability and clinical decision making: The impact of judgment error and bias. *Clinical Psychology Review, 24*, 707–729.

Heilburn, K. (2001). *Principles of forensic mental health assessment*. New York: Kluwer Academic/Plenum Publishers.

Heilburn, K., Grisso, T., & Goldstein, A. M. (2009). *Foundations of forensic mental health assessment*. New York: Oxford University Press. 180pp.

Heilburn, K., Marczyk, G., & DeMatteo, D. (2002). *Forensic mental health assessment: A casebook*. New York: Oxford University Press.

Heilburn, K., Marczyk, G., DeMatteo, D., & Mack-Allen, J. (2007). A principles-based approach to forensic mental health assessment: Utility and update. In A. M. Goldstein (Ed.), *Forensic psychology: Emerging topics and expanding roles* (pp. 45–72). Hoboken, NJ: Wiley.

Heilburn, K., Marczyk, G., DeMatteo, D., Zillmer, E., Harris, J., & Jennings, T. (2003). Principles of forensic mental health assessment: Implications for neuropsychological assessment in forensic contexts. *Assessment, 10*, 329–343.

Heilburn, K., Warren, J., & Picarello, K. (2003). Third party information in forensic assessment. In A. M. Goldstein (Ed.), *Forensic psychology: Vol. 11 of handbook of psychology* (pp. 69–86). Hoboken, NJ: Wiley.

Kahn, J. P., & Langlieb, A. M. (Eds.). (2005). *Mental health and productivity in the workplace: A handbook for organizations and clinicians*. San Francisco: Jossey-Bass.

Kane, A. W. (2008). Forensic psychology, psychological injuries, and the law. *Psychological Injury and Law, 1*(1), 36–58. https://doi.org/10.1007/s12207-007-9000-1

Kemper, P., Tu, H. T., Reschovsky, J. D., & Schaefer, E. (2002). Insurance product design and its effects: Trade-offs along the managed care continuum. *Inquiry, 39*(2), 101–117.

Melhorn, J. M., & Ackerman, W. E. (Eds.). (2008). *Guides to the evaluation of disease and injury causation*. Chicago: American Medical Association.

Melton, G., Petrila, J., Poythress, N., & Slobogin, C. (2007). *Psychological evaluations for the courts: A handbook for mental health professionals and lawyers* (3rd ed.). New York: Guilford Press.

Mittenberg, W., Patton, C., Canyock, E. M., & Condit, D. C. (2002). Base rates of malingering and symptom exaggeration. *Journal of Clinical and Experimental Neuropsychology, 24*(8), 1094–1102.

National Business Group on Health (NBGH). (2007). *An employer's guide to behavioral health services*. Washington, DC: National Business Group on Health. 100pp.

Norquist, G. S., & Regier, D. A. (1996). The epidemiology of psychiatric disorders and the de facto mental health care system. *Annual Review of Medicine, 47*, 473–479.

Otto, R. K., Slobogin, C., & Greenberg, S. A. (2007). Legal and ethical issues in accessing and utilizing third-party information. In A. M. Goldstein (Ed.), *Forensic psychology: Emerging topics and expanding roles* (pp. 190–208). Hoboken, NJ: Wiley.

Pransky, G. S., Shaw, W. S., Franche, R. L., & Clarke, A. (2004). Disability prevention and communication among workers, physicians, employers, and insurers: Current models and opportunities for improvement. *Disability & Rehabilitation, 26*(11), 625–634.

Robinson, R. C., Gatchel, R. J., & Whitfill, T. (2005). Tailoring psychosocial treatment for patients with occupational disability. In I. Z. Schultz & R. J. Gatchel (Eds.), *Handbook of complex occupational disability claims: Early risk identification, intervention, and prevention*. New York: Springer Science + Business Media. 566pp.

Rogers, R. (Ed.). (1988). *Clinical assessment of malingering and deception*. New York: Guilford Press.

Rogers, R. (Ed.). (1997). *Clinical assessment of malingering and deception* (2nd ed.). New York: Guilford Press.

Rogers, R., & Bender, S. D. (2003). Evaluation of malingering and deception. In A. M. Goldstein (Ed.), *Forensic psychology: Vol. 11 of handbook of psychology* (pp. 109–132). Hoboken, NJ: Wiley.

Rohling, M. L., Binder, L. M., & Langhinrichsen-Rohling, J. (1995). Money matters: A meta-analytic review of the association between financial compensation and the experience and treatment of chronic pain. *Health Psychology, 14*, 537–547.

Schultz, I. Z., & Gatchel, R. J. (Eds.). (2005). *Handbook of complex occupational disability claims*. New York: Springer.

Simon, R., & Gold, L. (2004). Psychiatric diagnosis in litigation. In R. Simon & L. Gold (Eds.), *Textbook of forensic psychiatry*. Washington, DC: American Psychiatric Publishing.

Talmage, J. B. (2007). Failure to communicate: How terminology and forms confuse the work ability/disability evaluation process. *Journal of Insurance Medicine, 39*, 192–198.

Talmage, J. B., & Melhorn, J. M. (Eds.). (2005). *A physician's guide to return to work*. Chicago: American Medical Association.

Thompson, J., LeBourgeois, H., & Black, R. (2004). Malingering. In R. Simon & L. Gold (Eds.), *Textbook of forensic psychiatry* (pp. 427–448). Washington, DC: American Psychiatric Publishing.

Van Gorp, W. (2007). Neuropsychology for the forensic psychologist. In A. M. Goldstein (Ed.), *Forensic psychology: Emerging topics and expanding roles* (pp. 154–170). Hoboken, NJ: Wiley.

Wang, P. S., Demler, O., & Kessler, R. C. (2002). Adequacy of treatment for serious mental illness in the United States. *American Journal of Public Health, 92*(1), 92–98.

Warren, P. A. (2003). The evaluation of stress concerns in the workplace. *Duke University Return to Work Newsletter*.

Warren, P. A. (2009). Behavioral health as a causation issue in workers' compensation and disability claims. *IAIABC Journal, 46*(2), 17–56.

Warren, P. A. (2013a). Those who hesitate are lost: The case for setting behavioral health treatment and disability standards, part I. *Psychological Injury and Law, 6*(3), 183–195.

Warren, P. A. (2013b). Those who hesitate are lost: The case for setting behavioral health treatment and disability standards, part I. *Psychological Injury and Law, 6*(3), 196–207.

Warren, P. A., & Hubbard, J. D. (2006). The disability claims process and determining mental health diagnoses versus workplace dissatisfaction. *American Academy of Disability Evaluating Physicians, 5*(2), 13–24.

Warren, P. A., & Hubbard, J. D. (2008). *Psychosocial issues related to behavioral health disability claims*. Fort Dearborn National Insurance Company.

Weber, M. C. (2008). AAPL guideline for forensic evaluation of psychiatric disabilities: A disability law perspective. *Journal of the American Academy of Psychiatry and the Law, 36*(4), 558–562.

Weiner, I., & Hess, A. (Eds.). (2005). *The handbook of forensic psychology* (3rd ed.). New York: Wiley.
Wiley, S. D. (1998). Deception and detection in psychiatric diagnosis. *Psychiatric Clinics of North America, 21*(4), 869–894.
Young, G., Kane, A. W., & Nicholson, K. (2007). *Causality of psychological injury: Presenting evidence in court*. New York: Springer.

Chapter 4
Systemic-Caused Iatrogenic Behavioral Health Disability and Contradiction Between Diagnostic Systems

Pamela A. Warren

4.1 Contradictory Laws and Rules Contributing to Behavioral Health Disability

4.1.1 The American Disability Act and Its Revision

American Disability Act Amendments Act (ADAAA, P.L. 110–325, 2008) is another law that impacts on BH disability with unanticipated consequences. In 1990, the original American with Disabilities Act (1990) was voted into law as a means to protect those with disability and preserve their rights. The ADA was replaced by the ADAAA in 2008. ADAAA was expanded to broaden the disability law since it was determined that the ADA did not go far enough to protect those with disabilities. Moreover, it provided additional direction regarding the types of conditions that qualified under the law. Lastly, the ADAAA's purpose is to protect those with disabilities. This revision provided additional protection to those who were previously excluded under ADA.

After the ADAAA became mandated, many individuals with mental health conditions and continued to work, were now considered disabled under the ADAAA. The purpose of the ADAAA is to protect those with conditions that preclude them from working or provide job protection for those who continue working. This all-inclusive approach has lumped all mental health conditions together without consideration of severity of the specific condition. Without a doubt, there are individuals with serious mental health conditions, such as schizophrenia, intellectual development disorder, and severe traumatic brain injury who have considerable impairment in functioning and need ongoing support (ApA, 2013). However, this is not true to

P. A. Warren (✉)
Carle Physician Group and University of Illinois Medical School, Department of Psychiatry, Monticello, IL, USA

P. A. Warren (ed.), *Handbook of Behavioral Health Disability Management*,
https://doi.org/10.1007/978-3-319-89860-5_4

all mental health conditions. Instead, many individuals with valid psychological conditions continue to work.

In addition, the ADAAA provides instruction regarding episodic relapses of mental health conditions, and that when a relapse occurs, the person is considered disabled. However, ADAAA does not discuss how an individual may have recovered sufficiently to return to work (RTW) and is no longer disabled. This illustrates a problem with associating a mental health condition with permanent or even episodic impairment. The majority of those with mental health conditions, such as major depressive disorder (MDD), persistent depressive disorder, and one of the anxiety disorders, have effective evidence-based treatments to facilitate the individual's return to previous levels of functioning. With the majority of these conditions, impairment is not sustained, except for complex clinical scenarios, such as with comorbid physical and psychological conditions. With the ADAAA's stance on mental health disability, it artificially inflates US disability figures.

ADAAA also indicates that a disability "determination" can be made even in regard to "negative" effects of medication or treatment. This stance demonstrates a lack of understanding that negative treatment effects may temporarily occur as medications are being titrated. Typically, there are no known negative treatment side effects of the primary evidence-based psychological treatment, CBT, for the majority of psychological conditions. Thus, a negative connotation appears to be subjective in nature, based on perception, versus a more objective approach and recognition that psychological conditions are put into remission as a standard part of the treatment process.

Moreover, ADAAA notes that when an employer regards an individual as being impaired related to a valid or *perceived* impairment, then additional subjectivity is introduced into the disability determination process.

ADAAA also adds and indicates that traits and behaviors are not mental impairments. Instead, behaviors such as poor decision-making, chronic tardiness, and mood may be related to how the mental impairment is manifested. It is the psychological condition that causes substantial impairment in functioning. Moreover, ADAAA emphasizes that substantial limitation is compared to those in the general population *without* a mental health condition. However, this stance ignores that the majority of individuals *with* a mental health condition continue to function in the major activities of life. Consequently, it is a more effective approach to compare those individuals early in the treatment process to those who have received treatment and returned to the previous level of functioning because this is comparing functioning in a more homogenous manner.

To further compound the problem, ADAAA instructs that individuals must be evaluated for impairment when the condition is in its "natural state," meaning without consideration of treatment or other assistance. This is concerning because many individuals who apply for disability or ADAAA accommodations are already receiving professional treatment. It is not appropriate or ethical to terminate treatment solely to assess whether a sustained impairment in functioning exists. Furthermore, it *is* the evidence-based treatment that mitigates the psychological impairment and restores the individual to the previous level of functioning. The question that must be answered is whether substantial impairment in functioning continues to exist *despite* evidence-based treatment. ADAAA acknowledges that psychological conditions may be episodic, but does not have requirements in place to reevaluate psychological impairment in an ongoing manner. The disability determination process is not a one-and-done approach. By melding a scientific approach into any disability determination process, the more sensible method is to reevaluate the individual at specific points of treatment to reassess not whether a psychological condition is still present but whether there is any objectively determined psychological impairment in functioning that continues to exist.

Here is an illustration of this point. If an individual is determined to be nearsighted, the person is likely to have great impairment in functioning (e.g., seeing things clearly at a distance) and may have trouble completing some major activities of life, such as reading a chalkboard, driving, seeing people at a distance). However, when the person's vision is evaluated by an optometrist or ophthalmologist and the strength of the corrective lenses is determined, the person still has the impairment in vision, but *with* lenses, the impairment in functioning is mitigated. The person with glasses is now able to read at a distance and drive since the impairment in functioning has been appropriately treated. This type of process currently exists for many of those with mental health conditions so that restoration of functioning is the expected treatment outcome, not the exception. The problem is that it is not recognized in laws such as the ADAAA. The current gap in all disability determination processes is the absence of objective data in the assessment of whether objective and severe impairment in functioning exists with psychological conditions.

Thus, when a law, such as ADAAA broadens the definition too much, it can encourage disability claims that with no to little validity. Moreover, more people are considered disabled permanently since they may not function well in all aspects of life on a permanent basis. The ADAAA may have the unanticipated outcome of iatrogenic disability through its definitions of sustained problems in life (Warren, 2013a).

More recently, issues related to limits in length of leave as a reasonable accommodation are being decided in the court system. In *Hwang v. Kansas State Uni., 753 F.3d 1159 (10th Cir.* 2014*)*, it noted that "accommodations are all about enabling employees to work, not to not work." The Court further indicated that a person who "couldn't work at any point or in any manner for a period spanning more than six months…goes without saying that an employee who isn't capable of working for so long isn't an employee capable of performing a job's essential functions – and that requiring an employer to keep a job open for so long doesn't qualify as a reasonable accommodation." As time goes by, it is likely that the Court will provide further clarification regarding implications of ADAAA.

It is beyond the scope of this chapter to discuss the substantial nuances of the interaction between HIPAA, ADAAA, and other US laws and all of the clinical implications. Some of these issues are likely to be decided in future court proceedings. Instead, it is essential to note how laws, such as HIPAA and ADAAA, are interpreted and cause potential ethical and legal issues for all professionals. Moreover, professionals must be aware of these potential pitfalls and take steps to avoid them as much as possible. The savvy professional will also seek continuing professional education as well as obtain legal advice to best manage these issues.

4.1.2 The Health Insurance Portability and Accountability Act and Behavioral Health Disability

The Health Insurance Portability and Accountability Act of 1996 Public Law 104–191 (HIPAA) was made into law to protect patient data privacy and delineate security measures to be taken to guard medical information. It also protects individuals who may lose or change jobs so that they do not lose their insurance coverage. The Department of Health and Human Services (HHS) published the final Privacy Rule in December of 2000. It was later modified in August 2002. The privacy applies to three types of covered entities: health plans, healthcare clearing houses, and healthcare providers who provide treatment and electronically bill for their services. Compliance with the Privacy Rule was required in April 14, 2003.

HHS published the final Security Rule in February 2003. This rule provides national standards for protecting confidentiality, the integrity, and availability of electronically protected health information. On April 2005, full compliance with the security was required.

As part of the American Recovery and Reinvestment Act of 2009 (ARRA, 2009), the Health Information Technology for Economic and Clinical Health (HITECH) was established. HITECH is comprised of four final rules:

1. Final modifications to HIPAA Privacy, Security, and Enforcement Rules were made which made business associates of covered entities liable to HIPAA, further limited the use or disclosure of protected health information (PHI), expanded the individuals' rights to receive electronic copies of their health information and restrict disclosures for which the individual has paid for fully, modified a covered entity's notice of privacy practices, and adopted additional HITECH Act changes to the Enforcement Rule.
2. A final rule was added to change HIPAA's Enforcement Rule with higher penalties.
3. A final rule was issued on reach notification for unsecured protected health information.
4. A modification of HIPAA to prohibit most health plans from using or disclosing genetic information for underwriting purposes (Genetic Information Nondiscrimination Act (GINA, 2008), Pub. L. 110–233, 122 Stat. 881).

On the face of things, HIPAA rules provide a much higher degree of protection than previously existed. These rules appear to afford a greater opportunity to obtain healthcare insurance and to keep it if a person experiences life changes. Because of these changes, it is difficult to deny that the basic rules of HIPAA are not helpful to people having increased rights regarding their healthcare. However, some of

HIPAA's apparent intentions to legally protect people's healthcare may unintentionally ignore or exclude consideration of other types of laws, such as contractual law that frequently pertain to professionals working for a third party, such as an attorney or insurer, or interpret the rules more broadly than written.

The Office of Civil Rights (OCR), a part of HHS, enforces HIPAA Privacy and Security Rules. Frequently, OCR gathers information pertaining to potential HIPAA violations. In the majority of cases, OCR resolves HIPAA violations. However, if there is evidence of criminal violation, OCR may refer the case to the Department of Justice. Thus, HIPAA rules are being constantly interpreted and applied to specific situations, post hoc. The legal definition is Post hoc *ergo propter hoc* meaning "after this, therefore because of this" (Garner & Black, 2009). These ongoing post hoc determinations can, at times, place BH professionals in both in ethical and legal dilemmas. Thus, it is important to resolve these conflicts to reduce the professional liability. Once HIPAA became mandated, there was no other oversight of the law other than how the OCR interprets the law. There is no system of checks and balances in place to ensure that interpretation of HIPAA does not conflict with other laws. Professionals are instructed to follow HIPAA or the State law pertaining to mental health, whichever is more stringent. The OCR does consider Workers' Compensation (WC) laws as exceptions to HIPAA. Thus, the OCR recognizes that HIPAA is in conflict with those laws and that WC take precedence over HIPAA, while minimizing the general release of WC medical treatment information. Other laws, such as contract law, do not appear to be considered in regard to HIPAA. Thus, this lack of consideration of those laws can place a professional in ethical and legal conflict at times.

In regard to clinical psychologists, there are specific ethical principles that must be followed. Clinical psychologists who are members of the American Psychological Association (APA) must follow the Ethical Principles of Psychologists and Code of Conduct (2014). There are five general principles: (a) beneficence and nonmaleficence (to safeguard the rights of those with whom a psychologist works), (b) fidelity and responsibility (uphold professional standards of conduct, clarify professional roles, and manage conflicts to reduce harm), (c) integrity (promote "accuracy, honesty, and truthfulness" in professional work), (d) justice (promote fairness and justice as well as use reasonable judgment to reduce biases and boundaries of competency), and (e) respect for people's rights and dignity (respect the dignity of others as well as protect others' privacy and confidentiality).

More specifically, the American Psychological Association (2016) Ethical Standard 1.02 states that if a psychologist's ethical responsibilities conflict with "law, regulations, or other governing legal authority" then the psychologist must make the conflict known and take reasonable steps "to resolve the conflict consistent with the General Principles and Ethical Standards of the Ethics Code." Thus, the APA member is expected to follow the ethical standards to guide their professional behavior. This is an important point since it clarifies that the psychologist must maintain the ethical standards as a part of professional standards of care. Moreover, the ethical standards are enforceable rules pertaining to psychologists' conduct.

There are other ethical standards to provide further clarification of what potential conflicts psychologists must avoid as well (Caine, 2003; Pope & Vasquez, 2016).

Ethical Standard 3.04 instructs psychologists to avoid harm to all individuals and organizational clients. In other words, psychologists must carefully consider interactions with others in order to minimize any potential harm.

In Ethical Standard 3.05, psychologists are instructed to avoid multiple relationships. The first example of a potential ethical violation given is when the psychologist is already in one type of professional role with an individual (e.g., treating role) and then is simultaneously in another role with that person (e.g., the psychologists has agreed to evaluate the individual forensically). Dual relationships place the BH professional in problematic situations where she/he is likely to have competing ethical and legal obligations from with concurrent professional roles that may impair objectivity. An example of this is when a psychologist is clearly in a forensic role, such as being hired by an employer to evaluate one of its employees. The legal client is the employer, not the person who is being evaluated. This legal obligation is based on contractual law. Thus, the psychologist is legally obligated to maintain the employer's confidential records and communications, not the person who is being evaluated.

Additionally, the Ethical Standard 3.06 instructs psychologists to refrain from a professional role that either impedes their professional objectivity or exposes the person or organization with whom psychologists are working with to harm, such as with a conflict of interest. When this ethical standard is paired with 3.05, it provides further guidance that harm may result by blurring professional boundaries or by attempting to serve in multiple professional roles simultaneously. It makes clear that this is unethical professional behavior and may result in the psychologist being sanctioned by the State or APA Ethics Committees.

Furthermore, in Ethical Standard 3.07, psychologists are required to clarify their professional relationship/roles before any professional services are provided at the request of a third party. Consequently, the psychologist must inform the person or organization if the psychologist is a consultant, expert witness, in a treating or forensic role. Thus, this makes clear that a psychologist cannot be in both a treating role and a forensic role concurrently.

Taken together, these APA ethical standards provide clear and unequivocal rules regarding acceptable professional behavior and appropriate roles. The potential pitfalls of not following ethical standards may have legal consequences for psychologists, including disciplinary action by a State or a professional organization, such as the American Psychological Association.

In addition, there are other laws that provide clear language and instruction regarding types of professional services, such as contractual law. Contractual law, while not a constitutional right, is a part of the US legal system on which breaking the terms of the contract may result in harm or damage to the individual or entity who hired a professional. Additionally, contractual law has specific legal requirements that must be fulfilled for contracts to be satisfied. A contract's components are an offer (entering into a binding contract), acceptance (acceptance must mirror terms of the contract), consideration (payment), conditions (stipulates what the professional is to do), and breach (not completing the terms of the contract) remedies, and discharge of duty.

When a BH professional takes on an evaluative role at the request of a third party, such as an employer, then, the BH professional has entered into a legal contractual agreement with that entity. That professional has a fiduciary duty to that third party to represent that entity's interests above all others. Because of this fiduciary duty, a professional cannot have a conflict of interest that is in violation of the legal contract. One way that a conflict of interest can be avoided is to avoid taking on competing professional roles, such as to refrain from being in both a treating role and a forensic/independent evaluator of the person simultaneously. It is not possible to remain unbiased and satisfy a professional fiduciary duty while serving in two competing professional roles. More frequently, contracts also include a clause regarding confidentiality to protect the proprietary information of a person or organization from being obtained from others. If the professional behaves in a manner that is counter to the fiduciary duty, that professional is at risk for several types of damages: compensatory (monetary award), punitive (punishment beyond compensatory damages), and professional (e.g., malpractice lawsuit or loss of a professional license). This illustrates the seriousness of potential legal ramifications if the professional follows HIPAA over a professional fiduciary duty. In other words, HIPAA laws make it difficult to be in compliance with both HIPAA and professional fiduciary duties concurrently. Thus, if a professional serves in two competing roles, a professional cannot protect an individual's and an organization's confidentiality at the same time. If the professional attempts to do so, then the professional may be inappropriately in competing multiple professional relationships.

There is another complication that related to HIPAA. HIPAA states healthcare as: "Care, services, or supplies related to the health of an individual. It includes, but is not limited to…Preventative, diagnostic, rehabilitative, maintenance, or palliative care, and counseling, service assessment, or procedure with respect to the physical or mental condition, or functional status, of an individual or that affects the structure or function of the body" (U.S. Department of Health and Human Services, 45 C.F.R. 160.103). Some professionals (Bush & Heilbronner, 2012; Bush & Martin, 2008; Bush & Martin, 2010a, 2010b; Bush, Demarkis, & Rohling, 2017; Young et al., 2007; Connell and Koocher, 2003) opined that forensic services do not meet this requirement since it falls into a similar category such as Workers' Compensation laws. Moreover, there are competing interests of both the individual and a third party that cannot be met by a psychologist in multiple professional relationships. Typically, in forensic settings, a third party has hired the psychologist (American Psychological Association Specialty Guidelines for Forensic Psychology, 2013). Thus, this means that the psychologist or other treating professional will have access to the third party's confidential information. By entering into a contractual agreement, the psychologist is legally obligated to protect the third party's interests above all others.

Those that hold that forensic services are not covered under HIPAA provide several reasons to support this stance: there is no treating professional relationship, a third party hired the psychologist, there are binding contractual obligations that the psychologist must meet, the third party is the client, the forensic or independent role reduces bias and conflict, there is more objectivity in being in a non-treating role, the psychologist evaluation assists the "trier of fact", and this removes the psychologist from being in treating and independent roles simultaneously (e.g., unethical multiple relationships). It is for these reasons that forensic services are opined to not be healthcare services (Heilburn, 2001; Heilburn et al., 2002; 2003; 2007; 2009; Koocher et al., 2005; 2013; Koocher & Keith-Spiegel, 2016; Warren, 2013b; Weber, 2008; Weiner & Hess, 2005) .

Others assert that HIPAA makes explicit that forensic evaluations are healthcare and, thus, subject to the same HIPAA requirements as other healthcare records (Borkosky, 2012; 2013; 2014; Borkosky & Pellett, 2013; Borkosky & Smith, 2015; Borkosky, Pellett, & Thomas, 2013). Those who opine that forensic work is subject to HIPAA note the following reasons: no support in specific documents and guidelines reviewed that specifically noted that a third party is the client; that there is no support for a third party's controls of record release, psychologists are specifically noted within HIPAA as covered entities; and that there was no agreement among the few documents and guidelines reviewed that support the exclusion of forensic and independent evaluations from HIPAA. Moreover, supporters of forensic services being covered under HIPAA noted that APA ethical standards and records are in conflict in providing guidance.

However, there are problems with these assertions. Of note, there is no discussion by this opposing group regarding other salient laws, such as contract laws and the legal obligations imposed by these laws. Instead, the position is that HIPAA supersedes all other laws. It is important to note that a close review of the language in HIPAA indicates that if other State laws are more stringent, then they take prevalence over HIPAA. Moreover, HIPAA instructs that WC treatment and insurance record requests for billing for treatment and disability purposes are not covered under it. Taken as a whole, this suggests that there may be additional professional situations in which HIPAA does not apply as well. Furthermore, APA provides clear instruction admonishing psychologists to avoid being in dual professional relationships, and examples of these types of relationships were discussed earlier. Thus, the argument that APA ethical standards provide contradictory guidance is quickly demonstrated as inaccurate when the pertinent ethical standards are closely examined.

In any event, the wise professional will seek legal advice on how to best avoid some of the potential legal issues discussed here.

4.1.3 Contradictions Between US Diagnostic Criteria and Billing Codes and Global Criteria

There are currently two systems that are utilized in the USA for making professional diagnoses and the billing of professional services in the USA. The first system is the *Diagnostic and Statistical Manual* (*DSM*). The second is *International*

Classification of Diseases (*ICD*) which has its own diagnostic criteria and billing codes (WHO, 1992). The *ICD-10* developed by the World Health Organization is a separate set of diagnostic criteria covering both physical and mental health conditions. Outside of the USA, the *ICD* is the only system utilized by other countries. Thus, those countries have never had the difficulties experienced by employing one system for diagnostic purposes and another for billing purposes. The USA is the outlier when it comes to how mental health conditions are diagnosed and how they are billed.

The *DSM* underwent a massive revision recently. The result of the revision is the *DSM-5*. The *DSM* was developed by the American Psychiatric Association (ApA, 2013). The *DSM* provides the diagnostic criteria for current psychological conditions. Traditionally, the *DSM* diagnoses have been used to delineate psychological conditions from one another. Thus, BH professionals have long used *DSM* diagnoses to clarify the condition that is being treated. In the past, the *DSM* diagnosis was submitted for insurance billing. However, a problem existed since US BH professionals employed *DSM* codes and US insurers used the *ICD* codes. A clean alignment between *DSM* diagnostic criteria and codes and *ICD* diagnostic criteria and codes has never existed. In the past, *DSM* codes were converted via a crosswalk into an *ICD* codes for billing and insurance reimbursement purposes. If the *DSM* diagnosis was not found in the *ICD* code, then the billing and insurance professionals had to make a best guess about which billing code to use. Otherwise, those *DSM* diagnoses not found in the *ICD* system were frequently denied by insurers. Needless to say, because of the lack of absolute alignment between the two systems, the attempted utilization of them was awkward, at best.

When Congress made HIPAA law, it also mandated the usage of *ICD* codes to reduce the past billing issues and to ensure that *ICD* codes were used in both treatment and billing settings. *DSM-5* and *ICD-10* crosswalks of diagnostic codes were developed so that treating professionals submitted only *ICD-10* codes for billing purposes.

On October 1, 2015, the US Department of Health and Human Services required all treating professionals to transition to the *International Classification of Diseases, 10th Revision, Clinical Modification/Procedure Coding System* (*ICD-10-CM/PCS*) for all HIPAA-covered entities. The legally mandated usage of the *ICD-10* came about for several reasons; however, the primary reason was to standardize diagnostic and billing criteria and billing across for both treating professionals and insurers. It was effort to streamline the treatment and billing processes (Centers for Medicare and Medicaid Services, 2017).

However, there are issues that exist with this legally mandated approach (Department of Health and Human Services, Federal Register 45 CFR 160; 45 CFR 164, 2013). First, this transition caused unintentional confusion regarding the continued usage of the *DSM-5* for its diagnostic criteria for psychological conditions. Professionals who treat psychological conditions are trained to use the *DSM* as the authoritative reference for diagnostic criteria and for specific types of psychological conditions. The *DSM* has been employed as the sole diagnostic reference for decades. Professionals within the USA have not been trained to use the *ICD-10* diagnostic criteria. The *DSM-5* continues to be the primary diagnostic reference used by US treating professionals.

Second, the rest of the world uses the *ICD-10* codes exclusively for both diagnosis and billing purposes. Consequently, the US system still remains at odds with the rest of the world in how individuals with mental health conditions are diagnosed (*DSM* criteria) and how those services are billed (*ICD-10* codes).

Additionally, while the USA has just started using the *ICD-10 codes*, the rest of the world is getting ready to use the *ICD-11* codes that have recently been field-tested. This means that the USA will remain out of step with how other countries diagnosis psychological conditions.

Moreover, the diagnostic criteria for psychological conditions in the *DSM* and *ICD* are not completely analogous. Consequently, this can cause further confusion about the diagnostic criteria that are specific to a psychological condition.

Third, some *DSM* conditions have different *ICD* diagnostic criteria, such as those conditions related to pain conditions (e.g., somatoform disorder). Therefore, these diagnostic criteria leave treating professionals with a dilemma since they may have been providing treatment for a legitimate condition in the *DSM-IV-TR*, but that condition no longer exists in the *DSM-5*.

Finally, the *ICD* codes are modified from country to country. This is a long-standing practice. The primary argument for this is that it better aligns the *ICD* with a specific country's own mental health treatment. However, this begs the question of whether these diagnostic modifications are considerably different from country to country. If so, are these modifications substantial enough so that there is no longer agreement across the different modified *ICD* systems that are in existence? Substantial disagreement from one modified *ICD* system to another may have implications for both the research and treatment of psychological conditions.

The *DSM-5* revision resulted in either changed diagnostic criteria for several psychological conditions or removed them altogether. For example, Asperger's disorder was subsumed into autism spectrum disorder. Moreover, somatization disorder was changed to somatic symptom disorder. Consequently, some diagnoses no longer exist or are now diagnosed in a different manner than when the *DSM-IV-TR* was utilized. While this may not seem to be of much concern since *DSM-5* diagnostic codes are converted into *ICD-10* billing codes, it has created a conundrum professionally. There are *DSM-5* diagnostic conditions for which there are no equivalent *ICD* code. This leaves treating professionals in a quandary regarding how to make a diagnosis for a condition that *ICD-10* does not recognize and vice versa. Moreover, there is little overlap in the *DSM* diagnostic criteria and the *ICD's* diagnostic criteria. Since US BH professionals have used *DSM* diagnostic criteria throughout their careers, now they have to decide how to use the *DSM* diagnostic criteria with *ICD* diagnostic criteria. This can be particularly difficult since there is little alignment between the two systems and their diagnostic criteria. *ICD* codes have been required since 2003 as mandated by HIPAA. Consequently, *ICD* codes have been employed for electronic transactions for billing and reimbursement for over 10 years.

In addition, *CPT* (Current Procedural Terminology) codes have been developed by the American Medical Association (AMA, 2017). The *CPT* codes denote the type of service provided by the professional. Psychological *CPT* codes typically relate to either the face-to-face time spent providing professional services to an individual or the amount of time taken to complete a professional service, such as psychological test interpretation and reporting. What is important to know is that there is a critical relationship between and *ICD* code and a *CPT* code regarding whether the diagnosis supports the medical necessity of the treatment.

Equally important is that mental health professionals have typically employed *DSM* codes which are a part of their diagnostic and treatment processes. Moreover, professionals have come to believe that *DSM* codes are separate from *ICD* codes. Some of the issues and concerns related to changes of some psychological conditions were discussed earlier in this chapter. However, this belief regarding *DSM* and *ICD* differences is a misconception. The reason is that the majority of *DSM* diagnostic conditions have numeric codes which have corresponding *ICD* codes. When the *DSM-5* came into usage, it provided direction to the corresponding *ICD* diagnostic codes. Consequently, even if professional notes a *DSM* diagnostic code in treatment records, all *DSM* diagnostic codes are converted at the time of billing into the appropriate *ICD* billing code.

One final consideration with the *DSM* and *ICD* diagnostic codes relates to past research regarding conditions that are no longer found in either system, such as somatic symptom disorder. There is a large body of empirical research pertaining to somatization disorder. Now that this condition no longer exists, it begs the question of how to develop new treatment standards or best practice guidelines for the new condition of Somatic Symptom Disorder (SSD). Do professionals continue to provide the same types of treatments for SSD as those that were found effective for somatization disorder? Are other types of treatments more effective for SSD? While on the surface, this distinction may seem to be making a mountain out of a molehill. However, many States and the federal government legally mandate best practice standards. This is discussed in greater depth in Chap. 7. Consequently, when these State and federal laws legally require specific treatments for certain psychological conditions that no longer exist, this means that the laws are no longer aligned with current treatment standards. This is especially true for State and federal Workers' Compensation laws. Moreover, treatment guidelines and laws are not updated frequently to reflect these changes. Thus, this represents an additional quandary for professionals to provide empirically supported treatment, but also to provide treatment that is in deemed appropriate by these laws. Consequently, treating professionals must stay abreast of current treatment guidelines and be prepared to explain why specific treatments were provided. This does not mean that professionals should provide any type of treatment solely based on professional opinion alone. Instead, the wise professional stays abreast of potential treatment standards and legal issues. It is important to seek ongoing professional training to stay current on these types of changes. Additionally, it is essential to consult with attorneys in order to seek advice on how to best address potential pitfalls.

4.2 Conclusions

While many potential ethical and legal dilemmas exist in the mental health field, there are ways to better address these issues. In Chap. 5, strong, scientifically based strategies will be discussed in order to positively improve the BH treatment and disability process and, most importantly, to accurately assess the potential underlying BH concerns in order to facilitate the individual's return to health.

References

American Medical Association. (2017). Current Procedural Terminology; https://www.ama-assn.org/practice-management/cpt-current-procedural-terminology. Accessed June 5, 2017.

American Psychiatric Association. (2013). Diagnostic and statistical manual of mental disorders: DSM-5 .Washington. In *DC: American Psychiatric Association.*

American Psychological Association. (2013). Specialty guidelines for forensic psychology. *The American Psychologist, 68*, 7–19. https://doi.org/10.1037/a0029889.

American Psychological Association. (2016). Ethical Principles of Psychologists and Code of Conduct. Accessed September 1, 2017. http://www.apa.org/ethics/code/

American Recovery and Reinvestment Act of 2009 (ARRA), Pubic Law No. 111–5.

American with Disabilities Act Amendments Act (ADAAA). (2008). ADA Amendments Act of 2008. http://www.eeoc.gov/laws/statutes/ adaaa.cfm. ADAAA, P.L. 110–325, 2008.

Borkosky, B. (2012). Why forensic records are no longer "owned" by the referral source: Psychologists are required to permit patient access and release of forensic records. *The Florida Psychologist, 63*(8–9), 22–23. Retrieved from http://flapsych.com.

Borkosky, B. (2013). Patient access to records: The invisible confidentiality right. *National Psychologist, 22*, 9–10. Retrieved from http://bit.ly/19lsHZC.

Borkosky, B. (2014). HIPAA's patient access rights: What patients and providers need to know when patients want a copy of their records. Retrieved from http://bit.ly/1oMS4eG and http://bit.ly/1lKQ7Bl

Borkosky, B., & Pellett, J. M. (2013). Can FMHPs refuse to release records to evaluees because the records are "information compiled in reasonable anticipation of" litigation (as defined by HIPAA)? *American Journal of Forensic Psychology, 31*, 21–40.

Borkosky, B. G. & Smith, D. (2015). The risks and benefits of disclosing psychotherapy records to the legal system: What psychologists and patients need to know for informed consent. *International Journal of Psychiatry and Law*, 42-43(19–30). http://dx.doi.org/10.1016/j.ijlp.2015.08.003

Borkosky, B., Pellett, J. M., & Thomas, M. S. (2013). Are forensic evaluations "healthcare" and are they regulated by HIPAA? *Psychological Injury and Law, 7*(1), 1–8. https://doi.org/10.1007/s12207-013-9158-7.

Bush, S. S., Demarkis, G. J., & Rohling, M. L. (2017). *APA handbook of forensic neuropsychology*. Washington, D.C.: American Psychological Association.

Bush, S. S., & Heilbronner, R. L. (2012). The neuropsychological IME. In S. S. Bush & G. L. Iverson (Eds.), *Neuropsychological assessment of work-related injuries* (pp. 280–302). New York: Guilford Press.

Bush, S. S., & Martin, T. A. (2008). Confidentiality in neuropsychological practice. In J. A. M. Horton & D. Wedding (Eds.), *The neuropsychology handbook* (3rd ed., pp. 515–530). New York: Springer.

Bush, S. S., & Martin, T. A. (2010a). The ethical and clinical practice of disclose ng raw test data: Addressing the ongoing debate. *Applied Neuropsychology: Adult, 13*, 115–124. https://doi.org/10.1207/s15324826an1302_6.

Bush, S. S., & Martin, T. A. (2010b). Privacy, confidentiality, and privilege in for ensic neuropsychology. In A. M. Horton Jr. & L. C. Hartlage (Eds.), *The hand book of forensic neuropsychology* (2nd ed., pp. 235–244). New York: Springer.
Caine, E. D. (2003). Determining causation in psychiatry. In K. A. Phillips, M. B. First, & H. A. Pincus (Eds.), *Advancing DSM: Dilemmas in psychiatric diagnosis*. Washington, DC: American Psychiatric Association.
Centers for Medicare and Medicaid Services. https://www.cms.gov/Medicare/Coding/ICD10/. Accessed July 1, 2017.
Connell, M. A., & Koocher, G. P. (2003). HIPAA and forensic practice. *AP-LS News, 23*, 16–19. Retrieved from http://bit.ly/1fG57R1.
Department of Health and Human Services, Federal Register 45 CFR 160; 45 CFR 164, 2013. https://www.gpo.gov/fdsys/pkg/FR-2013-01-25/pdf/2013-01073.pdf. Accessed September 1, 2017.
Garner, B. A., & Black, H. C. (2009). *Black's law dictionary*. 9th ed. St. Paul, MN: West.
Genetic Information Nondiscrimination Act (GINA). (2008). Pub. L. 110–233, 122 Stat. 881).
Health Insurance Portability and Accountability Act of 1996 (HIPAA), Public Law No. 104–191.
Heilburn, K. (2001). *Principles of forensic mental health assessment*. New York: Kluwer Academic/Plenum Publishers.
Heilburn, K., Grisso, T., & Goldstein, A. M. (2009). *Foundations of forensic mental health assessment*. New York: Oxford University Press. 180 pp.
Heilburn, K., Marczyk, G., & DeMatteo, D. (2002). *Forensic mental health assessment: A casebook*. New York: Oxford University Press.
Heilburn, K., Marczyk, G., DeMatteo, D., & Mack-Allen, J. (2007). A principles-based approach to forensic mental health assessment: Utility and update. In A. M. Goldstein (Ed.), *Forensic psychology: Emerging topics and expanding roles* (pp. 45–72). Hoboken, NJ: John Wiley & Sons.
Heilburn, K., Marczyk, G., DeMatteo, D., Zillmer, E., Harris, J., & Jennings, T. (2003). Principles of forensic mental health assessment: Implications for neuropsychological assessment in forensic contexts. *Assessment, 10*, 329–343.
Hwang v. Kansas State Uni., 753 F.3d 1159 (10th Cir. 2014).
Koocher, G. P., & Keith-Spiegel, P. (2016). *Ethics in psychology and the mental health professions* (4th ed.). Oxford: NY. Oxford University Press.
Koocher, G. P., Norcross, J. C., & Greene, B. A. (2013). *Psychologist' desk reference* (3rd ed.). Oxford, NY: Oxford University Press.
Koocher, G. P., Norcross, J. C., & Hill, S. S. (2005). *Psychologists' desk reference* (2nd ed.). Oxford, NY: Oxford University Press.
Pope, K.S. & Vasquez, M.J.T. (2016). Ethics in psychotherapy and counseling, 5th ed. Wiley & Sons, NJ: Hoboken.
U.S. Department of Health and Human Services., 45 C.F.R. 160.103
Warren, P. A. (2013a). Those who hesitate are lost: The case for setting behavioral health treatment and disability standards, part I. *Psychological Injury and Law, 6*(3), 183–195.
Warren, P. A. (2013b). Those who hesitate are lost: The case for setting behavioral health treatment and disability standards, part I. *Psychological Injury and Law, 6*(3), 196–207.
Weber, M. C. (2008). AAPL guideline for forensic evaluation of psychiatric disabilities: A disability law perspective. *Journal of the American Academy of Psychiatry and the Law, 36*(4), 558–562.
Weiner, I., & Hess, A. (Eds.). (2005). *The handbook of forensic psychology* (3rd ed.). New York: John Wiley & Sons.
World Health Organization. (1992). *The ICD-10 classification of mental and behavioural disorders: Clinical descriptions and diagnostic guidelines*. Geneva: World Health Organization.
Young, G., Kane, A. W., & Nicholson, K. (2007). *Causality of psychological injury*: Presenting evidence in court. New York: Springer.

Chapter 5
Effective Psychological Evaluation and Management of Behavioral Health Concerns

Pamela A. Warren

5.1 The Importance of Appropriate Psychological Evaluation of Behavioral Health Concerns

As noted in Chap. 2, there are multiple systemic issues that arise to negative impact on treatment and disability processes (Chellappa & Ramaraj, 2009; Dersh et al., 2005; Gerdtham & Johannesson, 2003; Otto, Slobogin, & Greenberg, 2007; Reed, Kihlstrom, & Messer, 2006; Rush et al., 2009; Schultz & Gatchel, 2005; Scott et al., 2007, 2009; Social Security Administration [SSA], 2008; Thompson, LeBourgeois, & Black, 2004; Trivedi et al., 2006; Van Gorp, 2007; Wang, Berglund, & Kessler, 2000; Wang, Demler, & Kessler, 2002; Warren, 2005; Warren & Hubbard, 2006; Weber, 2008). Fortunately, many of these issues can be addressed by making multiple changes within the current BH treatment and disability processes. Of note, BH professionals can play a particularly strong role in making substantial changes to serve as a catalyst for other fields to make similar changes. Much of the initial changes within the BH evaluation and treatment model will stem from addressing the current problematic evaluation issues by following the more standardized model that is taught in graduate and medical school. Thus, the focus will shift to address the specific elements of a standardized psychological evaluation. In this chapter, the current model will be discussed and then the efficacy of including additional components so that the current evaluation model allows for a more thorough evaluation of current functioning of the individual from a biopsychosocial basis (Warren, 2005, 2009; Warren & Hubbard, 2006).

P. A. Warren (✉)
Carle Physician Group and University of Illinois Medical School, Department of Psychiatry, Monticello, IL, USA

P. A. Warren (ed.), *Handbook of Behavioral Health Disability Management*,
https://doi.org/10.1007/978-3-319-89860-5_5

5.2 Current BH Evaluation Model

The current BH model has multiple standard components that are taught in graduate and medical training to complete a comprehensive and competent evaluation. These components are a comprehensive evaluation of the individual's current relationship status, past and current employment status, the presenting problem(s) that brought the individual into treatment, personal habits, coping strategies, social history, education history, psychological history, medical history, medications, mental status evaluation, diagnostic impressions, and summation and treatment recommendations. Additional required components that must be included in the BH evaluation process will be discussed as well. A brief overview of each component will be presented simply to ensure understanding of what is required in each section. However, it is not possible to present a comprehensive discussion of the intricacies of each component within the limited scope of this chapter (American Psychiatric Association [ApA], 2013; American Psychological Association [APA], 2009; Caine, 2003; Warren, 2009).

5.2.1 Relationship Status

This section is designed to gather information about whether the person is single or is involved in a relationship. Moreover, if the person is currently in a relationship, a careful probing of the quality of the relationship is made as well. Inquiries regarding the number of long-term relationships, including past marriages, are made to ascertain whether there are chronic issues within personal relationships. This is important because it establishes a potential pattern of difficulties within personal relationships that may mirror similar concerns with workplace communication. It is also important to ask about the person's current living conditions to establish if other people, including children, are living with the person seeking treatment. Thus, the BH evaluator is able to determine if there are problematic issues arising with personal relationships.

5.2.2 Employment Status

The BH professional should also ask about the individual's current employment status to determine if the person is employed. If unemployed, a thorough probing of the individual's perceptions of the contributory factors should be gathered. If employed, information regarding one's current job title, workplace duties, and any past or current workplace concerns is obtained. Moreover, a comprehensive review of the person's entire work history should be gathered and have the same type of information obtained for each position held. Catalysts for the person seeking a new job should be explored as well to ascertain whether potential concerns existed.

5.2.3 *Presenting Problem(s)*

A brief appraisal of the primary concerns that brought the individual to seek treatment is conducted. Although brief, the BH professional should try to note all of the concerns that initially brought the individual into treatment. This helps to provide an initial understanding to both the individual and the BH evaluator in specifying what particular issues are likely to be addressed in treatment. This does not mean that additional concerns cannot be added later but rather what the individual deems as problematic at the outset. This process also allows the BH evaluator to briefly assess the individual's insight, logic, and reasoning abilities as well as illuminates any deficiencies in recognizing serious, unidentified issues.

5.2.4 *Personal Habits*

With regard to the evaluation of personal habits, any underlying issues, such as sleep difficulties that leave the person feeling fatigued, illicit and inappropriate prescription drug usage which may be demonstrative of the person, self-medicating emotional issues or substance abuse, and dependence issues and heavy caffeine usage which may mimic symptoms of anxiety must be explored in order to rule in or rule out these concerns. The number and frequency of meals as well as the quality of the diet, in general, provide important information about whether there is a potential eating disorder, poor diet, or infrequent meals all of which can contribute to symptoms of low blood sugar, which may also mimic symptoms of an anxiety disorder, are important to ascertain. The objective determination of a true psychological disorder will be evaluated later through standardized psychological testing.

Additional areas that the BH evaluator should inquire about are tobacco usage, alcohol usage, and amount of exercise obtained during a normal week. Heavy tobacco usage can compromise physical health and thus impact on an individual's ability to function. Heavy alcohol usage can not only be a sign of abuse problem, but it is disruptive to the quality of sleep that one receives. In addition, the individual should be asked about current coping strategies in managing life stressors and whether these are deemed as effective at present. Deficits in coping mechanisms should be explored to understand the specific problems that the person perceives.

By gathering this type of information, it quickly allows the BH evaluator to identify positive habits and strategies, and those are clearly negative, such as alcohol and drug abuse and dependence. By inquiring about this aspect of the person's life, other salient treatment issues are identified and can be made part of the resulting treatment plan.

5.2.5 Social History

An individual's social history is appraised to learn about the person's upbringing, whether one's parents are alive, remained married, or divorced. Moreover, the number of siblings is identified as well. This process is designed to assess the family dynamics, regarding communication, interactions, and problems. Careful probing regarding the demonstration of affection, disciplinary action, and even how emotions were expressed within the family are pertinent to how the person currently functions. In addition, the BH evaluator should ask for information about where the person grew up and ascertain if the family moved frequently. If frequent moves are noted, then the BH evaluator should spend time in gathering information about catalysts that prompted the moves. Finally, the BH evaluator should ask about religious orientation and spiritual beliefs, as well as discern if there are cultural differences that may account for some of the purported concerns or problematic interactions.

5.2.6 Educational History

An assessment of the person's educational history to date is generally obtained by the BH evaluator. This provides a careful review of the person's scholastic career, particular academic strengths, learning difficulties, and degrees obtained. Moreover, it is a means for the BH evaluator to initially assess past performance in a setting in which one needed to learn new skills. While the information is subjective in nature, in some instances, it may be correlated with school records. The ability to learn and function in the past is a crucial piece of data to ascertain, since past behavior is one of the best predictors for future behavior and functioning (Kahn & Langlieb, 2005).

5.2.7 Past and Current Psychological History

The BH professional must determine if the individual has received professional BH care in the past. If so, then the information about the purpose of seeking treatment, the type of professional who provided the treatment, the specific treatment given, and the length of the treatment must be obtained. Moreover, it is important to assess what new skills were learned in the past treatment by the individual to better cope with a stressful situation or event. The BH professional should also ask if the treatment was helpful and if not, identify what were the barriers present to prevent an effective outcome.

Before initiating any professional treatment, the BH professional must also determine whether the person is currently involved in any other BH treatment at present. If so, it is essential to ask the individual to sign a release to permit professional collaboration as well as establish what each BH professional will and will not address in treatment to protect the individual from receiving counterproductive treatment. For example, the American Psychological Association (2014) requires psychologists to maintain appropriate professional boundaries and to take steps to ensure that inappropriate care (in this case, potential duplicate care) is not provided.

The BH professional must also evaluate the person's past history of physical, emotional, sexual, and substance abuse. Each of these instances is an important component to understand how the person has learned to interact in relationships, whether the person was allowed to set appropriate personal boundaries and the emotional sequelae from an abusive situation. Most importantly, this assists the BH professional in both understanding the individual's past history and how past behaviors may be impacting on the present, such as relationships and personal interactions with others (Gold et al., 2008; Goldstein, 2003a, 2003b; Melton, Petrila, Poythress, & Slobogin, 2007).

5.2.8 Medical History

A careful review of past and current medical conditions is another essential part of a comprehensive BH evaluation since it provides information about potential comorbid physical concerns that may be currently impacting on the individual's ability to function (Buist-Bouwman, de Graaf, Vollebergh, & Ormel, 2005; Campbell, Clauw, & Keefe, 2003; Dersh, Gatchel, Polatin, & Mayer, 2002; Dersh et al., 2005; de Waal et al., 2009; Disability Management Employer Coalition [DMEC], 2008, 2009; Evans et al., 2005; Fava et al., 2006; Gatchel, 2004; Kessler et al., 2006; Kessler & Frank, 1997; Kessler, Ormel, Dernier, & Stang, 2003, Kessler, Zhao, Blazer, & Swartz, 1997; Merikangas et al., 2007; Suls & Bunde, 2005; Warren, 2009). This is one means in which a BH evaluator assesses the biological component of the biopsychosocial model (Warren & Hubbard, 2008). Moreover, while a person may initially indicate that one does not have any health concerns, it is common for these concerns to become apparent when the person is asked about the medications currently being taken. The BH professional should also ask what specific professional is treating each concern and how frequently the person follows up with the TP (Simon & Gold, 2004). The individual should be asked to explain what treatment is being conducted, what is being learned to better manage current problematic issues, and what are the expected outcomes with treatment? Additionally, the BH professional should ask whether the person is complying with all treatment recommendations. At times, a person may pick and choose specific elements to follow, while ignoring other components. This inconsistent compliance can occur for many reasons, but importantly can be a cause of poor treatment outcomes. Thus, a means of cross-checking available to the BH professional is to correlate the person's verbal statements with other treatment records (ACOEM, 2006, 2008; American Medical Association [AMA], 2008; American Psychiatric Association, 13; Caine, 2003; Robinson, Gatchel, Whitfill, Schultz, & Gatchel, 2005).

5.2.9 Mental Status Evaluation

Typically, in the mental status evaluation (MSE), the BH professional asks the individual questions to assess the following, regarding multiple domains of cognitive and emotional functioning:

- *Appearance:* (a) level of consciousness (e.g., awake, sedated), (b) age (whether the person appears to be one's stated age), (c) posturing, (d) abnormal physical traits, (e) grooming (e.g., the quality of one's hygiene), and (f) eye contact during the evaluation.
- *Activity:* (a) voluntary movement, (b) involuntary movement, (c) automatic movement, (d) tics, and (e) compulsions.
- *Mood and affect:* (a) mood is the individual's overall emotional state at the time of the evaluation, through self-report; (b) affect pertains to the clinical observations of the BH professional and is directly observed. However, it should be noted that an objective evaluation of mood will occur through standardized psychological testing to rule out perceptual bias.
- *Speech and language:* (a) fluency of speech, (b) comprehension, (c) repetition, (d) naming, (e) writing, (f) reading, (g) prosody (e.g., intonation, rate, and rhythm of speech), and (h) quality of speech.
- *Thought processes, thought content, and perception:* (a) Thought process directly relates to the spontaneous communication process in the evaluation process; (b) thought content pertains to specific types of spontaneous speech that may reveal delusions. Rumination, suicidal and homicidal ideation, as well as phobias to name a few concerns, and (c) perception pertains to whether the individual is experiencing hallucinations, depersonalization, derealization, and the like.
- *Cognition:* (a) orientation to time, date, place, and person, (b) attention and concentration, (c) short-term memory, (d) long-term memory, (e) a brief assessment of executive functioning, and (f) estimation of IQ.
- *Insights and judgment:* (a) insight is the self-awareness that one possesses regarding the full spectrum of reality, and (b) judgment is the process in which the person is able to appropriately assess different components of an issue (Koocher, Norcross, & Hill, 2005, pp. 7–12).

The *GAF* (Global Assessment of Functioning) score has been found to be problematic because it is left to the clinician's subjective opinion in assigning the specific rating without a means to verify this rating in an objective manner. Because of this, the *GAF* was removed from the *DSM-5*. Some of the reasons for the removal from the *DSM-5* are the clinician's estimation is an attempt to provide some type of subjective measurement of an individual's current level of functioning. But, the *GAF* rating system does not have any standardized means to reliably determine an individual's *GAF* from one professional to another. Consequently, the *GAF* rating is of relatively low value in the determination process of an individual's level of functioning (Warren, 2009).

5.2.10 Summation and Treatment Recommendations

This portion of the BH evaluation provides a summarization of the salient clinical concerns and issues to be addressed in the treatment process. While the individual should be asked about desired end goals for treatment, the BH professional must also note whether there are potential issues such as motivation and compliance, inability to come regularly to treatment which will negative impact on the treatment process and outcome. A specific initial treatment plan should be outlined and tailored to treat the identified *DSM-5* (2013) diagnosis(es). It is the *DSM-5* diagnosis that determines the type of professional treatment conducted since there are many scientifically based treatments that effectively facilitate the return to the previous level of functioning (American Psychiatric Foundation [APF], 2005).

By presenting the standardized model (APA, 2009) that is taught in graduate or medical training, it allows both other BH clinicians as well as other non-BH professionals to understand the typical process that should occur. Moreover, this permits a means to note deficiencies in the BH professional evaluation process when a more superficial evaluation or even no evaluation is completed. While many BH professionals do follow such an evaluation process, there is a considerable number who do not. Unfortunately, this creates problems within the BH treatment and disability processes, in terms of poor quality of professional treatment, increased costs, and potentially, unnecessary, and inappropriate identification of an individual as being disabled.

In a greatly simplified overview of the BH assessment model, BH professionals must evaluate the person from multiple aspects of the person's life, health, psychological, cognitive, emotional, and psychosocial factors to determine the appropriate diagnosis and then treatment. This type of evaluation corresponds with the biopsychosocial model accepted in the medical and BH fields. In addition, BH impairment in functioning is multifactorial in nature (Gatchel, 2004). Consequently, the evaluation must appropriately evaluate each aspect of salient functioning with this comprehensive evaluation model. When this is not done by BH professionals, it further compounds the lack of translation to biopsychosocial functioning and makes the process vulnerable to indirect professional conclusions being drawn regarding the person's ability to function, legal causality, and an arbitrary categorization of work or non-work-related causation to the application of the BH treatment system. This leads to the current problems of frustration and misconceptions about appropriate BH treatment (Bruns & Disorbio, 2005). In order for a BH professional to attempt to answer the issue of causality, it is incumbent upon the other individuals involved in the disability process, employee/claimant, employer, families, coworkers, treating professionals, insurers, and attorneys, to recognize:

1. The difference between impairment and disability
2. What constitutes appropriate roles for the treating and evaluating professional

3. The essential criteria of an accurate diagnosis, appropriate best-practice standard-based treatment
4. The expectation of setting return to work (RTW) as a treatment goal
5. The high probability in remission of the majority of psychological disorders and reduction in objectively determined impairment
6. The ultimate goal of the BH treatment process is to restore the person to one's previous level of functioning

This last aspect is of particular importance because if the TP is for treating the person to restore to one's previous level of functioning, then it may potentially reduce the monetary award or benefits paid to the individual from either a legal procedure, the workers' compensation, or the disability claim systems (Kahn & Langlieb, 2005; Melhorn & Ackerman, 2008; Warren, 2009).

5.3 Additional Assessment Components to Add to the BH Evaluation

5.3.1 Military History

The information about an individual's military history is another means to assess the person's ability to function in a highly structured setting and in which teamwork is the norm. A careful evaluation of the length of time in the military, beginning and ending rank, special distinctions or awards, as well as the manner in which one terminated one's career in the military (e.g., retirement, honorable or dishonorable discharge) are all meaningful aspects to address in the psychological evaluation. Because military service, typically, is organized with numerous supervisors, sustained difficulties should be noted since this may be an example of previous communication or behavioral difficulties.

5.3.2 Legal History

The BH professional should inquire about the person's past legal history. For example, information about lawsuits, arrests, and imprisonment are quite important to know before beginning professional treatment. For example, if the person is involved in a workers' compensation claim, the BH clinician must be aware of this since the probability of the professional's records being requested by the individual's attorney and/or being asked to give professional opinion in a deposition is high. Moreover, the BH professional should make note of the name of the person's attorney to ensure that records are released to this professional and not to the attorney defending the business or insurer. A careful evaluation of the reasons behind any legal concerns to address what prompted the legal action as well as the outcome should also be obtained.

5.3.3 *Disability History*

A review of the individual's current disability history is important to ascertain how long the person was off work and how the RTW and any accommodations were addressed. The BH evaluator must ask about current barriers that the person perceives to either staying at work (SAW) or returning to work (RTW) (ACOEM, 2006). Coupled with this, it is important to ask about how the person spends a typical day to reveal if any significant portions of the day are spent in which the person is inactive. Moreover, this allows the BH professional a chance to compare activities of daily living (ADLs) to similar workplace responsibilities. This is essential because with reported BH impairment issue, if a person is able to complete a set of cognitive activities in one setting, then it is exceedingly rare for the individual to not be able to do so in another setting (Warren, 2013a, b).

The BH evaluator must also ascertain whether the person has a past disability history. Aspects such as the reason for the disability leave, length of the leave, types of treatment obtained, and how the RTW process was addressed is essential to note. Frequently, if the person is in the midst of a disability claim that is protracted, the individual may have obtained an attorney for legal representation. The professional evaluator should collect the person's attorney's name for future reference, in case the evaluator's records are requested. This helps the evaluator to avoid inappropriately releasing potential protected health information (PHI). In all instances for release of information, it is critical that the professional obtain a signed release from the person to be evaluated. While HIPAA (1996) ARRA (2009) does allow for information to be released to insurers for the claim management process, this does not necessarily release the BH professional from all legal responsibilities (both state-mandated and HIPAA-related) to release minimally required information. Thus, a signed release ensures that the individual being evaluated is aware and gives permission for the evaluation and treatment information to be released and to a specific party (Kemper et al., 2002; Lerner & Henke, 2008; MacDonald-Wilson, Rogers, & Anthony, 2001; Melhorn & Ackerman, 2008).

5.3.4 *Evaluation for Potential Medicalized Issues, Malingering, and Symptom Exaggeration*

The BH evaluator should also take note of potential issues that may contribute to the individual's perception of impairment, such as self-report of excessive stress, job dissatisfaction, job security, workplace conflict, marital discord, workplace performance, motivational concerns, and inappropriate workplace behavior, such as harassment of others or criminal action. While all of these psychosocial issues may negatively impact on a true psychological disorder, none are actual *DSM-5* diagnoses. Instead, these common occurrences are in everyday life, with the exception of criminal action which is dealt with by the legal action and procedures. Consequently, the BH evaluator should note each type of psychosocial issues without rendering an opinion, until objective standardized testing has confirmed or ruled out the concern noted (Barsky & Borus, 1995).

It is essential to note that the AMA (2008) has stipulated that the assessment of symptom exaggeration and malingering must occur as a routine component of the evaluation of an individual, in particular when it is related to disability assessment. Therefore, this must occur by all professionals evaluating BH disability issues as a required component in the assessment process. Moreover, because empirical research has identified a high prevalence of both symptom exaggeration and malingering (30–40%) in disability and contested injuries and illnesses, it is imperative for all professionals involved in both the treatment and disability management continuum to evaluate for these potential concerns (AMA, 2008; American Psychiatric Association, 2013; Aronoff et al., 2007; Barsky, 2002; Binder & Rohling, 1996; Caine, 2003; Gerdtham & Johannesson, 2003; Grant & Robbins, 2005; Gros, Antony, McCabe, & Swinson, 2009; Hamm, Reiss, Paul, & Bursztajn, 2007; Hutter, Scheidt-Nave, & Baumeister, 2009; Iverson, 2007; McCracken & Gatchel, 2000; Melton et al., 2007; Mittenberg, Patton, Canyock, & Condit, 2002; Rogers, 1988, 1997; Rogers & Bender, 2003; Rohling, Binder, & Langhinrichsen-Rohling, 1995; Wiley, 1998).

5.3.5 Collaborative Communication and BH Referrals

The BH professional should make every effort to obtain the TP(s)' evaluation, assessment, and treatment records. This will require a signed release from the person with the reported BH concern, indicating the approval for the release. As with the workplace documentation, information obtained should be noted in the finalized report as well as any unfulfilled requests. The BH professional should note whether there is clear evidence of active collaborative communication among all TPs and note any deficiencies in that regard. It is important for TPs to collaborate with the evaluating BH professional so that if treatment will occur, it can be coordinated and optimized. Moreover, this ensures that TPs understand what specific concerns are being treated by other TPs. This also allows TPs to discuss any differences in a *DSM-5* diagnosis(es) since the diagnosis drives what type of professional treatment will be given. Further, it allows for observation whether a RTW goal has been set and if the individualized transitional RTW plan has been discussed with the individual and the workplace. Lastly, this allows a BH professional to ascertain whether the person appears to have complied fully with treatment recommendations or if issues of noncompliance may exist (Pransky, Shaw, Franche, & Clarke, 2004; Talmage, 2007; Warren, 2009).

Questions that an evaluating BH professional should ask of other TPs are as follows:

1. What are the specific reasons that you are providing treatment to this individual?
2. What is the specific *DSM-5* diagnosis(es) that you have made?
3. What sources of corroborative information and documentation have you used to verify the individual's perceptions?
4. Have you completed any psychological testing?
5. If so, what tests were employed and what were the results, including validity indices, base rates, and T-scores?
6. If not, why?
7. What specific treatment are you providing?
8. How long have you been treating the individual?
9. Has the individual to whom you're providing treatment made progress? If so, how has this been determined? If not, how has this been determined?
10. If so, what is the anticipate goal? If not, why not?
11. Are there other TPs who are providing concurrent treatment?

With regard to referrals, if the TP is the referring professional, it is important to discuss with the TP the reasons for the referral and what specific issues the TP views will be assisted by the referral. The BH evaluator should note the discussion as well as what issues will be addressed and what specific questions regarding psychological functioning will be answered (APA, 2001, 2002, 2007a, 2007b, 2014).

If the referral source is not a treating professional, but an employer, attorney, or insurer, then a discussion to delineate the appropriate professional boundaries, types of information to be explored and gathered, and limitations of information that may be obtained must occur. In addition, if treatment will be needed, then, the anticipated length of treatment should be noted (both are determined only after the BH evaluation has taken place), (Heilbrun, 2001; Heilbrun, Marczyk, & DeMatteo, 2002; Heilbrun, Marczyk et al., 2003; Heilbrun, Marczyk, DeMatteo, & Mack-Allen, 2007; Heilbrun, Grisso, & Goldstein, 2009; Heilbrun, Warren, & Picarello, 2003; Kahn & Langlieb, 2005; Talmage, 2007; Talmage & Melhorn, 2005).

In conclusion, there are specific questions that the BH professional should ask of the referral sources:

1. What are the specific reasons that you are referring this individual?
2. What are the specific questions that you want to have answered regarding the current level of functioning?
3. Can you send corroborative documentation or data? If yes, what types and how will it be sent? Whether or not corroborating documentation is sent, it should be noted in the professional records.

4. Who are the TPs from whom the individual has already received professional treatment for the reported concern?
5. Can the TP's records (both medical and psychological) be sent for review? If not, the BH professional should note this in the records. If yes, then the BH professional notes the type of records to be received.
6. Can workplace documentation be sent for review? The BH professional should note if workplace documentation is to be received and the types of information being provided. The lack of workplace documentation must also be documented.
7. Are there potential legal issues concerning this referral?
8. If so, has the individual obtained an attorney?
9. If so, who is the attorney representing the referral source?
10. Is the purpose of the requested referral for the professional evaluation strictly for treatment, or will an independent evaluation be completed? This allows the BH professional to set clear professional boundaries and expectations at the beginning of contact as to what role the BH professional will take.

5.3.6 Corroborating Documentation and Data

It is essential for the BH evaluator to obtain as much collaborative information as possible regarding the issues that the person with the reported BH concern has noted. Examples of collaborative information are workplace documentation, review of other TPs' treatment records, and medical records. Workplace documentation and medical records will be discussed further (ACOEM, 2006; AMA, 2008; Lerner & Henke, 2008; Melhorn & Ackerman, 2008).

Workplace documentation is simply the documentation of current job title, written job responsibilities, current supervisor, length of employment, internal departmental transfers, name of the current department, job performance evaluations, workplace attendance records, past and current disability records, workplace disciplinary records, workplace advancement and recognition, and if legally allowed, direct communication with the employer. It should be noted that this listing is not all-inclusive nor is always possible to obtain all workplace documentation. Despite this, it is important to request as much information and documentation as possible. In addition, requests that were not fulfilled should be noted in the finalized report (ACOEM, 2006, 2008; Lerner & Henke, 2008; Warren, 2009).

A trend that has been ascertained has been the aspect of the BH professional utilizing one set of standards to determine treatment when the individual presents with personal issues and a different set of professional standards when the workplace is the primary issue. Interestingly, Weinstein (1969) observed a trend of some psychiatric patients improving, while others did not. He called this the "illness process." Weinstein noted a series of discrete steps that led from the individual's subjective distress (e.g., anxiety and depression) which led to the "emergence of

Table 5.1 A 40+ year old recognized formula from psychiatric literature

(a) Personality difficulties + (b) troubled life situation = (c) unacceptable disability
(c) Unacceptable disability + (d) accidents, illness, alcoholism, etc. = (e) acceptable disability

Weinstein (1969)

stress-related sanctioned disability." An example of this would occur if the patient/applicant presented with personal difficulties and a troubled life situation; this typically was viewed in Weinstein's model as an unacceptable cause of disability. The rationale was it was viewed that the individual could conceivably make changes to better one's life. However, Weinstein observed that if the person presented with personal difficulties, a troubled life situation, and either alcoholism, an illness, injury, or as the result of an accident, then the BH professional tended to label the person as disabled. Weinstein held that BH health professionals must help the individual seeking assistance in learning positive coping strategies in either instance, not just the second example. In this way, the individual is taken out of the sanctioned disability model and taught to return to life and all of its challenges fully (Table 5.1).

When BH clinicians do not assist their clients or patients in learning to adapt to life and work situations or to problem-solve effectively, then the professional is utilizing one's own subjective opinions versus appropriate clinical evaluation protocol, standardized and diagnostic criteria, and evidenced-based treatment (Grove, Zald, Lebow, Smitz, & Nelson, 2000; Harding, 2004). This results in questionable clinical opinions and inappropriate psychological care (National Business Group on Health [NBGH], 2007; Surgeon General's Report, 1999). Weinstein opined that BH professionals have contributed to the development and persistence of disability in the manner in which clients or patients were facilitated through the disability process, with being placed on permanent disability as the ending point. It is a major cause of iatrogenic BH disability (AMA, 2008).

There are several ways to avoid this problematic approach. First, it is important to remember that in both instances of acceptable and unacceptable disability that Weinstein noted, the primary role of the BH professional is to help the individual learn to cope with the situation and how to live life as active as possible in order to preserve physical and emotional functioning. Second, it is essential to ensure that the appropriate psychological diagnosis is made and is documented in the records. If the professional does not note this information, then the lack of appropriate documentation leaves the BH professional vulnerable to legal issues, such as insufficient documentation to support the resulting psychological services, and makes it likely that the applicant will have a disability claim denied because of poor documentation. This results in unnecessary increased costs and leaves the BH professional vulnerable to legal challenges of misrepresentation and malpractice. Third, the BH professional must be clear as what the precise professional role that the professional is in during the BH disability process. Specifically, the BH professional avoids being in the dual role of TP and evaluating professional simultaneously. When the BH professional takes this approach, then s/he has a strong sense of the legal implications of causation of disability, makes the distinction between impairment and disability, and thoroughly understands the complexities of the biopsychosocial evaluation and treatment model for psychological disorders. A simple means to point the BH professional in the right direction is to remember that psychological impairment must meet two criteria: (1) psychological impairment is the objective loss of psychological function; and (2) it may represent a limitation. Limitation is (a) something an individual cannot do because of functional loss *or* (b) something a person should not do because of realistic harm to self or others as determined by the comprehensive BH evaluation and standardized psychological testing. This is called psychological determination (Gold et al., 2008; Heilbrun, 2001; Heilbrun et al., 2009, 2002, 2007; Heilbrun, Marczyk et al., 2003; Heilbrun, Warren et al., 2003; Young, Kane, & Nicholson, 2007).

On the other hand, BH disability is a non-standardized term loosely employed by various organizations and laws as is taken generally to mean the loss of the ability to perform a defined role (e.g., a work role) because of medical or psychological circumstances as noted in Chap. 2. This issue of disability is one that all BH professionals are asked to answer during their careers. However, it is important to keep in mind that the ability to function, in this case, the ability to work primarily represents contractual and legal constructs. Importantly, it is not an issue decided by the BH professional but a legal and contractual agreement between the employer and the employee, in some instances and in legal procedures in other situations. Therefore, in most instances, BH professionals will not be deciding the issue of psychological disability but instead will be evaluating whether objective impairment actually exists, and if so, in what capacity is the individual limited in functioning. However, in those instances where the BH professional attempts to answer the BH disability question on a BH disability application, one should be aware and consider the risks of the legal consequences for practicing beyond one's area of professional competency, such as not being licensed as an attorney (Gold et al., 2008; Heilbrun, 2001; Heilbrun et al., 2009, 2002, 2007; Heilbrun, Marczyk et al., 2003; Heilbrun, Warren et al., 2003).

Medical records, both past and present, should be obtained in order to evaluate the types of professionals who provided treatment, diagnoses provided, types of treatment conducted, MRI, CT, blood work, and other test results. This allows the BH evaluator to understand the biological component of the issues that may contribute to the person's current level of functioning (Gold et al., 2008; Heilbrun, 2001; Heilbrun et al., 2009, 2002, 2007; Heilbrun, Marczyk et al., 2003; Heilbrun, Warren et al., 2003).

5.3.7 Standardized Psychological Testing

As was noted in Chap. 2, it is common among TPs to administer screening tools, such as the Beck Depression Inventory, surveys, or fill-in-the-blank questionnaires to gather information from an individual with a reported BH concern. However, these current standards in the evaluation of impairment in behavioral health functioning specifically note that this is inappropriate because of the limitations in such tools to fully and objectively evaluate current functioning (AMA, 2008; Warren, 2009). Instead, objective standardized psychological and, in many instances, psychological test batteries are the current gold standard to complete this type of objective evaluation of the person. Moreover, at present, there is no single standardized psychological test that evaluates all psychological, cognitive, and emotional domains related to functioning at this time. Instead, the current practice standard is to administer a minimum of two standardized psychological tests specific to the deficit being reported. There is a more complete discussion of psychological testing in Chap. 4 that will address specific types of standardized tests to employ, how these types of tests are useful in the evaluation of malingering, symptom exaggeration, and in separating psychosocial issues from true psychological disorders. However, it was important to note the required component of objective, standardized psychological testing, as a part of the BH evaluation to more objectively evaluate the individual's reported concerns in a comprehensive manner. By doing so, this helps to overcome the issues of the professional and the person's biases regarding the diagnosis and impairment (Grove et al., 2000; Harding, 2004).

It is important to note that any reporting of test data must include a synthesis of all test data, not just the data that appear to support a reported concern. This is following appropriate reporting of psychological testing data that is in compliance with the American Psychological Association (APA)'s The Standards for Educational and Psychological Testing (2001, 2002, 2007a, 2007b, 2014, 2016). All professionals who conduct psychological testing, including those who are not members of the APA, are still bound to follow these standards. Psychological testing is generally under the auspices of the American Psychological Association. This organization determines the general standards for appropriate psychological testing. Moreover, most objective, standardized psychological tests have strict limitations in who may purchase and administer them. Furthermore, all standardized psychological tests must be developed and administered in accordance with these rules.

5.3.8 Appropriate Documentation Regarding Potential Limitations in Objective Impairment in Functioning

The APA's testing standards (2014) and the AMA's *Guides to the Evaluation of Permanent Impairment* (6th ed.) (2008) require any professional who conducts standardized psychological testing to report all scores in the finalized evaluation report. The specific questions regarding the individual's current level of functioning are answered at this point. Any reported impairment must be supported by objective psychological testing results, not simply by clinical opinion because of the inherent bias that occurs with clinical opinion. By following this process, any psychological disorder or impairment in functioning is either confirmed or ruled out through more objective means.

Many professionals tend to report individual test scores as "proof of impairment." However, all test scores are required to be noted in any documentation in order to make a careful and balanced professional summarization regarding functioning. The APA (2014) also requires all professionals to write the finalized report in a language that avoids professional terminology and jargon and more in a manner so that the average layperson can understand it. Any noted diagnosis must be an actual *DSM-5* diagnosis since this is the current practice standard and has specific criteria to be met that will be understood across all BH professionals. Furthermore, it is the *DSM-5* diagnosis that determines the appropriate treatment, particularly the specific evidence-based treatment (Warren, 2009). Lastly, it is important to be mindful that a diagnosis does not necessarily equate an impairment (American Psychiatric Foundation, 2005).

5.3.9 Drawing on the Strength of Scientifically Based Treatments of BH Concerns

It is important to note that the majority of psychological disorders have not been found to result in permanent impairment in functioning. The American Psychiatric Foundation's Partnership for Workplace Mental Health (2005) came to the same conclusion independently and noted that the reported inability to work must be considered a crisis and requires immediate, intensive treatment by all TPs. The APF also pointed out that there are currently multiple professional treatments that have been empirically supported to quickly restore the individual to one's previous level of functioning. For example, Major Depressive Disorder (MDD), one of the most common psychological disorders that may cause temporary impairment in functioning, has been examined through two well-known series of empirical research, STAR*D (Sequenced Treatment Alternatives to Relieve Depression) (Sinyor et al., 2009) and TIMA (Texas Implementation of Medication Algorithms) (Suehs et al., 2008). The results of STAR*D research in which individuals were treated for 16 weeks revealed: "In conclusion, about half of participants in the STAR*D study became symptom-free after two treatment levels. Over the course of all four treatment levels, almost 70% of those who did not withdraw from the study became symptom-free." The TIMA series of research demonstrated similar results and emphasized intensive care, including hospitalization if the person was unable to function. Thus, this briefly demonstrates just one psychological disorder that can be treated effectively in order to restore the individual to one's previous level of functioning. The key aspects emphasized are quick intensive treatment that is focused on optimizing medication levels quickly over a short period of time. It is important to note that there are similar scientifically based treatments for many other psychological disorders. Thus, if an individual is not improving over time, it may be necessary to examine whether medications should be increased, patient compliance, and perhaps, supplementing the current medication with other appropriate medications to positively augment the response to treatment.

5.3.10 *Appropriate Treatment Goals (Including RTW)*

If professional BH treatment is provided, then the RTW goal must be set as a required part of treatment. The APF (2005) emphasized that with the current empirically based treatments, the likelihood of permanent impairment with an objectively determined psychological disorder is rare and that a RTW is the norm. Therefore, it is essential to set the expectation from the start of treatment, including in the evaluation that the anticipated treatment outcome is either SAW or RTW, if true impairment in functioning is found.

As a part of treatment, it is important to educate the individual about a diagnosis after it has been objectively confirmed or ruled out. For those individuals with an objectively determined diagnosis, the BH professional should discuss what constitutes the current state-of-the-art, scientifically based treatment, what are the particular components involved in the treatment that the individual will need to take an active role in treatment, including homework assignments and increasing physical activity, anticipated treatment milestones so that progress can be noted, and if there needs to be additional collaboration with another BH professional, such as a psychiatrist to prescribed medications, if necessary (ACOEM, 2006; Warren, 2009).

The APF (2005) also noted that although most individuals who have been off work may experience anxiety about returning to the workplace, this is a normal reaction, and the TP should not take as a reason for the individual to not return to the workplace. Instead, the BH professional can note this ahead of time to desensitize the individual, and so that it is understood that this is a normal response, and to better help the person to identify ways in which to cope with the return.

5.4 The Behavioral Health Return-to-Work Process

After an individual has received appropriate, evidence-based treatment and is ready to return to the workplace, the BH professional can help in guiding the person through the process by first obtaining a signed release to talk with the Human Resource (HR) department. Most BH professionals do not follow this step, and it can make for an uneven transition by lack of communication to clarify the process and to have the employer become involved. Instead, by the BH professional talking with the HR, a clear line of communication is obtained. This allows for the development of a short-term, graduated RTW plan to be put into place. Moreover, the HR department can discuss the specifics of the RTW plan with the individual's supervisor as a means to ensure that all parties understand the proposed process. This alleviates the full burden of the RTW transition being placed on the individual who is returning to work and also helps the BH professional address any questions that the employer may have (Warren, 2009).

A common graduated RTW program that the author has successfully employed is outlined in Table 5.2.

Table 5.2 Example of a return-to-work program for behavioral health concerns

Name of employee, HR representative, and immediate supervisor
Return to work at 2 h a day for approximately 1 week
Employee will work 4 h a day for approximately 2 weeks
Employee will work 6 h a day for approximately 2–3 weeks
Employee returns to working a full day

5.4.1 Workplace Accommodations for Behavioral Health Concerns

There are times when workplace accommodations may greatly facilitate the individual's RTW sooner. However, it is still important to be aware that simply asking for accommodations does not necessarily ensure that accommodations will be provided by the employer. Frequently, well-meaning professionals and individuals will cite the Americans with Disabilities Amendments Act (ADAAA, 2008), which went into effect on January 1, 2008 and protects individuals against discrimination in the following areas of age, disability, equal pay, genetic information, national origin, pregnancy, race, retaliation, sex, and sexual harassment, as the basis for accommodations. But, it is important to know that although there are changes in the Act to allow for broader coverage, there are still limitations in requiring employers to make accommodations.

The US Equal Employment Opportunity Commission (EEOC, 2009) provides this brief guidance:

> The law (ADAAA) requires an employer to provide reasonable accommodation to an employee or job applicant with a disability, unless doing so would cause significant difficulty or expense for the employer.
>
> A reasonable accommodation is any change in the work environment (or in the way things are usually done) to help a person with a disability apply for a job, perform the duties of a job, or enjoy the benefits and privileges of employment. Reasonable accommodation might include, for example, making the workplace accessible for wheelchair users or providing a reader or interpreter for someone who is blind or hearing impaired.
>
> An employer doesn't have to provide an accommodation if doing so would cause undue hardship to the employer. Undue hardship means that the accommodation would be too difficult or too expensive to provide, in light of the employer's size, financial resources, and the needs of the business. An employer may not refuse to provide an accommodation just because it involves some cost. An employer does not have to provide the exact accommodation the employee or job applicant wants. If more than one accommodation works, the employer may choose which one to provide.

The ADAAA's current definition of disability is,

"In order to be protected, a person must be qualified for the job and have a disability as defined by the law."

A person can show that he or she has a disability in one of three ways:

- A person may be disabled if he or she has a physical or mental condition that substantially limits a major life activity (such as walking, talking, seeing, hearing, or learning).
- A person may be disabled if he or she has a history of a disability (such as cancer that is in remission).
- A person may be disabled if he is believed to have a physical or mental impairment that is not transitory (lasting or expected to last 6 months or less) and minor (even if he does not have such an impairment).

It is important to be cognizant that based on the current body of empirical research regarding scientifically based treatment, most true psychological disorders do not result in permanent impairment in functioning; thus, most requested accommodations are likely to be temporary in nature. Some exceptions to this are likely to occur with those individuals who have been diagnosed with Schizophrenia, traumatic brain injury (moderate to severe), and Bipolar Disorder that are unresponsive to treatment (Schretlen et al. 2007; Schretlen, Munro, Anthony, & Pearlson, 2003). Examples of accommodations related to true psychological disorders, as defined in the *DSM-5* (2013), are (1) working part time until medication has been optimized; (2) working in a different department with reduced work demands, until the disorder has been stabilized; and (3) taking breaks that allow the individual to take a walk in order to obtain some physical exercise during the workday as a means to reduce physiological symptoms of an anxiety disorder. It must be emphasized that the ADAAA is still very new, and it will be shaped over time by various legal challenges. Moreover, there are some situations where the Family and Medical Leave Act (2009) will be more appropriate to utilize than the ADAAA. Each Act has its own set of rules and regulations. Thus, it is important for all professionals to become educated regarding the specific requirements and limitations with each law. Moreover, when there is a question pertaining to a specific issue with an employee, an employer should seek legal consultation to ensure appropriate guidance in sound decision-making in the workplace.

5.5 Conclusion

While this chapter provides guidance about appropriate evaluation of objectively determined psychological impairment in functioning, there are several other groups of professionals typically involved in this process. Other professionals are typically physicians, such as occupational medicine physicians, psychiatrists, rehabilitation clinicians, nurse case managers, insurers, and attorneys. Each type of professional has a unique role in the BH disability process. The remaining chapters will discuss how BH concerns usually occur within each profession, how they are identified and managed, common problems that arise, as well as how to better address these issues to bring positive change (Centers for Disease Control and Prevention, 2008; National Center for Injury Prevention and Control, 2006).

References

American College of Occupational and Environmental Medicine's Stay-at-Work and Return-to-Work Process Improvement Committee, Christian, J., Martin, D., Brown, D., Colledge, A., Gean, C., et al. (2006). Introduction to ACOEM's new work disability prevention guideline: "Preventing needless work disability by helping people stay employed". *Journal of Occupational and Environmental Medicine, 48*(9), 972–987.

American College of Occupational and Environmental Medicine (ACOEM). (2008). *Occupational medicine practice guidelines: Evaluation and management of common health problems and functional recovery in workers* (3rd ed.). Beverly Farms, MA: OEM Health Information Press.

American Educational Research Association, the American Psychological Association, and the National Council on Measurement in Education. (2014). *Standards for educational and psychological testing* (3rd ed.). Washington, DC: American Educational Research Association, the American Psychological Association, and the National Council on Measurement in Education.

American Medical Association. (2008). *Guides to the evaluation of permanent impairment* (6th ed.). Chicago: American Medical Association.

American Psychiatric Association. (2013). *Diagnostic and statistical manual on mental disorders, fourth edition, text revision (DSM-V)*. Washington, DC: American Psychiatric Association Press.

American Psychiatric Foundation, Partnership for Workplace Mental Health. (2005). *Assessing and treating psychiatric occupational disability, executive report*. Washington, DC: American Psychiatric Association.

American Psychological Association. (2001). APA's guidelines for test user qualifications: An executive summary. *The American Psychologist, 56*(12), 1099–1113.

American Psychological Association (2016). *Ethical Principles of Psychologists and Code of Conduct*. Accessed September 1, 2017. http://www.apa.org/ethics/code/

American Psychological Association. (2007a). *Recent developments affecting the disclosure of test data and materials: Comments regarding the 1996 statement on the disclosure of test data* (pp. 1–7).

American Psychological Association. (2007b). Record keeping guidelines. *The American Psychologist, 62*, 993–1004.

American Psychological Association. (2009). *Guidelines and principles for accreditation of programs in professional psychology* (pp. 1–38). Washington, DC: American Psychological Association.

American Recovery and Reinvestment Act of 2009, (ARRA), Pub. 111–5

American with Disability Act Amendments Act of 2008, PL 110-325 (S 3406) September 25, 2008.

Aronoff, G. M., Mandel, S., Genovese, E., et al. (2007). Evaluating malingering in contested injury or illness. *Pain Practice, 7*(2), 178–204.

Barsky, A. J. (2002). Forgetting, fabricating, and telescoping: The instability of medical history. *Archives of Internal Medicine, 162*, 981–984.

Barsky, A. J., & Borus, J. F. (1995). Somatization and medicalization in the era of managed care. *JAMA: The Journal of the American Medical Association, 274*, 1931–1934.

Binder, L. M., & Rohling, M. L. (1996). Money matters: A meta-analytic review of the effects of financial incentives on recovery after closed head injury. *The American Journal of Psychiatry, 153*, 7–10.

Bruns, D., & Disorbio, J. M. (2005). Chronic pain and biopsychosocial disorders. *Practical Pain Management, 5*(7), 2–9.

Buist-Bouwman, M. A., de Graaf, R., Vollebergh, W. A. M., & Ormel, J. (2005). Comorbidity of physical and mental disorders and the effect on work-loss days. *Acta Psychiatrica Scandinavica, 111*(6), 436–443.

Caine, E. D. (2003). Determining causation in psychiatry. In K. A. Phillips, M. B. First, & H. A. Pincus (Eds.), *Advancing DSM: Dilemmas in psychiatric diagnosis*. Washington, DC: American Psychiatric Association.

Campbell, L. C., Clauw, D. J., & Keefe, F. J. (2003). Persistent pain and depression: A biopsychosocial perspective. *Biological Psychiatry, 54*, 399–409.

Centers for Disease Control and Prevention. (2008). *Behavioral risk factor surveillance system prevalence data*. Atlanta, GA: CDC.

Centers for Disease Control and Prevention; National Center for Injury Prevention and Control. (2006). *Web-based Injury Statistics Query and Reporting System (WISQARS)*. Retrieved from http://www.cdc.gov/ncipc/wisqars/default.htm

Chellappa, P., & Ramaraj, R. (2009). Depression, homocysteine concentration, and cardiovascular events. *JAMA: The Journal of the American Medical Association, 301*(15), 1542.

de Waal, M. W., Arnold, I. A., Spinhoven, P., et al. (2009). The role of comorbidity in the detection of psychiatric disorders with checklists for mental and physical symptoms in primary care. *Social Psychiatry and Psychiatric Epidemiology, 44*(1), 78–85.

Dersh, J., Gatchel, R. J., Polatin, P., & Mayer, T. (2002). Prevalence of psychiatric disorders in patients with chronic, work-related musculoskeletal pain disability. *Journal of Occupational and Environmental Medicine, 44*, 459–468.

Dersh, J., Polatin, P., Leeman, G., Gatchel, R. J., Gatchel, R., & Schultz, I. Z. (Eds.). (2005). *Secondary gains and losses in the medicolegal setting. Handbook of complex occupational disability claims: Early risk identification, intervention, and prevention* (pp. 421–441). New York: Springer Science + Business Media. xv, 566pp.

Disability Management Employer Coalition. (2008). *DMEC 2008 employer behavioral risk survey*. San Diego: Disability Management Employer Coalition.

Disability Management Employer Coalition. (2009). *Tools of the trade: A compilation of programs and processes for the absence, disability, health and productivity professional*. San Diego: Disability Management Employer Coalition.

Evans, D. L., Charney, D. S., Lewis, L., et al. (2005). Mood disorders in the medically ill: Scientific review and recommendations. *Biological Psychiatry, 58*, 175–189.

Family and Medical Leave Act (RIN 1215-AB35), January 16, 2009.

Fava, M., Rush, A. J., Alpert, J. E., et al. (2006). What clinical and symptom features and comorbid disorders characterize outpatients with anxious major depressive disorder: A replication and extension. *Canadian Journal of Psychiatry, 51*(13), 823–835.

Gatchel, R. J. (2004). Comorbidity of chronic mental and physical health conditions: The biopsychosocial perspective. *The American Psychologist, 59*, 792–805.

Gerdtham, U. G., & Johannesson, M. (2003). A note on the effect of unemployment on mortality. *Journal of Health Economics, 22*, 505–518.

Gold, L. H., Anfang, S. A., Drukteinis, A. M., et al. (2008). Guideline for forensic evaluation of psychiatric disability. *The Journal of the American Academy of Psychiatry and the Law, 36*(Suppl 4), S3–S50.

Goldstein, A. M. (Ed.). (2003a). *Forensic psychology: Vol. 11 of Handbook of psychology*. Hoboken, NJ: Wiley.

Goldstein, A. M. (2003b). Overview of forensic psychology. In A. M. Goldstein (Ed.), *Forensic psychology: Vol. 11 of Handbook of psychology* (pp. 3–20). Hoboken, NJ: Wiley.

Grant, B. L., & Robbins, D. B. (2005). Disability and workers' compensation. In J. P. Kahn & A. M. Langlieb (Eds.), *Mental health and productivity in the workplace: A handbook for organizations and clinicians* (pp. 347–368). San Francisco: Jossey-Bass.

Gros, D. F., Antony, M. M., McCabe, R. E., & Swinson, R. P. (2009). Frequency and severity of the symptoms of irritable bowel syndrome across the anxiety disorders and depression. *Journal of Anxiety Disorders, 23*(2), 290–296.

Grove, W. M., Zald, D. H., Lebow, B. S., Smitz, B. E., & Nelson, C. (2000). Clinical versus mechanical prediction: A meta-analysis. *Psychological Assessment, 12*(1), 19–30.

Hamm, R. M., Reiss, D. M., Paul, R. K., & Bursztajn, H. J. (2007). Knocking at the wrong door: Insured workers' inadequate psychiatric care and workers' compensation claims. *International Journal of Law and Psychiatry, 30*, 416–426.

Harding, T. P. (2004). Psychiatric disability and clinical decision making: The impact of judgment error and bias. *Clinical Psychology Review, 24*, 707–729.

Heilbrun, K. (2001). *Principles of forensic mental health assessment*. New York: Kluwer/Plenum.

Heilbrun, K., Grisso, T., & Goldstein, A. M. (2009). *Foundations of forensic mental health assessment* (xi, 180 pp). New York: Oxford University Press.

Heilbrun, K., Marczyk, G., & DeMatteo, D. (2002). *Forensic mental health assessment: A casebook*. New York: Oxford University Press.

Heilbrun, K., Marczyk, G., DeMatteo, D., & Mack-Allen, J. (2007). A principles-based approach to forensic mental health assessment: Utility and update. In A. M. Goldstein (Ed.), *Forensic psychology: Emerging topics and expanding roles* (pp. 45–72). Hoboken, NJ: Wiley.

Heilbrun, K., Marczyk, G., DeMatteo, D., et al. (2003). Principles of forensic mental health assessment: Implications for neuropsychological assessment in forensic contexts. *Assessment, 10*, 329–343.

Heilbrun, K., Warren, J., & Picarello, K. (2003). Third party information in forensic assessment. In A. M. Goldstein (Ed.), *Forensic psychology: Vol. 11 of Handbook of psychology* (pp. 69–86). Hoboken, NJ: Wiley.

Hutter, N., Scheidt-Nave, C., & Baumeister, H. (2009). Health care utilisation and quality of life in individuals with diabetes and comorbid mental disorders. *General Hospital Psychiatry, 31*(1), 33–35.

Iverson, G. L. (2007). Identifying exaggeration and malingering. *Pain Practice, 7*(2), 94–102.

Kahn, J. P., & Langlieb, A. M. (2005). *Mental health and productivity in the workplace: A handbook for organizations and clinicians*. San Francisco: Jossey-Bass.

Kemper, P., Tu, H. T., Reschovsky, J. D., & Schaefer, E. (2002). Insurance product design and its effects: Trade-offs along the managed care continuum. *Inquiry, 39*(2), 101–117.

Kessler, R. C., Akiskal, H. S., Ames, M., et al. (2006). Prevalence and effects of mood disorders on work performance in a nationally representative sample of U.S. workers. *American Journal of Psychiatry, 163*(9), 1561–1568.

Kessler, R. C., & Frank, R. G. (1997, July). The impact of psychiatric disorders on work loss days. *Psychological Medicine: A Journal of Research in Psychiatry and the Allied Sciences, 27*(4), 861–873.

Kessler, R. C., Ormel, J., Dernier, O., & Stang, P. E. (2003). Co-morbid mental disorders account for the role impairment of commonly occurring chronic physical disorders: Results from the National Comorbidity Survey. *Journal of Occupational and Environmental Medicine, 45*, 1257–1266.

Kessler, R. C., Zhao, S., Blazer, D. G., & Swartz, M. (1997). Marvin prevalence, correlates, and course of minor depression and major depression in the national comorbidity survey. *Journal of Affective Disorders, 45*(1–2), 19–30.

Koocher, G. P., Norcross, J. C., & Hill, S. S. (2005). *Psychologists' desk reference* (2nd ed.). Oxford, NY: Oxford University Press.

Lerner, D., & Henke, R. M. (2008). What does research tell us about depression, job performance, and work productivity? *Journal of Occupational and Environmental Medicine, 50*(4), 401–410.

MacDonald-Wilson, K., Rogers, E. S., & Anthony, W. A. (2001). Unique issues in assessing work function among individuals with psychiatric disabilities. *Journal of Occupational Rehabilitation, 11*(3), 217–232.

McCracken, L. M., & Gatchel, R. J. (2000). The magnification of psychopathology sequelae associated with multiple chronic medical conditions. *Journal of Applied Biobehavioral Research, 5*(1), 92–99.

Melhorn, J. M., & Ackerman, W. E. (Eds.). (2008). *Guides to the evaluation of disease and injury causation*. Chicago: American Medical Association.

Melton, G., Petrila, J., Poythress, N., & Slobogin, C. (2007). *Psychological evaluations for the courts: A handbook for mental health professionals and lawyers* (3rd ed.). New York: Guilford.

Merikangas, K. R., Ames, M., Cui, L., et al. (2007). The impact of comorbidity of mental and physical conditions on role disability in the US adult household population. *Archives of General Psychiatry, 64*, 1180–1188.

Mittenberg, W., Patton, C., Canyock, E. M., & Condit, D. C. (2002). Base rates of malingering and symptom exaggeration. *Journal of Clinical and Experimental Neuropsychology, 24*(8), 1094–1102.

National Business Group on Health. (2007). *An employer's guide to behavioral health services* (p. 100). Washington, DC: National Business Group on Health.

Otto, R. K., Slobogin, C., & Greenberg, S. A. (2007). Legal and ethical issues in accessing and utilizing third-party information. In A. M. Goldstein (Ed.), *Forensic psychology: Emerging topics and expanding roles* (pp. 190–208). Hoboken, NJ: Wiley.

Pransky, G. S., Shaw, W. S., Franche, R. L., & Clarke, A. (2004). Disability prevention and communication among workers, physicians, employers, and insurers: Current models and opportunities for improvement. *Disability and Rehabilitation, 26*(11), 625–634.

Reed, G. M., Kihlstrom, J. F., & Messer, S. B. (2006). What qualifies as evidence of effective practice? In J. C. Norcross, L. E. Beutler, & R. F. Levant (Eds.), *Evidence-based practice in mental health: Debate and dialogue on fundamental questions* (pp. 13–55). Washington, DC: American Psychological Association.

Robinson, R. C., Gatchel, R. J., Whitfill, T., Schultz, I. Z., & Gatchel, R. J. (Eds.). (2005). *Tailoring psychosocial treatment for patients with occupational disability. Handbook of complex occupational disability claims: Early risk identification, intervention, and prevention* (pp. 151–163). New York: Springer Science + Business Media. xv, 566 pp.

Rogers, R. (Ed.). (1988). *Clinical assessment of malingering and deception*. New York: Guilford.

Rogers, R. (Ed.). (1997). *Clinical assessment of malingering and deception* (2nd ed.). New York: Guilford.

Rogers, R., & Bender, S. D. (2003). Evaluation of malingering and deception. In A. M. Goldstein (Ed.), *Forensic psychology: Vol. 11 of Handbook of psychology* (pp. 109–132). Hoboken, NJ: Wiley.

Rohling, M. L., Binder, L. M., & Langhinrichsen-Rohling, J. (1995). Money matters: A meta-analytic review of the association between financial compensation and the experience and treatment of chronic pain. *Health Psychology, 14*, 537–547.

Rush, A. J., Warden, D., Wisniewski, S. R., et al. (2009). STAR*D: Revising conventional wisdom. *CNS Drugs, 23*(8), 627–647.

Schretlen, D. J., Cascella, N. G., Meyer, S. M., et al. (2007). Neuropsychological functioning in bipolar disorder vs. schizophrenia. *Biological Psychiatry, 62*(2), 179–186.

Schretlen, D. J., Munro, C. A., Anthony, J. C., & Pearlson, G. D. (2003). Examining the range of normal intra-individual variability in neuropsychological test performance. *Journal of the International Neuropsychological Society: JINS, 9*, 864–870.

Schultz, I. Z., & Gatchel, R. J. (Eds.). (2005). *Handbook of complex occupational disability claims*. New York: Springer.

Scott, K. M., Bruffaerts, R., Tsang, A., et al. (2007). Depression-anxiety relationships with chronic physical conditions: Results from the World Mental Health Surveys. *Journal of Affective Disorders, 103*, 113–120.

Scott, K. M., Von Korff, M., Alonso, J., et al. (2009). Mental-physical co-morbidity and its relationship with disability: Results from the World Mental Health Surveys. *Psychological Medicine, 39*(1), 33–43.

Simon, R., & Gold, L. (2004). Psychiatric diagnosis in litigation. In R. Simon & L. Gold (Eds.), *Textbook of forensic psychiatry*. Washington, DC: American Psychiatric Publishing.

Sinyor, M., Schaffer, A., & Levitt, A. (2009). The sequenced treatment alternatives to relieve depression (STAR*D) trial: a review. *Canadian Journal of Psychiatry, 55*(3), 126–135.

Social Security Administration. (2008). *Research, statistics, & policy analysis annual statistical report on the social security disability insurance program, 2007*. Baltimore: Social Security Administration.

Suehs, B., Argo, T.R., Bendele, S.D., Crismon, M.L., Trivedi, M.H., & Kurian, B. (2008). *Texas medication algorithm project procedural manual*. Texas Department of State Health Services.

Suls, J., & Bunde, J. (2005). Anger, anxiety, and depression as risk factors for cardiovascular disease: The problems and implications of overlapping affective dispositions. *Psychological Bulletin, 131*, 260–300.

Surgeon General's Report (1999), United States. Office of the Surgeon General (1999). *Mental Health*. Rockville, VA. National Institute of Mental Health.

Talmage, J. B. (2007). Failure to communicate: How terminology and forms confuse the work ability/disability evaluation process. *Journal of Insurance Medicine, 39*, 192–198.

Talmage, J. B., & Melhorn, J. M. (Eds.). (2005). *A physician's guide to return to work*. Chicago: American Medical Association Press.

The Health Insurance Portability and Accountability Act of 1996 (HIPAA) Pub. Law No. 104–191. (1996)

Thompson, J., LeBourgeois, H., & Black, R. (2004). Malingering. In R. Simon & L. Gold (Eds.), *Textbook of forensic psychiatry* (pp. 427–448). Washington, DC: American Psychiatric Publishing.

Trivedi, M. H., Rush, A. J., Wisniewski, S. R., et al. (2006). Factors associated with health-related quality of life among outpatients with major depressive disorder: A STAR*D report. *The Journal of Clinical Psychiatry, 67*(2), 185–195.

U.S. Equal Employment Opportunity Commission. (2009). Notice concerning the Americans with disability act amendments act of 2008. Retrieved December 1, 2009, from http://www.eeoc.gov/laws/statutes/adaaa_notice.cfm

Van Gorp, W. (2007). Neuropsychology for the forensic psychologist. In A. M. Goldstein (Ed.), *Forensic psychology: Emerging topics and expanding roles* (pp. 154–170). Hoboken, NJ: Wiley.

Wang, P. S., Berglund, P., & Kessler, R. C. (2000). Recent care of common mental disorders in the United States: Prevalence and conformance with evidence-based recommendations. *Journal of General Internal Medicine, 15*(5), 284–292.

Wang, P. S., Demler, O., & Kessler, R. C. (2002). Adequacy of treatment for serious mental illness in the United States. *American Journal of Public Health, 92*(1), 92–98.

Warren, P. A. (2005). *The management of workplace mental health issues and appropriate disability prevention strategies*. San Diego: Work Loss Data Institute.

Warren, P. A. (2009, Fall). Behavioral health as a causation issue in workers' compensation and disability claims. *IAIABC Journal, 46*(2), 17–56.

Warren, P. A. (2013a). Those who hesitate are lost: The case for setting behavioral health treatment and disability standards, part I. *Psychological Injury and Law, 6*(3), 183–195.

Warren, P. A. (2013b). Those who hesitate are lost: The case for setting behavioral health treatment and disability standards, part I. *Psychological Injury and Law, 6*(3), 196–207.

Warren, P. A., & Hubbard, J. D. (2006). The disability claims process and determining mental health diagnoses versus workplace dissatisfaction. *American Academy of Disability Evaluating Physicians, 5*(2), 13–24.

Warren, P. A., & Hubbard, J. D. (2008). *Psychosocial issues related to behavioral health disability claims*. Dearborn National Insurance Company.

Weber, M. C. (2008). AAPL guideline for forensic evaluation of psychiatric disabilities: A disability law perspective. *Journal of the American Academy of Psychiatry and the Law, 36*(4), 558–562.

Weinstein, M. R. (1969). The disability process: Contributions of service agencies to client disabilities. *Comprehensive Psychiatry, 10*(5), 398–405.

Wiley, S. D. (1998). Deception and detection in psychiatric diagnosis. *The Psychiatric Clinics of North America, 21*(4), 869–894.

Young, G., Kane, A. W., & Nicholson, K. (2007). *Causality of psychological injury: Presenting evidence in court*. New York: Springer.

Chapter 6
Assessment of Psychosocial Contributions to Disability

Daniel Bruns and Pamela A. Warren

6.1 Introduction

Disability has traditionally been defined in terms of the biomedical model, where an individual's limitations were seen as being the product of objectively verifiable physical problems. More recently though, disability has been redefined in terms of functionality within a social context (Pledger, 2003). The emphasis of new conceptualizations of disability is that in addition to the individual's physical limitations, disability is also influenced heavily by the ecology of the psychosocial environment. "This disability paradigm maintains that disability is a product of the intersection of individual characteristics (e.g., conditions or impairments, functional status, or personal and socioeconomic qualities) and characteristics of the natural, built, cultural, and social environments"(U.S. Department of Education & Rehabilitation Research, 2009, p. 2). Consequently, determining that a person is disabled cannot be made by assessing the person in isolation, without consideration of the social environment (Jette & Badley, 2000). Thus, disability is best understood as a biopsychosocial phenomenon that combines biological, psychological, and social elements.

D. Bruns (✉)
Health Psychology Associates, Greeley, CO, USA
e-mail: daniel.bruns@healthpsych.com

P. A. Warren
Carle Physician Group and University of Illinois Medical School, Department of Psychiatry, Monticello, IL, USA

P. A. Warren (ed.), *Handbook of Behavioral Health Disability Management*,
https://doi.org/10.1007/978-3-319-89860-5_6

6.2 Biopsychosocial Aspects of Disability

Biopsychosocial disorders arise out of an interaction between biological and psychosocial forces in a patient's life (Gallagher, 2004; Gatchel, 2004; Grace, 2000; Hyams, 2004; Ong & Keng, 2003; Turk & Okifuji, 2002). Although biopsychosocial disorders have often been discussed as if they were a single condition, more recently these disorders have been described as occurring in distinct forms and as having an identifiable natural history (Bruns & Disorbio, 2005). Consequently, the goal of the psychological evaluation of an individual with disability is to (1) review the individual's medical findings, with particular attention to any biological factors that may be a direct cause of impairment, (2) understand the individual's perception of and emotional reaction to the medical condition, (3) identify any psychological contributions to symptoms or disability, and (4) understand the meaning of this condition in the social context in which it occurs.

The fact that objective physical conditions can lead to disability is readily understandable. If a person's hand is traumatically amputated in an accident, the disabling consequences of this are obvious. In contrast, the psychosocial aspects of disability are often more difficult to assess, with the assessment of subjective psychological variables generally being the most challenging. Despite their subjective nature, however, psychosocial variables have a strong influence on disability.

Some psychosocial risk factors are objective in nature. For example, race has been found to predict outcomes from treatments for cancer (Terplan, Smith, & Temkin, 2009) and heart disease (Greene Jackson, Hamilton, Hutchinson, & Huber, 2009), presumably because race is associated with the quality of care received. Perhaps for similar reasons, low education has been found to be predictive of poor outcome from lumbar surgery (den Boer et al., 2006b). Other behaviors that bear on a person's health, such as smoking and diet, are also in principle objectively verifiable activities. However, a complication here is that in practice, the evaluator is dependent on patient reports to determine the presence of many of these risk factors, and unfortunately, patient self-reports are not always accurate. Consequently, many psychosocial variables that would appear to be objective in nature, in practice, are not. Because of this, one of the goals of the psychological evaluation of disability is to determine the extent to which a patient's self-reports might be inaccurate or biased.

Behavioral health disability may co-occur with medical conditions, and the interaction of behavioral and medical disorders may contribute to the disability. When this happens, it is sometimes referred to as a mind-body disorder. One proposed classification system for mind-body disorders employed a 2 × 2 matrix (Bruns & Disorbio, 2003, 2005). Based on this classification system, the first type of mind-body disorder would be an endogenous disorder. Endogenous disorders originate with biological processes. This injury or disease state once present directly alters brain functioning, and in so doing produces the psychological condition. For example, an adrenal tumor can produce abnormally elevated levels of epinephrine, which in turn can cause the patient to feel anxiety. Alternately, a traumatic brain injury can lead to personality change or to depression. In these cases, the biological state produced by the illness or injury has a direct impact on brain functioning and the associated psychological state.

The second type of mind-body disorder is a reactive disorder. Reactive disorders are those which occur when there is a psychological reaction to a biological state. For example, suppose a patient has had a lifelong habit of participation in heavy labor, until sustaining a foot injury that limits activity. In this case, injury to the foot has no direct effect on brain functioning. However, the mental reaction is not the product of a biological process, as the patient is reacting to the *meaning* of this career-ending injury. While the patient experienced an objective medical injury, there is no direct biological mechanism through which the injury to the foot produced depression. Instead, the depression results from how the patient construes the meaning of the foot injury. Thus, while in the case of endogenous disorders, the psychological condition is directly caused by biological processes, in the case of reactive disorders, it is psychological processes that produce the psychological symptoms. Examples of reactive disorders can include post-traumatic stress disorder, adjustment disorders, and major depression.

The third type of mind-body disorder is psychophysiological disorder. Psychophysiological disorders originate with psychological processes, which in turn can produce objectively observable medical symptoms. For example, a patient who is prone to generalized anxiety disorder may worry chronically, and this may manifest physically in the form of chronic muscular bracing, with palpable tension in the patient's neck and shoulders or elsewhere. Psychophysiological disorders may produce their physical symptomatology via a number of mechanisms, such as via the sympathetic nervous system, the adrenergic branch of the endocrine system, stress-related alterations of the inflammatory process, stress-related alterations in the immune system, and through stress-related changes of the microbiome in the gut. In each case, psychophysiological disorders begin with perceptions and cognitions, which then produce a variety of symptoms via medical states triggered by the stress-related physiological changes.

The fourth type of mind-body disorder is the somatizing disorder. In somatizing disorders, psychological processes give rise to the perception or report physical symptoms in the absence of objective pathophysiology. For example, a patient who is hypochondriacal and who is obsessively hypervigilant about disease may over-interpret minor or relatively normal symptoms as being indications of the presence of serious disease, and become subjectively convinced that a disease state does in fact exist. The patient may be so subjectively convinced of this as to be resistant to medical opinions to the contrary. In other cases, the report of physical symptoms can be associated with primary, secondary, or tertiary gain. Of these, secondary gain, or the presence of external reward for the symptom, is the one most commonly discussed. In contrast, primary gain is said to occur when there is an internal gain (e.g., the patient feels internally guilty about not engaging in a certain behavior, but uses an exaggerated physical symptom to internally justify the act, alleviating the guilt). Lastly, tertiary gain is said to occur when the gain is received for a loved one. For example, a parent could exaggerate or feign a physical symptom in order to justify staying at home with a special needs child. In tertiary care, the reward is received by someone else.

It should be noted that the mind-body disorders listed above are not mutually exclusive. Furthermore, traditional psychological diagnoses may fit into one category or the other depending on the particular manifestation of that condition. For example, the *DSM-5* Somatic Symptom Disorder can be either a reactive disorder or a somatizing disorder, depending on whether the pathophysiology is real or perceived. Similarly, a conversion disorder could involve a mechanism that is an objective psychophysiological disorder (a syncopal conversion seizure) or is a somatized perception of a symptom that has no objective basis.

The value of the biopsychosocial model is that it provides methods of generating alternate hypotheses with regard to why some patients don't get better. These hypotheses can provide alternate methods of intervention for complex patients.

6.2.1 Subjective Risk Factors for Disability

In contrast to objective risk factors, many psychological variables are inherently subjective in nature. Even so, these variables can have a profound influence on disability. Research by the World Health Organization (WHO) has used the concept of disability-adjusted life years (DALY) to assess the burden of disease, where one DALY represents 1 year of healthy life lost either to death or disability. Using DALY, WHO determined that in 2004, worldwide, the three disease states with the highest burden of disability were (1) respiratory infections, (2) diarrheal diseases, and (3) Major Depressive Disorder (MDD) (World Health Organization, 2008). This study ranked the disabling burden of depression worldwide as being greater than heart disease, HIV/AIDS, malaria, diabetes, and many other conditions. Furthermore, WHO projections are that by 2020, Major Depressive Disorder will be the second greatest source of disability (Murray & Lopez, 1997) and by 2030 will be the most disabling condition (World Health Organization, 2008). Unlike the other conditions noted above, however, the diagnosis of depression relies heavily on patient self-reports of subjective feelings and behavior.

Pain is also a subjective experience, which cannot be directly assessed. Pain is one of the most common reasons why people see physicians, with one study finding that 80% of patients presenting in office-based care had complaints of pain (Koch, 1986). Not surprisingly, chronic pain has been found to be one of the most expensive conditions in managed care (Disorbio, Bruns, & Barolat, 2006). Several studies have found that pain also tends to be associated with other unpleasant subjective experiences, such as depression (Campbell, Clauw, & Keefe, 2003; Fishbain, Cutler, Rosomoff, & Rosomoff, 1997; Polatin, Kinney, Gatchel, Lillo, & Mayer, 1993) and anxiety (Gureje, 2007, 2008; Roy-Byrne et al., 2008).

Even though pain is a subjective experience, reducing pain is a common goal for surgical interventions. The scientific standards for assessing the effectiveness of surgery for pain reduction were published in a consensus statement by Dworkin and colleagues (Dworkin et al., 2005) in a work called the Initiative on Methods, Measurement, and Pain Assessment in Clinical Trials (IMMPACT). The IMMPACT study recommended that all scientific studies of spinal surgery use five dimensions of medical treatment outcome that consisted of physical functioning, emotional functioning, level of pain, patient satisfaction (all of which are assessed predominantly by patient report), and adverse symptoms (which may be assessed by patient report). When considering the IMMPACT outcome variables, it is worth considering that pain is a subjective feeling, as is satisfaction with care. Additionally, functioning is behavior, and generally determinations of improvement of functioning are assessed by patient report and are dependent on behavioral adherence to exercises and physical therapies post surgery. Overall, it is evident that even though surgery is a biological treatment, determinations of medical treatment outcome and of disability are largely based on subjective report.

While most painful conditions are easily treated and resolve quickly, a small number of painful conditions are extremely expensive to treat. With regard to back injury, one study found that 10% of all cases accounted for 79% of all costs (Spengler et al., 1986), while another study concluded that 5% of cases led to 75% of all costs (Frymoyer & Cats-Baril, 1991). Similarly, a study in Quebec found that 7% of injured patients accounted for 76% of costs. As only 14% of the costs in the Quebec study were for medical care, though, it was concluded that these high costs were not driven by medical complexity, but rather by psychosocial complications (Spitzer, Leblanc, & Dupuis, 1987).

When objective, biomedical impairments are present, it would seem a reasonable assumption that they would be the primary determinants of disability, with psychosocial variables making a smaller contribution. However, this is often not the case. For example, Major Depressive Disorder is commonly associated with serious illness and injury. When depression co-occurs with a serious disease, such as heart disease or diabetes, it would be natural to assume that the physical disease state is the primary cause of disability. However, an international study performed by WHO found that disability was more closely associated with psychopathology than physical disease severity. Overall, it was concluded that impairments of emotion, motivation, and cognition were more powerful determinants of functional disability than the physical disease status itself (Ormel et al., 1994).

If we consider patients with spinal injuries, MRI studies are often used to assess objective pathophysiology. However, a number of studies have shown that positive MRI findings are common in individuals who are symptom-free (Jensen et al., 1994). In contrast, psychological testing has been found to be more predictive than MRI with regard to predicting future disability (Carragee, Alamin, Miller, & Carragee, 2005; Carragee, Barcohana, Alamin, & van den Haak, 2004). Another study found that physical pathology accounted for only 10% of disability 1 year after the evaluation while psychosocial variables could account for 59% of the disability (Burton, Tillotson, Main, & Hollis, 1995). Consistent with this, a prospective study showed that patients who were satisfied with their care were significantly more likely to go on to have a good treatment outcome (Butler & Johnson, 2008). These findings have led the American Medical Association to conclude the following in its *Guides to the Evaluation of Permanent Impairment* (Rondinelli, Genovese, Brigham, & American Medical Association, 2008):

> The traditional and outdated biomedical approach assumes that all pain symptoms have a specific physical cause, and attempts to eradicate the cause directly, by rectifying the presumed pathophysiology. However, chronic pain can rarely be understood by linear, nociceptive mechanism… There is often an absence of a documentable relationship between pain and pathophysiology (p. 32).

Research on the relationship between pain and disability has found that pain levels were more closely associated with disability and patient satisfaction with care than were objective physical impairments (Chiu, Lam, & Hedley, 2005). Other studies have also found strong correlations between subjective pain reports and disability (Fejer & Hartvigsen, 2008; Koho, Aho, Watson, & Hurri, 2001), and that pain was associated with a decreased willingness to use muscles forcefully, which potentially could impact one's overall level of disability (Ylinen et al., 2004). Lastly, research has also shown that the tendency to seek medical care is strongly impacted by societal attitudes and patient demands (Barsky & Borus, 1995; Proctor, Mayer, Gatchel, & McGeary, 2004).

Given this biopsychosocial nature of pain, it has been recommended that treating physicians should more strongly consider the conservative, multidisciplinary treatment approaches that include medical management, physical therapy, and behavioral interventions and avoid unnecessary surgical procedures when possible. Given that surgery always carries a certain degree of risk, it was concluded by one study that by taking a conservative approach, the level of physician-caused disability could be reduced (Aronoff & Livengood, 2003). Consistent with this, a recent study found that intensive multidisciplinary rehabilitation was as effective for nonradicular back pain as was a lumbar fusion (Chou et al., 2009), while other studies have shown that using case managers to address psychosocial and other complications can improve return to work (Butler, Johnson, & Gray, 2007; Tompa, de Oliveira, Dolinschi, & Irvin, 2008). Overall, multidisciplinary treatment is widely regarded as a first-line treatment for chronic pain.

6.3 The Assessment of Psychological States Leading to Disability

The assessment of subjective psychological states is inherently difficult. Of course, one can simply ask the patient how he or she feels and record the answer, but there are two general problems with this. First of all, patients may lack insight into their psychological status and are thus unable to answer certain questions. If patients do not know what depression is, they cannot say if they are depressed. Second, even if patients do have adequate insight, they may be motivated somehow to bias their reports of information. In some cases, out of guilt or shame, patients may minimize their psychological difficulties. In other cases, however, especially when there are incentives to do so, patients may magnify their symptomatic complaints.

The AMA Guides to the Evaluation of Permanent Impairment (Rondinelli et al., 2008) discusses the dilemma that disability ratings in the past have been too dependent on the subjective impressions of the patient, and has suggested instead that disability be assessed by physician ratings. However, this is not much better, as when performing these ratings, the professional is still heavily dependent on patient report. For example, consider the assessment of depression. According to the *DSM-5* (American Psychiatric Association, 2013), Major Depressive Disorder (MDD) is defined as the daily or almost daily presence of five or more of the following symptoms: depressed moods, markedly diminished interest in activities, decrease or increase in appetite or significant weight loss, insomnia or hypersomnia, psychomotor agitation or retardation, fatigue, feelings of worthlessness or guilt, indecisiveness, diminished ability to think, or recurrent thoughts of death. Furthermore, diagnosis of MDD requires that the above subjective difficulties give rise to either significant distress or impairment in social, occupational, or other functioning. Upon inspecting the diagnostic criteria mentioned above, it is evident that a professional performing a disability rating would remain heavily dependent upon patient reports to make many determinations. For example, determinations about feelings of fatigue, appetite, recurring thoughts, or feeling worthless are diagnostic criteria dependent on patient report.

It could be argued that in theory, the above determinations about depression could be made primarily by the objective observations of a professional. In reality though, this is not possible. The diagnostic criteria of MDD require that the patient have some of the above symptoms for much of the day, almost every day. This would require a degree of professional observation that is completely impractical. If for some reason though, it were economically warranted to pay a professional to observe a patient for days at a time, this would still not resolve the problem. A professional could try to assess a feeling such as appetite by observing eating behaviors. However, these behaviors are largely under the voluntary control of the patient and could be altered as desired. Intensity of libido might be judged by sexual behaviors, but observing this is not ethically allowed. Thus, for a myriad of reasons, we must turn to patient report to assess important subjective variables, such as appetite, libido, pain, depression, and anxiety. Unfortunately, patients may be unable or unwilling to accurately report these subjective states. In some cases, the patient may be motivated to intentionally supply false information. While the subjective contributions to biopsychosocial disorders and to disability are so important that they cannot be dismissed, the assessment of these subjective traits remains challenging. Fortunately though, there is a means of addressing this problem.

6.4 Psychometric Assessment and Disability

Psychometrics is the scientific method used to measure subjective psychological human abilities, traits, and experiences. This includes inferred traits such as intelligence or personality, subjective experiences, such as emotions, thoughts, and memories, and physical symptoms, such as pain or fatigue. Psychometrics involves the systematic analysis of overt human behavior as a means of assessing unobservable psychological attributes (Furr & Bacharach, 2008). The observed behaviors may include memory tasks, problem solving, verbal reports, responses to paper-and-pencil questionnaires, or motor behaviors (e.g., drawing a picture). From a careful scientific analysis of the data gathered, underlying attributes can be inferred and measured.

Although psychometrics sounds mysterious, it is a science that Western society has come to rely on heavily. Perhaps the most common example of this is that on almost every edition of the news on television, the results of a poll are reported. Scientific surveys, which employ psychometric principles, have an established ability to accurately predict the sentiments of a population, with a known degree of error. In a manner analogous to the way that scientific questioning of voters can assess their subjective opinions and predict voting behavior, standardized psychometric instruments can assess subjective states that predict disability in patients. Psychometric tests are often employed to assess psychological (e.g., depression or personality) or neuropsychological (e.g., memory or reasoning) constructs. Additionally though, they can also be used to assess a patient's perception of physical abilities, health behaviors, or symptoms (e.g., measures of physical functioning like the Oswestry Disability Index (Fairbank & Pynsent, 2000) or the Dialysis Symptom Index (Weisbord et al., 2004)). Overall, psychometric tests can be used for a variety of purposes. These uses include: (1) diagnostic classification; (2) description of patient traits or characteristics; (3) intervention planning; (4) tracking changes in symptoms, beliefs, or behaviors over time; and (5) prediction of future thoughts, feelings, behaviors, or events, including satisfaction with care or treatment outcome (Turner, DeMers, Fox, & Reed, 2001).

One of the important contributions of psychometric assessment is not only to measure *whether or not* a condition like depression is present but also to assess *the degree* to which it is present. For example, the National Comorbidity Study found that between 2001 and 2003, 20% of the population from 18 to 54 years of age had received some sort of treatment for an emotional disorder. However, only about half of those that received treatment had disorders that met the diagnostic criteria for a mental disorder (Kessler, Chiu, Demler, Merikangas, & Walters, 2005). This research suggests that a low level of psychological distress and other conditions is common in the healthy population. Consequently, during a disability evaluation, it becomes important to determine (1) whether or not depressive or other symptoms are present, and (2) whether or not these symptoms are indicative of commonly occurring mild adjustment difficulties, or a more serious psychological condition that could contribute to disability. The advantage of a psychometric measure of depression is that it can return a percentile rank, thus more precisely and reliably quantifying the degree of depression that is present.

Despite the advantages of the biopsychosocial model, integrating psychological concepts into the biomedical model can be daunting. Those who do not adopt an integrated biopsychosocial model of disability, though, are at risk for oscillating between biomedical and psychological reductionism. On the one hand, using biomedical reductionism, it could be argued that depression or anxiety can "really" be reduced to a purely physical disease state, defined by aberrant levels of serotonin, norepinephrine, or other neurotransmitters, and that the subjective experience is irrelevant. Alternately, for those patients who complain of disabling symptoms that are medically improbable, psychological reductionism can be employed: "Your symptoms aren't real. They are all in your head." Neither type of reductionism though can fully explain the spectrum of variables that lead to disability. In contrast, the strength of the biopsychosocial approach is that it attempts to bring together these disparate biological, psychological, and social aspects of the human condition under one umbrella and, in this manner, can achieve greater explanatory power.

The biopsychosocial assessment of patients is a challenging task. Despite this, multiple evidence-based medical guidelines recommend a biopsychosocial approach (American College of Occupational and Environmental Medicine, 2008a; Colorado Division of Workers' Compensation, 2017; Hegmann, 2017; Work Loss Data Institute, 2009). With regard to performing the best possible assessments of the psychosocial aspects of disability, the following suggestions are made.

6.5 An Introduction to Psychological Testing Concepts

Psychometric questionnaires vary greatly with regard to what they are intended to assess and the degree to which they have met accepted psychometric standards. While a very large number of psychometric questionnaires are available, not all measures are equal, and many are not appropriate for clinical assessment. Standardized psychometric tests differ substantially from informal questionnaires. The definitive standard for determining whether or not a questionnaire can be regarded as a "standardized test" is a work called the *Standards for Educational and Psychological Testing* (American Educational Research Association, American Psychological Association, National Council on Measurement in Education, Joint Committee on Standards for Educational, and Psychological Testing (U.S.), 1999). In addition to meeting the criteria specified by the *Standards*, others have suggested that a standardized psychological test should also have been reviewed by the *Mental Measurements Yearbook* (American College of Occupational and Environmental Medicine, 2008b; Mitrushina, Boone, & D'Elia, 1999) and have generated publications in peer-reviewed journals (Mitrushina et al., 1999).

How good are psychometric tests? A systematic review of the literature reviewed 125 meta-analyses on test validity and 800 samples used for multimethod assessment (Meyer et al., 2001). This study reached the following conclusions:

1. There is strong evidence that psychological tests can validly measure their intended constructs.
2. Psychological test validity is comparable to medical test validity.
3. Psychological tests are a distinct assessment method that can provide a unique source of information.
4. Psychological tests can provide information that cannot be gained by interview alone.

The Meyer study concluded that psychometric tests are the scientific equal of medical tests. Beyond this, however, in some studies, psychometric tests were better predictors of medical outcome than standard medical assessment techniques. For example, as noted previously, studies have found that psychological variables were (a) better than either MRIs or discography in predicting future back pain disability (Carragee et al., 2005), (b) stronger contributors to disability than was disease severity (Ormel et al., 1994), and (c) able to predict delayed recovery without using medical diagnostic information (Gatchel, Polatin, & Mayer, 1995).

Overall, standardized tests offer an efficient means of gathering information about psychological, social, and medical variables. Standardized psychometric tests can help the disability evaluator by (a) providing a means to quantify a patient's subjective reports in a manner that an interview cannot, (b) helping to control for a patient's tendency to exaggerate or minimize symptoms, and (c) evaluating the individual in a standardized way that reduces the effect of biases on the part of the professional. Thus, psychometric tests can be an important part of a thorough assessment and facilitate the evaluation of the patient in a comprehensive manner.

6.5.1 What Is a Standardized Test?

The defining features of a standardized test are listed in Table 6.1. While this information is known by psychologists, it is offered here as it is not common knowledge among members of other professions. It is important to recognize that many commonly used questionnaires (such as the Oswestry and the Zung Depression Scale) are not standardized. The *Standards* indicate that while such measures may work well in research settings, only standardized tests should be used for clinical assessments. It could be countered, "How can you say that Test XYZ should not be used clinically? It has been used in numerous research studies. Isn't that enough?"

To illustrate the effects of lack of standardization, consider the 0–10 pain rating scale. It has been noted that this scale has literally thousands of variations, with no agreed upon definition of what a pain level of 10 is, no agreed upon time frame (e.g., pain right now versus usual pain or worst pain), or pain location (overall pain versus back pain or headaches) (American College of Occupational and Environmental Medicine, 2008b). Because of these problems, Turk and Melzack (1992) stated:

> The appropriateness of norms of tests has rarely been considered in the pain literature. In the absence of normative information, the raw score on any test is meaningless. To observe that a patient with a migraine headache scores a 10 on a Visual Analog Scale (VAS) of intensity conveys little or no information.

Another problem with nonstandardized measures is that users sometimes modify them. For example, the Oswestry Disability Index has been modified multiple times. Further, some of the modifications have been done carelessly, as some published versions of the Oswestry contain misprints, and others omit the scoring system altogether (Fairbank & Pynsent, 2000). The practice of modifying questionnaires serves to create nonequivalent forms of the measure, and this negates any standardization a test may have had.

Table 6.1 Defining features of a standardized test

Test-retest reliability (stability)	The degree to which a scale produces consistent results, e.g., if a test is given twice in a short time frame, the results should be very similar
Internal reliability (homogeneity)	The degree to which the items of a scale all assess the same thing
Validity	The extent to which a test or scale actually measures what it purports to measure, e.g., if a test of depression includes items about weight change, loss of libido, and fatigue, to what extent is it measuring the effects of illness or medication side effects as opposed to depression
Standard test materials and methods	Standardized tests reduce error by having standardized materials, administration procedure, instructions, scoring, and interpretation methods
Norms	The scores of a reference group to which a patient's score is compared. The closer the norm group is to the patient's status and situation, the more relevant the information
Standardized score	A score, such as IQ score or a T-score, that compares an individual's score to the normal distribution of scores occurring in the norm group. For example, an IQ of 115 and a T-score of 60 both indicate scores one standard deviation above the mean of the norm group and at the 84% percentile relative to that group
Test manual and documentation	A standardized test has a manual that documents the following:
	Purpose and uses of test
	Standardized instructions and scoring
	Standardized score interpretation
	Documentation of test norms and norm groups
	Documentation of test reliability and validity
	Documentation of test development process
Validity measures	A measure employed on some clinical tests that attempts to assess whether a *particular subject's responses* are valid, as opposed to being the product of faking, exaggerating, minimizing, illiteracy, or random responding

The lack of standardization is compounded when a test is informally translated into a different language. For example, one unauthorized Spanish translation of the Beck Anxiety Inventory in use with Spanish speakers translated the item "dizzy or light-headed" as "dizzy or light on hooves." This poor translation is worsened by the fact that the phrase "light on hooves" is a figure of speech in Spain and Puerto Rico that implies promiscuity (Artiola i Fortuny & Mullaney, 1997). This type of mistranslation would be comical, if not for the fact that this measure could be used for clinical decision-making.

It would be a mistake to say informal or nonstandardized questionnaires are without value. In research settings, nonstandardized questionnaires are frequently used and modified to address particular research questions. This is a perfectly acceptable practice in research, where the task at hand is to compare groups of patients. In contrast, clinical assessment is fundamentally different. In clinical assessment, the scores of one individual are assessed to determine if they are unusual enough to cause concern or suggest alterations to the treatment regimen. This is a much more

Table 6.2 Types of biopsychosocial interactions

Mechanism of mind-body connection		Origin of disorder	
		Biological processes	Psychological processes
		Endogenous psychological disorders	Psychophysiological disorders
Connection between physical and mental symptoms accomplished via biological mechanism	Sample types	Depression due to hypothyroidism; personality change due to brain injury	Tension headaches, stress-related hypertension, irritable bowel syndrome
	Mechanism	Illness or injury has direct effect on brain processes involving emotion, cognition, or personality	Stress-related chronic autonomic arousal or unhealthy behaviors lead to measureable organic changes
	Example	Patient becomes short-tempered and impulsive due to brain injury	Autonomic arousal leads to palpable muscle tension and to chronic muscle pain; autonomic arousal and functional gastric pain
	Psychological treatment	Psychological support, disease management, compensatory strategies, address lifestyle changes (e.g., diet, exercise, smoking cessation)	Stress management, biofeedback, relaxation training, behavioral treatment to reduce distress and make lifestyle changes (e.g., work habits, exercise)
	Medical treatment	Appropriate medical treatment for illness/injury, medication as needed for depression or anxiety, or to stabilize central nervous system	Medications (e.g., anxiolytics, antidepressants, muscle relaxants, or beta blockers) to interrupt the "fight or flight" response

		Reactive psychological disorders	Somatizing disorders
Connection between physical and mental symptoms accomplished via psychological mechanism	Sample types	Injury or illness with reactive depression	Somatic symptom disorders, somatization, conversion disorders, factitious disorders
	Mechanism	Emotional reaction to an objective organic problem	Misperception of or exaggerated report of physical symptoms that can be psychologically but not biologically explained
	Example	Patient suffers a disabling injury and reacts with depression; patient is diagnosed with a terminal condition and has an anxiety attack	Unrecognized severe anxiety manifests with palpitations and is perceived as a cardiac condition; symptom magnification to gain disability status
	Psychological treatment	Psychological support, address anxiety and depression, symptom management, and facilitate lifestyle changes (e.g., diet, exercise, smoking cessation)	Psychotherapy to address underlying somatized concerns, psychological management of primary, secondary or tertiary gain
	Medical treatment	Appropriate medical treatment for illness/injury, medication as needed for reactive depression or anxiety	Medication for any underlying and somatized depression or anxiety

Adapted from Bruns and Disorbio (1996), used with permission challenging task. As noted in Table 6.1, this cannot be accomplished unless we know that the test (1) is a valid measure of what we want to assess, (2) is a reliable measure, (3) has standardized materials and scoring methods, and (4) has standardized scores based on norms that will allow the identification of unusual scores.

6.5.2 Validity Assessment

Part of human nature is that for a variety of reasons, patients may sometimes answer questions or respond to test items in aberrant ways. During a disability evaluation, a patient may be consciously or unconsciously incentivized to provide distorted or blatantly false information, and in so doing, invalidate the results. These incentives could include the presence of primary gain (e.g., a person enjoys being a patient or being in a hospital), secondary gain (e.g., the patient will receive monetary rewards for being disabled or opioids for being in pain), or tertiary gain (e.g., the patient realizes with somewhat misguided altruism that being disabled would make it possible to spend more time with one's child, which would benefit the child). Beyond the effects of these sorts of incentives, there are a number of other types of aberrant responding that could also invalidate a psychometric test's results. These include a reluctance to reveal private information, confusion, illiteracy, careless responding due to fatigue, lack of motivation, or response sets.

A response set is a tendency to respond to a psychometric test in a manner that is independent of the test items. For example, the response set of acquiescence involves the tendency to agree with anything, regardless of content. In contrast, social desirability is a response set where a person is always prone to choose the most socially desirable response, while a response set called "primacy" involves a tendency to choose the first alternative that is presented. Overall, subjects prone to response sets are not really responding to the content of the test item, but rather to an incidental feature of the test or test administration, and this undermines the validity of their test results.

To control for various sorts of threats to validity, many psychological tests employ validity indices. When validity indices are lacking, the test administrator may not be able to determine if the test taker is underreporting or exaggerating responses, responding randomly, influenced by a response set, or responding in other aberrant ways. The use of validity measures is an important control when assessing the subjective reports of patients in the clinical setting. Through the use of these measures, it is possible to better assess the accuracy of the patient's self-report of abilities and subjective experiences.

In general, there are two types of validity measures: psychological and neuropsychological. Psychological validity measures assess traits such as the tendency to conceal embarrassing information (defensiveness), exaggerate positive traits, or aberrant responding due to response sets, illiteracy, or random responding. Psychological validity scales assess the validity of symptom reports related to subjective psychological difficulties, such as depression, post-traumatic stress disorder, or pain. In contrast, neuropsychological validity scales assess the motivation to give best effort during the assessment of challenging mental tests, such as the measures of reasoning and memory. Neuropsychological validity scales assess the validity of symptom reports related to mental functions, such as cognition, memory, and perception, especially with regard to brain injury or disease.

An interesting study employed a factor analytic method to mathematically identify the patterns of biased reporting while taking psychological tests. This method identified four patterns of biased reports, which were (1) the underreporting of psychological symptoms, (2) the over reporting of "neurotic" and vague illness symptoms, (3) insufficient cognitive effort, and (4) the over reporting of psychotic or bizarre symptoms (Nelson, Sweet, Berry, Bryant, & Granacher, 2007). Biased reporting may go beyond the reports of current symptoms. Studies have shown that in addition to exaggerating present symptomatology, biased reporting can also involve exaggerating how much better one was in the past (Greiffenstein, Baker, & Johnson-Greene, 2002; Mittenberg, DiGiulio, Perrin, & Bass, 1992).

All major psychological tests, such as the BHI 2, MBMD, MCMI-IV, MMPI-2, MMPI-2-RF, and PAI, include multiple measures of validity (see Appendix 1). In contrast, brief psychological tests generally do not have validity measures. The exceptions to this are the P3, which has a measure of bizarre responding, and the BBHI 2, which includes assessments of exaggerating, minimizing, random responding, and psychosis. In a nutshell, validity measures on these tests are looking for statistically implausible reports. This could involve implausibly low reports of emotional distress (e.g., patient claims to have never been mad or had sad feelings), implausibly high levels of bizarre psychological symptoms (e.g., patient complains of a far higher level of bizarre symptoms than do patients with paranoid schizophrenia), or high levels of diffuse physical symptomatology that are difficult to explain medically.

The psychological test that has generated the most research on malingering is the MMPI-2. The current MMPI-2 computerized report incorporates nine separate validity measures, each of which has specific purposes, strengths, and weaknesses (Arbisi & Butcher, 2004). The new MMPI-2-RF (revised form) has similar, shortened versions of eight of the MMPI-2 validity scales (Ben-Porath & Tellegen, 2008), but has to date less research on this topic. While the MMPI tests include measures to assess a wide variety of invalid test protocols, much attention has focused on the Fake Bad Scale (FBS), which has been extensively researched (Nelson, Sweet, & Demakis, 2006). Some have been critical of this scale, saying that the scale is "likely to classify an unacceptably large number of individuals who are experiencing genuine psychological distress as malingerers" (p. 473) (Butcher, Arbisi, Atlis, & McNulty, 2003). This underscores the fact that a score on any single psychometric measure of validity, while useful, is not sufficient to declare a person to be a malingerer, but rather needs to be interpreted within the context of other test scores, clinical observations, and the patient's history.

Assessing validity for neuropsychological conditions is somewhat different than psychological conditions. In general, it is not possible to fake good on a neuropsychological test (e.g., an individual with dementia cannot pretend to be intellectually gifted). In contrast, neuropsychological tests are very vulnerable to faking bad: All a patient has to do is to not try very hard, or say, "I don't know." To control for this, symptom validity tests (SVTs) are used to assess motivation during neuropsychological test administration.

The Word Memory Test (WMT) is a commonly used SVT. The WMT is called a "forced choice test," and it operates in the following manner. A testing subject is first shown a list of words. After a delay, the subject is shown two words, and asked to choose which one of these was seen previously. Using this method, a person with no verbal memory ability at all would be expected to get about 50% correct just by guessing. In theory, to get a score below chance levels such as 25% correct, a subject must remember the right answer and choose the opposite one. The Test of Memory Malingering (TOMM) is similar to the WMT, but has the patient choose which of two pictures was previously seen, while the Computerized Assessment of Response Bias uses a similar procedure using the memory of numbers. Of these, research suggests that the WMT may be the strongest single measure (Gervais, Rohling, Green, & Ford, 2004).

In contrast, the Validity Indicator Profile (VIP) takes a somewhat different approach to validity assessment using a performance curve (Frederick, Crosby, & Wynkoop, 2000). On the VIP, the test subject is given both vocabulary and math items of varying difficulty in random order. In theory, a test subject who is capable of performing at the ninth grade level should score highly on items up to that level and progressively worse on items with a 10th, 11th, and 12th grade difficulty. This pattern of progressively increasing error rate is difficult to fake, however, and subjects who fail a large number of easy items while getting much harder items correct obtain profiles suggestive of poor motivation to perform (Frederick & Bowden, 2009; Frederick & Crosby, 2000).

Overall, psychological and neuropsychological tests employ a variety of validity measures intended to assess how a particular test subject approached the testing. There are a variety of reasons why a particular test may not be valid, though. Consequently, multiple measures of validity should be used (Lynch, 2004). When multiple measures of validity are administered, though, some of them may suggest that the results are valid, while others do not. This is not a contradiction, though, as each of these measures may assess a different aspect of valid test performance, and together these provide for a more accurate assessment of a patient's test-taking behaviors.

6.5.3 Malingering, Exaggeration, and Denial

Sometimes, there are incentives for a patient to appear disabled. In disability settings, one of the principal uses of test validity measures is to detect malingering or exaggeration. Malingering is defined by the *DSM-5* as "the intentional production of false or grossly exaggerated physical or psychological symptoms, motivated by external incentives such as avoiding military duty, avoiding work, obtaining financial compensation, evading criminal prosecution, or obtaining drugs" (p. 726).

According to the *DSM-5*, probable malingering exists when two or more of the following four conditions are present: (1) the patient presents in a medical/legal context; (2) there is a marked discrepancy between claimed disability and objective findings; (3) the patient exhibits a lack of cooperation with testing or treatment (a malingerer may avoid diagnostic evaluations that would fail to support the symptomatic complaints or treatment for which a genuine condition might respond); and (4) the patient has an antisocial personality disorder (American Psychiatric Association, 2013).

Studies have shown that psychological conditions can be easily faked (Hall, 2007) and that compensation for disability is associated with increased reports of symptoms (Binder & Rohling, 1996; Rohling, Binder, & Langhinrichsen-Rohling, 1995). Despite this, the prevalence of malingering remains controversial. The most extensive review to date of pain-related malingering reviewed 68 studies and estimated that malingering was present in 1.25–10.4% of patients with chronic pain (Fishbain, Cutler, Rosomoff, & Rosomoff, 1999). In contrast, some more recent studies have suggested that there may be a 30–40% incidence of malingering of pain, emotional distress, or cognitive symptoms in patients who were litigating or seeking benefits (Aronoff et al., 2007; Mittenberg, Patton, Canyock, & Condit, 2002). Variations in estimates of the prevalence of malingering may be explained in part by the fact that a recent study found that the prevalence of malingering was observed to increase along with the degree of potential for financial gain. Consequently, in situations where a high potential for financial gain was present, such as in federal litigation, the prevalence of malingering could be significantly higher. This phenomenon could help to explain wide variations in estimates of the prevalence of malingering (Bianchini, Curtis, & Greve, 2006).

The *DSM-5* and *ICD-10* both note that prior to diagnosing malingering, other psychiatric explanations must be ruled out. These alternative explanations include factitious disorders, somatic symptom or disorders (e.g., somatic symptom disorders, somatization, conversion disorder, pain disorder), or psychosis with somatic delusions (American Psychiatric Association, 2013). In contrast to malingering, where symptoms are feigned in the pursuit of some kind of external reward or secondary gain, in factitious disorders, symptoms are produced for primary gain. As noted above, in factitious disorders, a patient reports symptoms without any intent of external reward such as a disability settlement. Instead, in factitious disorders, the individual reports symptoms because he or she wants to be a patient (Wise & Ford, 1999). Thus, while a healthy patient may aspire to have a career, a factitious patient wants nothing more than to be a patient, even to the point of turning down a monetary settlement if it would jeopardize patient status. In some cases, factitious symptoms are feigned. In other cases though, patients with factitious disorders may actually self-induce a medical condition (such as by drinking a toxic substance or rubbing fecal material into a wound) in order to gain patient status (Mailis-Gagnon, Nicholson, Blumberger, & Zurowski, 2008).

Malingering must also be distinguished from disorders which involve somatizing, which includes Somatoform, Somatic Symptom and related disorders. Somatoform disorders are psychiatric conditions listed by *DSM-IV-TR* and *ICD-10*, where psychological difficulties are expressed in a somatic form. In Somatoform Disorders, the individual is typically unaware of any relationship between physical symptoms and his or her psychological status and is not in voluntary control of the physical symptoms (American Psychiatric Association, 2000). In the *DSM-5* Somatic Symptom Disorders, physical symptoms may or may not have an objective basis. In this disorder, the reported physical symptoms are associated with "excessive thoughts, feelings, or behaviors" (American Psychiatric Association, 2013). Somatizing disorders may involve both the exaggeration of physical symptoms and the simultaneous denial or minimization of psychological distress or dysfunction. This, in fact, is the core of somatizing: denied psychological difficulties unconsciously manifest themselves as inflated complaints of physical symptoms (Ford, 1986). An example of this would be a patient who denies being anxious, but continues to interpret a pounding heart as a deadly sign of a heart attack, even after this has been medically ruled out. In other cases, the patient may actively conceal psychological difficulties, out of the fear that if they were reported, the physical symptoms would be taken less seriously. Malingering is also distinguished from psychophysiological disorders, as stress and physiological arousal can sometimes lead to objective medical difficulties (Bruns & Disorbio, 2005, 2009) such as stress-related hypertension (Pickering, 2001).

Finally, malingering must be distinguished from exaggerating. Patients with objective physical difficulties may exaggerate the report of associated symptoms for a variety of reasons. Exaggeration can be related to personality type, depressive negativism, a cry for help, or out of a patient's perception that the physician is trivializing the reported symptoms (Iverson, 2007). Cognitive styles such as catastrophizing may also increase symptom reports (Sullivan et al., 2001). Further, one of the effects of litigation is that both sides may make biased or exaggerated statements as part of the adversarial process (Bornstein Whisenhunt, Nemeth, & Dunaway, 2002). While malingering involves the intentional report of information that is either a gross exaggeration or patently false, mild exaggeration is common and can occur for many reasons other than malingering.

Even when malingering is not judged to be present, environmental incentives can affect the treatment outcome. For example, research has shown that patients are less likely to recover from a back injury if they are in a lawsuit for that injury (Rohling et al., 1995). Similar studies have found that litigation is associated with poor outcome from treatment for head injury (Binder & Rohling, 1996) and for vocational rehabilitation (Lysgaard, Fonager, & Nielsen, 2005). Similarly, if a patient receives insurance compensation for disability (such as from the workers' compensation system), this has also been found to be associated with a poor prognosis for treatment (Bernard, 1993; Deyo, Mirza, Heagerty, Turner, & Martin, 2005; Epker & Block, 2001; Glassman et al., 1998; Greenough, Taylor, & Fraser, 1994; Groth-Marnat & Fletcher, 2000; Klekamp, McCarty, & Spengler, 1998; Mannion & Elfering, 2006; Taylor et al., 2000). In general, research suggests that when patients are paid or hope to be paid for having symptoms, their symptoms are less likely to get better.

Overall, malingering is not a medical or psychiatric condition. In the case of disability determinations, malingering is an illegal, fraudulent act, which has consequences under both criminal and civil law. Thus, for a medical professional to label someone a "malingerer" is not an act of diagnosis, but is rather rendering a verdict. As stated by Mendelson and Mendelson (Mendelson & Mendelson, 2004), "In our view, the ultimate issue of the veracity of the plaintiff is for the Court to decide, and epithets such as "malingerer" have no place in reports prepared for legal purposes by health care professionals" (p. 423).

6.5.4 Psychosocial Predictors of Poor Treatment Outcome and Disability

Research has shown that psychosocial variables can predict the outcome of certain medical treatments. In clinical settings, the practice that has received the most attention is the use of psychological evaluations prior to a variety of invasive procedures and other treatments for pain and injury. This practice has been judged valuable enough that in several jurisdictions, laws and regulations mandate the use of the biopsychosocial model, and that psychological evaluations are performed prior to various medical procedures (California Division of Workers' Compensation, 2009; Colorado Division of Workers' Compensation, 2017).

A substantial body of research has focused on predicting the outcome of invasive procedures such as spinal cord stimulation (SCS) (Burchiel et al., 1996; Heckler, Gatchel, Lou, Whitworth, Bernstein, & Stowell, 2007; Giordano & Lofland, 2005a) and spinal surgery (Block, Gatchel, Deardorff, & Guyer, 2003; Block, Ohnmeiss, Guyer, Rashbaum, & Hochschuler, 2001; Boersma & Linton, 2005; DeBerard, Masters, Colledge, & Holmes, 2003; den Boer, Oostendorp, Beems, Munneke, & Evers 2006; den Boer et al. 2000b; Epker & Block, 2001; Gatchel, 2001; Gatchel & Mayer, 2008; Gatchel, Mayer, & Eddington, 2006; Hagg, Fritzell, Ekselius, & Nordwall, 2003; LaCaille, DeBerard, Masters, Colledge, & Bacon, 2005; Schofferman, Anderson, Hines, Smith, & White, 1992). Several studies have found that psychosocial factors were successful in predicting the results of invasive surgical procedures correctly 80–85% of the time (Block et al., 2001; Giordano & Lofland, 2005b). Psychological evaluation prior to various invasive procedures is now recommended by multiple evidence-based medical guidelines (American College of Occupational and Environmental Medicine, 2008b; Work Loss Data Institute, 2008; Colorado Division of Workers' Compensation, 2017). With regard to outcome from back surgery, a systematic review found nine variables that were consistently associated with poor surgical outcome. These variables were depression, anxiety, somatization, pain, job dissatisfaction, functioning, days away from work, low education, and passive coping (den Boer et al., 2006a, 2006b).

The psychological assessment of patients is often portrayed as a counterpoint to biomedical assessment. For example, prior to various invasive procedures, a patient may be referred for both a medical opinion and a presurgical psychological evaluation as well. More recently though, one study noted that this approach is not consistent with the biopsychosocial perspective, as this type of evaluation should be approached as a single multidisciplinary assessment process (Bruns & Disorbio, 2009). This study concluded that both evidence and opinion were converging on a set a variables for biopsychosocial assessment. These variables were organized into a graphical paradigm called the vortex paradigm. The vortex paradigm (Bruns & Disorbio, 2009, 2014, 2015) conceptualizes intractable medical conditions such as chronic pain as being precipitated by the cumulative effect of biological, psychological, and social risk factors. In a manner similar to the way heart disease can be predicted by a multivariate equation that includes cholesterol, age, blood pressure, diabetes, genetics, etc., the vortex paradigm conceptualizes disability as a biopsychosocial phenomenon and holds that disabling conditions can be predicted by a multivariate equation that includes biological severity, depression, catastrophizing, drug abuse, personality disorder, job dissatisfaction, childhood trauma, secondary gain, etc. The vortex paradigm would posit that biological, psychological, and social variables may all contribute to the onset of an injury or illness. Once present, a significant biological condition may have direct psychological and social consequences, and these may interact with the patient's pre-existing biological, psychological, and social strengths and vulnerabilities. As the level of biopsychosocial risk factors increases, the risk of decompensation (a "downward spiral") into a disabling chronic condition increases. This paradigm suggests numerous falsifiable hypotheses that can be tested by multivariate methods (Fig. 6.1) and was adopted by the ACOEM/MDA Guidelines Chronic Pain Medical Treatment Guidelines (Hegmann, 2017).

In the vortex paradigm, risk factors were classified into two different levels, being either primary/"exclusionary risk factors" or secondary/"cautionary risk factors." Primary risk factors (e.g., dangerousness to self or others, psychosis, severe psychopathology) were thought to be so severe that the presence of one could by themselves would exclude a patient from consideration for surgical intervention, (Table 6.3) while the number of less severe "cautionary risks" were believed to increase the risk that the patient would not respond to the medical treatment (Table 6.4). This approach identifies statistically unusual complaints of problematic symptoms, which in past research were found to be associated with poor treatment outcomes. The identified risk factors were then assessed using standardized psychometric measures, the Battery for Health Improvement 2 (Bruns & Disorbio, 2003) and the shorter Brief Battery for Health Improvement 2 (Disorbio & Bruns, 2002). The US national norms for the prevalence of these risk scores were obtained, with the subjects being both community members, and injured patients with a variety of diagnoses being treated in a variety of treatment settings. The norms obtained from these samples allowed the calculation of a risk score percentile rank, which was used to establish empirical benchmarks for patient reports of behaviors and subjective symptoms (Bruns & Disorbio, 2009).

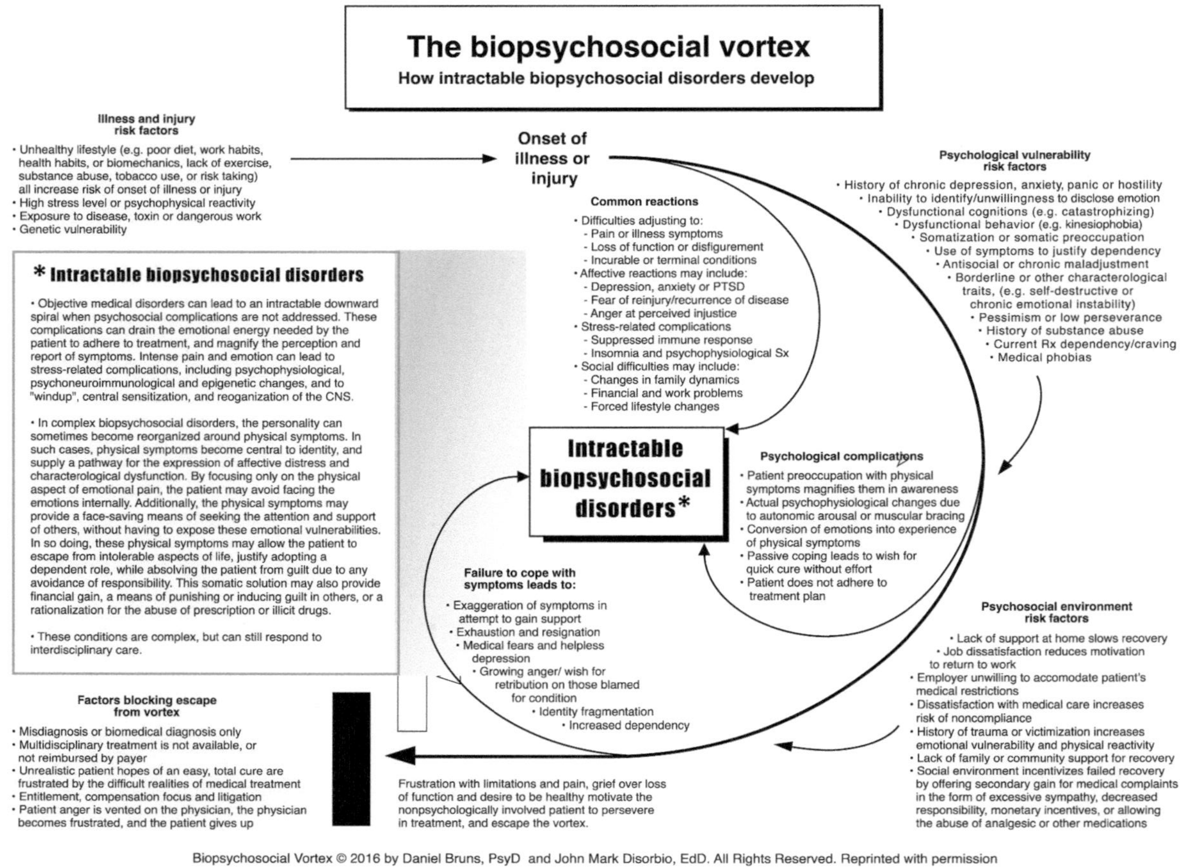

Fig. 6.1 Biopsychosocial vortex

Table 6.3 Primary (aka "exclusionary") risk factors

Type of risk		
Affective	Active suicidal urges	
	Active homicidal urges	
	Severe depression	
	Severe anxiety (generalized, panic, PTSD, med. Phobia/death fears, etc.)	
	Severe anger	
	Mood elevation/mania	
Other psychological risks	Psychosis/delusions/hallucinations	
	Active substance abuse	
	Somatization	
	Pain-focused somatoform disorder	
	Severe personality disorder	
	Extremely poor coping	
	Severe social isolation, family dysfunction, or current severe abuse	
Social	Litigation for pain and suffering, and pain-related treatment	
	Intense doctor/patient conflict	
Biological	*Pain*	Extraordinary pain reports
		Dysfunctional pain cognitions
		Extreme, invariant pain
		Extreme pain sensitivity
	Exam	Medically impossible symptoms
		Gross inconsistencies among objective findings, symptom reports, and patient behavior
		Falsifying information, malingering, or factitious symptoms
		Inability to cooperate with treatment due to cognitive or other problems
	History	Same treatment failed multiple times in past
		Abuse of prescription medications, violation of opioid contracts
		History of gross noncompliance
	Science	Evidence that the proposed medical treatment would be injurious or ineffective given the circumstances

Adapted from Bruns and Disorbio (2009). Used with permission

Using this approach, extreme exclusionary risk factor scores that were observed in less than 1% of a national sample of patients in rehabilitation were developed. In contrast, less extreme cautionary risk factor scores that were observed in only 16% of the national sample of patients in rehabilitation (one standard deviation above the mean) were developed. These risk scores demonstrated a test-retest reliability of 0.85–0.90, with no significant race or gender bias. Evidence of validity was based on the analyses of both community subjects and ten patient groups. The community norms allowed for the comparison of a patient's score to healthy persons in the community, which makes possible an assessment as to the degree to which a particular patient's condition differs from that of the typical healthy person. In contrast, the patient norms allow the identification of unusual patients, who report a level of symptomatic complaints that differs from that of the typical patient (Bruns & Disorbio, 2009).

Table 6.4 Secondary (aka "cautionary") risk factors

Type of risk		
Affective	Depression	
	Anger	
	Anxiety (fears, phobias, PTSD, etc.)	
Psychological vulnerability	History of substance of abuse	
	Personality disorder	
	Cognitive disorder or low education	
	Poor coping	
	Diffuse somatic complaints	
Social	Conflict with physicians	
	Job dissatisfaction	
	Family dysfunction	
	Hx abuse	
	Workers' compensation	
	Compensation focus	
	Represented by attorney	
Biological	*Pain and disability*	Extreme pain
		Dysfunctional pain cognitions
		Pain sensitivity
		Pain invariance
		Diffuse pain
		Pain >2 years
		Unexplained disability
	Exam	Degree to which patient does not meet medical criteria for procedure
		No medical necessity of procedure to preserve life or function
		Destructive/high risk elective medical procedure
		Procedure specific risks: smoking, diet, attitude toward implant, etc.
	History	Similar procedure failed previously
		No response to any treatment
		History of no adherence to conservative care
		No objective medical findings
	Science	Insufficient evidence that the proposed medical treatment would be effective

Adapted from Bruns and Disorbio (2009). Used with permission

The convergent model was then applied to multiple patient groups, which were back surgery patients, upper extremity surgery patients, patients with head injuries, patients with acute injuries in physical therapy, patients in multidisciplinary treatment, and patients with chronic pain. Across these multiple groups, elevated levels of the exclusionary and cautionary risk factors were found to be consistently associated with subjective dissatisfaction with care and with an objective outcome measure: unemployment (Bruns & Disorbio, 2009).

Although it was initially defined primarily by the chronic back pain literature, supportive results from the other groups in this study suggest that this method may have broad applicability. This assumption has some intuitive appeal: Regardless of a patient's medical condition, if the patient is reporting the presence of exclusionary risk factors (e.g., active suicidality, chronic intoxication, psychosis, or violent tendencies), it seems reasonable to assume that such traits could potentially compromise a patient's ability to adhere to a broad range of medical treatments. Similarly, if the patient reports the presence of cautionary risk factors, such as depression or job dissatisfaction, it seems reasonable to assume that this could potentially impact the patient's ability to return to work. Overall, this approach demonstrates how the careful application of psychometric methods can begin to contribute to the scientific assessment of psychosocial variables that contribute to disability (Bruns & Disorbio, 2009).

6.5.5 When to Administer Psychological Tests

Like a medical test, psychological tests should not be used indiscriminately, but should rather be used as indicated by specific clinical findings. Typical reasons that individuals are referred for psychological testing are:

- Suspected current psychological disorder.
- Known history of psychological disorder.
- Physical symptom complaints continue in the absence of supportive medical findings.
- Extreme or impossible symptomatology is reported.
- Lack of motivation in treatment is observed or suspected.
- Low treatment adherence or motivation.
- Medically unexplained levels of disability.
- Psychosocial issues appear to be impeding progress in treatment.
- Assessing primary, secondary, or tertiary gain issues.
- Psychosocial concerns or conflicts at home, work, or in the medical setting.

6.5.6 Test Selection

When psychological tests are used, the clinician (usually a psychologist) is responsible for the selection and use of appropriate test instruments that adequately and objectively assess the desired clinical concerns. As readers may not be familiar with commonly used psychometric tests, an appendix of commonly used tests is attached (Appendix 1). The goal of this appendix is to provide information that will promote the understanding of the psychometric assessment process. The tests listed here consist of psychometric tests commonly used to assess a variety of concerns that occur with disability, and which are also used to assess patients prior to certain medical procedures. A caveat that should be noted here is that while disability is widely regarded as being a biopsychosocial phenomenon, the interrelationships among biological, psychological, and social variables are complex, and high quality research demonstrating the relationship between selection of appropriate psychological tests must be left to the examiner.

Standardized psychological tests are developed and normed for specific clinical populations and concerns, and the instruments listed in Appendix 1 are grouped with similar tests for comparison, and basic information about each test is provided. With regard to test selection, no single psychological test adequately measures all psychological or cognitive domains of functioning. Consequently, some have recommended the use of a minimum of two standardized tests to measure the targeted clinical concerns (American College of Occupational and Environmental Medicine, 2008b). If two psychometric measures developed in different ways produce the same findings, this provides a higher degree of confidence in the results. However, multiple psychological tests should not be given without consideration of the referral questions to be answered or psychological concerns that need to be ruled in or ruled out.

Lastly, in the evaluation of disability, distinguishing an enduring trait from a temporary state is an important determination, as it cannot be assumed that the findings of an evaluation held true in the past or will continue to hold true in the future. Instead, the meaning of the test scores must be interpreted in the light of the referral questions, patient history, other test findings, the interview, and behavioral observations.

6.6 Testing the Biopsychosocial Model

The vortex paradigm would predict that biopsychosocial factors are strong contributors to medical disability. This hypothesis was tested by one large study, which predicted that the use of the biopsychosocial model could control medical expenditures while reducing disability. This study examined a system that employed the biopsychosocial model to treat pain-related disability. Data was collected prospectively from 1992 to 2007 in 45 US states for regulatory purposes. These data summarized the medical treatment and disability costs of 520,314 injured workers in Colorado (whose treatment was regulated by a biopsychosocial law) and an estimated 28.6 million injured workers nationally. As no other state was regulated by a biopsychosocial law, the Colorado workers' compensation system constituted a legislative natural experiment, where a treatment group was created by legally enforceable medical treatment guidelines. These guidelines mandated that all patients suffering from chronic pain should undergo both a comprehensive psychological evaluation and interdisciplinary treatment.

When the system of biopsychosocial laws in Colorado was created, initial concern was that by adding psychological services, the medical costs would be increased. Additionally, it was feared that psychological treatments may "coddle" chronic pain patients, increasing their disability. The data suggest that the reverse happened. The results of this study were that in the 15 years following the implementation of the reform, the inflation of medical costs in Colorado workers' compensation was only one third that of the national average, while the rate of inflation of indemnity/disability costs were only one fourth of the national average. This saved Colorado an estimated $859 million on patients injured in 2007 alone (Bruns, Mueller, & Warren, 2012). These savings were believed to occur for two reasons.

First of all, the effect of patient selection using psychological principles for surgeries may have worked to reduce the prevalence of ineffective surgery. Secondly, it may have served to increase the frequency of psychological treatments, which data shows are effective treatments for pain. In fact, when the MDA Guidelines reviewed 364 treatments for chronic pain, using the same empirical methodology, only 2 medical treatments were supported by more evidence than cognitive behavioral therapy. In contrast to the medical treatments though, cognitive behavioral therapy has no risk of mortality, no side effects, and involves little burden to the patient. With regard to relative cost, it was estimated that for patients suffering from low back pain, behavioral therapies may be as effective as surgical intervention, but surgery cost 168 times more than the behavioral treatment (Bruns et al., 2012).

6.7 Conclusions

Disability is a complex biopsychosocial phenomenon, which is determined by objective medical tests, by patient behavior, and by subjective psychological variables, such as pain, MDD, and cognition. Of these, patient behavior and self-reports are strongly influenced by psychosocial variables. Consequently, when evaluating patients for disability, psychosocial aspects of the condition must be assessed. The assessment of these psychosocial aspects relies, to a considerable degree, on the self-reports of the patient and the patient's willingness to perform on testing. Consequently, it is important to establish the veracity of the patient's subjective reports and the motivation to perform, especially when there are incentives for a patient to appear disabled. To this end, the inclusion of validity measures should be an integral part of the disability evaluation.

In the clinical setting, it has been said, "To have great pain is to have certainty. To hear that another has pain is to have doubt" (p. 7) (Scarry, 1985). This creates a dilemma for the disability evaluator, who is left with the responsibility of listening to a patient's reports and discerning the extent to which a disabling condition is present. To address this, perhaps the best advice is to follow the Russian maxim cited by President Reagan to General Secretary Gorbachev at the end of the Cold War: "Dovorey no provorey; Trust, but verify" (Reagan, 2009).

When properly performed, psychological testing can play a critical role in biopsychosocial assessment, by screening for psychiatric diagnoses and identifying psychosocial contributions to disability. This increases the chances of developing an effective multidisciplinary plan for addressing the totality of the patient's concerns, removing roadblocks to recovery, and decreasing disability. In this way, psychological testing can make a significant contribution to the assessment and treatment of patients with disabling conditions.

Appendix: Psychometric Assessment Tools

The tests listed below are for informational purposes only, and this is not an exhaustive list. The final decision about which tests to use must be left to the evaluator. Within each section, tests are listed in alphabetical order.

Assessment task	Test	Notes[a]	Description
Brief assessments of emotion	*These tests are useful when the assessment of a patient's emotional status is desired*		
	BDI II	S J B G	*Beck Depression Inventory II*: Well-researched measure of depression, widely used clinically and in research. A brief measure that assesses a broad range of cognitive, affective, and physical depressive symptoms. 21 items, 1 scale, no validity measures. 5 min, hand scoring, computerized scoring and report
	BSI 18	S J B G N	*Brief Symptom Inventory 18*: Brief measure of depression, anxiety, and somatization. Community and cancer patient norms. 18 items, 3 scales, no validity measures, computerized scoring and report, and hand scoring. 2–3 min
	CES-D	J G	*Center for Epidemiological Studies Depression Scale*: Brief measure of depression that has been widely used in research. Assesses depression without reliance on physical symptoms, reducing the risk of false positive findings. No norms. 20 items, 1 scale, no validity measures, 3 min, hand scoring
	HDI	J G	*Hamilton Depression Inventory*: Brief measure of depression, widely used in research. Assesses a broad range of cognitive, affective, and physical depressive symptoms. Uses community norms. 23 items, 1 scale, fifth grade reading level, no validity measures, 5 min. A variation of this is the *Hamilton Rating Scale*, which is a 17 or 21 item measure filled out by the professional
	STAI	S J B G N	*State-Trait Anxiety Inventory*: Well-researched measure of both anxious states and anxious tendencies. A brief measure that assesses a broad range of cognitive, affective, and physical anxiety symptoms. Community norms. 40 items, 2 scales, no validity measures, 8–10 min

Assessment task	Test	Notes[a]	Description
	Zung	J G	*Zung Depression Scale*: Brief measure of depression that has been widely used in research. A brief measure that assesses a broad range of cognitive, affective, and physical depressive symptoms. Uses cutoff scores, not norms. 20 items, 1 scale, no validity measures, 5 min, hand scoring
Brief assessment of pain and functioning	*These tests are useful when the assessment of a patient's ability to function is desired*		
	BPI-SF	S J G	*Brief Pain Inventory Short Form*: Assesses pain, pain variation, and pain distribution through drawing. Also assesses degree to which pain interferes with functioning. Used in pain research, no norms. 20 items, multiple measures, no validity measures, 4–6 min
	Oswestry	J G	*Oswestry Low Back Pain Disability Questionnaire*: Commonly used measure of functioning in research studies is known to be sensitive to assess change. Original version has been shown to be an effective research outcome measure, multiple modified versions, and no norms. 20 Items, 1 scale, no validity measures, 4–5 min
	PROMIS *PDQ*	S J N J G	*Patient-Reported Outcomes Measurement Information System*: A set of measures developed by US Department of Health and Human Services that assesses physical, mental, and social health in adults and children across all conditions *Pain Disability Questionnaire*: Brief tool that appears to be a sensitive measure of disability associated with pain. 15 items, 1 scale, no norms, no validity measures, 3–4 min
	Roland and Morris	J G	*Roland and Morris Disability Questionnaire*: Commonly used measure of functioning in research studies is known to be able to assess change in functioning. Original version is a frequently used research outcome measure.
			24 items, 1 scale, no norms, no validity measures, 4–5 min
			Translated into Arabic, Chinese, Croatian, Czech, Danish, Dutch, English, Flemish, French, German, Greek, Hindi, Hungarian, Iranian, Italian, Japanese, Kannada, Korean, Marathi, Norwegian, Polish, Portuguese, Romanian, Russian, Spanish, Swedish, Tamil, Telugu, Thai, Tunisian, Turkish, and Urdu, *3–4 min*

Assessment task	Test	Notes[a]	Description
	SF 36-V2	S J G N	*Short Form 36 Questionnaire Version 2*: Overall assessments of physical and mental health. Function scale is the strongest and it assesses subjective reports of impairment. Has scoring software. Original SF 36 is less well standardized. SF 36-V2 has an improved administration format, norms, and standardized scores. 36 items, 8 scales, no validity measures, 6–8 min
			Translated into English, Spanish, German, French, Chinese, Japanese, and for persons from the following countries: Armenia, Bangladesh, Brazil, Bulgaria, Cambodia, Croatia, Czech Republic, Finland, Greece, Hungary, Iceland, Israel, Korea, Latvia, Lithuania, Poland, Portugal, Romania, Russia, Singapore, Slovak Republic, Tanzania, Turkey, Wales (UK), and Vietnam
	MPQ-SF	J B G	*McGill Pain Questionnaire Short Form*: Assesses sensory, affective, and evaluative dimensions through the use of verbal descriptors of pain experience as opposed to pure pain intensity, no norms. 15 items, 2 scales, no norms, no validity measures, 3–5 min
			Translated into Amharic (Ethiopian), Arabic, Chinese, Czech, Danish, Dutch, English, Finnish, Flemish, French, German, Greek, Hungarian, Italian, Japanese, Norwegian, Polish, Portuguese, Slovak, Spanish, and Swedish
	NRS	J G	*Pain Numerical Rating Scale*: Ubiquitous pain rating scale is recommended by JCAHO. Extremely easy to use, usually administered verbally. Unstandardized test, with unknown number of variations. No agreement on scaling (e.g., 0–10 vs. 1–100), location (e.g., rating whole body vs. one body part) or time (e.g., right now vs. typical). No norms. *<1 min*
	VAS	J G	*Pain Visual Analog Scale*: Sensitive measure of pain used extensively in research. Unstandardized test, with unknown number of variations. No agreement on graphic format of test (e.g., length of line; does the line have numbers on it), location (e.g., rating whole body vs. one body part) or time (e.g., right now vs. typical). No norms. *<1 min*
Intermediate length assessments of pain and disability	*Intermediate length assessments of pain and disability*		

Assessment task	Test	Notes[a]	Description
	BBHI 2	S J B G N	*Brief Battery for Health Improvement 2*: Assesses depression, anxiety, somatization, pain, and function. Also has validity measures for minimizing, exaggerating, and random responding. Pain measures include pain intensity, distribution, and tolerability. Normed on both community sample and a rehabilitation sample. Computer scored. Has Spanish version. 63 items, 6 scales, 15 critical items, 1 validity measure, fifth grade reading level, *8–10 min*
	BPI	S J G	*Brief Pain Inventory-Long Form*: Assesses pain, pain variation, and pain distribution through drawing. Also assesses degree to which pain interferes with functioning. Includes demographic and medication short answer questions. *15–25 min*
	BSI	S J B G N	*Brief Symptom Inventory*: Brief assessment of a broad range of psychopathology, including somatization, depression, anxiety, hostility obsessive-compulsiveness, paranoid ideation, and psychoticism. 53 items, 12 scales, no validity measures, computerized scoring and report, 7–8 min
	P3	S J B G N	*Pain Patient Profile*: Measure of depression, anxiety, and somatization with chronic pain patient and community norm groups. Validity measure checks for random or bizarre responding. Has Spanish version. 44 items, 3 scales, 1 validity measure, computerized scoring and report, 12–15 min
Comprehensive assessment of psychopathology	*These tests are useful for the comprehensive assessment of psychopathology and were designed primarily for psychiatric patients*		
	MCMI IV	S J B G N	*Millon Clinical Multiaxial Inventory-IV*: Scales keyed to the *DSM-5*. Also has scales for *DSM-5* diagnoses of affective and psychotic disorders and for each form of personality disorder. Base rate scoring attempts to adjust test findings to approximate the actual base rates of psychological disorders in the psychiatric population. Has Spanish version. 175 items, 25 scales, 3 validity measures, critical items, computerized scoring and report, eighth grade reading level, 25–30 min
	MMPI-2	S J B G N	*Minnesota Multiphasic Personality Inventory-2*: Most researched psychological test, with well-established strengths and weaknesses. Over 100 scales and indices to assess a wide range of psychological conditions. Extensive validity assessment is valuable to assess conscious or unconscious exaggeration of reports. Has Spanish version. 567 items, 100+ scales and indices, critical items, computerized scoring and report, hand scoring, sixth grade reading level, 70–90 min

Assessment task	Test	Notes[a]	Description
	MMPI-2-RF	S J B G N	*Minnesota Multiphasic Personality Inventory 2 – Revised Form*: New version of MMPI-2 that has undergone radical revision to correct perceived MMPI-2 deficiencies. Extensive validity assessment is valuable to assess conscious or unconscious exaggeration of reports. May be stronger at psychiatric assessment, but some studies found it to be less capable when assessing somatoform disorders. (Butcher, Hamilton, Rouse, & Cumella, 2006; Thomas & Youngjohn, 2009) 338 items, 50 scales including 8 validity scales, critical items, fifth grade reading level 45–50 min
	PAI	S J B G N	*Personality Assessment Inventory*: A comprehensive personality test that is significantly shorter than the MMPI-2. Assesses a broad cross-section of affective, characterological, and psychotic conditions. Multiple validity measures. 340 items, 22 scales, including 4 validity scales, critical items, fourth grade reading level, 50–60 min
Comprehensive assessment of medical patients	*These are psychological tests designed specifically for the comprehensive assessment of medical patients*		
	BHI 2 and BHI 2 MIR	S J B G N	*Battery for Health Improvement 2*: Assesses broad range of psychological symptoms, characterological risks, social conflicts, coping, and physical symptoms, such as pain and disability complaints. Pain measures include pain intensity, pain distribution, pain intolerance, and dysfunctional pain cognitions. Normed on both community sample and a rehabilitation sample, plus has eight other reference groups, including chronic pain, head injury, and fake bad. Has three validity measures for minimizing, exaggerating and random responding. Has Spanish version. 217 items, 18 scales, including 3 validity measures, 40 subscales, 25 critical items, computerized scoring and report. Sixth grade reading level, 30–35 min *Battery for Health Improvement 2 Medical Intervention Risk report*: A separate test based on the BHI 2 items which assesses risk for poor response to surgery, rehabilitation, opioid and other habit forming medications, physical therapy, and other treatments. Has one validity measure for over or under reporting. Has Spanish version. 217 items, 7 scales, computerized scoring and report. Sixth grade reading level, 30–35 min

Assessment task	Test	Notes[a]	Description
	MBMD	S J B G N	*Millon Behavioral Medicine Diagnostic*: Assesses broad range of psychiatric and problematic behavioral comorbidities that may affect health management and compliance. Offers analysis of health habits, psychiatric indicators, coping styles, and stress moderators. Three validity scales were developed to detect exaggerating or minimizing of symptoms. Two patient norm groups, bariatric and chronic illness (heart disease, diabetes, HIV, neurological, and others). Has Spanish version. 165 items, 38 scales, 3 validity measures, computerized scoring, sixth grade reading level, 20–30 min
Assessment of malingering	*These tests are used solely to detect malingering*		
	CARB	S J B G N	*Computerized Assessment of Response Bias*: Used to assess whether an individual is falsifying symptoms of memory impairment. No norms
	Hare	S J B G N	*Hare Psychopathy Checklist – Revised*: The assessment can be used to help assess the degree to which an individual exhibits severe antisocial traits, in the form of a prototypical violent psychopath. May be useful if assessing patients who are making threats
	SIMS	S J B G N	*Structured Inventory of Malingered Symptomatology*: Used for both malingered psychopathology and neuropsychological symptoms
	TOMM	S J B G N	*Test of Memory Malingering*: Used to assess whether an individual is falsifying symptoms of memory impairment. No norms
	VIP	S J B G N	*Validity Indicator Profile*: Employs independent verbal and nonverbal subtests to assess the validity of the patient's reports. Computer scored. No norms
	WMT	S J B G N	*Word Memory Test*: Used to assess whether an individual is falsifying symptoms of verbal memory impairment. No norms
Assessment of cognitive ability	*These tests are measures of intelligence, memory, and cognitive processing ability*		
	GAMA	S J B G N	*Global Assessment of Mental Ability*: Culture-free measure of general intellectual ability. Based on the scores on four subtest scales: matching, analogies, sequences, and construction. Community norms. *25 min timed test*
	RBANS	S J B G N	*Repeatable Battery for the Assessment of Neuropsychological Status*: Measures neuropsychological status and cognitive decline in individuals who have experienced stroke, head injury, dementia, or neurological injury or disease. Community norms. *Less than 30 min*
	WASI	S J B G N	*Wechsler Abbreviated Scale of Intelligence*: An abbreviated measurement of adult intelligence in short and very short forms. *15 min for 2 subtests IQ. 30 min for 4 subtest IQ*

Assessment task	Test	Notes[a]	Description
	WAIS-IV	S J B G N	*Wechsler Adult Intelligence Scale-IV*: Common measure of adult intelligence assesses cognitive strengths and weaknesses. WAIS-IV and WMS-IV are the only conormed ability-memory instruments. *60–90 min*
	WMS-IV	S J B G N	*Wechsler Memory Scale-IV*: Measures visual and auditory memory, immediate versus delayed memory, and free recall versus cued recall as well as recognition. Normed on older adolescents and adults. *30–35 min*
	WRAT-4	S J B G N	*Wide Range Achievement Test-4*: Achievement test assesses basic academic skills of reading, spelling, and math, with norms to age 94. The test has been validated against multiple other cognitive psychological tests. *35–45 min*

[a]Notes: *S* standardized test materials, *N* norms, *J* peer-reviewed journal publications, *B* reviewed by Buros Institute, *G* noted in treatment guidelines

Colorado division of workers' compensation guideline – Approved measures for assessing functional changes improvement in treatment		
Name of test/site link body part description	Body part	Description
Neck Disability Index http://www.maic.qld.gov.au/forms-publications-stats/pdfs/NDI.pdf	Cervical spine	Ten questions addressing pain, personal care, headaches, and functional deficits
Simple Shoulder Test http://www.orthop.washington.edu/?q=patient-care/articles/shoulder/simple-shoulder-test.html	Shoulder	Shoulder function only
Quick DASH (Disabilities of the Arm, Shoulder, and Hand) http://dash.iwh.on.ca/quickdash	Upper extremity	Shoulder, elbow, and hand assessment
PREE – Patient-Rated Elbow Evaluation http://srs-mcmaster.ca/wp-content/uploads/2015/05/English-PREE.pdf	Elbow	Elbow joint specific
Hand/Wrist Symptom Severity Scale http://hqlo.biomedcentral.com/articles/10.1186/1477-7525-4-87	Hand/wrist	Hand and wrist specific
Oswestry Low Back Pain Disability Questionnaire http://www.rehab.msu.edu/_files/_docs/Oswestry_Low_Back_Disability.pdf	Lumbar spine	Functional questions with sleeping, lifting, walking, sitting, and standing
Quebec Back Pain Disability Scale https://www.tac.vic.gov.au/files-to-move/media/upload/quebec_scale.pdf	Spine	Functional and emotional questions
Dallas Pain Questionnaire http://www.rehabilities.com/index_htm_files/dallas.pdf	Spine	Chronic pain

Colorado division of workers' compensation guideline – Approved measures for assessing functional changes improvement in treatment		
Name of test/site link body part description	Body part	Description
Oxford Hip, Knee, Elbow, Shoulder, and Shoulder Instability Score www.orthopaedicscore.com	Hip, knee, shoulder, and elbow	Functional ADLs
LEFS (Lower Extremity Functional Scale) http://www.emoryhealthcare.org/physical-therapy/pdf/hip-lefs.pdf	Lower extremity	Disorders of one or both lower extremities, standing, walking, running (higher functioning)
Lower Limb Questionnaire http://www.aaos.org/research/outcomes/Lower_Limb.pdf	Lower extremity	Brief seven questions with ability to ambulate addressed (lower functioning)
Foot and Ankle Outcomes Questionnaire http://www.aaos.org/research/outcomes/Foot_Ankle.pdf	Foot and ankle	Lower extremity functional ADLs
SF-36 and SF-12 http://www.rand.org/health/surveys_tools/mos/mos_core_12item.html	Physical health	Assesses ADLs
FOTO – Focus on Therapeutic Outcomes, Inc. www.fotoinc.com	Various body parts	Functional ADLs specific to body part
BBHI 2 (Brief Battery for Health Improvement – 2nd Edition) www.pearsonclinical.com	Behavioral health	Measures pain, functioning, somatization, depression, anxiety; brief measure of risk factors for delayed recovery; two validity measures for exaggerating, minimizing, and random responding
DRAM (Distress and Risk Assessment Method) https://www.worksafe.qld.gov.au/__data/assets/pdf_file/0005/76883/distress-and-risk-assessment-method- dram1.pdf	Behavioral health	Measures depression and somatic symptoms of anxiety, risk factors commonly associated with chronic pain
CES-D (Center for Epidemiological Studies Depression Scale) http://cesd-r.com/	Behavioral health	Measures depression, 20 items
BDI II (Beck Depression Inventory – 2nd edition) www.psychcorp.com	Behavioral health	Measures depression, 21 items
PRIME-MD (Primary Care Evaluation for Mental Disorders) http://www.psy-world.com/prime-md_print1.htm	Behavioral health	Two components: paper and pencil screen for patient and follow-up interview by physician. Assesses mood, anxiety, somatoform tendencies, alcohol, and eating disorders

Colorado division of workers' compensation guideline – Approved measures for assessing functional changes improvement in treatment		
Name of test/site link body part description	Body part	Description
Zung Depression Inventory www.glaxowellcome.com	Behavioral health	Measures depression, brief measure
PHQ (Patient Health Questionnaire) and PHQ-9 www.phqscreeners.com	Behavioral health	Self-administered version of the PRIME-MD. Assesses mood, anxiety, somatoform tendencies, alcohol, and eating disorders

References

American College of Occupational and Environmental Medicine. (2008a). *Occupational medicine practice guidelines* (2nd Revised ed.). Beverly Farms, MA: OEM Press.

American College of Occupational and Environmental Medicine. (2008b). Chronic pain treatment guidelines. In K. Hegmann (Ed.), *Occupational medicine practice guidelines* (2nd ed.). Beverly Farms, MA: OEM Press.

American Educational Research Association, American Psychological Association, National Council on Measurement in Education, Joint Committee on Standards for Educational and Psychological Testing (U.S.). (1999). *Standards for educational and psychological testing*. Washington, DC: American Educational Research Association.

American Psychiatric Association. (2013). *Diagnostic and statistical manual of mental disorders : DSM-5* (5th ed.). Washington, DC: American Psychiatric Association.

American Psychiatric Association. Task Force on DSM-IV. (2000). *Diagnostic and statistical manual of mental disorders : DSM-IV-TR* (4th ed.). Washington, DC: American Psychiatric Association.

Arbisi, P. A., & Butcher, J. N. (2004). Psychometric perspectives on detection of malingering of pain: Use of the Minnesota Multiphasic Personality Inventory-2. *The Clinical Journal of Pain, 20*(6), 383–391.

Aronoff, G. M., & Livengood, J. M. (2003). Pain: Psychiatric aspects of impairment and disability. *Current Pain and Headache Reports, 7*(2), 105–115.

Aronoff, G. M., Mandel, S., Genovese, E., et al. (2007). Evaluating malingering in contested injury or illness. *Pain Practice, 7*(2), 178–204.

Artiola i Fortuny, L., & Mullaney, H. A. (1997). Neuropsychology with Spanish speakers: Language use and proficiency issues for test development. *Journal of Clinical and Experimental Neuropsychology, 19*(4), 615–622.

Barsky, A. J., & Borus, J. F. (1995). Somatization and medicalization in the era of managed care. *The Journal of the American Medical Association, 274*(24), 1931–1934.

Ben-Porath, Y. S., & Tellegen, A. (2008). *MMPI-2-RF™ manual*. Minneapolis, MN: University of Minnesota.

Bernard Jr., T. N. (1993). Repeat lumbar spine surgery. Factors influencing outcome. *Spine, 18*(15), 2196–2200.

Bianchini, K. J., Curtis, K. L., & Greve, K. W. (2006). Compensation and malingering in traumatic brain injury: A dose-response relationship? *The Clinical Neuropsychologist, 20*(4), 831–847.

Binder, L. M., & Rohling, M. L. (1996). Money matters: A meta-analytic review of the effects of financial incentives on recovery after closed-head injury. *The American Journal of Psychiatry, 153*(1), 7–10.

Block, A. R., Gatchel, R. J., Deardorff, W. W., & Guyer, R. D. (2003). *The psychology of spine surgery*. Washington, DC: American Psychological Association.

Block, A. R., Ohnmeiss, D. D., Guyer, R. D., Rashbaum, R. F., & Hochschuler, S. H. (2001). The use of presurgical psychological screening to predict the outcome of spine surgery. *The Spine Journal, 1*(4), 274–282.

Boersma, K., & Linton, S. J. (2005). Screening to identify patients at risk: Profiles of psychological risk factors for early intervention. *The Clinical Journal of Pain, 21*(1), 38–43. Discussion 69–72.

Bornstein, B. H., Whisenhunt, B. L., Nemeth, R. J., & Dunaway, D. L. (2002). Pretrial publicity and civil cases: A two-way street? *Law and Human Behavior, 26*(1), 3–17.

Bruns, D., & Disorbio, J. M. (1996). *Battery for Health Improvement Manual*. Minneapolis, MN: Pearson.

Bruns, D., & Disorbio, J. M. (2003). *Battery for health improvement 2 manual*. Minneapolis, MN: Pearson.

Bruns, D., & Disorbio, J. M. (2005). Chronic pain and biopsychosocial disorders: The BHI 2 approach to classification and assessment. *Practical Pain Management, 5*(7), 52–61.

Bruns, D., & Disorbio, J. M. (2009). Assessment of biopsychosocial risk factors for medical treatment: A collaborative approach. *Journal of Clinical Psychology in Medical Settings, 16*(2), 127–147.

Bruns, D., & Disorbio, J. M. (2014). The psychological evaluation of patients with chronic pain: A review of BHI 2 clinical and forensic interpretive considerations. *Psychological Injury and Law, 7*(4), 335–361. https://doi.org/10.1007/s12207-014-9206-y

Bruns, D., & Disorbio, J. M. (2015). The psychological assessment of patients with chronic pain. In T. R. Deer, M. S. Leong, & A. L. Ray (Eds.), *Treatment of chronic pain by integrative approaches: The American Academy of Pain Medicine textbook on patient management* (pp. xix, 325 pages). New York/Heidelberg/Dordrecht/London: Springer.

Bruns, D., Mueller, K., & Warren, P. A. (2012). Biopsychosocial law, health care reform, and the control of medical inflation in Colorado. *Rehabilitation Psychology, 57*(2), 81–97. https://doi.org/10.1037/a0028623

Burchiel, K. J., Anderson, V. C., Brown, F. D., et al. (1996). Prospective, multicenter study of spinal cord stimulation for relief of chronic back and extremity pain. *Spine, 21*(23), 2786–2794.

Burton, A. K., Tillotson, K. M., Main, C. J., & Hollis, S. (1995). Psychosocial predictors of outcome in acute and subchronic low back trouble. *Spine (Phila Pa 1976), 20*(6), 722–728.

Butcher, J. N., Arbisi, P. A., Atlis, M. M., & McNulty, J. L. (2003). The construct validity of the Lees-Haley Fake Bad Scale. Does this scale measure somatic malingering and feigned emotional distress? *Archives of Clinical Neuropsychology, 18*(5), 473–485.

Butcher, J. N., Hamilton, C. K., Rouse, S. V., & Cumella, E. J. (2006). The deconstruction of the Hy Scale of MMPI-2: Failure of RC3 in measuring somatic symptom expression. *Journal of Personality Assessment, 87*(2), 186–192.

Butler, R. J., & Johnson, W. G. (2008). Satisfaction with low back pain care. *The Spine Journal, 8*(3), 510–521.

Butler, R. J., Johnson, W. G., & Gray, B. P. (2007). Timing makes a difference: Early nurse case management intervention and low back pain. *Professional Case Management, 12*(6), 316–327. Quiz 328–319.

California Division of Workers' Compensation. (2009). *Chronic pain medical treatment guidelines*. From http://www.dir.ca.gov/dwc/DWCPropRegs/MTUS_Regulations/MTUS_ChronicPainMedicalTreatmentGuidelines.pdf http://www.dir.ca.gov/dwc/DWCPropRegs/MTUS_Regulations/MTUS_ChronicPainMedicalTreatmentGuidelines.pdf. Accessed 20 July 2009.

Campbell, L. C., Clauw, D. J., & Keefe, F. J. (2003). Persistent pain and depression: A biopsychosocial perspective. *Biological Psychiatry, 54*(3), 399–409.

Carragee, E. J., Alamin, T. F., Miller, J. L., & Carragee, J. M. (2005). Discographic, MRI and psychosocial determinants of low back pain disability and remission: A prospective study in subjects with benign persistent back pain. *The Spine Journal, 5*(1), 24–35.

Carragee, E. J., Barcohana, B., Alamin, T., & van den Haak, E. (2004). Prospective controlled study of the development of lower back pain in previously asymptomatic subjects undergoing experimental discography. *Spine, 29*(10), 1112–1117.

Chiu, T. T., Lam, T. H., & Hedley, A. J. (2005). Correlation among physical impairments, pain, disability, and patient satisfaction in patients with chronic neck pain. *Archives of Physical Medicine and Rehabilitation, 86*(3), 534–540.

Chou, R., Baisden, J., Carragee, E. J., Resnick, D. K., Shaffer, W. O., & Loeser, J. D. (2009). Surgery for low back pain: A review of the evidence for an American pain society clinical practice guideline. *Spine (Phila Pa 1976), 34*(10), 1094–1109.

Colorado Division of Workers' Compensation. Chronic Pain Task Force. (2017). Rule 17, Exhibit 9: Chronic pain disorder medical treatment guidelines: Colorado Department of Labor and Employment: Division of Worker Compensation.

Congressional Budget Office. (2012). *Policy options for the Social Security Disability Insurance program*. Retrieved from http://www.cbo.gov/sites/default/files/cbofiles/attachments/43421-DisabilityInsurance_screen.pdf

DeBerard, M. S., Masters, K. S., Colledge, A. L., & Holmes, E. B. (2003). Presurgical biopsychosocial variables predict medical and compensation costs of lumbar fusion in Utah workers' compensation patients. *The Spine Journal, 3*(6), 420–429.

den Boer, J. J., Oostendorp, R. A., Beems, T., Munneke, M., & Evers, A. W. (2006). Continued disability and pain after lumbar disc surgery: The role of cognitive-behavioral factors. *Pain, 123*(1–2), 45–52.

den Boer, J. J., Oostendorp, R. A., Beems, T., Munneke, M., Oerlemans, M., & Evers, A. W. (2006). A systematic review of bio-psychosocial risk factors for an unfavourable outcome after lumbar disc surgery. *European Spine Journal, 15*(5), 527–536.

Deyo, R. A., Mirza, S. K., Heagerty, P. J., Turner, J. A., & Martin, B. I. (2005). A prospective cohort study of surgical treatment for back pain with degenerated discs; study protocol. *BMC Musculoskeletal Disorders, 6*(1), 24.

Disorbio, J. M., & Bruns, D. (2002). *Brief battery for health improvement 2 manual*. Minneapolis, MN: Pearson.

Disorbio, J. M., Bruns, D., & Barolat, G. (2006). Assessment and treatment of chronic pain: A physician's guide to a biopsychosocial approach. *Practical Pain Management, 6*(2), 11–27.

Dworkin, R. H., Turk, D. C., Farrar, J. T., Haythornthwaite, J. A., Jensen, M. P., Katz, N. P., et al. (2005). Core outcome measures for chronic pain clinical trials: IMMPACT recommendations. *Pain, 113*(1–2), 9–19.

Epker, J., & Block, A. R. (2001). Presurgical psychological screening in back pain patients: A review. *The Clinical Journal of Pain, 17*(3), 200–205.

Fairbank, J. C., & Pynsent, P. B. (2000). The oswestry disability index. *Spine, 25*(22), 2940–2952. Discussion 2952.

Fejer, R., & Hartvigsen, J. (2008). Neck pain and disability due to neck pain: What is the relation? *European Spine Journal, 17*(1), 80–88.

Fishbain, D. A., Cutler, R., Rosomoff, H. L., & Rosomoff, R. S. (1997). Chronic pain-associated depression: Antecedent or consequence of chronic pain? A review. *The Clinical Journal of Pain, 13*(2), 116–137.

Fishbain, D. A., Cutler, R., Rosomoff, H. L., & Rosomoff, R. S. (1999). Chronic pain disability exaggeration/malingering and submaximal effort research. *The Clinical Journal of Pain, 15*(4), 244–274.

Ford, C. V. (1986). The somatizing disorders. *Psychosomatics, 27*(5), 327–331. 335–327.

Frederick, R. I., & Bowden, S. C. (2009). Evaluating constructs represented by symptom validity tests in forensic neuropsychological assessment of traumatic brain injury. *The Journal of Head Trauma Rehabilitation, 24*(2), 105–122.

Frederick, R. I., & Crosby, R. D. (2000). Development and validation of the validity indicator profile. *Law and Human Behavior, 24*(1), 59–82.

Frederick, R. I., Crosby, R. D., & Wynkoop, T. F. (2000). Performance curve classification of invalid responding on the validity indicator profile. *Archives of Clinical Neuropsychology, 15*(4), 281–300.

Frymoyer, J. W., & Cats-Baril, W. L. (1991). An overview of the incidences and costs of low back pain. *The Orthopedic Clinics of North America, 22*(2), 263–271.

Furr, R. M., & Bacharach, V. R. (2008). *Psychometrics: An introduction*. Los Angeles: Sage Publications.

Gallagher, R. M. (2004). Biopsychosocial pain medicine and mind-brain-body science. *Physical Medicine and Rehabilitation Clinics of North America, 15*(4), 855–882. vii.

Gatchel, R. J. (2001). A biopsychosocial overview of pretreatment screening of patients with pain. *The Clinical Journal of Pain, 17*(3), 192–199.

Gatchel, R. J. (2004). Comorbidity of chronic pain and mental health disorders: The biopsychosocial perspective. *The American Psychologist, 59*(8), 795–805.

Gatchel, R. J., & Mayer, T. G. (2008). Psychological evaluation of the spine patient. *The Journal of the American Academy of Orthopaedic Surgeons, 16*(2), 107–112.

Gatchel, R. J., Mayer, T. G., & Eddington, A. (2006). MMPI disability profile: The least known, most useful screen for psychopathology in chronic occupational spinal disorders. *Spine, 31*(25), 2973–2978.

Gatchel, R. J., Polatin, P. B., & Mayer, T. G. (1995). The dominant role of psychosocial risk factors in the development of chronic low back pain disability. *Spine, 20*(24), 2702–2709.

Gervais, R. O., Rohling, M. L., Green, P., & Ford, W. (2004). A comparison of WMT, CARB, and TOMM failure rates in non-head injury disability claimants. *Archives of Clinical Neuropsychology, 19*(4), 475–487.

Giordano, N., & Lofland, K. (2005a). A literature review of psychological predictors of spinal cord stimulator outcomes. *The Journal of Pain, 6*(3 Supplement), S67.

Giordano, N., & Lofland, K. (2005b). A literature review of psychological predictors of spinal cord stimulator outcomes. *American Pain Society 24th Annual Scientific Meeting*, Boston.

Glassman, S. D., Minkow, R. E., Dimar, J. R., Puno, R. M., Raque, G. H., & Johnson, J. R. (1998). Effect of prior lumbar discectomy on outcome of lumbar fusion: A prospective analysis using the SF-36 measure. *Journal of Spinal Disorders, 11*(5), 383–388.

Grace, V. M. (2000). Pitfalls of the medical paradigm in chronic pelvic pain. *Baillière's Best Practice & Research. Clinical Obstetrics & Gynaecology, 14*(3), 525–539.

Greene Jackson, D., Hamilton, P., Hutchinson, S., & Huber, J. (2009). The effect of patients' race on provider treatment choices in coronary care: A literature review for model development. *Policy, Politics & Nursing Practice, 10*(1), 40–63.

Greenough, C. G., Taylor, L. J., & Fraser, R. D. (1994). Anterior lumbar fusion. A comparison of noncompensation patients with compensation patients. *Clinical Orthopaedics and Related Research, 300*, 30–37.

Greiffenstein, M. F., Baker, W. J., & Johnson-Greene, D. (2002). Actual versus self-reported scholastic achievement of litigating postconcussion and severe closed head injury claimants. *Psychological Assessment, 14*(2), 202–208.

Groth-Marnat, G., & Fletcher, A. (2000). Influence of neuroticism, catastrophizing, pain duration, and receipt of compensation on short-term response to nerve block treatment for chronic back pain. *Journal of Behavioral Medicine, 23*(4), 339–350.

Gureje, O. (2007). Psychiatric aspects of pain. *Current Opinion in Psychiatry, 20*(1), 42–46.

Gureje, O. (2008). Comorbidity of pain and anxiety disorders. *Current Psychiatry Reports, 10*(4), 318–322.

Hagg, O., Fritzell, P., Ekselius, L., & Nordwall, A. (2003). Predictors of outcome in fusion surgery for chronic low back pain. A report from the Swedish Lumbar Spine Study. *European Spine Journal, 12*(1), 22–33.

Hall, R. C. (2007). Detection of malingered PTSD: An overview of clinical, psychometric, and physiological assessment: Where do we stand? *Journal of Forensic Sciences, 52*(3), 717–725.

Heckler, D. R., Gatchel, R. J., Lou, L., Whitworth, T., Bernstein, D., & Stowell, A. W. (2007). Presurgical Behavioral Medicine Evaluation (PBME) for implantable devices for pain management: A 1-year prospective study. *Pain Practice, 7*(2), 110–122.

Hegmann, K. (2017). Chronic pain guidelines. *MDGuidelines®. Occupational medicine practice guidelines: Evaluation and Management of Common Health Problems and Functional Recovery in Workers*. 3rd. Retrieved from www.mdguidelines.com

Hyams, J. S. (2004). Irritable bowel syndrome, functional dyspepsia, and functional abdominal pain syndrome. *Adolescent Medicine Clinics, 15*(1), 1–15.
Iverson, G. L. (2007). Identifying exaggeration and malingering. *Pain Practice, 7*(2), 94–102.
Jensen, M. C., Brant-Zawadzki, M. N., Obuchowski, N., Modic, M. T., Malkasian, D., & Ross, J. S. (1994). Magnetic resonance imaging of the lumbar spine in people without back pain. *The New England Journal of Medicine, 331*(2), 69–73.
Jette, A. M., & Badley, E. (2000). Conceptual issues in the measurement of work disability. In N. Mathiowetz & G. S. Wunderlich (Eds.), *Survey measurement of work disability: Summary of a workshop* (pp. 4–27). Washington, DC: National Academy Press.
Kessler, R. C., Chiu, W. T., Demler, O., Merikangas, K. R., & Walters, E. E. (2005). Prevalence, severity, and comorbidity of 12-month DSM-IV disorders in the National comorbidity survey replication. *Archives of General Psychiatry, 62*(6), 617–627.
Klekamp, J., McCarty, E., & Spengler, D. M. (1998). Results of elective lumbar discectomy for patients involved in the workers' compensation system. *Journal of Spinal Disorders, 11*(4), 277–282.
Koch, H. (1986). The management of chronic pain in office-based ambulatory care: National ambulatory medical care survey. In NDPN (Ed.), *Advance data from vital and health statistics* (pp. 86–1250). Hyattsville, MD: National Center for Health Statistics.
Koho, P., Aho, S., Watson, P., & Hurri, H. (2001). Assessment of chronic pain behaviour: Reliability of the method and its relationship with perceived disability, physical impairment and function. *Journal of Rehabilitation Medicine, 33*(3), 128–132.
LaCaille, R. A., DeBerard, M. S., Masters, K. S., Colledge, A. L., & Bacon, W. (2005). Presurgical biopsychosocial factors predict multidimensional patient: Outcomes of interbody cage lumbar fusion. *The Spine Journal, 5*(1), 71–78.
Lynch, W. J. (2004). Determination of effort level, exaggeration, and malingering in neurocognitive assessment. *The Journal of Head Trauma Rehabilitation, 19*(3), 277–283.
Lysgaard, A. P., Fonager, K., & Nielsen, C. V. (2005). Effect of financial compensation on vocational rehabilitation. *Journal of Rehabilitation Medicine, 37*(6), 388–391.
Mailis-Gagnon, A., Nicholson, K., Blumberger, D., & Zurowski, M. (2008). Characteristics and period prevalence of self-induced disorder in patients referred to a pain clinic with the diagnosis of complex regional pain syndrome. *The Clinical Journal of Pain, 24*(2), 176–185.
Mannion, A. F., & Elfering, A. (2006). Predictors of surgical outcome and their assessment. *European Spine Journal, 15*(Suppl 1), S93–108.
Mendelson, G., & Mendelson, D. (2004). Malingering pain in the medicolegal context. *The Clinical Journal of Pain, 20*(6), 423–432.
Meyer, G. J., Finn, S. E., Eyde, L. D., et al. (2001). Psychological testing and psychological assessment. A review of evidence and issues. *American Psychologist, 56*(2), 128–165.
Mitrushina, M. N., Boone, K. B., & D'Elia, L. (1999). *Handbook of normative data for neuropsychological assessment*. New York: Oxford University Press.
Mittenberg, W., DiGiulio, D. V., Perrin, S., & Bass, A. E. (1992). Symptoms following mild head injury: Expectation as aetiology. *Journal of Neurology, Neurosurgery and Psychiatry, 55*(3), 200–204.
Mittenberg, W., Patton, C., Canyock, E. M., & Condit, D. C. (2002). Base rates of malingering and symptom exaggeration. *Journal of Clinical and Experimental Neuropsychology, 24*(8), 1094–1102.
Mnookin, S., & World Bank Group, World Health Organization. (2016). *Out of the shadows: Making mental health a global development priority*. Geneva, Switzerland: World Health Organization.
Murray, C. J., & Lopez, A. D. (1997). Alternative projections of mortality and disability by cause 1990–2020: Global Burden of Disease Study. *Lancet, 349*(9064), 1498–1504.
Nelson, N. W., Sweet, J. J., Berry, D. T., Bryant, F. B., & Granacher, R. P. (2007). Response validity in forensic neuropsychology: Exploratory factor analytic evidence of distinct cognitive and psychological constructs. *Journal of the International Neuropsychological Society, 13*(3), 440–449.
Nelson, N. W., Sweet, J. J., & Demakis, G. J. (2006). Meta-analysis of the MMPI-2 fake bad scale: Utility in forensic practice. *The Clinical Neuropsychologist, 20*(1), 39–58.

Ong, K. S., & Keng, S. B. (2003). The biological, social, and psychological relationship between depression and chronic pain. *Cranio, 21*(4), 286–294.

Ormel, J., VonKorff, M., Ustun, T. B., Pini, S., Korten, A., & Oldehinkel, T. (1994). Common mental disorders and disability across cultures. Results from the WHO Collaborative Study on Psychological Problems in General Health Care. *The Journal of the American Medical Association, 272*(22), 1741–1748.

Pickering, T. G. (2001). Mental stress as a causal factor in the development of hypertension and cardiovascular disease. *Current Hypertension Reports, 3*(3), 249–254.

Pledger, C. (2003). Discourse on disability and rehabilitation issues. Opportunities for psychology. *The American Psychologist, 58*(4), 279–284.

Polatin, P. B., Kinney, R. K., Gatchel, R. J., Lillo, E., & Mayer, T. G. (1993). Psychiatric illness and chronic low-back pain. The mind and the spine–which goes first? *Spine (Phila Pa 1976), 18*(1), 66–71.

Proctor, T. J., Mayer, T. G., Gatchel, R. J., & McGeary, D. D. (2004). Unremitting health-care-utilization outcomes of tertiary rehabilitation of patients with chronic musculoskeletal disorders. *The Journal of Bone and Joint Surgery. American Volume, 86-A*(1), 62–69.

Reagan, R. (2009). *Remarks on signing the intermediate-range nuclear forces treaty, 1987.* From http://www.reagan.utexas.edu/archives/speeches/1987/120887c.htm. Accessed 13 Sep 2009.

Rohling, M. L., Binder, L. M., & Langhinrichsen-Rohling, J. (1995). Money matters: A meta-analytic review of the association between financial compensation and the experience and treatment of chronic pain. *Health Psychology, 14*(6), 537–547.

Rondinelli, R. D., Genovese, E., Brigham, C. R., & American Medical Association. (2008). *Guides to the evaluation of permanent impairment* (6th ed.). Chicago: American Medical Association.

Roy-Byrne, P. P., Davidson, K. W., Kessler, R. C., et al. (2008). Anxiety disorders and comorbid medical illness. *General Hospital Psychiatry, 30*(3), 208–225.

Scarry, E. (1985). *The body in pain: The making and unmaking of the world.* New York: Oxford University Press.

Schofferman, J., Anderson, D., Hines, R., Smith, G., & White, A. (1992). Childhood psychological trauma correlates with unsuccessful lumbar spine surgery. *Spine, 17*(6 Suppl), S138–S144.

Spengler, D. M., Bigos, S. J., Martin, N. A., et al. (1986). Back injuries in industry: A retrospective study. I. Overview and cost analysis. *Spine, 11*(3), 241–245.

Spitzer, W., Leblanc, F., & Dupuis, M. (1987). Scientific approach to the assessment and management of activity-related spinal disorders. A monograph for clinicians. Report of the Quebec Task Force on Spinal Disorders. *Spine (Phila Pa 1976), 12*(7 Suppl), S1–59.

Sullivan, M. J., Thorn, B., Haythornthwaite, J. A., et al. (2001). Theoretical perspectives on the relation between catastrophizing and pain. *The Clinical Journal of Pain, 17*(1), 52–64.

Taylor, V. M., Deyo, R. A., Ciol, M., et al. (2000). Patient-oriented outcomes from low back surgery: A community-based study. *Spine, 25*(19), 2445–2452.

Terplan, M., Smith, E. J., & Temkin, S. M. (2009). Race in ovarian cancer treatment and survival: A systematic review with meta-analysis. *Cancer Causes & Control, 20*(7), 1139–1150.

Thomas, M. L., & Youngjohn, J. R. (2009). Let's not get hysterical: Comparing the MMPI-2 validity, clinical, and RC scales in TBI litigants tested for effort. *The Clinical Neuropsychologist, 23*(6), 1067–1084.

Tompa, E., de Oliveira, C., Dolinschi, R., & Irvin, E. (2008). A systematic review of disability management interventions with economic evaluations. *Journal of Occupational Rehabilitation, 18*(1), 16–26.

Turk, D. C., & Melzack, R. (1992). Trends and future directions in human pain assessment. In D. C. Turk & R. Melzack (Eds.), *Handbook of pain assessment* (pp. 473–479). New York: Guilford Press.

Turk, D. C., & Okifuji, A. (2002). Psychological factors in chronic pain: Evolution and revolution. *Journal of Consulting and Clinical Psychology, 70*(3), 678–690.

Turner, S. M., DeMers, S. T., Fox, H. R., & Reed, G. (2001). APA's guidelines for test user qualifications: An executive summary. *The American Psychologist, 56*, 1099–1113.

U.S. Department of Education, Office of Special Education and Rehabilitative Services National Institute on Disability and Rehabilitation Research. (2009). *Long range plan: 1999–2003*. Washington, DC: U.S. Department of Education.

Weisbord, S. D., Fried, L. F., Arnold, R. M., et al. (2004). Development of a symptom assessment instrument for chronic hemodialysis patients: The dialysis symptom index. *Journal of Pain and Symptom Management, 27*(3), 226–240.

Wise, M. G., & Ford, C. V. (1999). Factitious disorders. *Primary Care, 26*(2), 315–326.

Work Loss Data Institute. (2008). *Official disability guidelines*. Encinitas, CA: Work Loss Data Institute.

Work Loss Data Institute. (2009). *Official disability guidelines*. Encinitas, CA: Work Loss Data Institute.

World Health Organization. (2008). *The global burden of disease: 2004 update*. Geneva, Switzerland: World Health Organization.

World Health Organization. (2016). *Global Health Estimates 2015: Disease burden by Cause, Age, Sex, by Country and by Region, 2000–2015*. Retrieved from Geneva: http://www.who.int/healthinfo/global_burden_disease/estimates/en/index2.html

Ylinen, J., Takala, E. P., Kautiainen, H., et al. (2004). Association of neck pain, disability and neck pain during maximal effort with neck muscle strength and range of movement in women with chronic non-specific neck pain. *European Journal of Pain, 8*(5), 473–478.

Chapter 7
Psychological Injury in the States and Federal Workers' Compensation Systems

Pamela A. Warren

7.1 Overview of the Workers' Compensation Systems

Although there are different regulations associated with each WC system, there are some commonalities across all systems. In the United States, both the States and federal WC systems were based on European social insurance. The UK and German laws have influenced the States and federal WC systems, respectively (Ranavaya & Rondinelli, 2000).

The British law influenced development of the States WC system. It is based on three pronged approach. The British WC system is based on no-fault principle. The Workers' Compensation Act became law in 1897. The British law views the social insurance system as elective, the administration of the work injury process is administered by a court system, and the insurance was provided by private companies (Elling, 1989).

The US federal WC system is influenced more by the German social insurance model. Germany was the first country to have a WC system. It began in 1884. The German WC system was built on the principle of "Rehabilitation vor Rente" with the focus on vocational retraining and rehabilitation before any pension. The primary philosophy is that work is vital to life. The German WC system is an exclusive remedy system, meaning it is the only system that addresses employees' workplace injuries. There is no access to tort remedy in its system. The German WC system accepts all treatment records as documentation of the reported injury and subsequent treatment. There is no mechanism in place to evaluate for fraud in this system. The financial contributions to the systems are shared by both employers and employee. This model requires German employees to pay for part of the treatment costs and that the administrative process was centralized (Howard, 2002).

P. A. Warren (✉)
Carle Physician Group and University of Illinois Medical School, Department of Psychiatry, Monticello, IL, USA

P. A. Warren (ed.), *Handbook of Behavioral Health Disability Management*,
https://doi.org/10.1007/978-3-319-89860-5_7

There are a few commonalities between the US States and federal WC systems. Each is a no-fault system. The term no-fault means that neither the employer nor employee can be found at fault for the workplace injury or illness. In this instance, the WC process is the exclusive remedy to receiving medical care and wage replacement after a workplace injury. There is a trade-off in that both the employer and employee are not found to be at fault for causing the workplace injury and so cannot make claims of the other party's blame for the injury. In order to receive the WC benefits, the employee relinquishes the right to sue the employer for tort of negligence. Recently, some State courts have found that the WC system is not the exclusive remedy when the employer violates safety regulations or where the employee is intentionally injured (Sengupta, Reno, Burton, & Baldwin, 2012).

The tort legal system is based on common law which hold that an event, situation, or person can cause another to suffer a loss or harm. An individual who is found to be responsible causing harm or loss to another person has legal liability (Henderson, Kysar, & Pearson, 2017). Usually, the tort system is not a part of the WC system. The only exception to this relates to railroad employees who are covered under the Federal Employers' Liability Act (FELA, 1908). FELA specifically allows railroad employees who are injured to recover monetary damages. Thus, FELA is a part of the tort legal system. FELA will be discussed later in Sect. 7.4.

In the United States, a State or federal WC claimant can access to the tort system only once all appeals within the State WC system are exhausted. At that point, WC laws no longer are applicable. Instead, tort laws apply in regard to liability for the reported injury. In the tort system, damages may be awarded to the prevailing party.

The WC no-fault system offers benefits to both employees and employers. Employees are able to receive timely medical care when injured in the workplace. In addition, the employee receives wage replacement for the time that she/he is either not able to work or is unable to resume all workplace responsibilities (e.g., light duties). Vocational rehabilitation and death benefits are also components of the WC system. Employers do not accept responsibility for the workplace injury and have limitations to the costs that they pay for workplace injuries. However, as mentioned earlier, recent court decisions in some States in which the state court decided that WC was not necessarily the exclusive remedy (Warren, 2016, 2017).

Conversely, there are potential downsides to the State WC systems. Employers are unable to indicate that the employee is at fault for the injury, even if the employee's behavior played a role in causing the injury. Employees receive a set amount for wage replacement that is based on each varying States' award schedules when a workplace injury occurs. Usually, the WC payment to the employee is not the same amount that is received for paid wages. Typically, the wage replacement amount is based on scheduled or unscheduled parts of the body. Scheduled awards are based on those body parts which are listed within a specific State's WC award schedules. Unscheduled awards may be given for those that are not listed in the schedule of awards. In some States, such as Illinois, an example of an unscheduled WC award is a workplace psychological injury claim (Warren, 2016, 2017).

While the federal WC system is wholly separate from the State WC systems, it too is a no-fault system (DFEC, DOL, n.d.; GAO-07-934SP; GAO-13-142R). All federal employees, except railroad employees, are covered under the *Federal Employees Compensation Act* (FECA). Moreover, the FECA WC system has its own schedule award system in which payment to the federal employee is based on loss of usage of parts of the body. The loss of usage and the percentage paid are calculated once the individual is evaluated for percentage of the loss of use. Loss of use is based on whether the person is determined to have permanent total impairment (e.g., can't work now or in the future) or partial loss of usage (e.g., may be able to work with changes in workplace duties) while the injury is being treated or after the person is determined to have reached maximum medical improvement (MMI) (GAO-13-142R).

Thus, it can be seen there are some initial commonalities in States and federal WC laws. For the sake of clarity, any usage of federal WC in the chapter refers to FECA. The FELA system will be discussed separately. Further exploration about commonalities in the WC claims processes will take place in the next section.

7.1.1 Commonalities in the WC Claims Processes

Both the States and federal WC systems have three types of claims that can be made. These types of claims are physical-mental (e.g., a physical injury causes a psychology injury), mental-physical (e.g., a work-related stressor or event causes a physical injury), and mental-mental (e.g., a work-related catalyst, such as stress, causes a psychological injury). An employee may file a claim after one of these types of claims occurs (Warren, 2016, 2017).

The process for initiation a claim is that the employee reports a workplace injury to the employer. The employer provides WC paperwork. In some States, the employee will need to be evaluated within a specific time period after the injury has occurred. The employer then turns the completed incident report paperwork into the WC insurer. The employer must also provide paperwork regarding the employee's rights and benefits under that WC system. In addition, the employer must also provide information regarding the employee's return to work. In addition, the employer must report workplace injuries to appropriate State WC boards and, in some instances, federal agencies (Tanabe, 2013; Warren, 2016, 2017).

The WC insurer will then make a determination whether to allow or deny the claim. If the WC insurer allows the claim, the employee decides whether to accept the insurer's the payment offer. However, the employee may also decide to negotiate for a lump-sum or structured settlement. If the WC insurer denies the claim, the employee can ask for the insurer to review information that is believed to be incorrect. The employee also has the option to request an appeal of a denial.

If the employee has been off of work due to a workplace injury or illness, there are specific actions the employee must take, such as attending schedule treatment appointments and complying with treatment recommendations to reduce any reported impairment. When an employee returns to work, she/he must notify the employer about the intent to return to work (RTW) as well as the WC insurer in writing. This provides a record of the employee's intent to return one's job.

Typically, those physical claims that do not have a reported psychological injury are managed in accordance with that specific State's award schedule. However, a WC claim with a purported psychological injury may be allowed in some States with specific restrictions. Because most State WC systems do not have psychology injuries as part of the award schedule, a workplace psychological injury that receives payments is called an unscheduled award. In many States, this means that the psychological injury is treated as an entire body injury versus the proportional parts of the body. In other words, the individual is viewed as being completely disabled and unable to work when a psychological injury is approved. The reasoning in the award schedules is in conflict with what is known about individuals who have a psychological condition (Warren, 2013a, 2013b, 2016, 2017). That is, the majority of individuals continue to work despite having a psychological condition. Moreover, with appropriate diagnosis and treatment, the majority return their previous level of functioning. Yet, most WC laws do not reflect this. ((85 O.S. Rules of the Workers' Compensation Court, Rule 20) *Commonwealth v. Lanigan*, 419 Mass. 15, 24–26 (1994); Bender, 2016; *Brown v. W.T. Martin Plumbing & Heating, Inc., 2013 VT 38* (June 21, 2013); *City of Owensboro v. Adams*, 135 S.W.3d. 446, 449-50 (Ky. 2004), (*MCLE Mass Workers' Comp*, 2nd ed., Chap.14, 2010); *Commonwealth v. Powell*, 450 Mass. 229, 238 (2007); Correio, 2015; Department of Labor, 2016; *Giaimo v. Florida Autosport, Inc.* 1D14-0077, 2014 WL 6679290 (Fla. 1st DCA, 11/26/14); *Ireton v. Horizon Mental Health Mgmt., LLC,* 2016 *Tenn.* Rolda v. Pitney Bowes (2001) 66 Cal. Comp. Cas 241).

Table 7.1 provides an overview of the similarities between the States and federal WC systems regarding different factors in comparison with FELA.

As can be seen, there are a number of commonalities in the State and federal systems, in terms of all WC systems are no-faults system. Moreover, all States and federal WC are legally mandated. In addition, all WC systems employ the usage of an award schedule, have similar types of claims, and have a process for adjudicating claims. However, considerable differences between the States and federal WC systems exist as well. Further discussion will take place in the next section to examine these differences (Bender, 2016; Kertay, Eskay-Auerbach, & Hyman, 2016; Warren, 2016, 2017).

7.2 Differences in States and Federal WC Systems Related to Workplace Psychological Injury Claims

While all States have a WC system, there are distinct differences from one State WC system to another as previously noted. Because of this, there is no standardization of the State WC laws or systems at present. This means that laws and rules vary widely from State to State. There is no common method or system of addressing

Table 7.1 Similarities in the WC systems

	State WC systems	Federal WC system (FECA)	FELA tort system
Mandatory coverage	Yes	Yes	No
No-fault system	Yes, although some State courts have allowed for suits outside of the WC system	Yes	No
Exclusive remedy	Yes, although some State courts have allowed suits outside of the WC system or when all WC appeals have been exhausted	Yes	No
Specific process for adjudicating WC claims	Yes	Yes	Yes
Specific WC laws addressing workplace injuries	Yes	Yes	No
Specific WC laws addressing workplace psychological injuries	Yes, in some, but not all States	Yes	No
Specific State or federal laws that require the usage of specific guide or treatment protocol related to workplace psychological injuries	Yes for some States which employ various editions of the American Medical Association's *Guides to Impairment in Functioning* (*Guides*) However, some States eschew the *Guides* altogether and use their own individually developed documentation process of substantiating psychological injury	Yes, FECA stipulates that the American Medical Association (AMA) *Guides, 6th edition*, must be used in the determination of psychological workplace injuries regarding the extent of impairment pertaining to functioning	No
Pays medical costs	Yes	Yes	Maybe
Pays wage replacement	Yes	Yes	Yes, but only if the railroad is found to be negligent
Pays for vocational rehabilitation	Yes	Yes	No
Pays death benefits	Yes	Yes	Yes
Award schedule	Yes	Yes	No
Types of claims allowed:			
Physical-mental	Yes	Yes	Yes
Mental-physical	Yes, but not in all States	Yes	Yes

(continued)

Table 7.1 (continued)

	State WC systems	Federal WC system (FECA)	FELA tort system
Mental-mental	Yes, but not in all States	Yes	Yes
Addresses psychosocial issues	No	No	No
The manner in which psychological injury is evaluated and assessed meets the current psychological standards of care	No	No	No

WC psychological injury claims. This becomes apparent in examining how States address WC psychological injuries (Warren, 2016, 2017).

As noted earlier, FECA covers all federal employees, except Railroad employees (U.S. Department of Labor, Office of Workers' Compensation Program, http://www.dol.gov/owcp/dfec/regs/compliance/ fecafact.htm n.d.; U.S. Department of Labor – Office of Workers' Compensation Programs (OWCP)-FECA, n.d. http://www.dol.gov/owcp/regs/compliance/ca_feca.htm).

This means that the same rules apply to the majority of federal employees regarding reported workplace psychological injuries. In addition, the US Department of Labor has a specific form related to psychiatry and psychological conditions that must be completed when filing a claim. It is a work capacity evaluation (OMB No.1240-0046). This forms focuses on the ability to work full time versus part time as well as if the person can work in another type of job. It emphasizes that the Office of Workers' Compensation Programs (FECA) focuses on reemployment, such as working in an alternative work location.

In the federal WC system, workplace psychological injuries must be reported, and the individual must be treated physicians (including family practice) and psychologists. Master's level professionals, including licensed clinical social workers, licensed professional counselors, nurse practitioners, and physician assistants, are not able to treat the individual unless supervised by a physician. In addition to reporting a psychological injury covered under FECA, federal employees may also file WC claims under the *Cutler Rule*.

With FECA claims, any treatment and documentation submitted regarding a workplace psychological injury must follow the American Medical Association's *Guides to the Evaluation of Permanent Impairment, 6th edition* (2008). There are several problems with this approach in that the *Guides*, 6th edition, are no longer aligned with current psychological standards of care. Specifically, the *Guides*, 6th ed., require a *DSM-IV-TR* diagnosis. The *DSM-IV-TR* (American Psychiatric Association, 2000) (ACOEM, 2008) is now obsolete in the psychological and psychiatric fields. Instead, the *DSM-5* (American Psychiatric Association (ApA), 2013) is the current diagnostic standard for psychological conditions in the United States. FECA asks for Global Assessment of Functioning (*GAF*) scores to complete each of the three measures used by the *Guides*, 6th ed., to determine a percentage of impairment in functioning for those individuals with psychological conditions. There are two issues with this: first, the *GAF* was removed from the *DSM-5* because it was determined to be too subjective of a measure (Aas, 2011, 2014; Bacon, Collins, & Plake, 2002; First, 2010; Gholizadeh, Malcarne, & Schatman, 2015; Ma, 2014; Vatnaland, Vatnaland, Friis, & Opjordsmoen, 2007); and second, the three measures employed for psychological impairment in the *Guides*, 6th ed., were altered arbitrarily without the benefit of going through validation and reliability processes (ACOEM, 2008; Warren, 2016). Consequently, it is not certain that any of the new measures actually measure the concerns they purport to measure. It is also not certain that the measures produce reliable (e.g., consistent) results when used. Thus, the inclusion of outdated psychological standards of care in the FECA disability process inappropriately allows a great deal of subjective information into the disability determination process (Ladou, 2009).

In addition, under the *Cutler Rule*, a federal employee who experiences emotional distress while carrying out normal workplace duties or is anxious about his or her ability to complete these duties may file a FECA claim. Thus, the federal WC system allows psychosocial issues (e.g., perceptions, beliefs, attitudes, job dissatisfaction, whether accurate or not) to be a reason for filing a WC claim. Empirical research has consistently found that psychosocial issues are subjective since they fluctuate so widely from person to person. Moreover, psychosocial issues, not physical or psychological conditions themselves, are primary causes of treatment failure and prolonged workplace absences. In addition, normal emotional responses are inappropriately elevated by attempting to say that normal responses are the equivalent as valid physical and psychological conditions by WC claimants and treating professionals alike. This is not accurate. When normal emotional responses are incorrectly said to cause impairment in functioning, this is called *medicalization* (Barsky, 2002; Barsky & Kaplan, 2007; Barth, 2012; Gatchel, 2013a; Grant & Robbins, 2003; Ramirez, Ekselius, & Ramklint, 2013).

By inappropriately allowing the inclusion of psychosocial issues, the current review of FECA beneficiaries consistently finds a great deal of fraud occurring in the federal WC system. The reason is that an employee can make claims of *feeling anxious* about ability to complete job duties *without any submitted documentation, such as standardized psychological testing* as it relates to the employee's actual ability to complete workplace responsibilities. The GAO noted that the federal system must provide greater oversight of FECA claims with greater case management of employees who have filed claims to ensure compliance with treatment and to develop a plan to return to work (GAO-13-142R; GAO-15-19; GAO-15-673T; GAO-16-375SP).

In Table 7.2, there are five distinct categories pertaining to WC psychological injury claims. This is some overlap between some of those categories. Some States either allow very limited specific psychological injury claims, or there is some overlap with one of the other categories regarding how a workplace psychological injury must occur in order to be compensable. These States are marked with an asterisk (Warren, 2016).

Table 7.2 Types of allowed States and federal workplace psychological injury claims

No allowance for mental-mental claims	Allowance for mental-mental claims only when circumstances occur beyond what is normally encountered	Allowance for mental-mental claims only when catalyst for injury occurs suddenly when working	Allowance of mental-mental claims with specific limitations	Allowance of mental-mental claims
Alabama Arkansas Connecticut[a] Florida Georgia Idaho Kentucky Montana Nebraska Nevada New Hampshire Ohio Oklahoma South Dakota Wyoming	Arizona Colorado[a] Illinois Iowa Louisiana[a] Maine Mississippi Missouri New Jersey New York North Carolina Oregon Pennsylvania Rhode Island South Carolina	Colorado[a] Louisiana[a] Maryland Tennessee Virginia FECA	Connecticut police and firefighters only Massachusetts District of Columbia	Alaska California Hawaii FELA[b]

[b]There is some overlap between categories. Thus, some States may appear in two categories
[b]FELA is not WC system. Instead, it is a tort-based legal system in which the employee must demonstrate railroad negligence

The first category lists those States that do not allow any mental-mental claims. The only exception is that Connecticut allows police and firefighters to file limited psychological injury claims (Bender, 2016; Larson, Larson, & Bender, 2016).

The second category notes States that allow psychological injury claims only when the catalyst for the claim is beyond what other employees in this claim have experienced. No workplace psychological injury claims may be filed if they relate to being fired, demoted, or moved to a different job or disciplinary action.

In the third category, States and federal government allow workplace psychological injury claims only if the impetus for the injury was severe and sudden. The reported injury must occur in the workplace. As with the second category, no workplace psychological injury claims may be filed related to being terminated, demoted, or moved to a different job or a disciplinary action (Warren, 2016, 2017).

The fourth category shows those States that allow workplace psychological injury claims but with specific limitations to either occupation or type of allowed psychological condition.

In the final category, three States allow workplace psychological injury claims to be made.

Some States also bar WC psychological claims that arise from personnel actions that result in an employee experiencing a psychological injury, unless the injury is related to an event that is not typical to the workplace. These types of claims are usually called mental-mental claims. These States which have specific limitations for these types of claims are Arkansas, Connecticut, Idaho, Massachusetts, Maine, Minnesota, Missouri, Nebraska, New Hampshire, Nevada, New York, Oregon, South Carolina, Tennessee, Texas, Utah, and Vermont.

In some States, a psychological diagnosis is required in submitting a WC mental injury claim. Those States which require a psychological diagnosis are Arkansas, Colorado, Florida, Idaho, Louisiana, Minnesota, Oklahoma, South Carolina, Washington, and Wyoming (Bender, 2016; Larson et al., 2016; Warren, 2016, 2017).

Eight States require a *Diagnostic and Statistical Manual* (*DSM*) (ApA, 2013) diagnosis. Those States are Arkansas, California, Florida, Idaho, Louisiana, Minnesota, Oklahoma, and Wyoming. This is important because the psychological diagnosis typically drives the type of treatment that the individual receives. A frequent cause of lack of improvement and poor treatment outcomes relates to vague "diagnoses" such as anxiety or depression. Both are laypeople's terms which are subjective in nature since people can perceive or define symptoms differently from others. Moreover, because "anxiety" and "depression" are simply symptoms, they lack diagnostic criteria. Therefore, when non-DSM "diagnoses" are provided by treating professionals, there are no standardized diagnostic criteria that are being employed by those professionals (Agency for Healthcare Research and Quality, 2016; Aronoff et al., 2007; Barth, 2012).

The following States require a psychologist or psychiatrist to diagnosis a workplace psychological injury for which a claim is submitted: Arkansas, Idaho, Louisiana, Minnesota, Oklahoma, and Wyoming (Hees, Nieuwenhuijsen, Koeter, Bultmann, & Schene, 2012; Heilbrun, Grisso, & Goldstein, 2009).

Other States have professional requirements for a workplace psychological injury diagnosis: Colorado requires either a licensed physician or psychologist; Connecticut requires licensed and board-certified mental health professionals; Florida requires psychiatrists only for WC psychological claims; South Carolina requires an authorized psychologist or psychiatrist, while Washington requires a licensed health-care professional with "appropriate training and experience" (Warren, 2016, 2017).

FECA stipulates that only physicians and clinical psychologists may provide documentation regarding the evaluation and treatment of a federal employee with a reported workplace psychological injury. FECA specifically notes that master's level professionals such as social workers are not able to submit documentation since they do not have the requisite training to do so (§8105. Total disability and §8106. Partial disability. (n.d.); Department of Labor, 1995, 2007, 2016).

By reviewing current State and federal WC laws, it is clear there is no standardization in how WC psychological injury is addressed within the States or federal WC systems. There are no common *DSM* diagnostic criteria required, except for a handful of States. There is also variability in the types of professionals who may submit documentation pertaining to a workplace psychological injury claim. In addition, because vague, non-standard diagnoses are introduced into the WC systems, it is not clear if a psychological condition actually exists or is merely the perception of the WC claimant or a subjective opinion of a treating professional. This introduces imprecision into the already highly imprecise WC systems. There are addition factors related the determination of workplace psychological injury that compound this problem further. These issues are discussed more fully in Sect. 7.4.

7.3 Federal Employers' Liability Act (FELA), the Railroad Retirement Board (RRB) and Railroad Employees

As noted earlier, all railroad employees are considered federal employees. However, they are not covered under FECA. Instead, the Federal Employers' Liability Act (FELA) is utilized for railroad employees with workplace injuries. FELA was enacted by Congress in 1908. FELA specifically excludes railroad employees from States' WC statutes.

If a railroad employee is injured on the job, that employee can initiate a lawsuit against the railroad carrier, its agents, or other employees if a sustained injury is due to negligence by the railroad. Thus, FELA claims differ from other types of WC claims since they are a part of the tort legal system. Lawsuits can be initiated in either the State or federal court systems. In order to sue the railroad, the employee must prove that injuries were related to the railroad's negligence. However, if the railroad violated a safety statute or safety regulation, then, congress imposed absolute liability on the railroad, without the employee needing to prove negligence. In addition, railroad employees have up to 3 years from the date of the injury to initiate a lawsuit.

In addition, FELA does not follow a benefit schedule like those that occur with State WC and FECA claims. Thus, FELA is not a traditional WC system. Any compensation received from a FELA claim is a much bigger monetary award than those associated with other WC systems (Federal Employers' Liability Act (FELA), 45 U.S.C. § 51 et seq. (1908)).

Typically, if a railroad employee is injured and receives medical treatment, bills for treatment must be sent to the railroad claim agent. This process is covered through the Railroad Retirement Board (RRB).

If a railroad employee becomes sick, the employee is required to use all accumulated sick time and vacation time for workplace absences. After both are exhausted, the employee can apply for short-term sickness benefits through the RRB. The short-term leave can be extended up to 12 months.

The RRB is a work benefit that has two tiers. Tier I is the equivalent of Social Security benefits. Tier II is a monetary supplement that is available to railroad employees only. In order to be eligible for RRB benefits, railroad employees accrue time credited by months in service. The minimum requirement for railroad employees for RRB benefits is 120 months (10 years) or 60 months (5 years), if work service was performed after 1995.

RRB benefits are available for any railroad employee who is sick or sustained work injuries, after meeting the minimum requirements of months in service. However, by law, the RRB is entitled to be recoup any benefits paid from judgments or settled lawsuits that were against the railroad or any third party. This is a lien that must be satisfied out of the monetary proceeds of any settlement. When a railroad employee is on disability, the employee is not credited with months in service during the length of the disability claim (RRB, 2009).

Railroad employees who have 240 months (20 years) and cannot perform any regular work duties may qualify for a disability annuity (retirement). In this instance, the railroad employee must submit medical documentation from licensed physicians to support the purported impairment in functioning. This type of disability is considered occupational disability (RRB, 2004).

In some instances, railroad employees are eligible for total disability benefits after accumulating 120 months in service (10 years). Total disability differs from occupational disability in that the railroad employee must demonstrate a permanent medical condition that prevents the employee from any substantial gainful employment (RRB, 2015). This means that the railroad employee not only cannot perform the regular railroad duties but cannot work in any other type of job, including non-railroad jobs (Federal Employers' Liability Act (FELA), 45 U.S.C. § 51 et seq. (1908)).

There are some of the same problematic issues that occur in the States and federal WC systems occur in the RRB disability process. There is considerable potential for individuals obtaining total disability improperly. Some of the problems that have been identified are that RRB disability claims are not adequately evaluated to ensure that claimants meet the program eligibility requirements (GAO-14-312). The Government Accountability Office (GAO-14-418) determined determined that the RRB employed the same criteria as the Social Security Administration (e.g., the physical or mental impairment must be present at least 1 year) but that claims were not reviewed until at least 1 year after the railroad employee was placed on disability. It was also found that the RRB lacked a means to evaluate accuracy and did not have a method to assess for potential fraud (GAO-15-535T, GAO-18-287).

7.4 Factors That Complicate WC Psychological Injury Claims in All WC Systems

There are several issues that muddle the determination of a workplace psychological injury in the States and federal WC systems. There is a lack of a standard definition regarding psychological injury and any subsequent impairment. In addition, the *Daubert* standard is not employed regarding documentation that is submitted to support the purported injury (*Daubert v. Merrell Dow Pharmaceuticals* (92-102), 509, U.S. 579 (1993); *Kumho Tire Co. v. Carmichael,* 526 U.S. 137 (1999); *General Electric Co. v. Joiner,* 522 U.S. 1136, 118 S. Ct. 512, 139 L Ed. 2d 508.).

There are clear differences between the legal versus psychological causation. Despite that most psychological conditions are brought into remission, there is an underlying assumption that a psychological condition can result in permanent disability. Finally, States and federal WC systems do not require comprehensive evaluation, assessment, and treatment that align with current psychological standards of care.

7.4.1 Defining Disability in the WC Systems

When looking at all 51 States and the federal WC laws, it is quickly observed that there is no standardization relating to defining disability, aside from "parts of a body." For example, usually each State and federal WC system has defined disability related to loss of usage of parts of the body, such as the hand, an arm, etc. Moreover, each system has its own formulas and percentages that are paid to an injured worker who has experienced loss of usage of a body part. In some instances, one system may pay more than another for the same injury solely because of the difference in how compensation for the loss is determined in another WC system (Bruns, Mueller, & Warren, 2010, 2012).

Loss of usage is also broken into three categories: *temporary total disability*, *permanent partial disability*, or *permanent total disability*.

In the WC systems, *permanent partial disability* is directly related to an individual being experiencing loss in arm, hands, legs, feet, or eyes. There are also combinations of using two combinations of these body parts. Usually, the individual is still able to use other limbs or parts of the body. *Temporary total disability* occurs when an injured employee is unable to work but on a temporary basis (Melhorn et al., 2013; Talmage, 2007).

When a person is determined to have *permanent total disability*, rigorous treatment is usually provided to rehabilitate the person, unless some type of catastrophic injury that results in permanent impairment occurred. Many individuals regain some functioning. When this occurs, the individual's functioning no longer meets the disability criteria for the permanent total disability definition (Melhorn et al., 2013). However, this applies primarily to physical injuries. Most WC psychological injuries are, by default, viewed as impacting on the individual's entire body (Escorpizo & Stucki, 2013). This means that in most WC systems, the individual is considered either temporary total disability or permanent total disability. This is because there is no analogous award schedule for psychological injuries (Hadjistavropoulos & Bieling, 2001; Hamm, Reiss, Paul, & Bursztajn, 2007; Warren, 2013a, 2013b, 2013c, 2016, 2017).

It is also important to note that WC award schedules do not have specific formulas or percentages related to psychological conditions and reported loss of functioning. In these instances, the three categories that apply to physical injuries and illnesses do not fit WC psychological injuries. These are addressed by some WC systems, such as Illinois, as calling the reported psychological injury, an unscheduled injury. Thus, it is an attempt to force workplace psychological injuries into the same types of categories as physical conditions (Gatchel, 2013b) .

However, there are problems with this approach. First, there is an assumption that physical and psychological conditions can be addressed in a similar manner. That is, the psychological conditions result in temporary total disability, permanent partial disability, or permanent total disability. This is not accurate since most psychological conditions are successfully treated with evidence-based treatments (Warren, 2013a, 2013b, 2013c, 2016, 2017). Therefore, the notion of permanent total disability for the majority of psychological conditions does not accurately reflect that remission is achieved with the majority of psychological conditions. Second, this line of reasoning is based on another faulty assumption, which is that when an event or situation occurs in the workplace and, then, any psychological condition that occurs afterward must be directly related to the workplace trigger. In other words, the exposure to the workplace incident caused the psychological condition. This is typically referred to as *causation*, which is discussed further in the next two sections.

7.4.2 Conflicts Between Legal Causation Versus Medical Causation Versus Psychological Causation

Legal procedures are generally concerned with the determination of fault or liability for a resulting injury. Typically, this determination process requires legal causation analysis. Attorneys are trained in this process. However, treating professionals, including psychologists and psychiatrists, are not. For treating professionals, the focus pertains to identifying the identification of a condition, the treatment of the condition, and the improvement of the individual's life (Heilbrun, Grisso, & Goldstein, 2009; Melhorn et al., 2013; Warren, 2013a, 2013b, 2013c; Young, Kane, Nicholson, & Shuman, 2007).

The WC claims and disability determination processes are also concerned with causation determination. This is because a workplace event must have occurred that produced the purported injury. If the workplace event caused the injury, then, the employee is entitled to WC benefits. Understandably, causation of an injury is frequently debated in any type of legal proceeding. If an impasse regarding causation occurs, typically, the both employer and employee hire attorneys to represent each party.

With WC claims, WC defense and plaintiff attorneys alike want to identify the most probable cause of the claimant's condition and demonstrate whether the condition is caused or is not caused by an event in the individual's workplace. Attorneys are most concerned with two types of causation. The first type of causation is called *cause-in-fact* which involves establishing the actual cause of the condition through the *but for* test. This relates to determining if the exposure to the workplace event or situation was a direct cause for the condition (Young et al., 2007). Frequently, this is established by the employee reporting an injury or accident to the employer. The employer usually receives some type of treatment (Warren, 2016). Thus, a timeline of the purported event and the employee's report of injury are critical to establishing legal causation.

The second type of causation is *proximate cause*. The closeness in time to the precipitating event is the primary component of this type of causation (Melhorn, 2013). An example of proximate cause is if a person is exposed to a workplace event or situation and, then, develops a psychological condition. The temporal relationship and the immediacy of the development of the condition serve as evidence of legal causation.

However, there are considerable differences in how legal causation is determined versus how mental health professionals view the development of a psychological condition. Psychologists and psychiatrists are interested in the examination of the individual regarding the complex interactions of medical, biological, emotional, cognitive, perceptional, intellectual, and environmental factors involved in the development of a psychological condition (Baumeister, Hutter, Bengel, & Harter, 2011; Baune, Caniato, Arolt, & Berger, 2009). This evaluative process involves examining not just a single event but rather careful probing of the individual's past and current history (Schultz, 2008, 2009; Schultz & Gatchel, 2015).

In addition, recent empirical research demonstrates that more than half of the psychological conditions, such as MDD, anxiety disorders, and substance abuse, begin in adolescence (Murphey, Barry, & Vaughn, 2013) by age 14. In addition, three-quarters of these conditions are present by age 24. Thus, this demonstrates that many psychological conditions begin earlier in life. These empirical findings must also be taken into consideration as part of the current psychological evaluation process as well as whether the individual received past psychological treatment.

Because of the complex interactions in the development of psychological conditions, psychologists and psychiatrist are interested in the identification of whether a psychological condition exists and if one exists, how to best treat it. Determination, in the legal sense of the word, does not routinely occur as part of the psychological evaluation process. Instead, treating professionals are interested in evaluating the individual from a biopsychosocial perspective. Empirical research has consistently demonstrated that there is a high comorbidity between physical and psychological conditions. Thus, if a physical condition is present, it is highly probable that a comorbid psychological condition is present as well (Baumeister et al., 2011; Baune et al., 2009; Bruffaerts et al., 2012; Dersh, Polatin, Leeman, & Gatchel, 2005; Druss et al., 2008; Druss & Walker, 2011; Gili et al., 2010; Laws & Colon, 2012; Preiss, Brennan, & Clarke, 2013; Roca et al., 2009; Warren, 2005, 2010). In addition, pain, mood, and sleep share the same neural pathways in the brain. Consequently, if one of these conditions is identified, it is important to evaluate and probe for the presence of the other conditions since psychological conditions can lead to poor sleep and increased perception of pain and vice versa.

Moreover, because the development of psychological condition is a complex one, it is frequently not possible to definitively say that a workplace event caused a psychological condition. This further complicates the legal determination process regarding a psychological condition arising from a single workplace event (Faust, Grimm, Ahern, & Sokolik, 2010; Faust & Ziskin, 2012; Walker, McGee, & Druss, 2015; Wang et al., 2010; Warren, 2013b).

Table 7.3 provides an overview of the legal, medical, and psychological causation determination processes. The differences between each causation process are noted.

In *medical causation*, the physician or other medical professional is asked to give an opinion that an event, such as a workplace accident, caused the workplace injury, such as a broken bone. However, physicians are not typically trained in the causa-

Table 7.3 Comparison of legal, medical, and psychological causation determination

	Causation across professions		
	Legal causation	Medical causation	Psychological causation
Training in causation analysis	Yes	No	No
Types of causation	(a) Cause-in-fact (b) Proximate cause	There may be a specific catalyst for medical causation, such as exposure to a toxic substance. Medical causation is not taught in medical school.	There is no specific catalyst for psychological causation, since most psychological conditions develop with complex physiological, cognitive, and psychological factors. Psychological causation is not taught in graduate school.
How causation is determined	(a) Cause-in-fact is based on whether a condition is caused by an event, action, or object. Cause-in-fact is determined by the *but for* test. If not for X, then Y would not have occurred (b) Proximate or legal causation is the primary situation, event, or behavior that directly results in the injury. The event occurred with foreseeable consequences and without intervention to prevent the injury by the defendant.	Medical causation relates to the physician who examines a person and determines whether a condition exists. If so, then, a diagnosis is made. For example, if a person is brought to the emergency department after being injured in the workplace, the physician will quickly gather information to assess the injury and to determine if further treatment is required. Examples of medical assessment are X-rays, CT scans, PET scans, MRIs, and blood assays. These types of assessments further confirm or rule out the presence of an underlying physical condition. Typically, the physician's assessment is found in the medical record. In the case of severe injury, the extent of the injury may be clearly determined. With mild injury, the extent of injury may not be fully evident.	Psychologists complete a comprehensive evaluation of an individual. This evaluation is based on a biopsychosocial perspective. That is, the assessment of the individual's physical and psychological history as well as the evaluation for potential psychosocial issues. Most psychological conditions do not result as a result of a single incident. Instead, there are complex interactions between multiple issues, such as biological, cognitive, perceptual, hormonal, physical, emotional, attitudinal, and individual biases, that interact throughout the individual's life time that may potentially result in that person developing a psychological condition. The majority of psychological conditions begin earlier in life around ages 14–24. The presence of a purported psychological condition must be assessed more objectively with standardized psychological testing. The psychological testing confirms or rules out psychological conditions. In addition, some psychological tests can identify the presence of psychosocial issues.

(continued)

Table 7.3 (continued)

	Causation across professions		
	Legal causation	Medical causation	Psychological causation
How attorneys ask the professional to answer the legal causation question	Attorneys generally ask questions framed in a yes/no or more probable than not.	Typically, both defense and plaintiff attorneys ask physicians to provide a professional opinion that a medical condition was more likely than not caused by exposure to a workplace incident.	Typically, both defense and plaintiff attorneys ask psychologists to provide a professional opinion that a psychological condition was more likely than not caused by exposure to a workplace incident.

tion analysis. Instead, they are trained to make a decision whether a condition exists or not. If a condition exists, then a diagnosis is made. For example, if the person is diagnosed with a fractured femur, then that person receives the appropriate treatment for the broken bone to heal it.

In WC claims, attorneys frequently ask for expert opinions from physicians regarding whether an injury is related to a workplace accident. After reviewing medical records, the physician is asked for his/her opinion regarding legal causation. In that situation, the physician is asked if she/he is "it is more probable than not" that a workplace event resulted in the injury. Usually, attorneys also ask about reasonable degree of medical certainty if, in this instance, the workplace accident caused the broken bone. It forces the physician to provide a simple yes or no answer to fit the legal causation question to establish cause of a purported injury.

When a psychological injury is reported, such as the employee reported developing major depressive disorder after a workplace accident, there can be as many as three types of causation: *legal*, *medical* (determination of if medical condition exists and the medical treatment to provide, if present), and *psychological* (determination of if a psychological condition exists and the psychological treatment is provided, if present) to be considered.

Attorneys tend to lump psychological causation in with medical causation. However, this is inaccurate. Many physicians receive minimal training regarding the diagnosis and treatment of psychological conditions. This lack of in-depth training tends to result in providing only those treatments that physicians are familiar with, such as medication. Empirical research confirms that most "psychological" treatment by non-psychiatrist medical providers tends to be in the form of medication only (Gilovich, Griffin, & Kahneman, 2002; Grove, Zald, Lebow, Snitz, & Nelson, 2000; Harding, 2004; Hofmann, 2016; Stolper et al., 2011). For example, when the individual comes to the physician and reports subjective symptoms that may be related to a psychological condition, the physician will complete a brief assessment which may or may not include the use of screening tools regarding the potential presence of a psychological condition. Many times, the physician's opinion is based on the individual's subjective self-report. After the physician decides that the person has a specific psychological condition, psychotropic medication is usually prescribed.

Frequently, physicians will opine that the individual needs to take time off from work to "recover." However, empirical research consistently demonstrates that being away from work or other normal activities of everyday life does not facilitate a person's recovery in the long run. Instead, when a person is off from work, physical and psychological deconditioning occur. Moreover, the person begins to identify work as the primary issue for the negative thoughts and feelings that are experienced (Barsky, 2002; Furlan et al., 2012; Jensen-Doss & Hawley, 2011; Mortelmans, 2013; Spengler et al., 2009; Wakefield, 2010).

Frequently, physicians are asked to render a medical opinion regarding legal causation of a reported psychological condition. When the average time that physicians spend with an individual (17.5 min), depending on the type of physician versus the time with individuals evaluated and treated by psychologists (45–55 min) and psychiatrists (20–32.7 min), is compared, it quickly becomes clear that an in-depth comprehensive evaluation and assessment cannot be completed by a general practice physician due to the limited available time. Yet, if a physician renders a medical opinion regarding a reported workplace psychological condition without the benefit of a thorough review of medical records and the lack of a careful evaluation, then, legal causation can be inappropriately established (Table 7.4).

Table 7.4 Comparison of professional time spent with patients

	General practitioner	Psychiatry	Psychology
Average appointment time spent with a patient	17.5 min	20–32.7 min	45–55 min
Average time spent with patient documentation	Roughly 2 h per every hour of direct patient care	Roughly 2 h per every hour of direct patient care	70 min for normal follow-up notes of all patients. 20+ min per consult documentation. 1.5+ h of test interpretation and report writing per each psychological test that was administered. Additional time for return phone calls, letters, and report writings
Average number of patients per day	20–27	14–20	7–9 patients
Length of consultation appointment	It depends on if the physician has allotted extra time beyond a normal patient appointment time slot	It depends on if the physician has allotted extra time beyond a normal patient appointment time slot. Many psychiatrists have 1 h consultation appointments	Typically, 1 to 1½ h If this is a disability evaluation, then, it may take 7–10 h which includes psychological testing time

When psychologists are asked by attorneys about legal causation, this is problematic for several reasons. First, psychologists and other behavioral health professionals are not trained in causation analysis. Without this type of training, it is common to not fully understand the complexities pertaining to causation analysis (Hamp et al., 2016).

Second, while attorneys are interested in a simple yes/no, more probable than not, or a reasonable degree of certainty answer regarding psychological causation, the issue is that psychological conditions do not simply develop in a purely linear fashion.

In reality, psychological causation is far more than difficult to establish definitively. The primary reason for this is that most psychological conditions do not necessarily develop immediately after a single event. As noted previously, there are complex interactions that occur in the development of a psychological condition. It can take months or years for many types of psychological conditions to develop. Thus, the careful review of existing medical and if available employment records must take place in order to more fully understand the individual's biopsychosocial history.

Further, it is now demonstrated through empirical research that most psychological conditions develop in adolescence (50%) and early adulthood (75%). Therefore, the probability that an individual was previously diagnosed with a psychological condition must be carefully assessed. Thorough assessment of the individual's past psychological history, the person's perception of whether past treatment was helpful, and any issues regarding treatment compliance must thoughtfully probed as well (Warren, 2013a, 2013b, 2016, 2017).

It is also important to consider the individual's co-workers who were exposed to the same workplace incident and whether there was any impact on the co-workers' functioning. This is a critical consideration for causation determination. The reason is that many States stipulate that the impetus for a claimed workplace psychological injury must be sudden and severe and is not something typically experienced as part of workplace duties. Thus, if the individual reports a psychological injury and, yet, co-workers continue to function at work, it is important to take into account whether a workplace event that is reported to cause a psychological injury is an unusual occurrence in the workplace.

When a person experiences a physical workplace injury, impairment in functioning may result. If impairment is present, it is observed in both the workplace and the individual's personal life. This is because impairment in functioning does not occur selectively, such as in only some settings. Valid impairment in functioning occurs across all aspects of life, no matter the setting. This is also true for valid psychological impairment in functioning. A common observation in WC claims is that some professionals opine that a psychological injury results in impairment in functioning in the workplace only. In reality, psychological impairment relates to specific types of cognitive functioning, such as short- and long-term memory, attention, decision-making, speaking, perceptual, and processing speed, among others, and is not specific to one environment, such as the workplace. Instead, valid psychological impairment in functioning occurs across all areas of the individual's life. The report of profound cognitive impairment requires extensive assessment of the reported deficits with neuropsychological testing. This type of test battery sorts out whether reported cognitive deficits objectively exist or are subjectively perceived (Akobeng, 2007; American Educational Research Association, American Psychological Association, and National Council on Measurement in Education, 2014; Heilbrun et al., 2009; Iverson, 2007; Naglieri, 2009; Stejskal, 2013).

Even if a psychological condition, such as Major Depressive Disorder (MDD), is determined to objectively exist, it does not mean that impairment in functioning exists as well. A diagnosis is the starting point for the psychological assessment process. This means that psychological testing is completed to confirm or rule out whether the condition exists and its severity. Moreover, most standardized psychological tests can identify the presence of both personality disorders and psychosocial issues (Warren, 2013a, 2013b, 2016, 2017).

Many personality disorders reflect the individual's weak self-concept, a tendency to express negative emotions in an uncontrolled manner, as well as a reduced capacity to adapt to others interpersonally. Those with personality disorders frequently have clear, long-standing patterns of disruptive behavior in the workplace and other settings. Personality disorders have specific *DSM* diagnostic criteria.

In contrast, psychosocial issues do not represent a condition or disorder. Instead, they are attitudes, beliefs, thoughts, and perceptions that are subjective in nature. This variation is due to the differences how one person perceives an event versus how another person views the same event. Psychosocial issues lack diagnostic criteria. This is because they are under voluntary control. Thus, psychosocial issues are not valid conditions (Hinkka, Kuoppala, Väänänen-Tomppo, & Lamminpää, 2013; Hofmann, 2016; Kahn & Langlieb, 2003; Warren, 2016, 2017).

In addition, it is essential to evaluate for symptom exaggeration (which is usually a person strongly endorsing valid symptoms that are experienced) versus malingering (e.g., conscious deception in which the person is falsely endorsing symptoms of a condition). Empirical research has consistently demonstrate 30–40% malingering for disability claims. This higher potential of fraud requires that all professionals do not rely on their opinion alone to determine whether a person is malingering since a professional opinion alone is wrong 50% of the time. Instead, malingering must be ruled out with the usage of a standardized psychological testing battery which has measures for test effort (Aronoff et al., 2007; Dersh et al., 2005; Flatten, 2013a, 2013b, 2013c; Iverson, 2007; Mittenberg, Patton, Canyock, & Condit, 2002).

Consequently, these additional factors further complicate the psychological causation determination process. In order answer fully and accurately, the professional must account for each of these factors and explain why these factors do not play a role in the individual's development of a psychological condition. If the professional does not do so, then, she/he is merely offering a professional opinion that may be colored by the professional's own perceptions and biases (Ropponen et al., 2012; Samuelsson, Ropponen, Alexanderson, & Svedberg, 2013a, 2013b) .

Frequently, the most honest and accurate answer regarding whether a psychological condition was caused by a workplace event was the direct cause of the psychological condition is "maybe." Then, an explanation of the multiple factors that are involved can take place. Otherwise, the professional who voices an opinion without this consideration is in danger of moving away from the current psychological standards of care and what is presently accepted within the scientific field of psychology (e.g., the *Daubert* standard). This type of professional opinion is vulnerable to a *Daubert* challenge. When a professional's opinion is challenged in legal proceedings because it does not meet current professional standards of care, such as in psychology, then all testimony by that professional is stricken from the court records.

When a professional loses a *Daubert* challenge, then credibility is lost. Moreover, a record of the professional losing the *Daubert* challenge is maintained and is discoverable in the future. Consequently, there are considerable consequences to those professionals who stray from current professional standards of care in their evaluation, treatment, and testimony of individuals with reported impairment in functioning (Kilgour, Kosny, Akkermans, & Collie, 2015; Kosny, MacEachen, Ferrier, & Chambers, 2011).

The *Daubert* standard and its utilization in WC settings are now explored in the next section.

7.5 Lack of Utilization of the *Daubert* Standard in WC Settings

The *Daubert* standard is currently used in tort legal proceedings. Under the *Daubert* standard, any professional testimony given is required to be based on five components:

(a) All presented evidence and data must be objective and reliable (e.g., valid and reliable in regard to psychological standards). This means that subjective information or opinion cannot be presented as evidence.
(b) All methodology employed by the professional must be peer-reviewed and published.
(c) All methodology used by the professional must have known potential rate of error that is known and controlled.
(d) Standards exist and are utilized by the professional in regard to the used techniques.
(e) The methodology is generally accepted within the appropriate scientific and professional field.

The *Evidence Rule 702* (2011) was later amended so that any professional testimony provided must be based on sufficient facts and date, reliable methods are employed, and the method application relates directly to the facts of the legal proceeding (*Daubert v. Merrell Dow Pharmaceuticals (*1993*)*, *General Electric Company v. Joiner (1997)*, *Kumho Tire Company v. Carmichael*; Young et al., 2007).

While the *Daubert* standard is used in State and federal tort legal procedures, it is not employed in WC procedures at present. Because the *Daubert* standard is not employed in WC, inappropriate professional treatment and professional testimony are frequently allowed that do not meet the current standards of psychological care to substantiate claims of a workplace psychological injury. Types of inappropriate professional documentation and testimony include imprecise diagnoses (e.g., non-*DSM* diagnoses), nonevidenced-based treatments, and inadequate documentation that do not objectively support the reported psychological injury. In addition, the majority of States do not stipulate specific types of professionals (e.g., psychologists and psychiatrists) who must treat individuals who report workplace psychological injuries. Therefore, many professionals, such as licensed clinical counselors and licensed social workers, are inappropriately allowed to submit documentation in support of a psychological injury claim. The reason that this is problematic is that those individuals do not have the same type of rigorous training and are not able to conduct the requisite standardized psychological testing. This results in much of the submitted documentation being based on the claimant's self-report and the professional's opinion alone (Warren, 2013a, 2013b).

Further examination of the effect of this inappropriate documentation and testimony inclusion results in legal causation being established based on subjective information. As discussed earlier, the development of a psychological condition is rarely straightforward with a single, identifiable cause (Grant & Robbins, 2003). In looking at empirical research, it is known that some individuals may be genetically predisposed to develop a psychological condition (Warren, 2005). Some psychological conditions, such as MDD *may* be more prevalent with gender, but gender alone does not cause a psychological condition (Kahn & Langlieb, 2003). One of the most intriguing and important empirical findings is that the majority of individuals who are exposed to traumatic event recover. Moreover, those individuals return to their previous level of functioning (Pflantz & Heidel, 2003). Finally, because there are multiple misattributions of causation, it is imperative for the professional to exclude primary gain, secondary, misperceptions, and malingering to routinely occur in the WC psychological injury evaluation process (Grant & Robbins, 2003; Parry, 2010; Parry & Drogin, 2007; Warren, 2013a, 2013b).

In general, the *Daubert* standard is not readily utilized in the State or federal WC claims or injury causation processes. This is because there are specific WC laws that apply instead. Recently though, this has changed in Florida, Kentucky, Massachusetts, and Oklahoma. All of these States now require that any provided documentation pertaining to the evaluation and treatment of individuals who have submitted WC claims must meet the *Daubert* standard. Thus, this is some movement toward the removing subjective and imprecise information from the WC process (*Giaimo v. Florida Autosport, Inc. 1D14-0077,* 2014 *WL 6679290 (Fla. 1st DCA, 11/26/14), City of Owensboro v. Adams, 135 S.W.3d. 446, 449-50 (Ky. 2004), (MCLE Mass Workers' Comp, 2nd ed., Chap.14,* 2010*), (85 O.S. Rules of the Workers' Compensation Court, Rule 20) Commonwealth v. Lanigan, 419 Mass. 15, 24–26 (*1994*); Commonwealth v. Powell, 450 Mass. 229, 238 (*2007*)*).

This move by those States is particularly salient because if the individual has exhausted the WC appeal process, the injured employee can appeal WC rulings in either the State Circuit or State Supreme Courts systems. Once the appeal enters either of these court systems, then the *Daubert* standard is applied to *all* submitted professional documentation and testimony. Thus, all previous documentation and testimony is scrutinized once again and if lacking in meeting the *Daubert* standard, it is stricken from consideration of the claim. This lack of consistent scientific standards in the WC causation determination process seems an obvious place to start to remove imprecision from it. However, there are other steps that must take place as well. These will be explored in the next section.

7.6 Evidence-Based Remedies to Address Current Deficiencies with Reported Workplace Psychological Injuries

There are a number of professional treatment guidelines that include duration guidelines as well. The professional treatment guidelines typically are developed by having multiple experts in that field review high-quality research to establish empirically supported best practice standards that should guide the treatment of a condition. Duration guidelines relate to how long a condition is typically present when treated appropriately. Duration guidelines have long been used in the insurance industry for case management purposes. In other words, duration guidelines spell out what normally occurs with a specific condition, such as usual symptoms, typical recovery estimates based on mild, moderate, and severe impairment in functioning. These estimates are used in terms of payment for disability benefits but also a general overview of when the person may be able to return to work.

While opponents opine that treatment guidelines oversimplify the assessment and treatment of all types of conditions, this determination was made by reviewing just a few studies. They report that guidelines are given too much weight when it comes to the treatment and claims approval processes. These concerns are voiced as though empirical findings are being employed inappropriately. However, this process of empirical research innovations being melded into professional standards of care is not new. Research is usually conducted to assess current treatment standards as well as to develop new methods to treat conditions. Thus, empirical research does not occur in a vacuum, but, with the purpose to move science and clinical practice forward. In an ideal world, professionals stay abreast of research to readily incorporate improvements in treatment. However, this does not occur. Thus, there is inconsistency in professional treatment that is provided, in particular in with psychological conditions.

When professionals provide less than optimal care than this can result in professionally caused poor treatment outcomes. This is called *professional iatrogenic disability*. It is caused in one of two ways. The first instance of professionally caused iatrogenic disability relates to the harm that can occur by an overt action by the professional, such as misdiagnosing a condition, providing the wrong treatment, or prescribing the wrong medication. This is particularly important in regard to psychological conditions. If a professional does not follow professional standards of care, such as utilizing standardized psychological testing to confirm or rule out a psychological condition, but merely opines that the condition exists, then the person may receive a medication for a condition that does not exist or may receive the wrong medication for the wrong condition. It is the diagnosis that drives the type of evidence-based treatment that a person receives. By employing empirically supported treatment, the individual has the best opportunity to return to the previous level of functioning once more. Moreover, empirical research has demonstrated that although some psychological conditions may go into remission without treatment, there are permanent changes that occur within brain structures that place the individual at much higher risk for relapse (Heilbrun et al., 2009; Jensen-Doss & Hawley, 2010; Maffeo, 1990).

The second manner in which well-meaning professionals may cause iatrogenic disability is when those professionals convey that the person is disabled or that the workplace is the source of the individual's concerns. Treating professionals play a considerable role in shaping patient beliefs, attitudes, and expectations regarding recovery and the return to work. When a treating professional tells a person she/he is disabled, then this conveys the message that the person will not recover and should not work. In regard to psychological conditions, there are very few conditions that are permanent and result in sustained impairment in functioning. Some conditions are Schizophrenia, dementia, or the cognitive impairment caused by a severe traumatic brain injury that can result in significant impairment in functioning permanently. However, other conditions, such as Major Depressive Disorder, anxiety disorders, or Post-Traumatic Stress Disorder, do not. This listing is not meant to be all inclusive. Instead, it is meant to demonstrate that the majority of psychological conditions have empirically supported treatments that restore the individual's functioning once more. This means that it is highly unusual for most individuals to be permanently impaired from psychological conditions and can no longer engage actively in life again. Most individuals with psychological conditions continue to actively participate in life, including working (Warren, 2013a, 2013b).

The inclusion of empirically supported professional standards of care into the States and federal WC systems can be beneficial in two ways. First, by legally mandating empirically supported standards into WC laws, it serves to remove professional causes of disability. In addition, it removes the inclusion of junk science or substandard documentation that is currently allowed to support WC psychological disability claims. Second, the usage of empirically supported treatment guidelines in the WC systems regarding WC psychological injuries provides the current state-of-the-art treatment to reduce impairment in functioning and to facilitate the individual's return to the workplace (MacEachen, Kosny, Ferrier, & Chambers, 2010; Mallon, Grizzell, Holland, & Hodgson, 2015; Nielsen et al., 2013).

Another issue that must be addressed in all WC systems is to remove all obsolete psychological terminology and diagnostic criteria in WC laws that currently exist. For example, some States have not updated their WC laws to reflect that the *DSM-*

IV-TR is no longer used. The *DSM-5* has been in use since 2013 (ApA, 2013). Moreover, some psychological conditions have had changes in either diagnostic criteria, name of the condition itself has changed (e.g., Dysthymic Disorder), or have been removed from the *DSM-5* (e.g., *Somatoform Disorder*). Thus, WC laws are not updated frequently enough to reflect ongoing changes in the psychological standards of care. This puts treating professionals who are trying to provide treatment that meets best practice standards in a precarious position. This is because psychologists are instructed to not use obsolete psychological tests through the American Psychological Association's *Ethical Principles of Psychologists and Code of Conduct, also called Code of Ethics* (see Chap. 5, Warren, 2016), and to provide treatment that meets current standards of care (Sects. 4.01, 2.03, and 4.04, Warren, 2016). Consequently, a psychologist or other treating professionals who provide documentation that meets current standards must recognize that the documentation may not meet those specific WC laws which stipulate the use of outdated methods to support psychological injury claims. In that instance, psychologists are obligated to make known the conflict between the psychologist's ethical obligation following APA *Code of Ethics*, pertaining to psychological testing and treatment standards and the WC law, exists. This must take the form of a detailed discussion in written form when evaluation and treatment documentation is submitted pertaining to WC psychological injury claims. Regardless of the specific WC system law, the psychologist is still ethically bound to follow appropriate psychological standards (GAO-07-943SP; GAO-15-593SP; Wickizer et al., 2011).

The most immediate manner in which to initiate profound change in all WC systems and laws is to legally mandate the *Daubert* standard in all professional documentation and testimony pertaining to WC injury claims. By doing so, this sets the same standard that is utilized in the tort system regarding the submission of documentation and testimony that meets standards of psychological care. Moreover, once a WC claimant has exhausted all appeals in a specific WC system, then that person can appeal to that State's or federal tort system to appeal the WC decision pertaining to the WC claim. However, all professional documentation will be reexamined to ensure that it meets the *Daubert* standard (Shaw 2016).

By including the *Daubert* standard across the legal system, consistency is essential to ensure that the imprecision currently exists in the WC systems is removed and professional documentation and testimony meets current standards of care. Through making this change, a higher degree of objectivity occurs. This is because there is melding of current standards of care into the legal decision-making process. This is done regularly with WC physical injury claims. The time has come to do the same with WC psychological injury claims as well. Only then will the inaccuracy and subjectivity that exist at present in the WC disability determination processes be addressed. The stakes are high for all parties. When the *Daubert* standard is legally mandated into the WC systems, it assists all parties involved in the WC disability processes to make more even-handed decisions that are in agreement with current psychological standards of care.

7.7 Conclusion

There are two primary WC systems in the United States: States and federal. Each system is entirely separate from any other WC system and governed by an individual set of statutes. Psychological injury is allowed in some States, while not in others. The States and federal WC system statutes do not align with current standards of psychological care. This allows a great deal of imprecision and lack of standardization into the WC claims processes. This leads to increased costs for open-ended workplace leave and for inappropriate claims of the existence of permanent psychological conditions with the majority of psychological injury claims.

Railroad employees are covered by FELA, which is a tort-based system. Psychological injury claims are allowed in the tort legal system. Because FELA is a tort-based system, any submitted documentation regarding workplace psychological injury must already meet the Daubert standard.

All WC systems have too much imprecision in the evaluation of purported psychological and claims process. A highly effective manner to address this imprecision is to include the *Daubert* standard in States and FECA WC pertaining to reported workplace psychological injury.

References

(85 O.S. Rules of the Workers' Compensation Court, Rule 20) *Commonwealth v. Lanigan*, 419 Mass. 15, 24–26 (1994).

§8105. Total disability and §8106. Partial disability. (n.d.). *U.S. Department of Labor – Office of Workers' Compensation Programs (OWCP) – Division of Federal Employees' Compensation (DFEC) – Federal Employees' Compensation Act*. Retrieved from http://www.dol.gov/owcp/dfec/regs/statutes/feca. htm#8105

Aas, I. M. (2011). Guidelines for rating Global Assessment of Functioning (GAF). *Annals of General Psychiatry, 10*(1), 2. https://doi.org/10.1186/1744-859x-10-2

Aas, I. M. (2014). Collecting information for rating global assessment of functioning (GAF): Sources of information and methods for information collection. *Current Psychiatry Reviews, 10*(4), 330–347.

Agency for Healthcare Research and Quality. (2016). *Library of Resources for Mental Health | Agency for Healthcare Research & Quality*. Retrieved from https://www.ahrq.gov/professionals/clinicians-providers/ehclibrary/mentalhealth/index.html

Akobeng, A. K. (2007). Understanding diagnostic tests 1: Sensitivity, specificity and predictive values. *Acta Paediatrica, 96*(3), 338–341.

American Educational Research Association, American Psychological Association, and National Council on Measurement in Education. (2014). *Standards for educational and psychological testing* (3rd ed.). Washington, DC: American Educational Research Association.

American Psychiatric Association. (2000). *Diagnostic and statistical manual of mental disorders: DSM-IV-TR*. Washington, DC: American Psychiatric Association.

American College of Occupational and Environmental Medicine (ACOEM). (2008). *Occupational medicine practice guidelines: Evaluation and management of common health problems and functional recovery in workers* (3rd ed.). Beverly Farms, MA: OEM Health Information Press.

American Psychiatric Association. (2013). *Diagnostic and statistical manual of mental disorders: DSM-5*. Washington, DC: American Psychiatric Association.

Aronoff, G. M., Mandel, S., Genovese, E., Maitz, E. A., Dorto, A. J., Klimek, E. H., et al. (2007). Evaluating malingering in contested injury or illness. *Pain Practice, 7*(2), 178–204.

Bacon, S. F., Collins, M. J., & Plake, E. V. (2002). Does the Global Assessment of Functioning assess functioning? *Journal of Mental Health Counseling, 24*, 202–212.

Barsky, A., & Kaplan, S. A. (2007). If you feel bad, it's unfair: A quantitative synthesis of affect and organizational justice perceptions. *Journal of Applied Psychology, 92*(1), 286–295. https://doi.org/10.1037/0021-9010.92.1.286

Barsky, A. J. (2002). Forgetting, fabricating, and telescoping: The instability of medical history. *Archives of Internal Medicine, 162*, 981–984.

Barth, R. J. (2012). Determining injury-relatedness, work-relatedness, and claim-relatedness. *AMA Guides Newsletter.*

Baumeister, H., Hutter, N., Bengel, J., & Härter, M. (2011). Quality of life in medically ill persons with comorbid mental disorders: A systematic review and meta-analysis. *Psychotherapy and Psychosomatics, 80*(5), 275–286. https://doi.org/10.1159/000323404

Baune, B. T., Caniato, R. N., Arolt, V., & Berger, K. (2009). The effects of dysthymic disorder on health-related quality of life and disability days in persons with comorbid medical conditions in the general population. *Psychotherapy and Psychosomatics, 78*(3), 161–166. https://doi.org/10.1159/000206870

Bender, M. (2016). *Workers' compensation index* (12th ed.). CA: Matthew Bender.

Brown v. W.T. Martin Plumbing & Heating, Inc., 2013 VT 38 (June 21, 2013).

Bruffaerts, R., Vilagut, G., Demyttenaere, K., Alonso, J., AlHamzawi, A., Andrade, L. H., et al. (2012). Role of common mental and physical disorders in partial disability around the world. *The British Journal of Psychiatry, 200*(6), 454–461. https://doi.org/10.1192/bjp.bp.111.097519

Bruns, D., Mueller, K., & Warren, P. A. (2010). A review of evidence-based biopsychosocial laws governing the treatment of pain and injury. *Psychological Injury and Law, 3*(3), 169–181.

Bruns, D., Mueller, K., & Warren, P. A. (2012). Biopsychosocial law, health care reform, and the control of medical inflation in Colorado. *Rehabilitation Psychology, 57*(2), 81–97.

City of Owensboro v. Adams, 135 S.W.3d. 446, 449-50 (Ky. 2004), (*MCLE Mass Workers' Comp*, 2nd ed., Chap.14, 2010).

Commonwealth v. Powell, 450 Mass. 229, 238 (2007).

Correio, R. F. (2015). *California: Rolda reloaded: A creative approach to the dual causation elements of the Rolda multi-level analysis*. Retrieved from https://wwwlexisnexis.com/legalnewsroom/workers-compensation/b/recent-cases-news-trends-developments/archive/2015/01/16/california-rolda-reloaded-a-creative-approach-to-the-dual-causation-elements-of-the-rolda-multi-level-analysis.aspx?Redirected=true

Daubert v. Merrell Dow Pharmaceuticals (92-102), 509, U.S. 579 (1993).

Department of Labor. (1995). *Part 2 – Claims*. Retrieved from http://www.dol.gov/owcp/dfec/regs/compliance/DFECFolio/ FECA-PT2.pdf

Department of Labor. (2007). *Injury compensation for federal employees*. Retrieved from http://www.dol.gov/owcp/dfec/regs/compliance/DFECFolio/agencyhb.pdf

Department of Labor. (2016). *United States Department of Labor*. Retrieved from https://www.dol.gov/

Dersh, J., Polatin, P., Leeman, G., & Gatchel, R. (2005). Secondary gains and losses in the medicolegal setting. In I. Z. Schultz & R. J. Gatchel (Eds.), *Handbook of complex occupational disability claims* (pp. 421–443). New York: Springer.

Division of Federal Employees' Compensation (DFEC). (n.d.). *U.S. Department of Labor – Office of Workers' Compensation Programs (OWCP) – Division of Federal Employees' Compensation (DFEC) Federal employees' compensation act*. Retrieved from http://www. dol.gov/owcp/dfec/regs/statutes/feca.htm

Division of Federal Employees' Compensation (DFEC) CA-11 When Injured at Work Information Guide for Federal Employees. (n.d.). *U.S. Department of Labor – Office of Workers' Compensation Programs (OWCP) – Division of Federal Employees' Compensation (DFEC) – Compliance – CA-11 When Injured at Work Information Guide for Federal Employees*. Retrieved from http://www.dol.gov/owcp/dfec/regs/compliance/ca-11.htm

Druss, B. G., Hwang, I., Petukhova, M., Sampson, N. A., Wang, P. S., & Kessler, R. C. (2008). Impairment in role functioning in mental and chronic medical disorders in the United States: Results from the National Comorbidity Survey Replication. *Molecular Psychiatry, 14*(7), 728–737. https://doi.org/10.1038/mp.2008.13

Druss, B. G., & Walker, E. R. (2011). *Mental disorders and medical comorbidity* (Research Synthesis Report 21). Retrieved from Robert Wood Johnson Foundation website: http://www.rwjf.org/en/library/research/2011/02/mental-disorders-and-medical-comorbidity.html

Elling, R. H. (1989). Workers' health, safety, and compensation in historical and cross-national perspective: An overview. *Annals of the New York Academy of Sciences, 572*, 240–255. https://doi.org/10.1111/j.1749-6632.1989.tb13610.x.

Escorpizo, R., & Stucki, G. (2013). Functioning and disability definitions. *Encyclopedia of Pain*, 1329–1335. https://doi.org/10.1007/978-3-642-28753-4_1121

Faust, D., Grimm, P. W., Ahern, D. C., & Sokolik, M. (2010). The admissibility of behavioral science evidence in the courtroom: The translation of legal to scientific concepts and back. *Annual Review of Clinical Psychology, 6*, 49–77. https://doi.org/10.1146/annurev.clinpsy.3.022806.091523

Faust, D., & Ziskin, J. (2012). *Coping with psychiatric and psychological testimony*. New York: Oxford University Press.

Federal Employers' Liability Act (FELA), 45 U.S.C. § 51 et seq. (1908).

First, M. B. (2010). Paradigm shifts and the development of the diagnostic and statistical manual of mental disorders: Past experiences and future aspirations. *The Canadian Journal of Psychiatry, 55*, 692–700.

Flatten, M. (2013a). *Disability can be easy street for federal bureaucrats* (p. 3). Washington, DC: Washington Examiner.

Flatten, M. (2013b). *Experts say fraud rampant in federal worker disability program* (p. 3). Washington, DC: Washington Examiner.

Flatten, M. (2013c). *Paralysis in congress keeps federal worker disability fraudsters cashing the checks* (p. 3). Washington, DC: Washington Examiner.

Furlan, A. D., Gnam, W. H., Carnide, N., Irvin, E., Amick, B. C., DeRango, K., et al. (2012). Systematic review of intervention practices for depression in the workplace. *Journal of Occupational Rehabilitation, 22*, 312–321.

Gatchel, R. J. (2013a). Disability assessment, psychological/ psychological evaluation. *Encyclopedia of Pain*, 993–995. https://doi.org/10.1007/978-3-642-28753-4_1122

Gatchel, R. J. (2013b). The biopsychosocial model of chronic pain. *Chronic Pain*, 5–17. https://doi.org/10.2217/ebo.13.469

General Electric Co. v. Joiner, 522 U.S. 1136, 118 S. Ct. 512, 139 L Ed. 2d 508.

Gholizadeh, S., Malcarne, V. L., & Schatman, M. E. (2015). Ethical quandaries for psychologists in workers' compensation settings: The GAF gaffe. *Psychological Injury and Law, 8*(1), 64–81.

Giaimo v. Florida Autosport, Inc. 1D14-0077, 2014 WL 6679290 (Fla. 1st DCA, 11/26/14).

Gili, M., Comas, A., García-García, M., Monzón, S., Antoni, S., & Roca, M. (2010). Comorbidity between common mental disorders and chronic somatic diseases in primary care patients. *General Hospital Psychiatry, 32*(3), 240–245. https://doi.org/10.1016/j.genhosppsych.2010.01.013

Gilovich, T., Griffin, D. W., & Kahneman, D. (2002). *Heuristics and biases: The psychology of intuitive judgement*. Cambridge, UK: Cambridge University Press.

Grant, B. L., & Robbins, D. B. (2003). Disability and workers' compensation. In *Mental health and productivity in the workplace: A handbook for organizations and clinicians* (pp. 347–368). San Francisco: Jossey-Bass.

Grove, W. M., Zald, D. H., Lebow, B. S., Snitz, B. E., & Nelson, C. (2000). Clinical versus mechanical prediction: A meta-analysis. *Psychological Assessment, 12*(1), 19–30.

Hadjistavropoulos, T., & Bieling, P. (2001). File review consultation in the adjudication of mental health and chronic pain disability claims. *Consulting Psychology Journal: Practice and Research, 53*(1), 52–63.

Hamm, R. M., Reiss, D. M., Paul, R. K., & Bursztajn, H. J. (2007). Knocking at the wrong door: Insured workers' inadequate psychiatric care and workers' compensation claims. *International Journal of Law and Psychiatry, 30*, 416–426.

Hamp, A., Stamm, K., Lin, L., & Christidis, P. (2016). *2015 APA survey of psychology health service providers*. APA Center for Workforce Studies. Retrieved October 30, 2017.

Harding, T. P. (2004). Psychiatric disability and clinical decision making: The impact of judgment error and bias. *Clinical Psychology Review, 24*, 707–729.

Hees, H. L., Nieuwenhuijsen, K., Koeter, M. W., Bultmann, U., & Schene, A. H. (2012). Towards a new definition of return to work outcomes in common mental disorders from a multi-stakeholder perspective. *PLoS One, 7*(6), e39947.

Heilbrun, K., Grisso, T., & Goldstein, A. M. (2009). *Foundations of forensic mental health assessment*. New York: Oxford University Press.

Henderson, J. A., Kysar, D. A., & Pearson, R. N. (2017). *The torts process* (9th ed.). Frederick, MD: Wolters, Kluwver, Aspen Casebook.

Hinkka, K., Kuoppala, J., Väänänen-Tomppo, I., & Lamminpää, A. (2013). Psychosocial work factors and sick leave, occupational accident, and disability pension. *Journal of Occupational and Environmental Medicine, 55*(2), 191–197.

Hofmann, B. (2016). Medicalization and overdiagnosis: Different but alike. *Medicine, Health Care, and Philosophy, 19*, 253–264.

Howard, C. (2002). Workers' compensation: Federalism, and the heavy hand of history. *Studies in American Political Development, 16*(S), 28–47. https://doi.org/10.1017/S0898588X02000020

Ireton v. Horizon Mental Health Mgmt., LLC, 2016 Tenn.

Iverson, G. L. (2007). Identifying exaggeration and malingering. *Pain Practice, 7*(2), 94–102.

Jensen-Doss, A., & Hawley, K. M. (2010). Understanding barriers to evidence-based assessment: Clinician attitudes toward standardized assessment tools. *Journal of Clinical Child and Adolescent Psychology, 39*(6), 885–896. https://doi.org/10.1080/15374416.2010.517169

Jensen-Doss, A., & Hawley, K. M. (2011). Understanding clinicians' diagnostic practices: Attitudes toward the utility of diagnosis and standardized diagnostic tools. *Administration and Policy in Mental Health and Mental Health Services Research, 38*(6), 476–485. https://doi.org/10.1007/s10488-011-0334-3

Kahn, J. P., & Langlieb, A. M. (2003). *Mental health and productivity in the workplace: A handbook for organizations and clinicians*. San Francisco: Jossey-Bass.

Kertay, L., Eskay-Auerbach, M., & Hyman, M. (2016). *AMA guides to navigating disability benefit systems: Essentials for the health care professional*. Chicago: American Medical Association.

Kilgour, E., Kosny, A., Akkermans, A., & Collie, A. (2015). Procedural justice and the use of independent medical evaluations in workers' compensation. *Psychological Injury and Law, 8*(2), 153–168.

Kosny, A., MacEachen, E., Ferrier, S., & Chambers, L. (2011). The role of health care providers in long term and complicated workers' compensation claims. *Journal of Occupational Rehabilitation, 21*(4), 582–590. https://doi.org/10.1007/s10926-011-9307-3

Kumho Tire Co. v. Carmichael, 526 U.S. 137 (1999).

Ladou, J. (2009). Federal employees' compensation act. *International Journal of Occupational and Environmental Health, 15*(2), 180–194.

Larson, A., Larson, L. K., & Matthew Bender (Firm). (2016). *Larson's workers' compensation law*. New York: Matthew Bender.

Laws, C., & Colon, D. (2012). *Comorbidities in workers' compensation*. Available at https://www.ncci.com/documents/Research-BriefComorbidities-in-Workers-Compensation-2012.pdf

Ma, H. (2014). Collecting information for rating global assessment of functioning (GAF) sources of information and methods for information collection. *Current Psychiatry Reviews, 10*(4), 330–347.

MacEachen, E., Kosny, A., Ferrier, S., & Chambers, L. (2010). The "toxic dose" of system problems: Why some injured workers don't return to work as expected. *Journal of Occupational Rehabilitation, 20*(3), 349–366.

Maffeo, P. A. (1990). Substantiating psychological injury under the federal employees' compensation act. *Behavioral Sciences & the Law, 8*(4), 435–445.

Mallon, T. M., Grizzell, T., Holland, L., & Hodgson, M. (2015). Managing federal workers' compensation injuries and costs. *Journal of Occupational and Environmental Medicine, 57*, S12–S19. https://doi.org/10.1097/jom.0000000000000410

Melhorn, J.M., Talmage, J.T., Hyman, M.H. (2011). *AMA guides to the evaluation of work ability and return to work (2nd ed.)*. American Medical Association. Chicago, IL.

Melhorn, J.M., Talmage, J.T., Ackerman, W.E., Hyman, M.H. (2013). *AMA guides to disease and injury causation (2nd ed)*. American Medical Association. Chicago, IL.

Mittenberg, W., Patton, C., Canyock, E. M., & Condit, D. C. (2002). Base rates of malingering and symptom exaggeration. *Journal of Clinical and Experimental Neuropsychology (Neuropsychology, Development and Cognition: Section A), 24*(8), 1094–1102.

Mortelmans, K. (2013). Return-to-work in sick-listed employees with major depressive disorder. *TBV – TIJDSCHRIFT VOOR BEDRIJFS- EN VERZEKERINGSGENEESKUNDE, 21*(8), 384–384. https://doi.org/10.1007/s12498-013-0177-9

Murphey, D., Barry, M., & Vaughn, B. (2013). *Mental health disorders* (1st ed. [ebook], pp. 1–6). Available at: http://www.childtrends.org/wp-content/uploads/2013/03/Child_Trends-2013_01_01_AHH_MentalDisordersl.pdf. Accessed 15 July 2017.

Naglieri, J. (2009). Psychometric issues in the assessment of impairment. *Assessing Impairment*, 49–57. https://doi.org/10.1007/978-1-387-87542-2_5

Nielsen, M., Madsen, I., Bultmann, U., Christensen, U., Diderichsen, F., & Rugulies, R. (2013). Encounters between workers sick-listed with common mental disorders and return-to-work stakeholders. Does workers' gender matter? *Scandinavian Journal of Public Health, 41*, 191–197.

Parry, J. (2010). *Civil mental disability law, evidence and testimony: A comprehensive reference manual for lawyers, judges and mental disability professionals*. Chicago: American Bar Association, Commission on Mental and Physical Disability Law.

Parry, J., & Drogin, E. Y. (2007). *Mental disability law, evidence, and testimony: A comprehensive reference manual for lawyers, judges, and mental disability professionals*. Washington, DC: American Bar Association, Commission on Mental and Physical Disability Law.

Pflanz, S. E., & Heidel, S. H. (2003). Psychiatric causes of workplace problems. In J. P. Kahn & A. M. Langlieb (Eds.), *Mental health and productivity in the workplace: A handbook for organizations and clinicians* (pp. 276–296). San Francisco, CA, US: Jossey-Bass.

Preiss, K., Brennan, L., & Clarke, D. (2013). A systematic review of variables associated with the relationship between obesity and depression. *Obesity Reviews, 14*(11), 906–918. https://doi.org/10.1111/obr.12052

Ramirez, A., Ekselius, L., & Ramklint, M. (2013). Axis IV – Psychosocial and environmental problems – In the DSM-IV. *Journal of Psychiatric and Mental Health Nursing*. https://doi.org/10.1111/jpm.12009

Ranavaya, M. I., & Rondinelli, R. D. (2000). The major US disability and compensation systems: Origins and historical overview. In R. D. Rondinelli & R. T. Katz (Eds.), *Impairment rating and disability evaluation* (pp. 3–16). Philadelphia: WB Saunders Co.

Roca, M., Gili, M., Garcia-Garcia, M., Salva, J., Vives, M., Garcia Campayo, J., et al. (2009). Prevalence and comorbidity of common mental disorders in primary care. *Journal of Affective Disorders, 119*(1–3), 52–58. https://doi.org/10.1016/j.jad.2009.03.014

Rolda v. Pitney Bowes, Inc. (2001) 66 Cal. Comp Cases 241. Labor Code Section 3208.3.

Ropponen, A., Svedberg, P., Huunan-Seppala, A., Koskenvuo, K., Koskenvuo, M., Alexanderson, K., et al. (2012). Personality traits and life dissatisfaction as risk factors for disability pension due to low back diagnoses: A 30-year longitudinal cohort study of Finnish twins. *Journal of Psychosomatic Research, 73*(4), 29–294.

Samuelsson, A., Ropponen, A., Alexanderson, K., & Svedberg, P. (2013a). A prospective cohort study of disability pension due to mental diagnoses: The importance of health factors and behaviors. *BMC Public Health, 13*(1), 621. https://doi.org/10.1186/1471-2458-13-621

Samuelsson, A., Ropponen, A., Alexanderson, K., & Svedberg, P. (2013b). Psychosocial working conditions, occupational groups, and risk of disability pension due to mental diagnoses: A cohort study of 43,000 Swedish twins. *Scandinavian Journal of Work Environmental Health, 39*(4), 351–360.

Schultz, I. Z. (2008). Disentangling the disability quagmire in psychological injury: Part 1–disability and return to work: Theories, methods, and applications. *Psychological Injury and Law, 1*, 94–102.

Schultz, I. Z. (2009). Determining disability: New advances in conceptualization and research. *Psychological Injury and Law, 2*(3–4), 199–204.

Schultz, I. Z., & Gatchel, R. J. (2015). *Handbook of return to work: From research to practice*. Boston: Springer.

Sengupta, I., Reno, V. P., Burton, J. F., Jr., & Baldwin, M. L. (2012). *Workers' compensation: Benefits, coverage, and costs, 2010*. National Academy of Social Insurance, August 2012. Available at SSRN: https://ssrn.com/abstract=2131336

Shaw, L. (2016). Working with stakeholders in return to work processes: Multisystem interactions. *Handbooks in Health, Work, and Disability*, 327–336. https://doi.org/10.1007/978-1-4899-7627-7_18

Spengler, P. M., White, M. J., Egisdottir, S., Maugherman, A. S., Lampropoulos, G. K., Walker, B. S., et al. (2009). The meta-analysis of clinical judgment project: Effects of experience on judgment accuracy. *The Counseling Psychologist, 37*(3), 350–399. https://doi.org/10.1177/0011000006295149

Stejskal, W. J. (2013). Psychological testing in workplace disability evaluations. In L. H. Gold & D. L. Vanderpool (Eds.), *Clinical guide to mental disability evaluations* (pp. 127–154). New York: Springer.

Stolper, E., Van de Wiel, M., Van Royen, P., Van Bokhoven, M., Van der Weijden, T., & Dinant, G. J. (2011). Gut feelings as a third track in general practitioners' diagnostic reasoning. *Journal of General Medicine, 26*(2), 197–203.

Talmage, J. B. (2007). Failure to communicate: How terminology and forms confuse the work ability/disability evaluation process. *Journal of Insurance Medicine, 39*, 192–198.

Tanabe, R. P. (2013). *Workers' compensation laws: As of January 2013*. Cambridge, MA: Workers Compensation Research Institute. International Association of Industrial Accident Boards and Commissions &Workers Compensation Research Institute.

U.S. Department of Labor – Office of Workers' Compensation Programs (OWCP) – Division of Federal Employees' Compensation (DFEC) Compliance – Federal Employees' Compensation Act. (n.d.). Retrieved from http://www.dol.gov/owcp/dfec/regs/compliance/ fecafact.htm

U.S. Department of Labor – Office of Workers' Compensation Programs (OWCP) – FECA. (n.d.). Retrieved from http://www.dol.gov/owcp/regs/compliance/ca_feca.htm

U.S. Government Accountability Office. (2007). *Modernizing federal disability policy (GAO-07-934SP)*. Retrieved from U.S. Govt. Accountability Office website: http://www.gao.gov/products/ GAO-07-934SP

U.S. Government Accountability Office. (2012). *Federal employees' compensation act: Analysis of proposed changes on USPS beneficiaries (GAO-13-142R)*. Retrieved from http://www.gao.gov/products/GAO-13-142R

U.S. Government Accountability Office. (2014a). *Enhanced policies and management focus needed to address potential physician-assisted fraud (GAO-15-19)*. Retrieved from http://gao.gov/assets/670 /666830.pdf

U.S. Government Accountability Office. (2014b). *Railroad retirement board: Total and permanent disability program at risk for improper payments*.

U.S. Government Accountability Office. (2014c). *Retirement security: Oversight of the national railroad retirement investment trust. (GAO-14-312)*. Retrieved from http://gao.gov/products/GAO-14-312

U.S. Government Accountability Office. (2015a). *Railroad retirement board: Actions needed to reduce continued risk of fraud and improper payments (GAO-15-535T)*. Retrieved from http://www.gao. gov/products/GAO-15-535T

U.S. Government Accountability Office. (2015b). *A framework for managing fraud risks in federal programs (GAO-15-593SP)*. Retrieved from United States Government Accountability Office website: http://www.gao.gov/products/GAO-15-593SP

U.S. Government Accountability Office. (2015c). *Disability insurance: Preliminary observations on overpayments and beneficiary work reporting (GAO-15-673T)*. Retrieved from http://www.gao. gov/products/GAO-15-673T

U.S. Government Accountability Office. (2016). *2016 annual report: Additional opportunities to reduce fragmentation, overlap, and duplication and achieve other financial benefits (GAO-16-375SP)*. Retrieved from http://www.gao.gov/products/GAO-16-375SP#mt= e-report

U.S. Government Accountability Office. (2018) Railroad retirement board: *Actions needed to improve the effectiveness and oversite of continuing disability reviews*. (GAO-18-287). Retrieved from http://www.gao.gov.products/GAO-18-287.

U.S. Railroad Retirement Board. (2004). *General conditions under which a person is entitled to a railroad retirement employee annuity. Form G-177*. http://www.rrb.gov

U.S. Railroad Retirement Board. (2009). *Employee disability benefits. Form RB-1d*. http://www.rrb.gov

U.S. Railroad Retirement Board. (2015). *How works affects your disability annuity. Form AB-31 (12-15)*. http://www.rrb.gov

Vatnaland, T., Vatnaland, J., Friis, S., & Opjordsmoen, S. (2007). Are GAF scores reliable in routine clinical use? *Acta Psychiatrica Scandinavica, 115*(4), 326–330.

Wakefield, J. C. (2010). Misdiagnosing normality: Psychiatry's failure to address the problem of false positive diagnoses of mental disorder in a changing professional environment. *Journal of Mental Health, 19*(4), 337–351. https://doi.org/10.3109/09638237.2010.492418

Walker, E. R., McGee, R. E., & Druss, B. G. (2015). Mortality in mental disorders and global disease burden implications. *JAMA Psychiatry, 72*(4), 334. https://doi.org/10.1001/jamapsychiatry.2014.2502

Wang, P. S., Sergio, A., AlHamzawi, A. O., Alonso, J., Andrade, L. H., Angermeyer, M. C., et al. (2010). Treated and untreated prevalence of mental disorders: Results from the World Health Organization World Mental Health (WMH) surveys. In: *Oxford textbook of community mental health*. doi:https://doi.org/10.1093/med/9780199565498.003.0027.

Warren, P. A. (2005). *The management of workplace mental health issues and appropriate disability prevention strategies*. Encinitas, CA: Work Loss Data Institute.

Warren, P. A. (2010). *Behavioral health disability: Innovations in prevention and management*. New York: Springer.

Warren, P. A. (2013a). Those who hesitate are lost: The case for setting behavioral health treatment and disability standards, part I. *Psychological Injury and Law, 6*(3), 183–195. https://doi.org/10.1007/s12207-013-9163-x

Warren, P. A. (2013b). Those who hesitate are lost: The case for setting behavioral health treatment and disability standards, part II. *Psychological Injury and Law, 6*(3), 196–207. https://doi.org/10.1007/s12207-013-9164-9

Warren, P. A. (2013c). Those who hesitate are lost: The case for setting behavioral health treatment and disability standards, part III. *Psychological Injury and Law, 6*(3), 208–214. https://doi.org/10.1007/s12207-013-9169-4

Warren, P. A. (2016). The usage of the *AMA Guides* for the determination of psychological injury within the state and federal workers' compensation systems. *Psychological Injury and Law, 9*(4), 313–340. https://doi.org/10.1007/s12207-016-9273-3

Warren, P. A. (2017). Imprecision in the evaluation of workers' compensation psychological injury claims. *AMA Guides Newsletter, May/June,* 4–12 and 16.

Wickizer, T., Franklin, G., Fulton-Kehoe, D., Gluck, J., Mootz, R., Smith-Weller, T., et al. (2011). Improving quality, preventing disability and reducing costs in workers' compensation healthcare: A population-based intervention study. *Medical Care, 49*(12), 1105–1111.

Young, G., Kane, A. W., Nicholson, K., & Shuman, D. W. (2007). *Causality of psychological injury: Presenting evidence in court*. New York: Springer.

Chapter 8
Psychiatric Issues in Behavioral Health Disability

Bettina B. Kilburn

8.1 Epidemiology and Prevalence of Psychological and Behavioral Health Concerns in Psychiatry

8.1.1 Psychiatry as a Medical Specialty

Psychiatrists are physicians (Doctors of Medicine or Doctors of Osteopathy) who specialize in the prevention, diagnosis, and treatment of mental, addictive, and emotional disorders, for example, psychoses, depression and other mood disorders, anxiety disorders, substance abuse disorders, developmental disabilities, sexual dysfunctions, and adjustment reactions (Reed, 2005). Psychiatrists have received specialized training in the biological, psychological, and social components of illness and can order laboratory tests and prescribe medications, as well as evaluate and treat psychological and interpersonal problems. Psychiatrists also intervene with individuals and families who are coping with crises and other problems. Psychiatric training includes broad skills in psychiatric and medical diagnosis, formal psychotherapies, and psychopharmacology. Some psychiatrists have received further training in more specialized areas such as psychoanalysis, alcohol and substance abuse, geriatrics, neuropsychiatry, or forensic psychiatry.

In real practice, many individuals with treatable mental disorders do not necessarily receive specialty psychiatric or other mental health evaluation and care. A study of a large national sample ($n = 77{,}183$) examined the healthcare visits made by individuals who self-reported significant symptoms of depression and found that only 14.3% of their total healthcare visits were to specialty mental health professionals, such as psychiatrists, psychologists, or mental health social workers (Druss, Rosenheck, Sledge, 2000). Another study of general medical, high-utilizing patients in primary healthcare clinic (patients who made an average of 15 visits and 15

B. B. Kilburn (✉)
Disability Research and Consulting, LLC, Atlanta, GA, USA

P. A. Warren (ed.), *Handbook of Behavioral Health Disability Management*,
https://doi.org/10.1007/978-3-319-89860-5_8

telephone calls to the clinic during the course of a year) found that at some point in their lives, 83.5% of those high utilizers had suffered from a psychiatric condition for which they had not received appropriate diagnosis or treatment. The most common disorders were Major Depressive Disorder, Dysthymic Disorder, Generalized Anxiety Disorder, and Somatization Disorder (Katon et al., 1990). Some researchers have estimated that half of all visits to primary care doctors result from symptoms unexplained by a physical illness but often associated with a psychiatric condition, most frequently a mood or anxiety disorder (Kroenke & Mangesldorff, 1989). Even after extensive medical evaluation, mental disorders are not often diagnosed or treated (Barsky, Delamanter, & Orav, 1999).

8.1.2 Psychiatry and Behavioral Health Disability

Each year, millions of American workers develop health problems that may prevent them from reentering the workforce, temporarily or permanently. In most cases, employees are able to stay at work or return to work after a brief recovery period. However, approximately 10% of these workers incur significant work absences and/or life disruptions that can lead to prolonged or permanent withdrawal from the workforce (ACOEM, 2006). During this non-working period, these individuals are described as "disabled," and many become involved in one or more of the existing disability systems and laws, for example, sick leave, workers' compensation, short-term disability, long-term disability, Social Security Disability Insurance, or the Americans with Disabilities Act (ADA). The estimated cost of disability benefits paid under all these systems exceeds $100 billion (ACOEM, 2006). As noted earlier in this book, mental health issues are involved in the largest portion of disability claims made.

The National Institute of Mental Health estimates that 1 in every 20 adults will be depressed in any given year, and the World Health Organization predicts that major depressive disorder will be the second leading cause of disability by 2020 (NIMH, 2001). A study using the National Comorbidity Survey Replication stimated that approximately half of the Americans will meet the criteria for a mental disorder at some point in their lives (Kessler et al., 2005).

The economic, social, and quality-of-life burdens of untreated or undertreated mental disorders are tremendous. Without appropriate intervention, mental disorders can be as debilitating as any chronic major illness (Lepine, 2002; Simon, 2003). Some rank Major Depressive Disorder as the third leading cause of loss measured in quality-adjusted life years (QALYs), after arthritis and heart disease and ahead of chronic lung disease, diabetes, stroke, and cancer. In particular, Major Depressive Disorder that co-occurs with a nonpsychiatric medical illness is a significant "compounder" of debility (Lecrubier, 2001; Simon et al., 2000; Unutzer et al., 1997). Major Depressive Disorder can significantly increase the rehospitalization rate and mortality rate of cardiac patients (Allison et al., 1995). It is associated with poor glycemic control and increased risk of complications in diabetics (Egede, 2004; Lustman, Griffith, & Clouse, 1997).

The economic costs of mental disorders go well beyond the direct cost of treatment for them, their compounding of direct healthcare costs for co-occurring medical conditions, and the costs of disability claims paid. Psychiatric disorders generate substantial indirect costs related to unemployment, absenteeism, and lack of productivity at work. Major Depressive Disorder (MDD) is one of the top five issues associated with work loss and presenteeism (an ill employee working at less than full capacity) (Kessler et al., 2001; Rossi, 2001). American employers spend at least an estimated $33 billion yearly related to indirect costs of MDD alone (Greenberg et al., 1996).

For the psychiatrist, the extent and impact of mental disorders, co-occurring conditions, disability issues, and economic and other costs have significant implications. By providing effective and collaborative treatment, aimed at maintaining and restoring function, the psychiatrist is in a position to improve an individual's overall health function by many measures, increase quality of life for mentally ill individuals and families, and impact the multidimensional costs of mental illness.

8.2 The Usual Treatment Process and the Role of the Psychiatrist

8.2.1 The Traditional Treatment Approach and the Paradigm Shift

Traditional medical thinking is that recovery from illness or injury requires work and withdrawal from work. Traditional psychiatric thinking has been consistent with this approach, particularly if the psychiatrist thinks his or her patient needs to "be away from" the demands of a stressor, such as his or her work situation, in order to recover from a mental illness. In recent years, this paradigm has begun to shift, as psychiatrists and other medical professionals recognize that people recover better and faster if they stay active and engaged in life as much as possible during episodes of illness, including period(s) of mental illness (Gerdtham & Johannesson, 2003; Harris et al., 2005; Krause et al., 2001). Disrupting a worker's daily life with unnecessary prolonged work absence can cause unnecessary and significant harm to his or her well-being and detract from robust recovery. While on extended disability status, many individuals lose social relationships with coworkers, the self-respect associated with earning a living, and a major part of their identity – their occupation or vocation. Recent research confirms that workers receiving disability benefits recover less quickly and with poorer clinical outcomes than those with the same conditions who do not receive disability benefits, and that people who never lose time from work have better outcomes than people who lose some time from work (Bartley, 1994; Harris et al., 2005; Jin, Shah, & Svoboda, 1995).

8.2.2 The Usual Treatment Process

As noted below (see Sect. 8.4.1), an individual may enter the psychiatric treatment process in a number of ways. If another provider, such as a primary care physician or non-physician mental health provider has already seen the patient, he or she may intend that the psychiatrist provide consultation or that the psychiatrist is to be the (new) primary source of mental health treatment. It is important that the psychiatrist have a clear understanding of his or her intended role. For example, if the psychiatrist is the primary mental healthcare provider, will the psychiatrist be the only provider prescribing psychotropic medications? Will the primary care physician enforce this if the patient misses psychiatric appointments but contacts the primary care physician for medication refills? If the referral source is a psychotherapy provider, does he or she plan to continue the patient's participation in psychotherapy with him or her?

The psychiatrist may spend 60–90 min on an initial clinical evaluation. The purposes of a general psychiatric evaluation (see Sect. 8.3.1) include establishing a psychiatric diagnosis and formulating a treatment plan, taking into account other professionals who may already be involved in the patient's treatment. To reach these aims, several evaluative sessions may be needed.

Once the psychiatrist establishes a diagnosis, the treatment plan should include determining the treatment setting, establishing and maintaining a therapeutic alliance, monitoring the patient's psychiatric status and safety, providing education to patients and families, enhancing treatment compliance (see Sect. 8.7.3), and working with patients to address early signs of relapse (American Psychiatric Association (APA), 2006). The APA has developed, updated, and published evidence-based guidelines specific to many mental disorders (APA, 2003–2016). The presence of a co-occurring substance abuse disorder, personality disorder, or medical condition impacts the treatment planning for any mental disorder.

"Split treatment," in which a psychiatrist's primary role is medication management while another mental health provider serves as a psychotherapist, is frequent in mental health treatment. This offers the advantage of enhanced monitoring of issues such as malingering, compliance, etc., gives each provider another set of "eyes and ears" for observations, and gives clear definition to the psychiatrist's role. However, the prescription of psychotropic medications carries with it psychotherapeutic implications and vice versa, making it critical that in a "split" treatment context, psychiatrist and psychotherapist are in agreement on their approaches and goals. "Split" treatment has the potential disadvantages of mixed communication to the patient and inconsistent (and therefore ineffective) treatment, especially if the psychiatrist and psychotherapist do not see themselves as a team. If more than one clinician is involved in providing the care, it is essential that all treating clinicians have sufficient ongoing contact with the patient and with each other to ensure that relevant information is available to guide treatment decisions.

For many disorders, especially if the psychiatrist is prescribing psychotropic medications, he or she will see the patient more frequently during the initial phase of treatment. For example, many antidepressant medications take 4–8 weeks to achieve moderate to full response. During this time, the psychiatrist may see the patient every 2 weeks to monitor response and side effects. If the patient has not responded or cannot tolerate side effects, the psychiatrist will reevaluate the treatment. Once a patient is responding to medication, the frequency of visits often decreases to once monthly or less often, while the psychiatrist makes further adjustments and then transitions the patient to a maintenance treatment schedule of once every 2–3 months.

The usual treatment process does not necessarily take into account that inability to work is a psychiatric crisis, one that demands an immediate and focused response from mental health providers (see Sect. 8.4.3) (American Psychiatric Foundation, Partnership for Workplace Mental Health, 2005). As do other psychiatric crises, inability to work due to mental disorder requires immediate and intensive treatment to prevent or minimize loss of function and/or to restore function. Immediate and intensive crisis-oriented treatment, rather than treatment every few weeks or months as per the usual treatment process, is indicated until the crisis is resolved and work function is stable or restored. Specific treatment considerations are discussed in Sect. 8.9.

8.2.3 Avoiding Dual Roles

If an individual has filed a disability or workers' compensation claim, a non-clinical third party, such as the Social Security Administration, insurer, or an attorney representing the individual ("claimant"), may ask a psychiatrist to evaluate the person independently (to perform an independent medical examination or "IME") at some point during the adjudication of the claim. A claims payer may also ask a psychiatrist to review available records for the purpose of determining the extent of functional capacity and/or impairment the records support, and/or answering other specific questions. When he or she is acting in any of these situations, the psychiatrist is applying his or her scientific and clinical expertise in a *legal* context and by definition is acting in a forensic role (AAPL, 2005).

Psychiatrists who take on a forensic role for the patients they are treating may adversely affect the therapeutic relationship with them. There are multiple reasons why a dual treatment and forensic relationship are not advisable. Psychiatry has delineated the conflicts inherent in the dual role to a greater extent than have other medical and surgical specialties (Morgan, 2006; Reid, 1993; Starsburger, Gutheil, & Brodsky, 1997). The purpose and goals of the treating psychiatrist are fundamentally different from those of the psychiatrist in a forensic role.

The treating provider has fiduciary and ethical obligations to the patient, which demand that he or she place the patient's interests before all else. In a treatment relationship, the patient has a right to rely on this attitude in the healthcare provider during (*and after*) the treatment relationship. The patient has the right to expect a single, private treatment role from his or her psychiatrist. This right is a cornerstone of the patient's ability to engage in treatment fully, free of concerns about future divulging of confidences, betrayal, or exploitation. On the contrary, the forensic consultant's responsibilities are to objectivity. Both the law and professional ethics demand that the forensic professional be objective in both commission and omission; he or she has no obligation to the claimant, litigant, or "evaluee" (and does not refer to that person as his or her "patient") (Starsburger et al., 1997).

A treating psychiatrist who endeavors to fulfill the conflicting duties to the primacy of the patient's interest *and* the objectivity that the forensic role demands is attempting an extraordinarily difficult, if not impossible, task. Having spent many hours (perhaps dozens or hundreds) working with a patient, sometimes quite intimately, a psychiatrist, understandably, often feels a personal affinity for that patient's viewpoint. There is thus a danger of *intentional* bias toward the patient. Separate from the psychiatrist's conscious awareness of a duty or wish to act in the patient's interest, he or she should be keenly aware of the obligation to "do no harm" to the patient. Even if a psychiatrist attempts to be objective in forensic reports or testimony, there is a danger of *unintended* bias toward the patient.

On a practical level, forensic evaluations often require examination of corroborative information and/or interview of corroborative sources, exposing information to third party or public scrutiny or subjecting the evaluee and the treatment process itself to cross-examination. The conflicts inherent in the differing clinical and forensic roles may also undermine the credibility of the forensic evaluation and the practitioner. For these reasons, treating psychiatrists should generally *avoid* performing forensic evaluations of their patients or acting as expert witnesses for their patients (AAPL, 2005, italics mine).

8.2.4 The Treating Psychiatrist as "Advocate"

Serving as an advocate, especially for rights of the mentally ill and the destigmatization of mental illness, has long been a part of the traditional role for the psychiatrist in many settings. The treating psychiatrist may see his or her role in relation to the disability claimant as one of advocating on behalf of the claimant against a system or insurer who is "denying benefits" to which the claimant is "entitled," "discriminating" against the claimant, etc. In fact, the psychiatrist's duty is to his or her patients, for whose health and interests he or she must advocate. However, advocating for the claimant's health and interests does not equate to advocating for benefit payments and need not involve an adversarial posture. It also does not mean advocating for whatever the claimant wants. Frequently, being a mental health advocate means promoting full participation in work and in other life activities, in the patient's interests.

8.2.5 *Defining "Disability"*

When dealing with a psychiatric disability claimant, the treating psychiatrist's understanding of his or her role can impact the course of treatment significantly. A narrow working understanding of "disability" may limit the treating psychiatrist's ability to evaluate and treat the claimant in a way that maintains and/or restores his or her functional capacity.

In real terms, disability is complex and involves far more than the presence of symptoms and findings that the psychiatrist treats. Beyond the presence of an illness that the psychiatrist can diagnose and treat, disability is a complex psychosocial process to which many factors contribute. These include but are not limited to an individual's values and beliefs, the role of illness in the individual's childhood and family experience, the meaning of mental illness to the individual, the individual's relationship to his or her employer, occupational alternatives available to the individual, the individual's financial situation and economic issues (such as the local economy and incentives associated with illness and disability), the motivation and ethics of the treating healthcare professional(s), the quality of mental health treatment and case management provided, workplace accommodations made by the employer, and the employer's policies, practices, culture, and values. From the perspective of the disability systems and insurers, contractual or rule definitions of disability are also complex and represent some attempts to capture the complexity of disability by including specific definitions of terms such as "total disability," "continuous disability," "own occupation," "any occupation," "gainful employment," etc.

Because of the multifaceted nature of disability and also for practical reasons, it is not helpful or appropriate for either the treating psychiatrist to "determine disability." The full complexities of disability and contractual and rules determination are beyond the skills and training of most psychiatrists. The primary role for the treating psychiatrist is to engage the claimant in treatment that facilitates functional recovery.

8.2.6 *Challenges for the Treating Psychiatrist*

Few physicians receive substantive training in disability prevention and management. And most medical schools and residency specialty training programs have not integrated evaluation and restoration of function into their curricula. Yet the average psychiatrist who treats working age adults may be asked to complete multiple forms and letters to employers and payers on a monthly or even weekly basis and is by definition a participant in the behavioral health disability process. The treating psychiatrist is often time pressed and wishes to focus on "treating the patient" rather than devoting time (for which he or she is not usually compensated) and energy to a process he or she does not fully understand. The following sections will clarify important aspects of the process for the treating psychiatrist and will provide some foundation and practical information to help the treating psychiatrist in his or her work in empowering maintenance and restoration of function for mentally ill patients.

8.3 Determining Current Psychiatric Functioning

8.3.1 The General Psychiatric Evaluation

While others may have evaluated an individual prior to him or her seeing a psychiatrist (see Sects. 8.4.1 and 8.4.2), it is vital that the psychiatrist, who has both general medical and specific mental health skills, performs a full psychiatric evaluation. Domains of the psychiatric evaluation include reason for the evaluation; history of the present illness; past psychiatric history; history of alcohol and other substance use; general medical history; developmental, psychosocial, and sociocultural history; occupational and military history; legal history; family history; review of symptoms; physical examination; mental status examination; functional assessment; diagnostic tests; and observations derived/observed during the interview process (APA, 2006). A general psychiatric evaluation has as its central component a face-to-face interview with the patient. Although medical technology has advanced tremendously and has increased the amount of laboratory and neuroimaging information available to assist psychiatrists in making more accurate diagnoses and developing more specific treatment plans for patients, these tests cannot supplant the importance of gathering critical data via the traditional psychiatric interview (Hales, Yudofsky, & Gabbard, 2008).

One of the primary aims of the psychiatric evaluation is to establish a psychiatric diagnosis. The current *Diagnostic and Statistical Manual of Mental Disorders* (*DSM-5*) is a categorical classification that divides mental disorders into types based on defining features (APA, 2013), and many of the defining features are symptom based and time defined. For example, the criteria for a major depressive episode include the presence of five or more specific symptoms during *the same 2-week period*, and the essential feature of generalized anxiety disorder is excessive anxiety and worry (apprehension and expectation), occurring more days than not *for a period of at least 6 months*. Therefore, the psychiatrist may spend much of the interview time obtaining the history of present illness – a detailed history of specific symptoms and their severity and time course – from the patient. Information related to the other historical domains help the psychiatrist to place the patient's symptoms in cultural, medical, and environmental context.

A review of systems helps the psychiatrist to identify whether the patient has symptoms that suggest an undiagnosed medical illness that may be causing or contributing to psychiatric symptoms or whether the patient is experiencing side effects from medications or other treatments. Whether the psychiatrist or another medical professional performs the physical examination, the presence of abnormalities, especially in the patient's general appearance, vital signs, skin, or neurological status, should prompt further investigation. It is important to detect nonpsychiatric disorders that present with psychiatric symptoms. For example, thyroid disorders, anemias, other endocrine and metabolic abnormalities, neurological disorders, other illnesses, or medication side effects can cause symptoms that masquerade as a depressive, anxiety, or thought disorder.

The mental status examination (MSE) is a core skill of psychiatrists and qualified mental health professionals and is a key part of the initial psychiatric assessment in any setting. MSE is a systemic collection of data based on the observation of the patient's behavior during the interview and before and after the interview while the patient is in the psychiatrist's view. Responses to specific questions are an important part of the MSE, particularly in the assessment of cognitive function (Trzepacz & Baker, 1993). Analogous to the physical examination for nonpsychiatric conditions, the purpose of the MSE is to obtain *evidence* of current mental disorders that the patient may be experiencing. Furthermore, the MSE provides *evidence* of the patient's insight, judgment, and abstract reasoning, which informs decisions about treatment choice and setting. The core elements of the MSE are general appearance and behavior, characteristics of speech, mood and affect (including stability, range, congruence, and appropriateness of affect), thought processes (including the presence of recurrent or persistent themes and whether the thought processes are coherent), thought content (including the presence of abnormalities such as delusions, ideas of reference, overvalued ideas, ruminations, obsessions, compulsions, and phobias), thought of harm directed to self or others, perceptual disturbances (the presence of hallucinations, illusions, derealization, or depersonalization), sensorium and level of cognitive function (orientation, attention, concentration, registration, short- and long-term memory, fund of knowledge, level of intelligence, drawing, abstract reasoning, and executive functioning), and level of judgment and insight.

It is vital that the psychiatrist distinguish between the patient's symptoms (*the patient's self-report*) and the psychiatrist's *findings and observation*. For example, a claimant may self-report forgetfulness or difficulty paying attention or concentrating (*symptoms*) and/but may or may not complete specific MSE tasks of attention, concentration, or memory (such as serial arithmetic or object recall) well (*findings*). Beyond the MSE, additional *observations* derived from the interview process include whether the patient is exaggerating symptoms, whether he or she appears to provide accurate information, and whether particular questions evoke hesitation or signs of discomfort (Hales et al., 2008). Instruments such as the Beck Depression Inventory (BDI), the Beck Anxiety Inventory (BAI), Hamilton Depression Scale (HDS, HAM-D, HRSD, or HDRS), and the Hamilton Anxiety Scale (HAS, HAM-A, or HARS) are validated *self-report* inventories that may help the clinician assess the severity of depressive or anxiety *symptoms* but are not *findings and observations*.

DSM-5 introduces Level 1 and Level 2 crosscutting symptom measures. The Level 1 crosscutting symptom measure is an informant-related measure that assesses mental health domains that are important across psychiatric diagnoses. It can help clinicians identify additional areas of inquiry that may have significant impact on the individual's treatment and prognosis. In addition, the clinician can use the measure to track changes in an individual's symptom presentation over time. Level 2 crosscutting symptom measures provide one method of obtaining more in-depth information on potentially significant symptoms to inform diagnosis, treatment planning, and follow-up. Much of current clinical practice depends primarily on an individual's "subjective" reports of symptom experience. However, those reports alone don't define functionality; they must be integrated with findings and observations (sometimes referred to as "objective data")[1] to build a foundation from which a psychiatrist can begin to build an occupational functional assessment. These include the results of properly interpreted psychological tests apart from those based on self-report, as discussed elsewhere in this book (the Chap. 6 on psychological testing).

8.3.2 *The Psychiatric General Functional Assessment*

Although treating psychiatrists in general understand the psychiatric evaluation process and the mental status very well, very often they do not understand, or they have not been trained to understand, functional status. In practice, neither a general functional assessment nor an occupational functional assessment is a consistent domain of an initial psychiatric evaluation (American Psychiatric Foundation, Partnership for Workplace Mental Health, 2005). If a psychiatrist performs a functional evaluation, often it is limited to evaluating the degree to which the patient can perform the physical activities of daily living (such as eating, toileting, transferring, bathing, and dressing) or can perform the instrumental activities of daily living (such as driving; using public transportation; taking medications as prescribed; shopping, managing finances; keeping house; communicating by mail, phone, or email; and caring for dependents) (Hales et al., 2008). The categorical and dimensional approach to psychiatric diagnosis in *DSM-5* gives attention to the various mental disorders and general medical conditions, to psychosocial and environmental problems, and to an individual's level of functioning.

---

[1] Often in relation to mental health disability, entities distinguish between "subjective" data (what the patient or claimant reports) and "objective" data (clinician findings and observations, as well as laboratory and imaging data.) This can connote minimizing the "subjective" data as "less real" than objective data. Therefore this author and others prefer the distinction of "self reported" data (for which the patient or claimant is the source) and "findings and observations (for which the mental health professional is the source).

8.3.3 The Psychiatric Occupational Functional Assessment

As noted previously, psychiatrists should consider it a crisis when an individual leaves work due to a mental health condition. A crisis situation requires that the psychiatrist must secure an assessment of the scope, range, and severity of the patient's functional abilities and impairments *as they pertain to the claimant's occupation* as the basis for treatment and return-to-work planning. The starting point for this assessment is the psychiatrist's findings and observations, as opposed to the patient's self-reported symptoms, as described above. *Symptoms in and of themselves* are not *impairments*. Furthermore, while accurate diagnosis is vital to appropriate treatment, the presence of a *diagnosis* is not itself an *impairment* (ACOEM, 2006).

Once the psychiatrist has identified and defined findings and observations, the psychiatrist should identify the individual's specific functional capacity. Based on the *findings and observations*, what can the person do today? What functional abilities are intact and which are limited? Which *findings and observations* support the capabilities and limitations? (For example, are there *findings* that indicate impairment in cognitive function? In affective stability? In basic functioning or social ability?) Has the patient's psychiatric condition made him or her so ill that he or she cannot maintain any focus and concentration, or organize information, or communicate appropriately socially in appearance, speech, or actions? If not, what can he or she do in his or her current condition? Can he or she comprehend and follow instructions, organize complex information, make effective decisions, organize and sustain energy, maintain stable relationships, and solve routine problems? What can the individual not do now that he or she could do previously? Are there any *medically based* restrictions – activities in which the patient should not engage because specific harm might occur? (For example, the individual has voiced credible threats toward self or others, or based on findings and observations, the psychiatrist has concerns about the safety of the patient's coworkers, the public, or the employing business.)

Next, the psychiatrist compares the demands of the patient's usual job with the individual's current functional capacities, limitations, and medically based restrictions with the demands of his or her usual job. To make this comparison, the psychiatrist must know the functional demands of the job, including what cognitive and social skills the job requires. For example, how important to the patient's work is his or her ability to comprehend and follow directions, perform simple and repetitive tasks, maintain a workplace appropriate to a given workload, supervise others, and interact with the public or with others internal or external to the business? Access to the person's job description is critical for this analysis. The end result of the occupational functional analysis is a definition of job duties the psychiatrist thinks the patient can perform, those which he or she thinks the patient cannot perform, and the specific *findings and observations* (taking into account the observations of the patient's function in job-like tasks such as managing finances; interacting in person, by phone, or in writing; working on a computer; organizing a daily plan; etc.) that are the basis for finding whether the patient is able to function or is impaired in each area.

In 2005, the Partnership for Workplace Mental Health, alongside the APA, convened the Taskforce on Disability and Return to Work to evaluate current clinical and employer practices; identify barriers; and develop a methodology that would routinely include treatment to preserve function, enhance stability, and facilitate return to work for employed individuals. As part of this work, the Taskforce developed a set of assessment tools and recommendations that are currently being pilot tested with a large employer in the Pacific Northwest.

For the psychiatrist, the occupational functional assessment forms the basis of incorporating a return-to-work plan into the overall treatment plan for the patient. If the psychiatrist performs an appropriate occupational functional assessment based on findings and observations and corresponding impairments – and does not base the occupational functional assessment solely or primarily on self-report of symptoms or on diagnosis – there may well be a difference between what the patient *says* he or she can and cannot do and what the psychiatrist believes that the patient can or cannot do. When this is the case, it is important that the psychiatrist consider the possibilities of medicalization (identifying everyday or life issues as medical concerns) or symptom exaggeration or malingering, which can complicate the mental health disability process. Section 8.5 addresses these issues.

8.4 The Psychiatric Referral and the Occupational Referral

8.4.1 The General Psychiatric Referral Process

An individual may enter the psychiatric treatment process in a variety of ways. Some individuals self-refer for evaluation and treatment. Other sources of referral include the primary care provider, a non-physician mental health provider (such as a psychologist or a social worker), or a clergy member. Entry into psychiatric evaluation and treatment related to a concern for mental health disability may also originate from the workplace.

8.4.2 The Occupational/Workplace Psychiatric Referral

Coworkers, managers, human resource personnel, and occupational health workers might notice signs of a potential mental health issue (Kahn, 2008). An employee may seem sad, withdrawn, angry, anxious, unmotivated, tired, or "out of it." His or her personality may change, and he or she may seem much more exaggerated, restrained, passive, or angry. He or she may express pessimistic, obsessive, overly insistent, or unrealistically positive or negative thoughts. Performance may have deteriorated, with errors or erratic behavior. Work relationships may have become more distant or difficult. Observations such as these should prompt thoughtful consideration and supportive conversation (Kahn, 2008). Where there is any question, or further concern, referral to appropriate resources is in order.

Occupational nurses and physicians, employee assistance program mental health specialists, psychologists, and social workers usually perform initial workplace-driven mental health evaluations. They may also formulate a differential diagnosis and provide treatment for mental disorders (Kahn & Aidinoff, 1999). Urgent psychiatric referral is indicated when there is evidence of risk of suicide or self-harm; risk of violence to others; marked symptoms of anxiety, depression, or psychosis; cognitive disorganization or acute cognitive changes; substance abuse; child abuse (for which appropriate notification of legal authorities is also required); and life issues or emotional crises requiring rapid and integrated management. Psychiatric referral may also be important in other situations, including the presence of a significant co-occurring medical condition, longer-term life issues, interpersonal or personality issues, inadequate response to nonpsychiatric treatment, need for reconsideration of or better definition of the diagnosis, need to reevaluate the treatment plan, the presence of heightened confidentiality issues, or the need for consultation on overall management (Kahn, 2008). The psychiatrist's combined medical and mental health skills and experience improve the likelihood of accurate diagnosis and effective treatment, and the psychiatrist can have more impact when referral occurs earlier in the process (Langlieb & Kahn, 2005).

8.4.3 The Occupational Psychiatric Referral in Practice

In practice, an occupational referral (and other referrals) may not occur promptly, and/or the psychiatrist may not receive all of the information he or she needs to initiate a general psychiatric evaluation or psychiatric functional assessment. The reason for the referral may be nonspecific, such as "psychiatric information" or "medication management." The historical information with regard to the domains of the general psychiatric evaluation (below) may not be included, in which case the psychiatrist spends much of the initial evaluation reconstructing the patient's history and then must spend additional or follow-up time on an occupational functional assessment. The referral may not include a job or occupational analysis or description, which is critical to the performance of the occupational functional assessment, discussed in detail below. The Partnership for Workplace Mental Health has identified inability to work as a psychiatric crisis, one that demands an immediate and focused response from mental health providers (American Psychiatric Foundation, Partnership for Workplace Mental Health, 2005). In order to provide an appropriate response to an individual in this psychiatric crisis, the psychiatrist must be able to perform an occupational functional assessment readily, and a job description is critical to this effort (see Sect. 8.3.3).

8.5 Medicalization

8.5.1 The Process of Medicalization and Psychiatric Context

"Medicalization (literally 'to make medical') describes a process by which non-medical problems become defined and treated as medical problems" (Conrad, 2007). There is an extensive body of analysis of medicalization; for nearly four decades, sociologists, anthropologists, bioethicists, physicians, and others have written about medicalization. Much writing about medicalization has been critical of the "over medicalization," of life processes such as menstruation, birth control, infertility, childbirth, menopause, aging, and death. But it is important to note that medicalization is a two-way process, in the sense that there can be both medicalization and demedicalization. For demedicalization to occur, the problem must no longer be described in medical terms, and medical treatments must no longer be deemed appropriate medical interventions (Conrad, 2007). In psychiatry, a classic example is homosexuality, which was officially demedicalized in the 1970s by APA. In a somewhat different vein, the disability movement has advocated, with partial success, for a demedicalization of disability and a reframing of it in terms of access and civil rights (Conrad, 2007).

During the past century, the trend has been to expand medicalization. Many social factors have encouraged this process, including the diminution of religion and abiding faith in science, rationality, and progress (strengthened by medicine's "great discoveries" of the late nineteenth and early twentieth centuries, including the "cause and effect" understanding of disease and the discoveries of insulin and penicillin), the American penchant for individual and technological solutions to problems, and a general humanitarian trend in Western societies (Conrad, 2007).

In psychiatry, there is controversy as to whether medicalization has gone too far in defining what mental illness is. In the early post-World War II years, psychiatrists began to "remedicalize" psychiatry in an attempt to extricate it from the prevailing attitude among psychoanalysts, who looked on a medical (non-psychodynamic) identification of mental illness with disdain (Chodoff, 2002). Successive editions of the *DSM* are the result of (re)medicalization, in which an atheoretical, symptom-based, and unpsychodynamic approach to diagnosis (and treatment) has become central to psychiatry. There is general acknowledgment that remedicalization has had a positive and invigorating effect on psychiatry and has led to more effective treatments. However, some believe that American psychiatrists "are running the risk of trying to medicalize not only psychiatry but the human condition itself…to apply a diagnostic label to various unpleasant or undesirable feelings or behaviors that are not readily distinguishable from the range of experiences that are often inescapable parts of being human" (Chodoff, 2002). *DSM-5* takes a more cautious approach to medicalization, allowing for cultural differences in defining what is normal and what is pathological. But there is still debate over whether creating a new series of "so-called behavioral addictions to shopping, sex, videogames, the Internet, and so on" will lead to the consequences of "inappropriately medicalizing behavioral problems, reducing individual responsibility, and complicating disability, insurance, and forensic evaluations" (Frances, 2009, Schatzberg, et al., 2009).

8.5.2 Overmedicalization in the Mental Health Disability Process

In the psychiatric disability process, the tendency of patients and many psychiatrists is toward "overmedicalization" – specifically the medicalization of "stress" or of issues such as job dissatisfaction, conflict at the workplace, marital difficulties, and non-work-related family care or other demands. While these issues have importance for treatment approaches, the psychiatrist should not identify these as functional mental health impairments.

"Stress" is a highly variable self-reported experience and not an objective finding. Both the workplace and the medical community overuse and underdefine the concept of "stress." "Stress" in and of itself is neither good nor bad. At its root, "stress" refers to the physiological reactions the human body makes in the face of a physical or mental challenge to the human body or mind and, therefore, can result from everyday life and workplace challenges. "Stress" is not a psychiatric condition or identified diagnosis.

With regard to the workplace, a "stressful" job means different things to different people. One individual may find the demands of a job overwhelming and feel that he or she cannot handle them; this person is likely to use absence from work as a way of coping. Another person may build healthy resistance to the demands of the same job. The former is more likely to seek "going on disability" as a way of dealing with "stress." It is very important that the psychiatrist not consider this as a mental health impairment. In my experience, I have seen psychiatrists complete "disability" forms identifying the claimant's impairment as "unable to handle stress" and recommend a restriction or limitation of "no work involving stress." In medicalizing stress, the psychiatrist is not acting in the patient's best interests. As noted already (Sect. 8.2.4), the mentally ill patient is more likely to recover more fully more quickly if he or she is active and engaged in life (and work) as much as possible. Furthermore, unless we return individuals with mental illness such as depression and anxiety to the workplace, they will *not* build resistance to everyday stressors and learn to cope and offset the impact of stressors on the body and mind (Sleeth, 2009). The psychiatrist may conclude that the stressors inherent in the patient's job are a poor fit for the patient's cognitive, emotional, and behavioral makeup – in which case the primary issue is poor job fit. Poor job fit is neither a psychiatric condition nor a psychiatric impairment. A mismatch between an individual's skills and temperament does not mean that the person is unable to work at his or her or another job. Also the mismatch does not respond to medical treatment; it may warrant human resource and/or vocational and career counseling efforts.

Other issues, such as job dissatisfaction, conflict at the workplace, marital difficulties, and non-work-related family care or other demands, may detract from an individual's enjoyment of work and/or his or her perception of what he or she is able to do. A dissatisfied worker is more likely than a fulfilled one to seek absence from work, including "going on disability." An individual may feel, understandably, that he or she does not have the physical or emotional energy to work and to deal with marital or family conflict or caretaking or other responsibilities at home. In many of these situations, the issue is not psychiatric impairment, as the patient may be able to engage in many activities requiring abilities similar to those he or she needs at the workplace, including engaging in socially appropriate interaction with others; maintaining a schedule of activities; performing tasks needing intact cognition; completing written, verbal, and email communication; handling interruptions and unexpected demands; etc. The issue may well be that the other demands consume the time, energy, and emotional resources that a person usually dedicates to the workplace; non-work activities in essence become the individual's "job." This issue, too, is not a psychiatric condition responsive to medical treatment; it may warrant human resource or similar efforts.

The assessment tools developed by the Taskforce on Disability and Return to Work, currently being pilot tested (Sect. 8.3.3), separate the duties the psychiatrist believes the patient cannot do from the duties the patient says he or she cannot do. If there is no specific *impairment* that the psychiatrist can define associated with the latter, the psychiatrist is asked to note whether the patient's self-report represents distress, time needed for other problems, or job conflict, thus separating these issues from *impairment* – and demedicalizing them.

8.6 Symptom Exaggeration and Malingering

8.6.1 Malingering and the Disability Process

According to medical anthropologists, individuals take on the "sick role" after becoming ill or injured (Twaddle, 1979). The sick role exempts people from their normal obligations, such as work, school, or parenting, while it also elicits care and concern from others. The mental health disability system provides the financial incentive of paid benefits, while at the same time exempting the person in the sick role from work responsibilities. Given the multidimensional incentives involved, the psychiatrist should consider the possibility of malingering any time a patient claims psychiatric disability (Samuel & Mittenberg, 2005).

It is estimated that malingering occurs in 7.5–33% of disability claimants (Binder, 1993; Frederick et al., 1994; Rogers, Harrell, & Liff, 1993; Trueblood & Schmidt, 1993). The financial costs of malingering are high. In the USA, "Fraud that broadly includes malingering costs the insurance industry $150 billion annually, increasing the cost of insurance by $150 billion" (Garriga, 2007). The *DSM-5* defines malingering as the intentional production of false or grossly physical or psychological symptoms, motivated by external incentives such as avoiding work or military duty, obtaining drugs or financial compensation, or evading criminal prosecution. The *DSM-5* further suggests that the mental health professional should suspect malingering strongly in the presence of any combination of the following: medicolegal context of the presentation (e.g., a disability evaluation or claim), a marked discrepancy between patient claims (self-report) and findings, lack of cooperation with evaluations or treatment, or presence of antisocial personality disorder. Antisocial personality disorder is not usually found in disability claimants, especially those with private disability policies – most likely because individuals need good employment capabilities and histories in order to obtain jobs in which they are eligible for such policies. However, the other three factors occur often (Samuel & Mittenberg, 2005).

8.6.2 Malingering and Psychiatric Disorders

Psychiatric disorders are notoriously easy for persons to malinger, as they are often defined by *self-reported* symptoms and histories. Additionally, malingering can coexist with psychiatric disorders. Individuals can have one psychiatric disorder and malinger by faking or exaggerating symptoms of other disorders. Likewise, an individual can have a psychiatric condition and exaggerate or fake the symptoms of that condition or the impact of the condition on his or her functioning. Any one of these constitutes malingering.

Studies have shown that the psychiatric interview is not an effective tool for detecting malingering. Psychiatrists detect approximately 50% of lies in interviews, which is no better than the percentage that would be discovered by chance (Ekman, 1985; Rosen et al., 2004). While lying or simulation do not equate directly to malingering, the studies indicate that psychiatrists cannot distinguish between genuine, fake, or exaggerated reports on the basis of the patient's demeanor. Techniques used to increase the accuracy of detecting malingering include using multiple sources of data, prolonged interviews, and psychological tests that assess effort or "faking" during test taking.

The primary mental disorder to consider in the differential diagnosis of malingering is factitious disorder, a somatic symptom and related disorder that *DSM-5* defines as "the falsification of medical or psychological signs and symptoms in oneself or others that are associated with the identified deception". Malingering is differentiated from Factitious Disorder by the intentional reporting of symptoms for secondary gain, for example money or time off work.

The psychiatrist may consider some other somatic symptom and related disorders, as defined in *DSM-5*, in the differential diagnosis. In somatic symptom disorder, there may be excessive attention and treatment seeking for perceived medical concerns, but there is no evidence that the individual is providing false information or behaving deceptively. Conversion disorder (functional neurological symptom disorder) is characterized by neurological symptoms that are inconsistent with neurological pathophysiology – without evidence of deceptive falsification of symptoms.

8.6.3 Psychiatric Response to Suspected Malingering

The psychiatrist may attribute suspected malingering to poor motivation or poor effort and/or medicalize it as part of the claimant's illness. This can occur for a variety of reasons, including fear of litigation, concern about error, and the pejorative nature of the term "malingering." However, misattribution of malingering is not in the patient's best interest. Malingering is *not* an illness or clinical disorder; therefore, evidence-based guidelines for its treatment have not been established. A malingering patient is less likely to experience iatrogenic symptoms and illness (e.g., side effects from medications) and more likely to engage in appropriate treatment for any accurately diagnosed conditions present if the psychiatrist presents to the patient the possibility of malingering in an empathetic, nonjudgmental, non-accusatory manner (Purcell, 2002). It is appropriate for the psychiatrist to include this possibility in a targeted discussion with the patient, which focuses on the psychiatrist's findings, observations of discrepancy between the claimant's self-report and the psychiatrist's findings, and the psychiatrist's emphasis on the importance of identifying and removing any and all barriers to the claimant's improved function. Many psychiatrists may suspect malingering but may lack the skills to evaluate malingering accurately. In those cases, it is appropriate for the psychiatrist to refer the patient for psychological testing and/or specialized psychological or psychiatric evaluation to address the concern, with honest discussion of the referral with the patient.

8.7 Patient Adherence Issues

8.7.1 Compliance and the Psychiatric Patient

The concept of "compliance" or "adherence" is highly important in all fields of medicine (Horwitz & Horwitz, 1993; Lerner, Gulick, & Dubler, 1998). Psychiatrists deal with complex compliance situations, which may involve nonadherence with specific therapy approaches (either in therapy with the psychiatrist or in split treatment), failure to keep appointments, and varying degrees of compliance with psychiatric medications. There is no universal definition of compliance, and even the language itself is somewhat controversial (Weiden & Rao, 2005). While most clinicians are comfortable with the term "noncompliance," some consider it to highlight a power imbalance between doctor and patient and to emphasize obedience in a way that is pejorative to patients. "Adherence" is used widely as a synonym for compliance. The proponents of "adherence" and "nonadherence" assert that these terms are free from the connotations of power imbalance and coercion that may freight "compliance" and "noncompliance." *DSM-5* uses terminology of "adherence." For the psychiatrist, nonadherence with psychiatric medications is one of the most common causes in "non response to treatment and is often not recognized by the psychiatrist" (Johnson, 1979), so this is the focus of this section. It is worth noting that according to some research, nonadherence may be the single greatest modifiable risk factor for unfavorable outcomes in psychopharmacology. For example, medication nonadherence is associated with significantly higher rehospitalization rates for depressive disorders, bipolar disorders, and schizophrenia (Pampallona et al., 2002; Sajatovic, Davies, & Hrouda, 2004; Weiden & Olfson, 1995).

The most common definition of nonadherence is a deviation from or cessation of a treatment recommended by the provider (Haynes, Taylor, & Sackett, 1979; Weiden & Rao, 2005). Nonadherence with treatment is not a mental disorder (*DSM-5*). However, it is a barrier to achieving desired treatment outcomes and as such warrants clinical attention when it occurs. "Nonadherence" assumes that the psychiatrist is prescribing the medication accurately and appropriately. In proposing a residency training curriculum for compliance, Reizen and Rao emphasize that when dealing with a "nonadherent" patient, the first question the psychiatrist should ask himself or herself is, "Is my treatment effective in the first place?" (Weiden & Rao, 2005). Misattributing the lack of adequate or expected response to a medication to nonadherence may prevent the psychiatrist from trying and finding more effective treatment for the patient. A good second question is, "Is the patient experiencing a relapse?" In some psychiatric conditions, a patient's insight and participation in treatment can deteriorate abruptly. A previously stable patient can become nonadherent, even if nonadherence is not the cause of the relapse.

8.7.2 Identifying Nonadherence

It has been estimated that the nonadherence rate for medication treatments of psychiatric disorders is well over 50% (Weiden & Rao, 2005). Furthermore, clinicians underestimate the extent of nonadherence in patients they are treating (Norell, 1981). Since the psychiatrist can expect nonadherence, it is appropriate for him or her to ask the patient about medication compliance in a routine and nonjudgmental manner. If the psychiatrist is non-threatening and curious, asking, for example, "Can you tell me about stopping your medication?", he or she makes it easier for the patient to respond truthfully. The psychiatrist should heighten his or her concern about possible nonadherence if there is an increase or decrease in reported side effects without any change in the psychotropic medication(s) or dose(s).

Beyond the clinical interview, other assessment methods can help the psychiatrist to determine whether the patient has been nonadherent. The psychiatrist may ask the patient to bring all medications, in their containers, to the appointment to facilitate a detailed review of the patient's medication practices. The psychiatrist may pursue other sources of information. These include interviewing those close to the patient (with the patient's consent), requesting pharmacy records, and/or considering blood levels when applicable. The psychiatrist should be aware of situations associated with nonadherence, which include changes in treatment environment (particularly when a patient is transitioning to a less structured setting), change in mental health provider(s), loss of a significant family or other personal relationship, and beginning or ending an important relationship (Weiden & Rao, 2005; Blackwell, 1976; Fenton, Blyler, & Heinssen, 1997; Perkins, 2002). Most of us who have been prescribed medications to take three or four times daily know how easy it is to forget one or more doses. It is critical that the psychiatrist distinguish between a patient's "inadvertent nonadherence" and a patient's intentional decision to "adjust" a dose or frequency of medication or to stop taking it altogether.

8.7.3 Treatment Approaches to Improve Adherence and Prevent/Reduce Nonadherence

There are a variety of theoretical perspectives that underlie approaches to improve adherence as an outcome (Barofsky, 1978; Eisenthal, Emery, & Lazare, 1979; Fishbein & Ajzen, 1975; Goldfinger, Hopkin, & Surber, 1984; Hall & Dornan, 1988; Moran, Freedman, & Sharfstein, 1984; Palardy et al., 1998; Soumerai et al., 1994). On a practical level, the two major areas of intervention likely to prevent or reduce nonadherence are maintaining the therapeutic alliance when addressing nonadherence and tailoring the medication treatment to the needs of the patient (Weiden & Rao, 2005).

In maintaining the therapeutic alliance, the psychiatrist should be aware that the patient's personal beliefs have a major influence on his or her adherence behavior. It is vital that the psychiatrist seek to understand the patient's point of view – what does the patient believe about the prescribed medication? Rather than "correcting" these, it is much more helpful for the psychiatrist to make an active effort to ensure that he or she understands the patient's beliefs and biases and to discuss them in a non-blaming way. It is important that the psychiatrist considers nonadherence as a treatment failure and not a patient failure and engages with the patient as a partner in achieving a good outcome.

When discussing the specifics of medication treatment with a patient, a psychiatrist is more likely to improve adherence if he or she offers information in the context of reducing the patient's distress (however the patient understands or experiences distress) rather than emphasizing decreasing target symptoms. The psychiatrist should consider the cognitive, social, time, and economic impact of the medication regimen as well as its impact on the patient's care/social network. The more "user friendly" and less complex the medication routine is, the more likely the patient is to follow it. In selecting a medication, the psychiatrist should make every attempt to minimize the side effects that would be of the greatest distress to the patient (e.g., drowsiness, "jitters," and weight gain) and should discuss this thoroughly with the patient – who may well be more concerned about side effects than about clinical efficacy.

8.8 Appropriate Documentation of Impairments and Limitations in Functioning

The psychiatric functional assessment, including identifying impairments and limitation in functioning, particularly occupational functioning, is discussed at length above (see Sect. 8.3.3). It is essential that the psychiatrist document the findings and observations, abilities and impairments that the findings and observation support, and occupational limitations based on the impairments – in one place for each visit. This allows the psychiatrist to track a patient's functional status regularly and facilitates both patient's and psychiatrist's focus on the goal of restoring function. Additionally, maintaining focused documentation enables the psychiatrist to communicate clearly with others involved in the patient's treatment.

Beyond being a helpful clinical tool, concise, focused functional documentation from the treating psychiatrist is immensely valuable to a psychiatrist involved in a forensic role in the patient's disability claim (see Sect. 8.2.3). As already noted, the psychiatrist in the forensic role has a duty to objectivity and, therefore, will appropriately give more weight to an analysis of impairments and limitations based on findings and observation than he or she will to self-report information or opinions based on self-report. For example, a psychiatrist completing a focused file review to determine whether the available records support occupational impairment will be highly focused on findings and observations and whether they are consistent with the impairments and restrictions/limitations proposed by the treating physician. It is in the patient's best interest for the treating psychiatrist to document this clearly and accurately. If the information is neither clear nor sufficient, it is likely that the review psychiatrist cannot determine what, if anything, the information supports in terms of functional and occupational capacity and impairment.

8.9 Treatment Outcomes: Strategies for Addressing Return to Work

The preceding sections have underscored the importance of the psychiatric functional assessment (see Sect. 8.3.3), coordination of treatment (see Sect. 8.2.2), avoiding medicalization (see Sect. 8.5.2), identifying and responding to malingering (see Sects. 8.6.2 and 8.6.3), and enhancing compliance (see Sect. 8.7.3). This chapter also emphasizes that true inability to work due to a psychiatric illness is a crisis warranting immediate and intensive intervention (see Sects. 8.2.2 and 8.4.3). While a psychiatrist may take all these to account and determine that the treatment of a patient follows evidence-based guidelines *and* is effective for that patient (see Sect. 8.7.1), it is not likely that the patient's return to work will occur solely as a result of these efforts. Treatment should include an explicit and clearly communicated goal of return to work. Because inability to work is a crisis, return-to-work function should be a top priority goal.

It is very important for the psychiatrist to understand that illness and impairment *can* coexist with adequate occupational function (American Psychiatric Foundation, Partnership for Workplace Mental Health, 2005). That is, a patient does not need to be 100% free of psychiatric symptoms, findings, or impairments in order to work. Many disability case managers have found that "People may *feel* they need to be 100% in order to return to work. But in reality, they can't really *be* 100% until they are back to work 100%" (Parker, 2009).

My colleagues and I have found several strategies helpful in achieving a return-to-work goal. When appropriate, we communicate to patients our belief that return to work is in the patient's best interests and clarify that it is our duty to advocate for those best interests. We engage patients in activities focused on the return-to-work goal, such as work hardening, communicating with the employer and human resources, etc. Work hardening, as defined by the American Physical Therapy Association, is a highly structured, goal-oriented, individualized intervention program designed to return the patient/client to work. Work hardening uses real or simulated work activities designed to restore physical, behavioral, and vocational functions (American Physical Therapy Association, 2009) (see Chap. 11). The psychiatrist can incorporate work hardening principles into mental health treatment by having a patient read successfully more challenging and technical material, complete email on a regular basis, or perform other tasks using the same abilities as those needed for his or her job. In discussing return to work, it is essential that the psychiatrist and the patient remain solution focused rather than barrier focused. For example, if a patient says that he or she cannot return to work until he or she feels 100% better, the psychiatrist can ask, "Did you ever work at less than 100%? What helped you then?" If a patient does not feel that he or she can return to the same boss or the same workload, the psychiatrist can engage the patient in a conversation on what *the patient* can do differently in terms of managing interactions, prioritizing the load, communicating his or her needs appropriately, etc. As a regular practice, we devote some of the face-to-face time to completing any forms required, to engage the patient in this process and as a practical time management approach.

While the psychiatrist can have significant impact on a patient-by-patient basis and can play a role in improving the mental health disability process, he or she is one part of a much larger system that includes employers, insurers, and many others, all of whom can help to build a better system and processes. It may help the psychiatrist to know that he or she is not alone in improvement efforts. Toward this end, the American College of Occupational and Environmental Medicine adopted a guideline in 2006, based on the work of the College's Stay-at-Work and Return-to-Work Process Improvement Committee (ACOEM, 2006). The Committee examined current stay-at-work and return-to-work processes, made recommendations to improve the processes, and examined current best practices and initiatives. Recommendations for insurers and employers included the following: revamp disability benefits systems to reflect the reality that restoring function is an urgent matter, given the short window of opportunity to normalize life; whenever possible, incorporate mechanisms into the stay-at-work and return-to-work process that prevent or minimize withdrawal from work; provide or pay for employee assistance and condition management services; inquire routinely into workplace social realities; develop and disseminate screening issues that flag workplace and social issues for investigation; perform prompt psychiatric assessments of workers with slower than normal recoveries; make payment for psychiatric treatment depending on evidence-based treatments with demonstrated effectiveness; educate healthcare providers about the financial aspects that can distort the disability process; compensate physicians for their time and effort in managing the stay-at-work and return-to-work processes; encourage programs that allow employees to take time off work without requiring a medical excuse; encourage employers, insurers, and benefits administrators to use communication methods that respect physicians' time; and standardize key information and processes.

Specific to psychiatry, in 2005, the Partnership for Workplace Mental Health convened a series of conferences with practicing psychiatrists, psychologists, employers, health plan representatives, members of the Social Security Administration, researchers, and other experts in the area of work disability/mental disorders to discuss the problem psychiatric occupational disability (American Psychiatric Foundation, Partnership for Workplace Mental Health, 2005). The Task Force made recommendations for clinicians and employers. Recommendations for employers included the following: establish policies and procedures to ensure that employees secure an accurate diagnosis and appropriate treatment plan, with an emphasis on a solid and objective assessment of the scope, range, and severity of functional impairment; require that their health/behavioral health/disability plan vendors use standardized functional assessment clinical tools (currently under pilot study; see Sect. 8.3.3); design their benefit plans in conjunction with their medical and disability providers to ensure that psychiatric conditions and disabilities, and physical disabilities with underlying psychiatric conditions, are treated by the appropriate mental health professional; intervene early in an employee's disability absence; and use a team-based approach to work (including the employee, treating provider(s), employer, EAP, and disability plan representatives).

Active discussions continue to take place across traditional boundaries, aimed at providing workers with health problems, including mental illness, with the care, support, and empowerment they need to own and promote their recoveries. The Work Fitness and Disability Roundtable is a community of professionals who share a commitment to preventing needless health-related job loss and work absence. Members represent a wide variety of disciplines, including medicine, psychology, human resources, law, media, theology, marketing, insurance, business, and finance. We work in multiple sectors of the economy, including healthcare delivery, managed care, insurance, NGOs, academia, community agencies, and government. The Roundtable has sparked additional efforts to engage employers, professionals, practitioners, and insurers in joint efforts. As a larger society, we benefit most when all individuals are engaged in the workforce to the best of their abilities.

Acknowledgments Each of us has the privilege of learning on the shoulders of others. In formulating this chapter, I have drawn deeply from the well of extensive research by many scholars and practitioners, to whom I am in great debt. Special thanks to Jennifer Christian, M.D., President and CMO of Webility Corporation and Founder of Work Fitness and Disability Roundtable and Jeffrey P. Kahn, M.D., CEO, WorkPsych Associates, Inc. for providing a wealth of foundational research and to Jeffrey Segal, M.D., J.D., F.A.C.S., CEO of Medical Justice, for invaluable assistance in defining and articulating the forensic psychiatric role.

References

Allison, T. G., Williams, D. E., Miller, T. D., et al. (1995). Medical and economic costs of psychologic distress in patients with coronary artery disease. *Mayo Clinic Proceedings, 70*, 734–742.

American Academy of Psychiatry and the Law. (2005). Ethics guidelines for the practice of forensic psychiatry. Available at www.aapl.org

American College of Occupational and Environmental Medicine (ACOEM). (2006). Preventing needless work disability by helping people stay employed. *Journal of Occupational and Environmental Medicine, 48*, 972–987.

American Psychiatric Association. (2003–2016). Clinical practice guidelines. https://www.psychiatry.org/psychiatrists/practice/clinical-practice-guidelines, accessed January 1, 2018

American Psychiatric Association. (2013). *Diagnostic and statistical manual of mental disorders, 5th edition*. Washington, D.C.: American Psychiatric Association

American Physical Therapy Association. (2009). Guidelines: occupational health physical therapy: work conditioning and work hardening programs. Available at www.apta.org

American Psychiatric Association. (2000). Diagnostic and statistical manual of mental disorders, 4th edition, text revision. In *Washington*. D.C: American Psychiatric Association.

American Psychiatric Association. (2006). *Practice guidelines for the treatment of psychiatric disorders, compendium* (p. 2006). Washington, D.C: American Psychiatric Association.

American Psychiatric Association. (2006). *Practice guidelines for the treatment of psychiatric disorders 2006. Condition specific guidelines updated through 2017*. Washington, D.C: American Psychiatric Association.

American Psychiatric Foundation, Partnership for Workplace Mental Health. (2005). Assessing and treating psychiatric occupational disability: new behavioral health functional assessment tools facilitate return to work. Available at www.workplacementalhealth.org

Barofsky, I. (1978). Compliance, adherence, and the therapeutic alliance: Steps in the development of self care. *Social Science and Medicine, 12*, 369–376.

Barsky, A. J., Delamanter, B. A., & Orav, J. E. (1999). Panic disorder patients and their medical care. *Psychosomatics, 40*, 50–56.

Bartley, M. (1994). Unemployment and ill health: Understanding the relationship. *Journal of Epidemiology and Community Health, 48*, 333–337.

Binder, L. M. (1993). *Portland digit recognition test manual*. Beaverton, OR: Laurence Binder.

Blackwell, B. (1976). Treatment adherence. *The American Journal of Psychiatry, 129*, 513–531.

Chodoff, P. (2002). The medicalization of the human condition. *Psychiatric Services, 53*, 627–628.

Conrad, P. (2007). *The medicalization of society: On the transformation of human conditions into treatable disorders*. Baltimore: Johns Hopkins University Press.

Druss, B. G., Rosenheck, R. A., & Sledge, W. H. (2000). Health and disability costs of depressive illness in a major US corporation. *The American Journal of Psychiatry, 157*, 1274–1278.

Egede, L. E. (2004). Diabetes, major depression, and functional disability among US adults. *Diabetes Care, 27*, 421–428.

Eisenthal, S., Emery, R., & Lazare, A. (1979). Adherence and the negotiated approach to parenthood. *Archives of General Psychiatry, 36*, 393–398.

Ekman, P. (1985). *Telling lies: Clues to deceit in the marketplace, politics, and marriage*. New York: Norton.

Fenton, W., Blyler, C., & Heinssen, R. (1997). Determination of medication compliance in schizophrenia: Empirical and clinical findings. *Schizophrenia Bulletin, 23*, 637–6510.

Fishbein, M., & Ajzen, J. (1975). *Belief, attitude, intention, and behavior*. Reading: Massachusetts.

Frances, A. (2009). A warning sign on the road to DSM-V: Beware of its unintended consequences. *Psychiatric Times, 26*(8), 1–9.

Frederick, R., Sargaty, S., Johnston, J. D., et al. (1994). Validation of a detour response bias on a forced-choice test of nonverbal ability. *Neuropsychology, 8*, 118–125.

Garriga, M. (2007). Malingering in the clinical setting. *Psychiatric Times, 24*(3), 1–4.

Gerdtham, U. G., & Johannesson, M. (2003). A note on the effect of unemployment on mortality. *Journal of Health Economics, 22*, 505–518.

Goldfinger, S. M., Hopkin, J. T., & Surber, R. W. (1984). Treatment resisters or system resisters?: Toward a better service system for acute care recidivists. *New Directions for Mental Health Services, 21*, 17–27.

Greenberg, P. E., Kessler, R. C., Nells, T. L., et al. (1996). Depression in the workplace: An economic perspective. In J. P. Feighner & W. F. Boyer (Eds.), *Selective serotonin re-uptake inhibitors: Advances in basic research and clinical practice*. New York: Wiley and Sons.

Hales, R. E., Yudofsky, S. C., & Gabbard, G. O. (2008). *The American psychiatric publishing textbook of psychiatry* (5th ed.). Arlington, VA: American Psychiatric Publishing.

Hall, J. A., & Dornan, M. C. (1988). What patients like about their medical care and how often they are asked: A meta analysis of the satisfaction literature. *Social Science and Medicine, 27*, 935–939.

Harris, I., Multford, J., Solomon, M., et al. (2005). Association between compensation status and outcome after surgery. *Journal of the American Medical Association, 293*, 1644–1652.

Haynes, R. B., Taylor, D. W., & Sackett, D. L. (1979). *Compliance in health care*. Baltimore: Johns Hopkins University Press.

Horwitz, R. I., & Horwitz, S. M. (1993). Adherence to treatment and health outcomes. *Archives of Internal Medicine, 153*, 1863–1868.

Jin, R. L., Shah, C. P., & Svoboda, T. J. (1995). The impact of unemployment on health: A review of the evidence. *Canadian Medical Association Journal, 153*, 529–540.

Johnson, D. A. W. (1979). Further observations on the duration of depot neuroleptic maintenance therapy in schizophrenia. *The British Journal of Psychiatry, 135*, 524–530.

Kahn, J. P. (2008). Diagnosis and referral of workplace depression. *Journal of Occupational and Environmental Medicine, 50*, 396–400.

Kahn, J. P., & Aidinoff, S. (1999). Occupational psychiatry and the employee assistance program. In J. Oher (Ed.), *The employee assistance handbook*. New York: Wiley and Sons.

Katon, W., Von, K. M., Lin, E., et al. (1990). Distressed high utilizers of medical care: DSM II diagnoses and treatment needs. *General Hospital Psychiatry, 12*, 355–362.

Kessler, R. C., Berglund, P., Demler, O., et al. (2005). Lifetime prevalence and age-of-onset distributions of DSM IV disorders in the National Comorbidity Survey Replication. *Archives of General Psychiatry, 62*, 593–602.

Kessler, R. C., Greenberg, P. E., Mickelson, K. D., et al. (2001). The effects of chronic medical conditions on work loss and work cutback. *Journal of Occupational and Environmental Medicine, 43*, 218–225.

Krause, N., Frank, J. W., Dasinger, L. K., et al. (2001). Determinants of disability and return to work after work-related injury and illness: Challenges for future research. *American Journal of Industrial Medicine, 40*, 464–484.

Kroenke, K., & Mangesldorff, A. D. (1989). Common symptoms in ambulatory care: Incidence, evaluation, therapy, and outcome. *The American Journal of Medicine, 86*, 262–266.

Langlieb, A. M., & Kahn, J. P. (2005). How much does quality mental health care profit employers? *Journal of Occupational and Environmental Medicine, 47*, 1099–1199.

Lecrubier, Y. (2001). The burden of depression and anxiety in general medicine. *The Journal of Clinical Psychiatry, 62*(Suppl 8), 4–9.

Lepine, J. P. (2002). The epidemiology of anxiety disorders: Prevalence and societal costs. *The Journal of Clinical Psychiatry, 63*(Suppl 14), 4–8.

Lerner, B. H., Gulick, R. M., & Dubler, N. N. (1998). Rethinking nonadherence: Historical perspectives on triple-drug therapy for HIV disease. *Annals of Internal Medicine, 129*, 573–578.

Lustman, P. J., Griffith, L. S., & Clouse, R. E. (1997). Depression in adults with diabetes. *Seminars in Clinical Neuropsychiatry, 2*, 15–23.

Moran, A. E., Freedman, R. I., & Sharfstein, S. S. (1984). The journey of Sylvia frumpkin: A case study for policy makers. *Hospital & Community Psychiatry, 35*, 887–893.

Morgan, H. (2006). A conflict of roles: Expert witness or treating physician? *SpineLine July/August, 2006*, 27–30.

National Institutes of Mental Health. (2001). Depression can break your heart. In *Available at.* www.nimh.gov

Norell, S. E. (1981). Accuracy of patient interviews and estimates of clinical staff in determining medication compliance. *Social Science and Medicine, 15*, 57.

Palardy, N., Greenberg, L., Ott, J., et al. (1998). Adolescents' health attitudes and adherence to treatment for insulin dependent diabetes mellitus. *Journal of Developmental and Behavioral Pediatrics, 19*, 31–37.

Pampallona, S., Bolini, P., Tibaldi, G., et al. (2002). Patient adherence in the treatment of depression. *British Journal of Psychiatry, 180*, 104–109.

Parker, J. (2009). Managing complex disability cases: A conversation about finding exceptions. *Back to Work: Disability Management and Return to Work Strategies in Canada, 13*(3), 6–7.

Perkins, D. O. (2002). Predictors of noncompliance in patents with schizophrenia. *The Journal of Clinical Psychiatry, 63*, 118–1121.

Purcell, T. B. (2002). Factitious disorders and malingering. In J. A. Marx, H. S. Robert, & R. M. Walls (Eds.), *Rosen's emergency medicine: Concepts and clinical practice* (5th ed.). St. Louis: Mosby.

Reed, P. (Ed.). (2005). *The medical disability advisor* (5th ed.). Westminster, CO: Reed Group, Ltd.

Reid, W. H. (1993). Law and psychiatry: Treating clinicians and expert testimony. *Journal of Practical Psychiatry and Behavioral Health, 4*, 1–3.

Rogers, R., Harrell, E. G., & Liff, C. D. (1993). Feigning neuropsychological impairment: A critical review of methodological and clinical considerations. *Clinical Psychology Review, 13*, 255–274.

Rosen, J., Mulsant, B. H., Bruce, M. H., et al. (2004). Actors' portrayals of depression to test interrater reliability in clinical trials. *The American Journal of Psychiatry, 161*, 1909–1911.

Rossi, A. S. (2001). *Caring and doing for others: Social responsibility in the domains of family, work, and community*. Chicago: University of Chicago Press.

Sajatovic, M., Davies, M., & Hrouda, D. R. (2004). Enhancement of treatment adherence among patients with bipolar disorder. *Psychiatric Services, 55*, 264–269.

Samuel, R. Z., & Mittenberg, W. (2005). Determination of malingering in disability determinations. *Primary Psychiatry, 12*(12), 60–68.

Schatzberg, A. F., Scully, J. H., Kupfer, D. J., & Regier, D. A. (2009). Setting the record straight: A response to Dr Frances' commentary on DSM-V. *Psychiatric Times, 26*(8, 1), 9–10.

Simon, G. E. (2003). Social and economic burdens of mood disorders. *Biological Psychiatry, 54*, 208–215.

Simon, G. E., Revicki, D., Heiligenstein, J., et al. (2000). Recovery from depression, work productivity, and health care costs among primary care patients. *General Hospital Psychiatry, 22*, 153–162.

Sleeth, J. (2009). Mental health, disability, and stress: What Selye and Mate can tell the human resources professional. *Back to Work: Disability Management and Return to Work Strategies in Canada, 13*(3), 8–9.

Soumerai, S., McLaughlin, T. J., Ross-Degnan, D., et al. (1994). Effects of limiting medicaid drug reimbursement benefits on the use of psychotropic agents and acute mental health services by patients with schizophrenia. *The New England Journal of Medicine, 331*, 650–655.

Starsburger, L. H., Gutheil, T. G., & Brodsky, A. (1997). On wearing two hats: Role conflict in serving as both therapist and expert witness. *The American Journal of Psychiatry, 154*, 448–456.

Trueblood, W., & Schmidt, M. (1993). Malingering and other validity considerations in the neuropsychological evaluation of mild head injury. *Journal of Clinical and Experimental Neuropsychology, 15*, 578–590.

Trzepacz, P. T., & Baker, R. W. (1993). *The psychiatric mental status exam*. Oxford, UK: Oxford University Press.

Twaddle, A. C. (1979). *Sickness behavior and the sick role*. Cambridge, MA: Schenkman Publishing.

Unutzer, J., Patrick, D. L., Simon, G., et al. (1997). Depressive symptoms and the cost of health services in HMO patients aged 65 years and older: A four year prospective study. *The Journal of the American Medical Association, 277*, 1618–1623.

Weiden, P., & Olfson, M. (1995). Cost of relapse in schizophrenia. *Schizophrenia Bulletin, 21*, 419–428.

Weiden, P., & Rao, N. (2005). Teaching medication compliance to psychiatric residents: Placing an orphan topic into a training curriculum. *Academic Psychiatry, 29*, 203–210.

Chapter 9
Behavioral Health and Occupational Medicine: Concepts

Garson M. Caruso

9.1 Introduction

Behavioral health (BH) issues play a widespread and crucial role in occupational and environmental medicine (OEM) but have long been underappreciated and often ignored. There are several major ways in which psychological issues impact the workplace:

- There are reciprocal effects between BH conditions and the workplace. Mental health disorders generate substantial direct and indirect costs to employers and may negatively affect worker productivity (e.g., presenteeism and absenteeism), contribute to or disrupt efficient and effective workplace function, and cause short- or long-term disability. Conversely, "stress" is a basic feature of work and may have positive or negative effects; workplace elements may contribute to exacerbation or provocation of pre-existing subclinical or clinical BH disorders.
- BH factors may strongly contribute to work-relevant conditions (WRCs). In this and the following chapter, work-related illness or injury (WRII) denotes a condition directly or indirectly caused, exacerbated, or aggravated by work activity or exposure. Examples include musculoskeletal trauma and other disorders, eye injuries, and BH concerns like untoward effects of excessive job stress. In contrast, WRC indicates a situation in which other influences (which may be pre-existing, coincident, or consequent and work-related or nonwork-related) complicate recovery from WRII (Burton, Kendall, Pearce, Birrell, & Bainbridge, 2009). Examples of such influences include substance dependence and abuse, occupational and nonoccupational (e.g., fibromyalgia) chronic pain syndromes, osteoarthritis (OA), and BH elements, including (1) appraisals, attitudes, beliefs, and expectations (AABEs) of all stakeholders; (2) individual characteristics of

G. M. Caruso (✉)
Occupational and Environmental Medicine, Mechanicsburg, PA, USA
e-mail: garson@gmcarusoconsulting.com

P. A. Warren (ed.), *Handbook of Behavioral Health Disability Management*,
https://doi.org/10.1007/978-3-319-89860-5_9

the affected worker (AW), including motivation and reward contingencies, learning, adverse childhood experiences (ACEs), perceived injustice (PI), and specific psychopathology; and (3) workplace elements.

- At least six domains of influence contribute to delayed or failed recovery and unnecessary disability (DFR/UD)[1] from both WRIIs and WRCs, including all the BH elements listed above, necessitating a biopsychosocioeconomic (BPSE) approach to understanding and managing these problems.
- BH components play a major role in administrative and clinical iatrogenicity (IAG) and the development and persistence of medically unexplained physical symptoms (MUPS), both of which can strongly alter the course of worker recovery and have a profound effect on the outcome of a worker condition.

The BH contribution to WRCs presents a major dilemma for workers' compensation (WC) and disability insurers who must often deal with influences (e.g., developmental and historical) which were and are largely out of their control. Although there is still a strong and appropriate emphasis on industrial causation (work relatedness) in WC systems, these conditions may adversely affect recovery and resumption of work activity regardless of industrial etiology and causation and thus need to be actively addressed. We can no longer selectively limit attention purely to "work-related" factors (Burton et al., 2009; Caruso, 2013). Overall, there is still a profound lack of recognition and management of these BH influences in OEM, for many reasons; this first of two chapters identifies and discusses some of the relevant considerations.

9.2 Behavioral Health Effects on the Workplace

BH disorders generate a high amount of direct and indirect (particularly productivity) costs for employers, may predispose AWs to WRII, have significant employment effects on individuals, and are a prominent comorbid feature of many "physical" WRCs.

- **Direct costs** of behavioral health disorders in the workplace comprise medical and indemnity expenses, including increased benefit utilization rates. Greenberg, Fournier, Sisitsky, Pike and Kessler (2015) estimated that depressive disorders alone directly cost the US economy $31.5 billion in 2000 (including suicide-related mortality costs). Olesen, Gustavsson, Svensson, Wittchen, Jönsson; CDBE2010 Study Group; and European Brain Council (2012) reported similar costs in the Europe Union-27 in 2010 of €194 billion.
- **Indirect costs** include productivity losses, predilection to WRII, and comorbidity. Greenberg et al. (2015) estimated that depressive disorders alone indirectly cost the US economy $51.5 billion. Birnbaum et al. (2010) found a linear

[1] These spheres of influence include administrative and medical factors, BH elements, personal and sociocultural influences, and systemic and workplace factors (Caruso et al. 2011).

relationship between MDD severity (mild, moderate, and severe) and employer burden (including mental health services utilization and costs and work performance) in the USA, estimating that monthly depression-related productivity losses were nearly $2 billion:

– Productivity losses include presenteeism and absenteeism, with the former generally considered to be a much greater contributor to lost work productivity due to BH disorders than the latter (Greenberg et al., 2003). Other indirect costs include turnover (e.g., recruitment, training, and salary for replacement workers); extended supplementary healthcare benefits; increased premium rates on worker's compensation and short- and long-term disability insurance; return-to-work accommodation; and administrative (e.g., supervisory time and claims administration) and business opportunity costs (Dyck, 2017). Further expenses include employee and family assistance plan (EFAP) use and those arising from workplace conflict and grievances, health and safety infractions, and human rights violations (Great-West Life, 2017).
– Workplace accidents are costly to employers both in terms of damage to or loss of equipment and product and temporarily or permanently reduced production (Hilton & Whiteford, 2010), with costs comparable to those of absenteeism and presenteeism (Wang et al., 2003). There is a strong relationship between BH disorders and incident commercial motor vehicle crashes (Hilton, Staddon, Sheridan, & Whiteford, 2009) and prevalence of occupational injury (Kim, 2008).
– There is a high degree of comorbidity between "physical" (e.g., cardiovascular, gastrointestinal, metabolic, neurological, and pulmonary) diseases and "psychiatric" illness (Henderson, Harvey, Overland, Mykletun, & Hotopf, 2011); Buist-Bouwman, de Graaf, Vollebergh, and Ormel (2005) found roughly additive (but not synergistic) effects between multiple physical and mood (but not substance abuse) disorders. Alavi, Makarem, Abbasi, Rahimi, and Mehrdad (2016) reported an association between upper extremity MSDs and psychiatric disorders, and Del Campo, Romo, de la Hoz, Villamor, and Mahíllo-Fernández (2017) documented increased risk of incident MSDs in healthcare workers with pre-existing anxiety and depression. There is also a high degree of co-occurrence among BH disorders; Greenberg et al. (2015) found that 62% of the total costs of MDD were attributable to anxiety, adjustment, and posttraumatic stress disorders and nonpsychiatric medical conditions such as chronic pain and sleep disturbance.

• BH disorders may exert multiple individual costs. They can decrease motivation and commitment, lead to poor decision-making, increase error rate, and increase interpersonal conflict and tension (Harnois & Gabriel, 2000). Barriers to competitive employment among those with behavioral health disorders include affective, cognitive, perceptual, and interpersonal impairment; symptoms which may inhibit obtaining and maintaining work; side effects of pharmacotherapy; and stigma and discrimination, including employer reluctance to hire or advance affected individuals (Waghorn & Lloyd, 2005). Underemployment in people with BH dysfunction has been repeatedly demonstrated (Dewa, McDaid, & Ettner, 2007).

9.3 Workplace Effects on Behavioral Health (and Other Disorders)

The net effects of the workplace on the individual depend upon a complex interaction of AABEs, personality, characteristics, motivation, and coping resources. Work-related stress may exacerbate or aggravate pre-existing anxiety, depressed mood, and other conditions and may precipitate new conditions, particularly in the presence of work-related illness or injury. Conversely, work has generally been shown to be beneficial to physical and behavioral health.

9.3.1 Work-Related Stress and Strain

Work-related stress may be best understood as a psychological state resulting from the interaction between the individual and their environment (Lazarus & Folkman, 1984), comprising three components: perceptual (how the individual recognizes a stressful situation), affective or emotional (how the individual experiences a stressful situation), and cognitive (how the individual response and attempts to cope with the experience) (Hassard et al., 2014). Responses to stress may be adaptive or positive (e.g., mobilization of energy or adoption of coping mechanisms, maintaining eustasis) or maladaptive or negative (causing strain or cacostasis; Chrousos, 2009). Common causes of negative stress at work include:

- Personal concerns: uncertainty about compensation, job security, and career advancement; lack of self-efficacy for job or task (insufficient training or experience) and difficulty in meeting new role requirements; excessively high or insufficient workload; lack of control over one's own or others' work activities
- Interpersonal concerns: poor working relationships, lack of support, frank conflict, harassment or bullying
- Management concerns: weak or ineffective management or overmanagement; confusing reporting lines; uncertainty about performance requirements and the future due to communications failures by management
- Cultural concerns: absence of safety focus or blame culture in the workplace
- Environmental concerns: suboptimal physical work environment

Strain generally refers to adverse physical and psychological effects of stress on the individual. Responses to strain may be physiological (e.g., cardiovascular disorders such as heart disease or high blood pressure or increased susceptibility to disease) or psychological, with the latter including affective effects like anxiety, boredom, depression, job dissatisfaction, and loss of self-esteem and behavioral manifestations such as aggressive behavior, substance abuse, poor performance, and job turnover (Thatcher & Miller, 2017).

9.3.2 Models of Work-Related Stress

There are four predominant models of work-related stress and its effects, all based on the relationship between the worker and the workplace:

- The demand-control-support model (Karasek & Theorell, 1990) postulates that work-related stress and strain are derived from situations in which the individual experiences high physical or psychological demand but limited decision latitude in terms of dealing with that demand, with the level of available social support either exacerbating (low support) or mitigating (high support) the strain.
- In the effort-reward imbalance model, stress and strain occur due to mismatch between intrinsic and extrinsic efforts at work activity and the concomitant rewards obtained by the individual (Siegrist, 2001).
- Per the person-environment fit model, stress and strain result from mismatch between an individual's capabilities (knowledge and skills) and demands placed upon them, as well as between needs (e.g., for interpersonal interaction) and actual attainment (Edwards, Caplan, & Harrison, 1998).
- The organizational justice model refers to the perceived fairness of rules, practices, and social norms within organizations. It includes distributive justice (allocation of benefits and resources), procedural justice (the methods and processes governing that distribution), and interactional justice (related to interpersonal relationships), with the latter comprising relational justice (the level of respect and dignity accorded to the worker by management) and informational justice (the adequacy and credibility of the information provided by management) (Harvey et al., 2017).

9.3.3 Negative Health Effects of Stress and Strain

Maintenance of physiological and psychological homeostasis in humans is a complex process involving the central and peripheral nervous systems (the latter acting principally through catecholamines and glucocorticoids), as well as cardiorespiratory, endocrine and metabolic, gastrointestinal, and immune function. Stress responses are affected by the individual's genetic variation, developmental history, nutrition, and stress experience (McEwen, 2007).

Acute stress can trigger allergic phenomena; angiokinetic disorders, such as migraine and blood pressure abnormalities; pain; gastrointestinal symptoms; and psychological disorders, including anxiety with panic attacks and psychotic episodes (Charmandari, Tsigos, & Chrousos, 2005). Chronic stress can contribute to cardiovascular, gastrointestinal, and sleep disorders; immune or metabolic dysfunction; and reproductive abnormalities (Franchimont, Kino, Galon, Meduri, & Chrousos, 2003). Psychobehavioral consequences of chronic stress result at least in part from homeostatic dysregulation and may include anorexia or hyperphagia; anxiety, cognitive dysfunction, and depressed mood; nonspecific symptoms such as fatigue; and chronic fatigue, fibromyalgia, obsessive-compulsive, panic, and posttraumatic stress disorders (Chrousos, 2009).

Stress responses are associated with physical and BH disorders and social consequences, including metabolic syndrome (Gimeno et al., 2010); neck and shoulder disorders (Kraatz, Lang, Kraus, Münster, & Ochsmann, 2013); shoulder, low back, and knee pain (Bernal et al., 2015); hypertension (Gilbert-Ouimet, Trudel, Brisson, Milot, & Vézina, 2014); anxiety and depressed mood and fibromyalgia (Nielsen, Magerøy, Gjerstad, & Einarsen, 2014); and compromise in the quality of relationships with spouse, children, and other family members (Amick & Mustard, 2005). Conversely, there is some evidence that higher levels of organizational justice may be protective from long-term sickness absence due to mental disorders (Elovainio et al., 2013) and disability pensioning from all causes (Juvani et al., 2016).

9.4 Beneficial Effects of Work in Behavioral Health Concerns

There is also strong evidence for the positive effects of work in both physical and psychological concerns. The classic monograph in this regard was by Waddell and Burton (2006), who provided extensive evidence up to that time that the overall effect was positive. Blustein (2008) reviewed the complex history of work in psychological theory and practice, supporting the critical role of work in psychological health, particularly for survival, providing individual satisfaction and accomplishment (self-determination), enhancing well-being, and promoting connection to the broader economic and social world (relatedness). van der Noordt, Ijzelenberg, Droomers, and Proper (2014) substantiated the benefits of employment, particularly for depressed mood and general mental health. Modini et al. (2016) observed that "… having a job is associated with a greater sense of autonomy, improved self-reported well-being, reduced depression and anxiety symptoms, increased access to resources to cope with demands, enhanced social status and unique opportunities for personal development and mental health promotion" (p. 335). Felhaber (2017) recently provided an excellent a review of the negative effects of worklessness.

9.5 Behavioral Health Influences on DRF/UD

9.5.1 Introduction

Most AWs experiencing WRII recuperate satisfactorily, often completely, but roughly 10% do not recover as expected. Delayed and failed recovery (DFR) refers to the persistence of symptoms and/or signs beyond an expected and medically reasonable time frame or failure to ever satisfactorily resolve complaints or physical findings and regain reasonable degree of function for given condition(s). Examples include many cases of prolonged postconcussion symptoms; most poorly defined musculoskeletal disorders (MSDs), such as "chronic sprain/strain" and "cumulative/repetitive "injuries"; and many instances of chronic pain disorders like "post-laminectomy syndrome." Unnecessary disability (UD) refers to medically avoidable limitation in the AWs' participation in work and/or daily living activity. There are three major areas of concern in DFR/UD:

- **Poor outcomes**, which include preventable morbidity (e.g., medication dependence and long-term decline in physical and mental health; Wilkinson & Marmot, 2003); suffering (e.g., pain, emotional distress, degradation of economic, family, and social quality of life, and loss of identity, self-worth, and social role; Coutu, Cote, & Baril, 2013); disability; and mortality (Loisel & Cote, 2013)
- **Excessive costs and inefficient resource allocation**, including personal, enterprise, and societal costs, with a Pareto distribution;[2] excess demand for and supply of unnecessary and sometimes counterproductive services; and markedly poorer outcomes in workers' compensation (WC) systems as opposed to group health (Cheriyan et al., 2015; Harris, Mulford, Solomon, van Gelder, & Young, 2005)
- **Disability creep**, which refers to increasing incidence and societal acceptance of unnecessary disability, including the gradual lowering of threshold of acceptability for "disability" (Aronoff, 1989, 1991); decrease in public tolerance of mild symptoms and "progressive medicalization of physical distress" (Barsky & Borus, 1995, p. 1931); increased perception of entitlement (Eberstadt, 2012); and encouragement of dependence on medical systems and care, with very few leaving benefits programs once they enter (Prins, 2013)

The following subsections briefly review the six domains of influence that contribute to DFR/UD and the consequent need for a biopsychosocioeconomic approach, discuss the psychological factors domain in more detail, and address the role of IAG and MUPS.

9.5.2 Domains of Influence, Complex Causality, and the BPSE Approach

9.5.2.1 Six Domains of Influence

DFR/UD result from a complex interaction of intrinsic and extrinsic influences on the AW (Caruso et al., 2011; Loisel et al., 2005)[3]:

[2] This includes disproportionate claim costs, with 7–8% of claims generating roughly 80–85% of costs (Kennedy 2016; Rosenblum 2016), and disparate cost generation by physicians, with 4–7% of physicians engendering 70–72% of costs (Bernacki, Tao, and Yuspeh, 2010; Wolfe 2013).

[3] Many of these considerations, especially AABEs, apply to other stakeholders as well as the AW, including family members and significant others, clinicians, allied health personnel, insurers, employers, regulators, and both plaintiff and defense attorneys.

- **Administrative and medical** This domain includes nonclinical (e.g., insurer) and clinical practices which may help or hinder recovery from WRII and WRCs.
- **Psychological** This category includes multiple behavioral health factors, such as AABEs, and is discussed in more detail in a later section.
- **Personal** This area includes individual factors associated with disability (e.g., age, gender, and race); education level and health literacy; behavior, particularly substance and tobacco abuse; and immediate familial and social influences, such as solicitous, enabling, and overprotective family members (Block, Ben-Porath, & Marek, 2013) or a history of a disability model in the family.
- **Sociocultural** This domain includes the effects of wider social influences including popular media and special interest groups and organizations.
- **Systemic** The systemic sphere includes several elements, including involvement in compensation systems; misaligned incentives; misplaced advocagenicity; and personal, local, and national economic factors.
- **Workplace** This purview includes multiple workplace effects, including culture; physical and psychological demands; work organization factors; training; communication; influence of co-workers and labor unions; and employer practices such as preplacement evaluation and proactive supervisor and worker training.

9.5.2.2 Complex Causality/Integration

DFR/UD is the result of multifactorial causation in each AW, with variable contributions from each of the above domains. Many of these elements have negative or positive valence (e.g., attitudes toward and beliefs about the employer, health system, and recovery; personal practices such as substance abuse; sociocultural influences on illness; and systemic factors such as attorney representation). These effects may be maladaptive, e.g., an external health locus of control (HLOC), or adaptive, e.g., a high degree of self-efficacy. They exert countervailing and compensating influences, and the overall outcome is a balance an integral of many forces (Melloh et al., 2009).

9.5.2.3 Biopsychosocioeconomic (BPSE) Approach

Current administrative and medical management in OEM, and WC and disability medicine, heavily emphasizes a classical biomedical (BM) approach, which assumes that discrete disease entities cause symptoms, which can then be diagnosed (often with the aid of complicated, expensive, and invasive testing) and then treated; this model presumes that pathology leads directly to impairment, functional limitation, and disability. This paradigm is both suitable and effective in most WC cases but likely contributes to DFR/UD in susceptible individuals. The BM approach does not include consideration of (1) human psychology and behavior, including biopsychology (especially neuroplasticity) and affective (emotional), behavioral, cognitive, or psychopathological concerns; (2) human sociology, including culture, financial and legal incentives, and competing priorities[4]; or (3) administrative and clinical problems with health service delivery (e.g., IAG) and MUPS. As Waddell and Aylward (2010) noted: "The crippling weakness of the medical model is that it does not include the patient or their unique human attributes and subjective experience" (p. 11).

Recognition of the BPSE nature of many OEM disorders has lagged many other fields of medicine, although many are properly viewed as biopsychosocial phenomena (Dersh, Gatchel, Mayer, Polatin, & Temple, 2006); examples include work-related upper extremity disorders, nonspecific low back pain, and many chronic pain syndromes, especially as experienced as delayed and/or failed recovery from relatively simple industrial illnesses and injuries. There is compelling evidence that overreliance on biomedical evaluation and intervention is suboptimal and iatrogenically harmful in these situations (Fava, Guidi, & Sonino, 2016; Waddell & Aylward, 2010) and that biopsychosocial and not biomedical interventions are both necessary and effective (Laisné, Lecomte, & Corbière, 2012; Schultz, Law, & Cruikshank, 2016). The BPSE model is discussed in greater depth in Chaps. 5, 6, and 7.

9.5.3 Psychological Influences on DFR/UD

All people have both inherited and acquired psychological characteristics, and although there are several domains of influence on DFR/UD as described above, psychological elements range widely across all of them and are arguably the most important single factor. In this context, the term "psychological" encompasses both psychophysiological and "pure" psychological effects, most of which overlap or are inextricably intertwined. The former include many genetic and epigenetic attributes which manifest as psychophysiological processes (e.g., neurologic, endocrine, and immune function; Rief & Barsky, 2005) and tendency toward neuroplasticity (Navarro, Vivó, & Valero-Cabré, 2007). The latter include cognition (AABEs); individual motivation, reward, and learning; developmental and environmental influences (ACEs and PI); psychopathology; and workplace factors, all of which have demonstrated associations with DFR/UD.

9.5.3.1 Appraisals, Attitudes, Beliefs, and Expectations (AABEs)

These cognitive factors are among the most potent influences on AW behavior and claim outcome. They shape individuals' perceptions, motivations, and values and exert a profound influence on their productivity, job satisfaction, and response to WRII, particularly expectations about illness or injury and the probability of recovery and the ability to return to premorbid function and to work (Gross & Battie, 2010;

[4] Christian (2017) added an economic dimension, which may become important in motivation and as a driver of behavior.

Iles, Davidson, & Taylor, 2008; Schultz, Crook, Meloche, Berkowitz, Milner, Zuberbier, & Meloche, 2004). Influences on AW cognitions include (1) developmental factors (e.g., cultural background, education, and childhood experience); (2) past experience with healthcare; (3) preparation for the WC experience within the workplace; (4) prior and present treatment accorded within medical and WC systems; (5) sociocultural influences (peer groups and popular media); and (6) legal representation (Gatchel & Gardea, 1999; Gatchel, Polatin, & Mayer, 1995). Once cognitions are developed, they may be very difficult to change (Rydell & McConnell, 2006).

Appraisals This refers to an individual's interpretation of new events and situations, assessment of those situations, and selection of appropriate response(s). These include perceptions and judgments about WRIIs and WRCs and the AW's own health condition, medical care, and treatment by employer and insurer under WC claim and severity and irreparability of injury-related losses, unfairness, and external attribution of blame (Sullivan et al., 2008). Keefe, Brown, Wallston, and Caldwell (1989) found that negative appraisal was a better predictor of low pain tolerance, depressed mood, and disability than disease activity or impairment.

Attitudes This term refers to feelings about persons, institutions, and events and mental predispositions to act (Halligan & Aylward, 2006). An important attribute of attitudes is valence (negativity or positivity); in this context, they may include those toward work, employers, the healthcare system, and WC and may strongly affect AW motivation for return to work (Franche & Krause, 2005).

Beliefs These are cognitive configurations about the nature of reality, including WRII and WC systems, which are used to make sense and to derive meaning from event and situations (Halligan & Aylward, 2006). They are developed through learning and experience, and shaped by cultural and societal factors and how individuals respond to the environment, although usually their formulation and expression are largely unconscious (Damasio & Eighth, 2000). Some erroneous illness beliefs (myths) which may contribute to eventual DRF/UD are:

1. Pain is equivalent to serious injury.
2. Work activity caused pain and/or serious injury and will make pain and/or serious injury worse.
3. Medical treatment and/or work absence is necessary for recovery.
4. A medical condition must be 100% resolved prior to return to work.
5. The AW is too ill, injured, or disabled to return to work and will experience pain or fatigue upon work resumption.
6. The AW cannot overcome and recover from the condition and will be forced into premature retirement (Kendall et al., 2009; Waddell, 2004).

Expectations Expectancies are a component of beliefs which relate to the future and what the individual anticipates will occur, such as with future treatment or regarding pain reduction and functional restoration (DeGood & Cook, 2011). Two forms of expectancy that are most relevant to the WC context are self-efficacy, which are convictions about one's own capacity to influence events or produce a desired result (Bandura, 1997), and outcome expectancy beliefs, which are anticipation that a given behavior or course of action will lead to a specific outcome. Shaw and Huang (2005) found that self-efficacy expectations in WC comprised both concerns about resuming physical activity and more complex return-to-work considerations (e.g., meeting role expectations). Turner et al. (2006) reported that worker recovery expectations and fear avoidance predicted work disability in cases of low back pain, and Laisne et al. (2012) found that AW expectations of recovery were the most consistent prognostic factor of work participation, disability, and pain outcomes.

There are three other important categories of AABEs relevant to DFR/UD:

- **Catastrophization (CAT) and fear avoidance (FA)** CAT is an irrational belief that anticipated or actual pain will result in both severe consequences and overall negative outcome (Quartana, Campbell, & Edwards, 2009). It is associated with delayed recovery and eventual disability (Ramirez-Maestre, Esteve, Ruiz-Párraga, Gómez-Pérez, & López-Martínez, 2017; Wertli et al., 2014), although these effects are still controversial (Lee et al., 2015; Valentin et al., 2016). FA is a behavioral expression of CAT (Vlaeyen & Linton, 2012), in which the following cascade occurs: the susceptible individual experiences pain with a high negative affectivity and threat → catastrophizing affective and pain-related fear → hypervigilance and autonomic arousal in response to further perceived threats of pain → (fear) avoidance of future activities → consequent disuse and depression → impairment and disability. The relationship between pain-related fear and eventual disability replicated in many studies (Leeuw et al., 2007; Zale, Lange, Fields, & Ditre, 2013).
- **Health locus of control (HLOC)** This refers to the extent to which the AW attributes their health to environmental factors and other external agents, or to their own actions (self-efficacy). An external locus is associated with sense of helplessness and worse functional outcomes (Wagner et al., 2014) and predicts poor outcome, for example, in chronic low back pain rehabilitation (Keedy, Keffala, Altmaier, & Chen, 2014). Conversely, self-efficacy is associated with better physical function and lower disability (Keedy et al., 2014) and return to work (RTW), with odds ratios up to 5.3 (Black, Keegel, Sim, Collie, & Smith, 2017).
- **Fallibility of human thought** This refers to cognitive errors of commission and omission which can occur in the normal course of human mental activity. There are multiple evidence lines: Lees-Haley et al. (1996, 1997) observed that insurance claimants reported marked differences between pre- and post-claim function, but that non-claimants reported no difference. Barsky (2002) found that insurance claimants underreported their pre-incident health history and overreported their post-incident history. Carragee (2008) and Don and Carragee (2009) indicated that 80% of claimants denied pre-existing conditions relevant to persistent neck/back pain, e.g., psych disorders or alcohol/drug abuse. To my knowledge, there is no direct evidence in the medical literature relating human fallibility to DFR/UD, but this phenomenon may be relevant in several ways, including (1)

AW AABEs, especially beliefs about their condition; (2) poor recall and/or bias, resulting in variable medical history as provided to successive practitioners (e.g., escalation of complaints as claims evolve), which may influence iatrogenicity; and (3) symptom extension (e.g., to the neck from distal UE injury) and expansion (e.g., numbness and tingling in addition to pain) due to learning and/or suggestibility.

9.5.3.2 Motivation/Reward/Learning

AW motivation and reward contingencies may act in contradictory ways, providing a stimulus for recovery from WRIIS and WRCs, or an impetus to seek secondary or tertiary gain. Choi, Asih, and Polatin (2016) provided an excellent analysis of gains and losses in the WC context, pointing out the complex balance and the roles of conscious and unconscious motivation. Wagner et al. (2014) concluded that "strong" evidence supported a lack of return-to-work motivation as a predictor for work disability.

Learning is an important component of the AW experience in WC and private insurance systems, contributing to UD, particularly under the influence of IAG:

- Claimants may consciously or unconsciously learn from interaction with healthcare and insurance personnel (Kosny et al., 2006) and the WC medicolegal system (which may extend to frank coaching by attorneys, physicians, and significant others).
- Claimants may experience "learned helplessness," or failure to pursue, utilize, and acquire adaptive responses (Mohanty, Pradhan, & Jena, 2015; Walker, 1992).
- Claimants may develop a learned dependence on healthcare systems, e.g., for opioids or unnecessary time away from work (i.e., secondary and tertiary gain).
- Classical and operant conditioning processes are operative in development and maintenance of chronic pain (Flor & Turk, 2013). An AW's pain and other behaviors may be reinforced by positive (e.g., personal attention or psychoactive medications) and negative (e.g., "sanctioned" release from unwanted work or home responsibilities) contingencies. AWs may learn to shape their behavior (pain and otherwise) in response to the perceived expectations of other stakeholders and contingent upon positive and negative rewards specific to the individual, including financial compensation.
- Aurbach (2015) described a process of "self-talk," in which the history of an AW's WRII and treatment becomes a script, self-belief becomes fixed, and the story takes on a life of its own.
- Any or all of these learning processes may contribute to symptom extension (e.g., generalization of discomfort proximally from a distal upper extremity to the neck) and expansion (e.g., from initial pain to numbness and tingling and/or weakness) due to suggestibility, learning, and/or coaching (although this situation may also involve a psychophysiological/neuroplastic component).

9.5.3.3 Adverse Childhood Experiences (ACEs)

ACEs include emotional, physical, or sexual abuse; emotional or physical neglect; and exposure to (growing up in) households with domestic violence, alcohol or drug abuse and/or mental illness, relational stress (e.g., separation or divorce), or criminal behaviors. The pathogenesis is complex but may involve chronic stress mediated by persistent epigenetic effects causing persistent hypercortisolism and proinflammatory cytokine production or represent delayed consequences of coping mechanisms (Anda, Butchart, Felitti, & Brown, 2010) or both; there is some evidence of permanent alteration in hypothalamic-pituitary-adrenal (HPA) axis function after significant ACEs (Chang et al., 2009). Schüssler-Fiorenza, Xie, and Stineman (2014) observed a strong graded (linear) relationship between ACEs and self-reported adult disability, and Austin, Herrick, Proescholdbell, and Simmons (2016) found significantly higher ACE exposure history in disabled adults, with high relative risks for poor physical and mental health.

9.5.3.4 Perceived Injustice (PI)

PI may include the AW's impression of low or unsatisfactory employer or co-worker support; poor treatment by a healthcare practitioner, employer, or insurer; or some form of injustice from family, significant others, friends, or society as a whole or may simply represent general disgruntlement and embitterment, possibly due to unfulfilled expectations of entitlement. The history of significant PI has been shown to predict greater pain severity and chronicity, more pain behavior, reduced function, and prolonged work disability (Scott et al., 2016) and adverse pain outcomes (Rodero et al., 2012). These factors may be more resistant to change than other pain-related psychosocial variables (Sullivan et al., 2008).

9.5.3.5 Psychopathology: Adjustment, Mood, and Personality (PD) and Somatic Symptom (SSD) Disorders

Many employed people may function in life and work despite having significant underlying psychopathology, even if they meet accepted diagnostic criteria (e.g., *DSM-5*; APA, 2013). Such conditions may be subclinical (and therefore undiagnosed and untreated) but allow function in a majority of aspects of work and daily life; those who are under treatment (e.g., psychotropic medication and psychotherapy) may have returned to premorbid levels of function. Still, these conditions may be strongly influential in the workplace:

- Sections 9.2 and 9.3 explored some relationships between psychopathology and WRII and comorbidity between "physical" and "psychiatric" illness.
- WRII may exacerbate pre-existing or precipitate new BH disorders. Dersh, Mayer, Theodore, Polatin, and Gatchel (2007) concluded that pre-existing psy-

chiatric illness was not a risk factor for development of work-related chronic spinal pain with disability, but rather that MDD was much more likely to occur after such work injuries. The stress of illness or injury may exacerbate such conditions to a level at which they become symptomatic or manifest in maladaptive behavior, with interference with recovery and rehabilitation; in addition, WRII may be a precipitating factor for MUPS.
- Various BH conditions are associated with DFR/UD in WRII and WC claims. Dersh et al. (2006) found that prevalence rates of anxiety, major depressive, substance abuse, and personality disorders were elevated above baseline population rates in patients with work-related chronic spine pain and disability. Chou and Shekelle (2010) reported higher likelihood ratios for development of chronic low back pain in patients with pre-existing psychiatric comorbidity, and Reme et al. (2011) found that anxiety and somatoform disorders were increased in chronic low back pain patients. Schultz et al. (2016) reviewed the medical literature relating psychiatric predictors (both mood and personality disorders) with occupational disability.

Specific psychopathologic conditions associated with DFR/UD include:

- **Adjustment disorders** These are defined as "psychological response to an identifiable stressor or stressors that result in the development of clinically significant emotional or behavioral symptoms" (APA, 2000). Both work-related and nonwork-related (i.e., contributing to WRCs) variants are probably the most common BH disorders seen by OEM physicians (van der Klink & van Dijk, 2003), and Chirico (2016) made a case for adjustment disorder as a chronic occupational disease.
- **Mood disorders (anxiety, depressed mood, and psychological distress)**[5] These conditions may contribute to WRCs, MUPS, or directly to DRF/UD. The prevalence of depressed mood is 7% in the general population, but 10–30% in chronic pain patients (Howe, Robinson, & Sullivan, 2015). Anxiety and depressed mood are associated with physical impairment and work disability and excess healthcare costs and mortality (Edwards, Dworkin, Sullivan, Turk, & Wasan, 2016). Dysthymia and Major Depressive, Panic, and Post-Traumatic Stress Disorders are associated with chronic pain and disability (Hees, Koeter, & Schene, 2012). Lee et al. (2015) found that psychological distress mediated the relationship between pain and disability. The effects of mood disturbance are probably bidirectional, both predating and then complicating WRII (i.e., causing WRC), and resulting from WRII (Dersh et al., 2007; Gatchel & Dougall, 2014). There is some controversy over these effects, e.g., Laisne et al. (2012) found no influence of MDDs in an extensive literature review.
- **Personality disorder** The essential features of these conditions are the presence of enduring pathological personality traits and impairment in personality func-

[5] Psychological distress refers to negative affect and mood and consequent emotional suffering, which may adversely impact work and daily living function without necessarily meeting criteria for diagnosis as a psychiatric disorder (Drapeau et al., 2012).

tioning, manifest as distorted thinking patterns, problematic emotional responses, poor impulse control, and interpersonal difficulties (APA, 2013). Tyrer (2014) made a case for the global influence of these conditions in OEM. Prevalence rates in the general population are 10–13%, but they are found in up to 70% of those with chronic disabling spine disorders (Dersh et al., 2006); they are strongly associated with acute and chronic low back pain (Polatin, Kinney, Gatchel, Lillo, & Mayer, 1993), sick leave and compensation (Gordon, Eisler, Gutman, & Gordon, 1991), chronic disability (Gatchel et al., 1995), deliberate job loss (Sansone & Wiederman, 2013), and disability pensioning (Ostby et al., 2014). A specific trait, neuroticism (a persistent tendency to experience negative affect or negative emotional state), is associated with development of MUPS (Rosmalen, Neeleman, Gans, & de Jonge, 2007) and has been shown to be associated with disability pensioning in twin studies (Gjerde et al., 2013; Ropponen et al., 2012). (In my experience as a WC medical director and disability case reviewer, I have found that PDs are often detected at formal psychological testing but routinely ignored as a contributor to the AW's overall condition.)

- **Somatic symptom disorder** A broad definition of somatization (introduced in *DSM-III* in 1980) is unconscious or conscious expression of mental phenomena as bodily symptoms, with exaggerated emphasis on bodily concerns, seeking of medical care, and impairment and disability (Dimsdale, 2018). A prominent feature of this phenomenon is a high number of medically unexplained symptoms, communicating an underlying psychological need that the individual cannot otherwise express. The term SSD replaced somatization in *DSM-5* (2013); the essential features of the new syndrome are 1) one or more somatic symptoms that are distressing and/or significantly disrupt daily life; 2) excessive thoughts, feelings, and/or behaviors related to symptoms or associated health concerns; and 3) chronicity, with at least one symptom persistent for at least 6 months. SSD and related terms (e.g., bodily distress disorder or BDD in *ICD-11*; Gureje & Reed, 2016) represent a gradual shift away from psychopathological emphasis to more neutral, non-etiological, and functional approach, based on a neutral and non-judgmental assessment of bodily symptoms only, and are intended as unifying concepts across multiple symptoms and syndromes (Budtz-Lilly et al., 2015). The concept of SSD may be helpful in dealing with MUPS in WC and disability claimants (Chap. 10).

9.5.3.6 Workplace Attributes

Several aspects of work and work organization have been identified as contributing to both WRCs and DFR/UD (Kristman et al., 2016). Ring et al. (2005, 2006) related psychological factors, including anxiety and depression, to idiopathic upper extremity pain, and in an extensive review involving only longitudinal studies, Hauke, Flintrop, Brun, & Rugulies (2011) concluded that work organization factors had a significant causal effect and increased risk of WRMSDs by 15–59%. Contributors to excessive work absence and disability include high physical demand, both in effort and pace, and suboptimal ergonomic considerations (Shaw et al., 2013; White et al., 2015); unbalanced elements of work organization, in the context of the models presented in Sect. 9.3.2 (Golubovich, Chang, & Eatough, 2014; Knardahl et al., 2017); and work-related personal factors such as perceived lack of social and managerial support (White et al., 2015) and low job satisfaction (Schultz et al., 2016).

9.5.4 *Iatrogenicity (IAG)*

The term "iatrogenic" originally referred to contribution to or causation of negative effects or outcomes by physicians; however, Batavia and Batavia (2004) argued that the term could and should be extended to all stakeholders in a particular medical situation (including employers, insurers, and others), any or all of whom might contribute (Illich, 2010; Null, Feldman, Rasio, & Dean, 2011). Administrative and medical iatrogenicity in occupational (including WC and disability) medicine is a complex psychosocial phenomenon involving most of the BH factors discussed in Sect. 9.5.3 and can have profound effects on the management and outcome of WRIIs and WRCs. There are four primary forms of IAG encountered in these fields: (1) medicalization, (2) inappropriate advocagenicity and nocebo effects, (3) focus on symptom relief (primarily pain) rather than function, and (4) unnecessary time delays in management. Loeser and Sullivan (1997) provided a unique and accurate summary of the role of physicians in this process, addressing "pseudodiagnosis and pseudodisability" in multiple medical specialties and "physician-generated disability" by many routes.

9.5.4.1 Medicalization

Medicalization refers to the perception or assumption that a bodily condition, behavior, or psychic state is a medical disorder and merits or needs medical treatment. Examples include common health problems (CHPs) like musculoskeletal (especially low back) pain; common mental health problems (CMHPs), such as anxiety and depressed mood, "stress," and periodic sleep disturbance (all of which may be normal human responses to WRII); and administrative and personnel issues (e.g., lack of private insurance, performance problems, or interpersonal conflicts). This practice may inaccurately and adversely shape an AW's appraisals of their medical condition and situation; attitudes toward treatment; beliefs (e.g., "something is really wrong"); and expectations of medical care and recovery (e.g., entitlement). Particularly in the WC context, it can and often does lead to unnecessarily prolonged, complicated, expensive, and ineffective treatment, including "Type II Medical Malpractice," i.e., "doing something to patients very well that was not needed in the first place" (Hadler, 2008, p. 20), including surgery (Stahel, Van der Heiden, & Kim, 2017), and eventual DFR/UD. Conrad (2007) estimated that medicalization accounted for $77B or almost 4% of direct healthcare costs in the USA in 2005.

9.5.4.2 Inappropriate Advocagenicity and Nocebo Effects

Advocagenicity refers to a disproportionate and often unquestioned bias toward the perceived or expressed needs or wants of the AW. The term was initially coined in reference to attorneys, particularly in WC claims (Lynch, Clay, Hegmann, Greaves, & Gold, 1998), but there is now good evidence that the actions and inactions of clinicians can have equally powerful effects (Kilgour, Kosny, McKenzie, & Collie, 2015a). This process may occur as an unintended consequence of routine interpersonal interactions and/or prolonged exposure to an adversarial claims process (Kilgour, Kosny, McKenzie and Collie (2015b), or by direct coaching, inappropriate medical practices (e.g., ordering of unsupported or excessive testing), or collusion between claimant and practitioner (Salmon, 2006). A particular example in WC claims is encouragement of the "sick" role by unnecessary and/or prolonged work restriction in the absence of clear medical indications. Attorney representation is associated with poorer physical and mental health outcomes in accident victims (Harris et al., 2008).

The converse of inappropriate advocagenicity is the nocebo effect, which technically refers to adverse effects of placebo, but encompasses negative influences of actions and words of healthcare practitioners and other stakeholders. Although much of the research in this area focuses on the effects of medications, Colloca and colleagues (2011; 2014a, b) have explored its effects on patient learning, particularly in chronic pain. Barsky (2017) discussed this phenomenon in direct relationship to patient experience of symptoms ("viscerosomatic amplification").

9.5.4.3 Symptom Vs. Functional Focus

This situation refers to inappropriate concentration on AW symptoms and attempts both to definitively identify their cause and to relieve them, as opposed to a more appropriate emphasis on functional restoration. Despite attempts by regulators and insurers to enforce "objectivity" in claimant evaluation and management, in current WC practice response to symptoms – with their inherently subjective component – remains firmly established as an end unto itself. Attempts at symptom eradication may lead to extended efforts to "find the anatomic pain generator" (so that a biomedical solution can be applied) and have become a focal point of treatment and desired outcome, when in fact a great deal of the symptoms encountered in WC may be medically unexplained, without a clear anatomic locus or rational treatment.

A related problem is the fear of missing organic (and potentially treatable) disease, which often drives intensive investigation by clinicians, although this concern has not been supported by recent investigations (Kooiman, Bolk, Rooijmans, & Trijsburg, 2004;

Stone et al., 2009). Extensive and unproductive workup and treatment is a particular problem in WC, for several reasons:

1. The assumption of a biomedical etiology and organic disease in most if not all cases
2. Nonmedical drivers, including claimant AABEs, clinician and attorney advocagenicity, and a relative lack of medical training and sophistication of employers and insurance adjusters
3. Generally ineffective cost and other constraints
4. Little appreciation for iatrogenic effects of excessive investigation, serially ineffective therapy, and prolonged case duration (especially with unnecessary activity limitation)

The symptom focus likely involves learning and reward contingencies and may reinforce psychological and psychosocial factors that lead to chronic pain states and disability; it may be used to justify excessive medical care and does not strongly contribute to meaningful improvement in function, e.g., return to work (Peat, 2008).

9.5.4.4 Time Delay

Unnecessarily prolonged work absence work can cause significant harm to an AW's well-being, due to physical, psychological, social, and vocational effects (Crichton, Stillman, & Hyslop, 2005), including increased mortality (Gerdtham & Johannesson, 2003). Physical deconditioning may result from FA and/or unnecessary activity limitation. Psychological deconditioning includes loss of identity and social relationships (Bartley, 1994) and may negatively affect appraisals and expectations (e.g., development of hopelessness and disability "mindset"). Recent research has shown that the brain undergoes large-scale neuroplastic changes in the shift from acute to chronic pain which occurs at 7–29 weeks post-injury (Hashmi et al., 2013), supporting expeditious management. Return-to-work probability is a function of time away from work (Waddell, 2004); longer durations of workers' compensation claims are associated with higher chronicity rates (Frank et al., 1998) and predict recurrence of the index condition (Wasiak, Verma, Pransky, & Webster, 2004). Bultmann and Brouwer (2013) described phase models for both development of disability and return to work, with implications for intervention and management.

9.5.4.5 Examples of Administrative and Clinical IAG

Administrative IAG may include:

- Excessive concern with procedural and legal aspects of claims, including pursuit of technicalities instead of simply doing the right thing for the AW in the situation; this includes focus on claim disposition and/or settlement even though outcome may not be sustainable, e.g., in cases in which the ATP erroneously places AW at MMI despite ongoing symptoms (Kilgour et al., 2015a, 2015b).

- Avoidable delay in case management, such as in approval of medications, diagnostics, therapy, and consultations (Sinnott, 2009).
- Failure to demand accountability from clinicians, including acceptance of poorly or unconsidered assumptions (e.g., regarding causation); lack of reasonably evidence-based justification for diagnostic and therapeutic interventions (e.g., treatment in response to symptoms as opposed to definable medical conditions); and poor medical documentation.

Clinical iatrogenicity may include:

- Medicalization of common health (CHPs) and mental health (CMHPs) problems, or nonmedical (e.g., administrative) concerns
- Failure to consider psychosocial aspects of a WRC, e.g., assumption of a "psychogenic" cause for symptoms, or of malingering
- Advocagenicity, including unreasonable focus on symptom (especially pain) relief vs. functional restoration (Turner et al., 2008; Wideman & Sullivan, 2011); providing long periods of unnecessary work disability (thus encouraging the "sick" role); and frank collusion (Salmon, 2006)
- Excessive diagnostic investigations, including exhaustive testing and overdiagnosis (Hill & Harris, 2008)
- Insufficient treatment planning without clear goals, particularly for functional restoration (anticipating the likely outcome of a claim as early as possible, e.g., recovery and RTW, vocational rehabilitation, or chronic pain management)
- Suboptimal management, including lack of adequate knowledge about treatment alternatives, and use of passive (e.g., excessive chiropractic therapy), addictive (unreflective use of opioids), or unnecessarily invasive (multiple pain management interventions without functional improvement) therapies

9.5.5 Medically Unexplained Symptoms (MUPS)

MUPS refer to "… physical symptoms persisting for more than several weeks and for which adequate medical examination has not revealed a condition that adequately explains the symptoms" (olde Hartman, Woutersen-Koch, & Van der Horst, 2013, p. 2). Examples include dizziness, lightheadedness, and visual and/or balance problems; pain anywhere in the body with no clear origin; or radicular symptoms (e.g., paresthesia) without signs. MUPS are often multiple and syndromic (collections of symptoms without objective findings),[6] with associated BH elements; the SPADE acronym encompasses essential features common to many patients, including sleep disturbance, pain, anxiety, depressed mood, and energy lack/fatigue (Kroenke, 2016). The symptoms are real, not primarily psychiatric, and may cause considerable distress and suffering (Barbour, 1995; Waddell, 2004). Evens, Vendetta,

[6] Examples include fibromyalgia, irritable bowel, and chronic pelvic pain syndromes; multiple chemical sensitivity; and idiopathic environmental intolerance.

Krebs, and Herath (2015) reviewed the history of these disorders and differentiation between functional and psychogenic neurologic symptoms.

MUPS are well established in general medicine, with prevalence of 16–53% in primary care (Burton, 2003; Kroenke 2014) and 30–52% in specialty care (Creed, Barsky, & Leiknes, 2011). They are much less well recognized in WC and disability, although the literature is growing: for example, Ihlebaek, Brage, and Eriksen (2007) found that sickness absence increased 65% in Norway between 1997 and 2003, with the most common reasons including anxiety, palpitations, sleep problems, and "tiredness"; Aamland, Malterud, and Werner (2012) described a linear correlation between increasing number of MUPS and sick leave days; and Rask et al. (2015) found that MUPS were associated with increased rates of long-term sickness absence and leave, unemployment, and new disability pension awards.

Causation of MUPS is complex, involving "pathophysiological responses to prolonged or severe mental and/or physical stress in genetically susceptible individuals" (Budtz-Lilly et al., 2015, p. 182). Symptoms result not from one specific disease process (an underlying assumption of the BM model), but rather from the interaction of various etiologic factors in different domains (e.g., the six spheres of influence described above) (Creed et al., 2011; Fink & Rosendal, 2015). Deary, Chalder and Sharpe, (2007) posited a behavioral/PPP model comprising (1) predisposing factors including a genetic, psychophysiological (particularly involving the HPA axis), individual (AABEs), and sociocultural diathesis; (2) precipitating elements including biological (e.g., physical injury) and psychological (e.g., emotional trauma) stressors; and (3) perpetuating features including psychophysiological, cognitive, behavioral (and learning), and sociocultural factors. Different components exert different levels of influence at different times and may be nonwork-related or work-related.

MUPS, especially pain, are at least partially mediated by central (CNS) and/or peripheral (PNS) nervous system sensitization, perhaps occurring in the precipitant phase. Neuroplasticity includes habituation (reduced response) and/or sensitization (increased response), and chronic pain syndromes result in part from increased activity in ascending (activating) and decreased activity in descending (inhibitory) pathways. In MUPS, these effects may result in persistent pain long after expected resolution; in addition, increased activation may result in heightened sensitivity to painful (hyperalgesia) and non-painful (allodynia) stimuli (explaining atypical symptoms), and decreased inhibition may result in both secondary (in neighboring dermatomes) and widespread (at remote sites) hyperalgesia (which may explain new symptoms and/or extension of symptoms to new body areas).

MUPS appear to be much more influential in OEM, at both subclinical and clinical levels, than currently appreciated or acknowledged. They may provide a credible explanation for mysterious persistent pain syndromes like "chronic sprain and strain," "cumulative trauma," "repetitive stress," and specific conditions like "failed back surgery syndrome."[7] The process may occur as follows (Caruso, 2013):

[7] These terms often appear to be used euphemistically when the clinician has no better descriptor for pain or other symptoms of uncertain etiology.

- A small proportion of AWs has significant predisposing (diathesis) factors which can contribute to MUPS (e.g., genetic/psychophysiological predisposition and BH elements such as AABEs, ACEs, and psychopathology). These may be subclinical and unsuspected prior to WRII or development of a WRC. (Although AWs often deny pre-existing complaints, symptoms may have been subclinical, or clinically present but subtle, and human memory is fallible.
- A precipitating situation or event occurs. This may involve medicalization of pre-existing CHPs, CMHPs, MUPS, or work-related influences like job dissatisfaction or PI to WRCs, with poor or no response to usual (BM) care. MUPS may develop either concurrently with or in response to legitimate WRII entailing some physical (particularly musculoskeletal) or psychological insult or appropriate treatment (e.g., low back surgery). Again, the resultant WRCs are often managed biomedically or overmanaged, with iatrogenic consequences, and some degree of CNS and/or PNS sensitization occurs.
- Both work- and nonwork-related perpetuating factors, particularly IAG, maintain and propagate the process.

9.6 The Psychological "Dilemma" in WC and Disability Systems

BH factors contributing to WRCs and to DFR/UD (e.g., psychological influences, IAG, and to some degree MUPS) pose a major dilemma for all stakeholders in WC and disability medicine. The "grand bargain" basis for WC calls for the employer (and insurer) to do what is needed to ameliorate WRIIs (Fishback & Kantor, 2000). However, as shown above, pre-existing and nonwork-related factors, including a psychophysiological diathesis and some of these BH elements, are clearly influential in a significant proportion of AWs. The precise mechanisms (not to mention interactions) of many contributors are unknown, and some may be of limited or no modifiability (e.g., HPA physiology). Administrative and medical IAG in WC systems is also generally "work-related," if it occurs in the service of a WC claim. All of these influences contribute to conversion of WRIIs (and in some cases CHPs and CMHPs) to very complex central and peripheral biopsychological disorders (WRCs). Regardless of precise causation, these contributing factors, and conditions, need to be addressed successfully, or many or most of these individuals are not going to (and do not) recover.

Obviously, industrial causality and apportionment are extremely problematic for employers and payers in these cases. How do we deal with WRCs, with substantial nonwork-related components, under current systems? How far can and should the employer and/or insurer go – or be expected to go – into the biopsychosocial realm to do this? We presently do not have good answers to these questions, and solutions to the dilemma involve several challenges:

- We need to develop a better understanding of how these complex influences might affect a given AW. There has been much progress over the past 10–20 years, with a great deal of research and some implemented programs (e.g., the Washington State Psychosocial Determinants Influencing Recovery [PDIR] program),[8] but our knowledge in this area and ability to apply it are still fragmented, and widespread appreciation of the influence of BH factors is still rudimentary among the most important stakeholders in these areas (AWs, clinicians, insurers, employers, and regulators).

- We need to better identify individuals with potentially influential BH factors, and thus at risk for DFR/UD, as early as possible, ideally from date of WC or disability claim filing, but as soon as possible in the case.
- We need to develop scientifically sound and ethically, legally, and practically effective methods of managing AWs with significant BH factors (and at risk of DFR/UD) and overcoming barriers to intervention. All stakeholders will have to decide their positions and approaches on this issue (which, along with case law, will likely constantly evolve) and determine how far and in what ways they are willing to go to address these situations. (For example, AWs may or may not want, or be compliant with, available treatment, and employers may balk at increased claim costs, although, as discussed in Chap. 10, this should be a cost-utility rather than pure cost decision.) Insurers should be the major drivers, as the principal payers and players, and will need to make very complicated decisions about acceptance of responsibility and cost utility of evaluation and treatment. In addition, increased consideration of BH factors in WC and disability may introduce new avenues to confound the ultimate goals of the WC process – rehabilitation of the AW and avoidance of unnecessary impairment and disability (e.g., by opportunistic AWs, clinicians, attorneys, and others.)

9.7 Why Aren't We Addressing Workplace BH Concerns More Effectively?

There are many reasons why we are not more actively using our substantial current knowledge of BH factors to improve WC care and disability prevention and management:

- **Lack of widespread awareness** There is a lack of widespread awareness and understanding of the strong influence and roles of psychophysiological and psychosocial factors such as those described above. Although this appears to be slowly improving, most of the people dealing with these problems currently have little or no comprehension of many of the factors involved.
- **Fear of psychology** This lack of knowledge may engender a wariness or frank fear of psychology. Behavioral health constructs and applications are generally less familiar (and thus more threatening) to both nonprofessional and professional stakeholders than biomedical concepts of symptoms, disease, and treatment.

[8] See http://www.lni.wa.gov/ClaimsIns/Files/OMD/MedTreat/2016PDIRResourceFinal.pdf

Employers and payers have a very legitimate concern about "buying" pre-existing (and possibly long-term and thus expensive) psychological conditions, which does occur much too often in current practice. However, Kertay (personal communication, 2017) has observed that there are distinct differences among psychological symptoms, psychological influences or factors, and psychopathology and that many if not most of the BH elements of interest to us are not psychological conditions, but rather symptoms or influences which act as barriers to recovery, which may be amenable to relatively simple intervention.

- **Stigma** This is not a new concept, but acquires enhanced significance in improved management of WRCs. Stigma regarding BH conditions involves perception (cues), stereotyping, prejudice, and discrimination (Corrigan, 2004) and may occur as social (prejudicial attitudes and differential behavior toward persons with BH disorders) or self-stigma (acceptance or internalization of perceptions of such bias). It includes both direct actions (e.g., exclusion of affected individuals from participation in normal life activities) and indirect effects (poor social support, decreased self-esteem and quality of life, and suboptimal vocational outcomes) (Yanos, Roe, & Lysaker, 2010).
- **Scientific denialism** There is an element of scientific denialism and rigid belief in and adherence to the BM approach, which may be based on lack of knowledge, or individual personality and approach to administrative or clinical practice. Many humans tend to continue doing the same thing despite contradictory evidence (Gorman & Gorman, 2017). Many of the psychological influences discussed above are basic to human nature and pre-existing in AWs (for example, the high baseline incidence of psychological disorders and MUPS in the general, non-WC population), and thus a widespread belief, particularly in the insurance industry, that many BH concerns are not "our fault" or our responsibility.
- **Inertia** There is a strong element of inertia and comfort with both administrative and clinical "business as usual" in WC, with a lack of compelling motivation to change, particularly in the face of the high volume and performance demands of current administrative and clinical practice; it is notoriously difficult to alter established patterns of thought and behavior (Bouton, 2014). Many of the BH influences discussed above are subclinical and unrecognized and/or unadmitted by the AW, and at least partially compensated, making them much more challenging to appreciate and incorporate into effective practice. There may also be a disconnect, and sometimes frank conflict, between clinical/medical and administrative/business considerations.
- **Dearth of practical interventions** There is a general lack of knowledge of how to approach and deal with psychosocial factors in occupational, WC, and disability medicine in practical, acceptable, and sustainable ways (Pransky, Loisel, & Anema, 2011). Many practitioners are intimidated by the complexity of these problems (Ramond-Roquin et al., 2014) and tend to fall back and rely upon and search for simple, monomodal solutions. Some BH interventions are still impractical in compensation settings, and there is still an excessive reliance on

largely ineffective BM interventions (and insufficient emphasis on functional rehabilitation).

- **Lack of resources** Even for those administrators and clinicians with some sophistication about BH influences, there is still a profound lack of resources to address the problem. Practical office-based clinical screening and insurer-based predictive models are in their infancy. Reliable, sophisticated, and effective psychological consultation and clinical care by practitioners trained and seasoned with WC and disability systems and claimants are not widely available (Langlieb & Kahn, 2005), and in my experience, many such specialists still take a strong advocagenic approach to the evaluation and treatment (Morgan, 2005).
- **Perceived cost** There are still major considerations of cost. Incorporation of BH elements (i.e., a BPSE approach) usually takes much more time and cognitive and emotional investment by all stakeholders than the BM model and cannot be adequately done under current remunerative practice (Kroenke, 2002). Although cost-utility rather than absolute cost approaches are more rational in this area, this perspective is not currently widespread (see Chap. 10).

9.8 Summary

BH issues are still poorly recognized and accepted in OEM, even though they have extensive impact in many aspects of the specialty. This chapter reviewed interdependent and reciprocal effects of BH and the workplace, including direct, indirect (productivity), and other costs, and effects of work-related stress. It discussed the multiple contributions of BH issues to delayed and failed recovery from work-related illness and injury and unnecessary work disability (DFR/UD), including the effects of administrative and clinical iatrogenicity. It explored the largely unrecognized but potentially significant role of medically unexplained physical symptoms (MUPS) in DFR/UD, how they constitute a major management dilemma for all stakeholders, and some reasons for the widespread reluctance to address these issues. Some conceptual and practical implications of these relationships, and recommendations for management, are presented in the next chapter.

References

Aamland, A., Malterud, K., & Werner, E. L. (2012). Phenomena associated with sick leave among primary care patients with medically unexplained physical symptoms: A systematic review. *Scandinavian Journal of Primary Health Care, 30*(3), 147–155. https://doi.org/10.3109/02813432.2012.704812

Alavi, S. S., Makarem, J., Abbasi, M., Rahimi, A., & Mehrdad, R. (2016). Association between upper extremity musculoskeletal disorders and mental health status in office workers. *Work, 55*(1), 3–11.

Amick, B. C., & Mustard, C. (2005). Chapter 27: Labour markets and health: A social epidemiological view. In S. Bianchi, L. M. Casper, & R. Berkowitz King (Eds.), *Work, family, health, and well-being*. Mahwah, NJ: Lawrence Erlbaum Associates.

Anda, R. F., Butchart, A., Felitti, V. J., & Brown, D. W. (2010). Building a framework for global surveillance of the public health implications of adverse childhood experiences. *American Journal of Preventive Medicine, 39*(1), 93–98. https://doi.org/10.1016/j.amepre.2010.03.015

APA. American Psychiatric Association. (2000). *Diagnostic and statistical manual of mental disorders: DSM-IV-TR* (4th ed.). Washington, DC: American Psychiatric Association.

APA. American Psychiatric Association. (2013). *Diagnostic and statistical manual of mental disorders* (5th ed.). Washington, DC: American Psychiatric Association.

Aronoff, G. M. (1989). The disability epidemic. *Clinical Journal of Pain, 5*(3), 203–204.

Aronoff, G. M. (1991). Chronic pain and the disability epidemic. *Clinical Journal of Pain, 7*(4), 330–338.

Aurbach, R. (2015). Better recovery through neuroscience: Addressing legislative and regulatory design, injury management and resilience. *Proceedings of the 2015 Injury Schemes Seminar*, Australian Actuaries Institute. http://www.uncommonapproach.com/docs/BetterRecoveryThroughNeuroscience.pdf. Accessed 29 April 2017.

Austin, A., Herrick, H., Proescholdbell, S., & Simmons, J. (2016). Disability and exposure to high levels of adverse childhood experiences: Effect on health and risk behavior. *North Carolina Medical Journal, 77*(1), 30–36. https://doi.org/10.18043/ncm.77.1.30

Bandura, A. (1997). *Self-efficacy: The exercise of control*. Gordonsville, VA: Worth Publishers.

Barbour, A. (1995). Caring for patients: a critique of the medical model. Stanford, CA. Stanford University Press.

Barsky, A. J. (2002). Forgetting, fabricating, and telescoping: The instability of the medical history. *Archives of Internal Medicine, 162*(9), 981–984.

Barsky, A. J. (2017, Oct 31). The iatrogenic potential of the physician's words. *Journal of the American Medical Association*. https://doi.org/10.1001/jama.2017.16216.

Barsky, A. J., & Borus, J. F. (1995). Somatization and medicalization in the era of managed care. *JAMA, 274*(24), 1931–1934.

Bartley, M. (1994). Unemployment and ill health: Understanding the relationship. *Journal of Epidemiology and Community Health, 48*(4), 333–337.

Batavia, A. I., & Batavia, M. (2004). Disability, chronic condition, and iatrogenic illness. *Archives of Physical Medicine and Rehabilitation., 85*(1), 168–171.

Bernacki, E. J., Tao, X., & Yuspeh, L. (2010). The impact of cost intensive physicians on workers' compensation. *Journal of Occupational and Environmental Medicine, 52*(1), 22–28. https://doi.org/10.1097/JOM.0b013e3181c91105

Bernal, D., Campos-Serna, J., Tobias, A., Vargas-Prada, S., Benavides, F. G., & Serra, C. (2015). Work-related psychosocial risk factors and musculoskeletal disorders in hospital nurses and nursing aides: A systematic review and meta-analysis. *International Journal of Nursing Studies, 52*(2), 635–648. https://doi.org/10.1016/j.ijnurstu.2014.11.003

Birnbaum, H. G., Kessler, R. C., Kelley, D., Ben-Hamadi, R., Joish, V. N., & Greenberg, P. E. (2010). Employer burden of mild, moderate, and severe major depressive disorder: mental health services utilization and costs, and work performance. *Depression and Anxiety, 27*(1), 78–89. https://doi.org/10.1002/da.20580

Black, O., Keegel, T., Sim, M. R., Collie, A., & Smith, P. (2017). The effect of self-efficacy on return-to-work outcomes for workers with psychological or upper-body musculoskeletal injuries: A review of the literature. *Journal of Occupational Rehabilitation*. https://doi.org/10.1007/s10926-017-9697-y

Block, A. R., Ben-Porath, Y. S., & Marek, R. J. (2013). Psychological risk factors for poor outcome of spine surgery and spinal cord stimulator implant: A review of the literature and their assessment with the MMPI-2-RF. *The Clinical Neuropsychologist, 27*(1), 81–107. https://doi.org/10.1080/13854046.2012.721007

Blustein, D. L. (2008). The role of work in psychological health and well-being: A conceptual, historical, and public policy perspective. *American Psychologist, 63*(4), 228–240. https://doi.org/10.1037/0003-066X.63.4.228

Bouton, M. E. (2014). Why behavior change is difficult to sustain. *Preventive Medicine, 68*, 29–36. https://doi.org/10.1016/j.ypmed.2014.06.010

Budtz-Lilly, A., Schröder, A., Rask, M. T., Fink, P., Vestergaard, M., & Rosendal, M. (2015). Bodily distress syndrome: A new diagnosis for functional disorders in primary care? *BMC Family Practice, 16*, 180–189. https://doi.org/10.1186/s12875-015-0393-8

Buist-Bouwman, M. A., de Graaf, R., Vollebergh, W. A., & Ormel, J. (2005). Comorbidity of physical and mental disorders and the effect on work-loss days. *Acta Psychiatrica Scandinavica, 111*(6), 436–443.

Bultmann, U., & Brouwer, S. (2013). Chapter 10: Individual-level psychosocial factors and work disability prevention. In P. Loisel, J. R. Anema, M. Feuerstein, E. MacEachen, G. Pranksy, & K. Costa-Black. (Co-Eds.) *Handbook of work disability prevention and management* (pp. 149–162). New York: Springer.

Burton, A. K., Kendall, N. A., Pearce, B. G., Birrell, L. N., & Bainbridge, L. C. (2009). Management of work-relevant upper limb disorders: A review. *Occupational Medicine (Lond), 59*(1), 44–52. https://doi.org/10.1093/occmed/kqn151

Burton, C. (2003). Beyond somatisation: A review of the understanding and treatment of medically unexplained physical symptoms (MUPS). *British Journal of General Practice, 53*(488), 231–239.

Carragee, E. J. (2008). Validity of self-reported history in patients with acute back or neck pain after motor vehicle accidents. *Spine Journal, 8*(2), 311–319.

Caruso, G. M., Barth, R. J., Christian, J., Goertz, M., Letz, G., Weiss, M.S., & Warren, P. A. (Co-Author). Kahn, J. P. & Talmage, J. B. (Panel Consultants). Harris, J. S. (Committee Consultant). (2011). "Chapter 5: Cornerstones of disability and management." In Hegmann, K. T. (Ed). Occupational medicine practice guidelines (3rd). Elk Grove Village, IL: American College of Occupational and Environmental Medicine (ACOEM).

Caruso, G. M. (2013). Biopsychosocial considerations in unnecessary work disability. *Psychological Injury and Law, 6*(3), 164–182. https://doi.org/10.1007/s12207-013-9162-y

Chang, L., Sundaresh, S., Elliott, J., Anton, P. A., Baldi, P., Licudine, A., et al. (2009). Dysregulation of the hypothalamic-pituitary-adrenal (HPA) axis in irritable bowel syndrome. *Neurogastroenterology and Motility, 21*(2), 149–159. https://doi.org/10.1111/j.1365-2982.2008.01171.x

Charmandari, E., Tsigos, C., & Chrousos, G. P. (2005). Neuroendocrinology of stress. *Annual Review of Physiology, 67*, 259–284.

Cheriyan, T., Harris, B., Cheriyan, J., Lafage, V., Spivak, J. M., Bendo, J. A., et al. (2015). Association between compensation status and outcomes in spine surgery: A meta-analysis of 31 studies. *Spine Journal, 15*(12), 2564–2573. https://doi.org/10.1016/j.spinee.2015.09.033

Chirico, F. (2016). Adjustment disorder as an occupational disease: Our experience in Italy. *International Journal of Occupational and Environmental Medicine, 7*, 52–57. https://doi.org/10.15171/ijoem.2016.716

Choi, Y., Asih, S. R., & Polatin, P. B. (2016). Chapter 4: Understanding motivation to return to work: The economy of gains and losses. In I. Z. Schultz & R. J. Gatchel (Eds.), *Handbook of return to work from research to practice* (pp. 67–80). New York: Springer.

Chou, R., & Shekelle, P. (2010). Will this patient develop persistent disabling low back pain? *Journal of the American Medical Association, 303*(13), 1295–1302. https://doi.org/10.1001/jama.2010.344

Christian, J. (2017). *Bio-Psycho-Socio-Economic Model (BPSE).* Praxis Partners. Key Concepts and Terms. http://www.webility.md/praxis/biopsychosocioeconomic.htm. Accessed 28 Oct 2017.

Chrousos, G. P. (2009). Stress and disorders of the stress system. *National Review of Endocrinology, 5*(7), 374–381. https://doi.org/10.1038/nrendo.2009.106

Colloca, L. (2014a). Placebo, nocebo, and learning mechanisms. *Handbook of Experimental Pharmacology, 225*, 17–35. https://doi.org/10.1007/978-3-662-44519-8_2

Colloca, L., & Grillon, C. (2014b). Understanding placebo and nocebo responses for pain management. *Current Pain and Headache Reports, 18*(6), 419. https://doi.org/10.1007/s11916-014-0419-2

Colloca, L., & Miller, F. G. (2011). The nocebo effect and its relevance for clinical practice. *Psychosomatic Medicine, 73*(7), 598–603. https://doi.org/10.1097/PSY.0b013e3182294a50

Conrad, P. (2007). *The medicalization of society: On the transformation of human conditions into treatable disorders*. Baltimore: The Johns Hopkins University Press.

Corrigan, P. (2004). How stigma interferes with mental health care. *American Psychologist, 59*(7), 614–625. https://doi.org/10.1037/0003-066X.59.7.614

Coutu, M. F., Cote, D., & Baril, R. (2013). Chapter 2: The work-disabled patient. In P. Loisel, J. R. Anema, M. Feuerstein, E. MacEachen, G. Pranksy, K. Costa-Black (Co-Eds.) *Handbook of work disability prevention and management* (pp. 15–30). New York: Springer.

Creed, F., Barsky, A., & Leiknes, K. A. (2011). Chapter 1: Epidemiology: Prevalence, causes and consequences. In F. Creed, P. Henningsen, & P. Fink (Eds.), *Medically unexplained symptoms, somatization, and bodily distress: Developing better clinical services* (pp. 1–42). Cambridge, UK: Cambridge University Press.

Crichton, S., Stillman, S., & Hyslop, D. (2005). *Returning to work after injury: Longitudinal evidence on employment and earnings*. Discussion Paper No. 1857. Bonn, Germany: Institute for the Study of Labor (IZA).

Damasio, A. R., & Eighth, C. U. (2000). Ariëns Kappers lecture. The fabric of the mind: A neurobiological perspective. *Progress in Brain Research, 126*, 457–467.

Deary, V., Chalder, T., & Sharpe, M. (2007). The cognitive behavioural model of medically unexplained symptoms: A theoretical and empirical review. *Clinical Psychology Review, 27*(7), 781–797.

DeGood, D. E., & Cook, A. J. (2011). Chapter 4: Psychosocial assessment: Comprehensive measures and measures specific to pain beliefs and coping. In D. C. Turk & R. Melzack (Eds.), *Handbook of pain assessment* (3rd ed., pp. 67–97). New York: Guilford Press.

Del Campo, M. T., Romo, P. E., de la Hoz, R. E., Villamor, J. M., & Mahíllo-Fernández, I. (2017). Anxiety and depression predict musculoskeletal disorders in health care workers. *Archives of Environmental and Occupational Health, 72*(1), 39–44. https://doi.org/10.1080/19338244.2016.1154002

Dersh, J., Gatchel, R. J., Mayer, T., Polatin, P., & Temple, O. R. (2006). Prevalence of psychiatric disorders in patients with chronic disabling occupational spinal disorders. *Spine, 31*(10), 1156–1162.

Dersh, J., Mayer, T., Theodore, B. R., Polatin, P., & Gatchel, R. J. (2007). Do psychiatric disorders first appear preinjury or postinjury in chronic disabling occupational spinal disorders? *Spine, 32*(9), 1045–1051.

Dewa, C. S., McDaid, D., & Ettner, S. L. (2007). An international perspective on worker mental health problems: who bears the burden and how are costs addressed? *Canadian Journal of Psychiatry, 52*(6), 346–356.

Dimsdale, J. E. (2018). *Overview of somatization. Merck Manual Professional Version*. http://www.merckmanuals.com/professional/psychiatric-disorders/somatic-symptom-and-related-disorders/overview-of-somatization. Accessed 7 Oct 2017.

Don, A. S., & Carragee, E. J. (2009). Is the self-reported history accurate in patients with persistent axial pain after a motor vehicle accident? *Spine Journal, 9*(1), 4–12. https://doi.org/10.1016/j.spinee.2008.11.002

Drapeau, A., Marchand, A., & Beaulieu-Prevost, D. (2012). Chapter 5: Epidemiology of psychological distress. In Labate, L. (Ed.) Mental illnesses – Understanding, prediction, and control. Rijeka, Croatia: Intech. http://cdn.intechopen.com/pdfs/25512/InTech-Epidemiology_of_psychological_distress.pdf. Accessed 25 Nov 2017.

Dyck, D. E. G. (2017). *Disability management: Theory, strategy, and industry practice* (6th ed.). North York, Ontario: LexisNexis.

Eberstadt, N. A. (2012). *Nation of takers: America's entitlement epidemic*. West Conshohocken, PA: Templeton Press.

Edwards, J. R., Caplan, R. D., & Harrison, R. V. (1998). Person-environment fit theory: Conceptual foundations, empirical evidence, and directions for future research. In C. L. Cooper (Ed.), *Theories of organizational stress* (pp. 28–67). Oxford, UK: Oxford University Press.

Edwards, R. R., Dworkin, R. H., Sullivan, M. D., Turk, D. C., & Wasan, A. D. (2016). The role of psychosocial processes in the development and maintenance of chronic pain. *Journal of Pain, 17*(9), T70–T92. https://doi.org/10.1016/j.jpain.2016.01.001

Elovainio, M., Linna, A., Virtanen, M., Oksanen, T., Kivimäki, M., Pentti, J., & Vahtera, J. (2013). Perceived organizational justice as a predictor of long-term sickness absence due to diagnosed mental disorders: Results from the prospective longitudinal Finnish public sector study. *Social Science & Medicine, 91*, 39–47. https://doi.org/10.1016/j.socscimed.2013.05.008

Evens, A., Vendetta, L., Krebs, K., & Herath, P. (2015). Medically unexplained neurologic symptoms: A primer for physicians who make the initial encounter. *The American Journal of Medicine, 128*, 1059–1064.

Fava, G. A., Guidi, J., & Sonino, N. (2016). The psychosomatic practice. *Acta Dermato-Venereologica, 96*(217), 9–13. https://doi.org/10.2340/00015555-2431

Felhaber, T. (2017). *The risks of worklessness*. Blog entry: This changed my practice. http://thischangedmypractice.com/author/taryl-felhaber/. Accessed 4 Nov 2017.

Fink, P., & Rosendal, M. (Eds.). (2015). *Functional disorders and medically unexplained symptoms: Assessment and treatment*. Aarhus, Denmark: Aarhus University Press.

Fishback, P. V., & Kantor, S. E. (2000). *A prelude to the welfare state: The origins of workers' compensation*. Chicago: University of Chicago Press.

Flor, H., & Turk, D. C. (2013). Chapter 18: Cognitive and learning aspects. In S. B. McMahon, M. Koltzenburg, I. Tracey, & D. C. Turk (Eds.), *Wall & Melzack's textbook of pain* (6th ed., pp. 256–272). Philadelphia: Elsevier Saunders.

Franche, R. L., & Krause, N. (2005). Readiness for return to work following injury or illness. In I. Schultz & R. J. Gatchel (Eds.), *Handbook of complex occupational disability claims* (pp. 67–92). New York: Springer Sciences+Business Media.

Franchimont, D., Kino, T., Galon, J., Meduri, G. U., & Chrousos, G. P. (2003). Glucocorticoids and inflammation revisited. NIH clinical staff conference. *Neuroimmunomodulation, 10*, 247–260.

Frank, J. W., Sinclair, S., Hogg-Johnson, S., Shannon, H., Bombardier, C., Beaton, D., & Cole, D. (1998, 16). Preventing disability from work related low-back pain. New evidence gives new hope—If we can just get all the players onside. *Canadian Medical Association Journal, 158*(12), 1625–1631.

Gatchel, R. J., & Dougall, A. L. (2014). Chapter 12: Psychosocial and psychiatric sequelae of chronic musculoskeletal pain and disability disorders. In R. J. Gatchel & I. Z. Schultz (Eds.), *Handbook of musculoskeletal pain and disability disorders in the workplace* (pp. 219–234). New York: Springer.

Gatchel, R. J., & Gardea, M. A. (1999). Psychosocial issues: Their importance in predicting disability, response to treatment, and search for compensation. *Neurology Clinics, 17*(1), 149–166.

Gatchel, R. J., Polatin, P. B., & Mayer, T. G. (1995). The dominant role of psychosocial risk factors in the development of chronic low back pain disability. *Spine, 20*(24), 2702–2709.

Gerdtham, U. G., & Johannesson, M. (2003). A note on the effect of unemployment on mortality. *Journal of Health Economics, 22*(3), 505–518.

Gilbert-Ouimet, M., Trudel, X., Brisson, C., Milot, A., & Vézina, M. (2014). Adverse effects of psychosocial work factors on blood pressure: Systematic review of studies on demand-control-support and effort-reward imbalance models. *Scandinavian Journal of Work, Environment, and Health, 40*(2), 109–132. https://doi.org/10.5271/sjweh.3390

Gimeno, D., Tabák, A. G., Ferrie, J. E., Shipley, M. J., De Vogli, R., Elovainio, M., et al. (2010). Justice at work and metabolic syndrome: The Whitehall II study. *Occupational and Environmental Medicine, 67*(4), 256–262. https://doi.org/10.1136/oem.2009.047324

Gjerde, L. C., Knudsen, G. P., Czajkowski, N., Gillespie, N., Aggen, S. H., Røysamb, E., et al. (2013). Genetic and environmental contributions to long-term sick leave and disability pension: A population-based study of young adult Norwegian twins. *Twin Research and Human Genetics, 16*(4), 759–766. https://doi.org/10.1017/thg.2013.36

Golubovich, J., Chang, C. H., & Eatough, E. M. (2014). Safety climate, hardiness, and musculoskeletal complaints: A mediated moderation model. *Applied Ergonomics, 45*(3), 757–766. https://doi.org/10.1016/j.apergo.2013.10.008

Gordon, R. E., Eisler, R. L., Gutman, E. M., & Gordon, K. K. (1991). Predicting prognosis by means of the DSM-III multiaxial diagnoses. *Canadian Journal of Psychiatry, 36*(3), 218–221.

Gorman, S. E., & Gorman, J. (2017). *Denying to the grave: Why we ignore the facts that will save us*. New York: Oxford University Press.

Great-West Life Centre For Mental Health in the Workplace. 2017. *Workplace strategies for mental health.* https://www.workplacestrategiesformentalhealth.com/job-specific-strategies/Considering-the-Costs. Accessed 29 Oct 2017.

Greenberg, P. E., Kessler, R. C., Birnbaum, H. G., Leong, S. A., Lowe, S. W., Berglund, P. A., & Corey-Lisle, P. K. (2003). The economic burden of depression in the United States: how did it change between 1990 and 2000? *Journal of Clinical Psychiatry, 64*(12), 1465–1475.

Greenberg, P. E., Fournier, A. A., Sisitsky, T., Pike, C. T., & Kessler, R. C. (2015). The economic burden of adults with major depressive disorder in the United States (2005 and 2010). *Journal of Clinical Psychiatry, 76*(2), 155–162. https://doi.org/10.4088/JCP.14m09298

Gross, D. P., & Battie, M. C. (2010). Recovery expectations predict recovery in workers with back pain but not other musculoskeletal conditions. *Journal of Spinal Disorders and Techniques, 23*(7), 451–456.

Gureje, O., & Reed, G. M. (2016). Bodily distress disorder in ICD-11: Problems and prospects. *World Psychiatry, 15*(3), 291–292. https://doi.org/10.1002/wps.20353

Hadler, N. M. (2008). *Worried sick: A prescription for health in an overtreated America*. Chapel Hill, NC: University of North Carolina Press.

Halligan, P., & Aylward, M. (Eds.). (2006). *The power of belief: Psychosocial influences on illness, disability, and medicine*. Oxford, UK: Oxford University Press.

Harnois, G. & Gabriel, P. (2000). *Mental health and work: Impact, issues, and good practices*. Geneva: WHO. http://www.who.int/mental_health/media/en/712.pdf. Accessed 7 Oct 2017.

Harris, I. A., Mulford, J., Solomon, M., van Gelder, J. M., & Young, J. (2005). Association between compensation status and outcome after surgery: A meta-analysis. *Journal of the American Medical Association, 293*(13), 1644–1652.

Harris, I. A., Young, J. M., Jalaludin, B. B., & Solomon, M. J. (2008). The effect of compensation on general health in patients sustaining fractures in motor vehicle trauma. *Journal of Orthopedic Trauma, 22*(4), 216–220. https://doi.org/10.1097/BOT.0b013e31815c11dc

Harvey, S. B., Modini, M., Joyce, S., Milligan-Saville, J. S., Tan, L., Mykletun, A., et al. (2017). Can work make you mentally ill? A systematic meta-review of work-related risk factors for common mental health problems. *Occupational and Environmental Medicine, 74*(4), 301–310. https://doi.org/10.1136/oemed-2016-104015

Hashmi, J. A., Baliki, M. N., Huang, L., Baria, A. T., Torbey, S., Hermann, K. M., et al. (2013). Shape shifting pain: Chronification of back pain shifts brain representation from nociceptive to emotional circuits. *Brain, 136*(Pt 9), 2751–2768. https://doi.org/10.1093/brain/awt211

Hassard, J., Teoh, K., Cox, T., Dewe, P. D., Cosmar, M., Grundler, R., et al. (2014). *Calculating the cost of work-related stress and psychosocial risks*. Luxembourg: Publications Office of the European Union. https://doi.org/10.2802/20493

Hauke, A., Flintrop, J., Brun, E., & Rugulies, R. (2011). The impact of work-related psychosocial stressors on the onset of musculoskeletal disorders in specific body regions: A review and meta-analysis of 54 longitudinal studies. *Work and Stress, 25*(3), 243–256. https://doi.org/10.1080/02678373.2011.614069

Hees, H. L., Koeter, M. W., & Schene, A. H. (2012). Predictors of long-term return to work and symptom remission in sick-listed patients with major depression. *Journal of Clinical Psychiatry, 73*(8), e1048–e1055. https://doi.org/10.4088/JCP.12m07699

Henderson, M., Harvey, S. B., Overland, S., Mykletun, A., & Hotopf, M. (2011). Work and common psychiatric disorders. *Journal of the Royal Society of Medicine, 104*(5), 198–207. https://doi.org/10.1258/jrsm.2011.100231

Hilton, M. F., Staddon, Z., Sheridan, J., & Whiteford, H. A. (2009). The impact of mental health symptoms on heavy goods vehicle drivers' performance. *Accident Analysis and Prevention, 41*(3), 453–461. https://doi.org/10.1016/j.aap.2009.01.012

Hilton, M. F., & Whiteford, H. A. (2010). Associations between psychological distress, workplace accidents, workplace failures and workplace successes. *International Archives of Occupational and Environmental Health, 83*(8), 923–933. https://doi.org/10.1007/s00420-010-0555-x

Howe, C. Q., Robinson, J. P., & Sullivan, M. D. (2015). Psychiatric and psychological perspectives on chronic pain. *Physical Medicine and Rehabilitation Clinics of North America, 26*(2), 283–300. https://doi.org/10.1016/j.pmr.2014.12.003

Ihlebaek, C., Brage, S., & Eriksen, H. R. (2007). Health complaints and sickness absence in Norway, 1996–2003. *Occupational Medicine (Lond), 57*(1), 43–49.

Iles, R. A., Davidson, M., & Taylor, N. F. (2008). Psychosocial predictors of failure to return to work in non-chronic non-specific low back pain: A systematic review. *Occupational and Environmental Medicine, 65*(8), 507–517.

Illich, I. (2010). *Limits to medicine: Medical nemesis: The expropriation of health*. London: Marion Boyars Publishers.

Juvani, A., Oksanen, T., Virtanen, M., Elovainio, M., Salo, P., Pentti, J., et al. (2016). Organizational justice and disability pension from all-causes, depression and musculoskeletal diseases: A Finnish cohort study of public sector employees. *Scandinavian Journal of Work, Environment, and Health, 42*(5), 395–404. https://doi.org/10.5271/sjweh.3582

Karasek, R. A., & Theorell, T. (1990). *Healthy work: Stress, productivity and the reconstruction of working life*. New York: Basic Books.

Keedy, N. H., Keffala, V. J., Altmaier, E. M., & Chen, J. J. (2014). Health locus of control and self-efficacy predict back pain rehabilitation outcomes. *The Iowa Orthopaedic Journal, 34*, 158–165.

Keefe, F. J., Brown, G. K., Wallston, K. A., & Caldwell, D. S. (1989). Coping with rheumatoid arthritis pain: Catastrophizing as a maladaptive strategy. *Pain, 37*(1), 51–56.

Kendall, N., Burton, A., Main, C., Watson, P., & on behalf of the Flags Think-Tank. (2009). *Tackling musculoskeletal problems: A guide for the clinic and workplace: Identifying obstacles using the psychosocial flags framework*. London: The Stationery Office.

Kilgour, E., Kosny, A., McKenzie, D., & Collie, A. (2015a). Healing or harming? Healthcare provider interactions with injured workers and insurers in workers' compensation systems. *Journal of Occupational Rehabilitation, 25*(1), 220–239. https://doi.org/10.1007/s10926-014-9521-x

Kilgour, E., Kosny, A., McKenzie, D., & Collie, A. (2015b). Interactions between injured workers and insurers in workers' compensation systems: A systematic review of qualitative research literature. *Journal of Occupational Rehabilitation, 25*(1), 160–181. https://doi.org/10.1007/s10926-014-9513-x

Kim, J. (2008). Psychological distress and occupational injury: Findings from the National Health Interview Survey 2000-2003. *Journal of Preventive Medicine and Public Health, 41*(3), 200–207.

Knardahl, S., Johannessen, H. A., Sterud, T., Härmä, M., Rugulies, R., Seitsamo, J., & Borg, V. (2017). The contribution from psychological, social, and organizational work factors to risk of disability retirement: A systematic review with meta-analyses. *BMC Public Health, 17*(1), 176. https://doi.org/10.1186/s12889-017-4059-4

Kooiman, C. G., Bolk, J. H., Rooijmans, H. G., & Trijsburg, R. W. (2004). Alexithymia does not predict the persistence of medically unexplained physical symptoms. *Psychosomatic Medicine, 66*(2), 224–232.

Kosny, A., Franche, R. L., Pole, J., Krause, N., Côté, P., & Mustard, C. (2006). Early healthcare provider communication with patients and their workplace following a lost-time claim for an occupational musculoskeletal injury. *Journal of Occupational Rehabilitation, 16*(1), 27–39.

Kraatz, S., Lang, J., Kraus, T., Münster, E., & Ochsmann, E. (2013). The incremental effect of psychosocial workplace factors on the development of neck and shoulder disorders: A systematic review of longitudinal studies. *International Archives of Occupational and Environmental Health, 86*(4), 375–395. https://doi.org/10.1007/s00420-013-0848-y

Kristman, V. L., Shaw, W. S., Boot, C. R., Delclos, G. L., Sullivan, M. J., Ehrhart, M. G., & Hopkinton Conference Working Group on Workplace Disability Prevention. (2016). Researching complex and multi-level workplace factors affecting disability and prolonged sickness absence. *Journal of Occupational Rehabilitation, 26*(4), 399–416.

Kroenke, K. (2002). Psychological medicine. *British Medical Journal, 324*(7353), 1536–1537.

Kroenke, K. (2014). A practical and evidence-based approach to common symptoms: A narrative review. *Annals of Internal Medicine, 161*(8), 579–586. https://doi.org/10.7326/M14-0461

Kroenke, K. (2016). Somatic symptoms deserve our attention. *Families, Systems, and Health, 34*(4), 330–333.

Laisné, F., Lecomte, C., & Corbière, M. (2012). Biopsychosocial predictors of prognosis in musculoskeletal disorders: A systematic review of the literature (corrected and republished). *Disability and Rehabilitation, 34*(22), 1912–1941.

Langlieb, A. M., & Kahn, J. P. (2005). How much does quality mental health care profit employers? *Journal of Occupational and Environmental Medicine, 47*(11), 1099–1109.

Lazarus, R. S., & Folkman, S. (1984). *Stress, appraisal, and coping*. New York: Springer Publishing Company.

Lee, H., Hübscher, M., Moseley, G. L., Kamper, S. J., Traeger, A. C., Mansell, G., & McAuley, J. H. (2015). How does pain lead to disability? A systematic review and meta-analysis of mediation studies in people with back and neck pain. *Pain, 156*(6), 988–997. https://doi.org/10.1097/j.pain.0000000000000146

Lees-Haley, P. R., Williams, C. W., & English, L. T. (1996). Response bias in self-reported history of plaintiffs compared with nonlitigating patients. *Psychological Reports, 79*(3 Pt 1), 811–818.

Lees-Haley, P. R., Williams, C. W., Zasler, N. D., Marguilies, S., English, L. T., & Stevens, K. B. (1997). Response bias in plaintiffs' histories. *Brain Injury, 11*(11), 791–799.

Leeuw, M., Goossens, M. E., Linton, S. J., Crombez, G., Boersma, K., & Vlaeyen, J. W. (2007). The fear-avoidance model of musculoskeletal pain: Current state of scientific evidence. *Journal of Behavioral Medicine, 30*(1), 77–94.

Loeser, J. D., & Sullivan, M. (1997). Doctors, diagnosis, and disability: A disastrous diversion. *Clinical Orthopedics and Related Research, 336*, 61–66.

Loisel, P., Buchbinder, R., Hazard, R., Keller, R., Scheel, I., van Tulder, M., & Webster, B. (2005). Prevention of work disability due to musculoskeletal disorders: The challenge of implementing evidence. *Journal of Occupational Rehabilitation, 15*(4), 507–524.

Loisel, P., & Cote, P. (2013). Chapter 5: The work disability paradigm and its public health implications. In P. Loisel, J. R. Anema, M. Feuerstein, E. MacEachen, G. Pranksy, & K. Costa-Black, (Co-Eds.) *Handbook of work disability prevention and management* (pp. 59–67). New York: Springer.

Lynch, N. T., Clay, R. L., Hegmann, K. T., Greaves, W. W., & Gold, J. A. (1998). Advocagenic illness: A new name for an old phenomenon. *Legal Medicine Perspectives, 5*(4), 1–2.

McEwen, B. S. (2007). Physiology and neurobiology of stress and adaptation: Central role of the brain. *Physiological Reviews, 87*, 873–904.

Melloh, M., Elfering, A., Egli Presland, C., Roeder, C., Barz, T., Rolli Salathé, C., et al. (2009). Identification of prognostic factors for chronicity in patients with low back pain: A review of screening instruments. *International Orthopedics, 33*(2), 301–313. https://doi.org/10.1007/s00264-008-0707-8

Modini, M., Joyce, S., Mykletun, A., Christensen, H., Bryant, R. A., Mitchell, P. B., & Harvey, S. B. (2016). The mental health benefits of employment: Results of a systematic meta-review. *Australasian Psychiatry, 24*(4), 331–336. https://doi.org/10.1177/1039856215618523

Mohanty, A., Pradhan, R. K., & Jena, L. K. (2015). Learned helplessness and socialization: A reflective analysis. *Psychology, 6*, 885–895.

Morgan, R. F. (2005). *The iatrogenics handbook*. Chico, CA: Morgan Foundation Publishers.

Navarro, X., Vivó, M., & Valero-Cabré, A. (2007). Neural plasticity after peripheral nerve injury and regeneration. *Progress in Neurobiology, 82*(4), 163–201.

Nielsen, M. B., Magerøy, N., Gjerstad, J., & Einarsen, S. (2014). Workplace bullying and subsequent health problems. *Tidsskrift for den Norske Lægeforening, 134*(12-13), 1233–1238. https://doi.org/10.4045/tidsskr.13.0880

Null, G., Feldman, M., Rasio, D., & Dean, C. (2011). *Death by medicine*. Mt. Jackson, VA: Praktikos Books.

olde Hartman, T. C., Woutersen-Koch, H., & Van der Horst, H. E. (2013). Medically unexplained symptoms: Evidence, guidelines, and beyond. British Journal of General Practice, 63(617), 625-6. https://doi.org/10.3399/bjgp13X675241.

Olesen, J., Gustavsson, A., Svensson, M., Wittchen, H. U., Jönsson, B., & CDBE2010 study group; & European Brain Council. (2012). The economic cost of brain disorders in Europe. *European Journal of Neurology, 19*(1), 155–162. https://doi.org/10.1111/j.1468-1331.2011.03590.x

Østby, K. A., Czajkowski, N., Knudsen, G. P., Ystrom, E., Gjerde, L. C., Kendler, K. S., et al. (2014). Personality disorders are important risk factors for disability pensioning. *Social Psychiatry and Psychiatric Epidemiology, 49*(12), 2003–2011. https://doi.org/10.1007/s00127-014-0878-0

Peat, G. (2008). Targeting treatment for non-specific musculoskeletal pain. *Pain, 139*(3), 483–484. https://doi.org/10.1016/j.pain.2008.09.002

Polatin, P. B., Kinney, R. K., Gatchel, R. J., Lillo, E., & Mayer, T. G. (1993). Psychiatric illness and chronic low-back pain. The mind and the spine–which goes first? *Spine (Phila Pa 1976), 18*(1), 66–71.

Pransky, G. S., Loisel, P., & Anema, J. R. (2011). Work disability prevention research: Current and future prospects. *Journal of Occupational Rehabilitation, 21*(3), 287–292. https://doi.org/10.1007/s10926-011-9327-z

Prins, R. (2013). Chapter 1: Sickness absence and disability: An international perspective. In Loisel, P., Anema, J. R., Feuerstein, M., MacEachen, E., Pranksy, G., Costa-Black, K. (Co-Eds.) *Handbook of work disability prevention and management* (pp. 3–14). New York: Springer.

Quartana, P. J., Campbell, C. M., & Edwards, R. R. (2009). Pain catastrophizing: A critical review. *Expert Review of Neurotherapeutics, 9*(5), 745–758. https://doi.org/10.1586/ern.09.34

Ramírez-Maestre, C., Esteve, R., Ruiz-Párraga, G., Gómez-Pérez, L., & López-Martínez, A. E. (2017). The key role of pain catastrophizing in the disability of patients with acute back pain. *International Journal of Behavioral Medicine, 24*(2), 239–248. https://doi.org/10.1007/s12529-016-9600-9

Ramond-Roquin, A., Bouton, C., Gobin-Tempereau, A. S., Airagnes, G., Richard, I., Roquelaure, Y., & Huez, J. F. (2014). Interventions focusing on psychosocial risk factors for patients with non-chronic low back pain in primary care–a systematic review. *Family Practice, 31*(4), 379–388. https://doi.org/10.1093/fampra/cmu008

Rask, M. T., Rosendal, M., Fenger-Grøn, M., Bro, F., Ørnbøl, E., & Fink, P. (2015). Sick leave and work disability in primary care patients with recent-onset multiple medically unexplained symptoms and persistent somatoform disorders: A 10-year follow-up of the FIP study. *General Hospital Psychiatry, 37*(1), 53–59. https://doi.org/10.1016/j.genhosppsych.2014.10.007

Reme, S. E., Tangen, T., Moe, T., & Eriksen, H. R. (2011). Prevalence of psychiatric disorders in sick listed chronic low back pain patients. *European Journal of Pain, 15*(10), 1075–1080. https://doi.org/10.1016/j.ejpain.2011.04.012

Rief, W., & Barsky, A. J. (2005). Psychobiological perspectives on somatoform disorders. *Psychoneuroendocrinology, 30*(10), 996–1002.

Ring, D., Kadzielski, J., Fabian, L., Zurakowski, D., Malhotra, L. R., & Jupiter, J. B. (2006). Self-reported upper extremity health status correlates with depression. *Journal of Bone and Joint Surgery American Version, 88*(9), 1983–1988.

Ring, D., Kadzielski, J., Malhotra, L., Lee, S. G., & Jupiter, J. B. (2005). Psychological factors associated with idiopathic arm pain. *Journal of Bone and Joint Surgery American Version, 87*(2), 374–380.

Rodero, B., Luciano, J. V., Montero-Marín, J., Casanueva, B., Palacin, J. C., Gili, M., et al. (2012). Perceived injustice in fibromyalgia: Psychometric characteristics of the injustice experience questionnaire and relationship with pain catastrophising and pain acceptance. *Journal of Psychosomatic Research, 73*(2), 86–91.

Ropponen, A., Svedberg, P., Huunan-Seppälä, A., Koskenvuo, K., Koskenvuo, M., Alexanderson, K., et al. (2012). Personality traits and life dissatisfaction as risk factors for disability pension due to low back diagnoses: A 30-year longitudinal cohort study of Finnish twins. *Journal of Psychosomatic Research, 73*(4), 289–294. https://doi.org/10.1016/j.jpsychores.2012.07.003

Rosmalen, J. G., Neeleman, J., Gans, R. O., & de Jonge, P. (2007). The association between neuroticism and self-reported common somatic symptoms in a population cohort. Journal of Psychosomatic Research, 62(3), 305-311.

Rydell, R. J., & McConnell, A. R. (2006). Understanding implicit and explicit attitude change: A systems of reasoning analysis. *Personality and Social Psychology Review, 91*(6), 995–1008.

Salmon, P. (2006). Chapter 9: Explaining unexplained symptoms: The role of beliefs in clinical management. In P. Halligan & M. Aylward (Eds.), *The power of belief: Psychosocial influences on illness, disability, and medicine* (pp. 137–160). Oxford, UK: Oxford University Press.

Sansone, R. A., & Wiederman, M. W. (2013). Losing a job on purpose: Relationships with borderline personality symptomatology. *Early Intervention in Psychiatry, 7*(2), 210–212. https://doi.org/10.1111/eip.12014

Schultz, I. Z., Crook, J., Meloche, G. R., Berkowitz, J., Milner, R., Zuberbier, O. A., & Meloche, W. (2004). Psychosocial factors predictive of occupational low back disability: Towards development of a return-to-work model. *Pain, 107*(1-2), 77–85.

Schultz, I. Z., Law, A. K., & Cruikshank, L. C. (2016). Prediction of occupational disability from psychological and neuropsychological evidence in forensic context. *International Journal of Law and Psychiatry, 49*(Pt B), 183–196. https://doi.org/10.1016/j.ijlp.2016.10.005

Schüssler-Fiorenza, R. S. M., Xie, D., & Stineman, M. (2014). Adverse childhood experiences and disability in U.S. adults. *Physical Medicine and Rehabilitation, 6*(8), 670–680. https://doi.org/10.1016/j.pmrj.2014.01.013

Scott, W., McEvoy, A., Garland, R., Bernier, E., Milioto, M., Trost, Z., & Sullivan, M. (2016). Sources of injustice among individuals with persistent pain following musculoskeletal injury. *Psychological Injury and Law, 9*, 6–15. https://doi.org/10.1007/s12207-015-9249-8

Shaw, W. S., & Huang, Y. H. (2005). Concerns and expectations about returning to work with low back pain: Identifying themes from focus groups and semi-structured interviews. *Disability and Rehabilitation, 27*, 1269–1281.

Shaw, W. S., Reme, S. E., Pransky, G., Woiszwillo, M. J., Steenstra, I. A., & Linton, S. J. (2013). The pain recovery inventory of concerns and expectations: A psychosocial screening instrument to identify intervention needs among patients at elevated risk of back disability. *Journal of Occupational and Environmental Medicine, 55*(8), 885–894. https://doi.org/10.1097/JOM.0b013e318289ee6c

Siegrist, J. (2001). A theory of occupational stress. In J. Dunham (Ed.), *Stress in the workplace* (pp. 52–66). London/Philadelphia: Whurr Publishers.

Sinnott, P. (2009). Administrative delays and chronic disability in patients with acute occupational low back injury. *Journal of Occupational and Environmental Medicine, 51*(6), 690–699. https://doi.org/10.1097/JOM.0b013e3181a033b5

Stahel, P. F., VanderHeiden, T. F., & Kim, F. J. (2017). Why do surgeons continue to perform unnecessary surgery? *Patient Safety in Surgery, 11*(1). https://doi.org/10.1186/s13037-016-0117-6

Stone, J., Carson, A., Duncan, R., Coleman, R., Roberts, R., Warlow, C., et al. (2009). Symptoms 'unexplained by organic disease' in 1144 new neurology out-patients: How often does the diagnosis change at follow-up? *Brain, 132*(Pt 10), 2878–2888. https://doi.org/10.1093/brain/awp220

Sullivan, M. J. L., Adams, H., Horan, S., Maher, D., Boland, D., & Gross, R. (2008). The role of perceived injustice in the experience of chronic pain and disability: Scale development and validation. *Journal of Occupational Rehabilitation, 18*(3), 249–261.

Thatcher, A. & Miller, K. *Stressor-(stress)-strain: Expanding on a name*. http://www.academia.edu/28090488/Stressor_-_stress_-_strain_expanding_on_a_name. Accessed 27 Oct 2017.

Tyrer, P. (2014). Personality disorders in the workplace. *Occupational Medicine, 64*(8), 566–568. https://doi.org/10.1093/occmed/kqu113

Turner, J. A., Franklin, G., Fulton-Kehoe, D., Sheppard, L., Wickizer, T. M., Wu, R., et al. (2006). Worker recovery expectations and fear-avoidance predict work disability in a population-based workers' compensation back pain sample. *Spine, 31*(6), 682–689.

Valentin, G. H., Pilegaard, M. S., Vaegter, H. B., Rosendal, M., Ørtenblad, L., Væggemose, U., & Christensen, R. (2016). Prognostic factors for disability and sick leave in patients with subacute non-malignant pain: A systematic review of cohort studies. *BMJ Open, 6*(1), e007616. https://doi.org/10.1136/bmjopen-2015-007616

van der Klink, J. J., & van Dijk, F. J. (2003). Dutch practice guidelines for managing adjustment disorders in occupational and primary health care. *Scandinavian Journal of Work, Environment, and Health, 29*(6), 478–487.

van der Noordt, M., Ijzelenberg, H., Droomers, M., & Proper, K. I. (2014). Health effects of employment: A systematic review of prospective studies. *Occupational and Environmental Medicine, 71*(10), 730–736. https://doi.org/10.1136/oemed-2013-101891

Vlaeyen, J. W., & Linton, S. J. (2012). Fear-avoidance model of chronic musculoskeletal pain: 12 years on. *Pain, 153*(6), 1144–1147. https://doi.org/10.1016/j.pain.2011.12.009

Waddell, G. (2004). *The back pain revolution* (2nd ed.). Edinburgh, Scotland: Churchill Livingstone.

Waddell, G., & Burton, A. K. (2006). *Is work good for your health and Well-being?* London: The Stationery Office.

Waddell, G., & Aylward, M. (2010). *Models of sickness and disability applied to common health problems*. London: Royal Society of Medicine Press.

Waghorn, G., & Lloyd, C. (2005). The employment of people with mental illness. *Advances in Mental Health, 4*(2), 129–171.

Wagner, S., White, M., Schultz, I., Murray, E., Bradley, S. M., Hsu, V., et al. (2014). Modifiable worker risk factors contributing to workplace absence: A stakeholder-centred best-evidence synthesis of systematic reviews. *Work, 49*(4), 541–558. https://doi.org/10.3233/WOR-131709

Walker, J. M. (1992). Injured worker helplessness: Critical relationships and systems level approach for intervention. *Journal of Occupational Rehabilitation, 2*(4), 201–209. https://doi.org/10.1007/BF01078998

Wang, P. S., Beck, A., Berglund, P., Leutzinger, J. A., Pronk, N., Richling, D., et al. (2003). Chronic medical conditions and work performance in the health and work performance questionnaire calibration surveys. *Journal of Occupational and Environmental Medicine, 45*(12), 1303–1311.

Wasiak, R., Verma, S., Pransky, G., & Webster, B. (2004). Risk factors for recurrent episodes of care and work disability: Case of low back pain. *Journal of Occupational and Environmental Medicine, 46*(1), 68–76.

Wertli, M. M., Eugster, R., Held, U., Steurer, J., Kofmehl, R., & Weiser, S. (2014). Catastrophizing-a prognostic factor for outcome in patients with low back pain: A systematic review. *Spine Journal, 14*(11), 2639–2657. https://doi.org/10.1016/j.spinee.2014.03.003

White, M. I., Wagner, S. L., Schultz, I. Z., Murray, E., Bradley, S. M., Hsu, V., et al. (2015). Non-modifiable worker and workplace risk factors contributing to workplace absence: A stakeholder-centred synthesis of systematic reviews. *Work, 52*(2), 353–373. https://doi.org/10.3233/WOR-152134

Wilkinson, R., & Marmot, M. (2003). *Social determinants of health: The solid facts* (2nd ed.). Copenhagen, Denmark: World Health Organization.

Wolfe, K. (2013). *Study finds less than 7% of medical providers in WC generate over 70% of costs.* http://medmetrics.blogspot.com/2013/06/study-finds-less-than-7-of-medical.html. Accessed 30 April 2017.

Yanos, P. T., Roe, D., & Lysaker, P. H. (2010). The impact of illness identity on recovery from severe mental illness. *American Journal of Psychiatric Rehabilitation, 13*(2), 73–93. https://doi.org/10.1080/15487761003756860

Zale, E. L., Lange, K. L., Fields, S. A., & Ditre, J. W. (2013). The relation between pain-related fear and disability: A meta-analysis. *Journal of Pain, 14*(10), 1019–1030. https://doi.org/10.1016/j.jpain.2013.05.005

Chapter 10
Behavioral Health Disability and Occupational Medicine: Practices

Garson M. Caruso

10.1 Introduction

The previous chapter outlined major considerations in the interface between occupational and environmental medicine (OEM) and behavioral health (BH), including mutual and reciprocal influences of BH and the workplace; comorbidity of physical and BH concerns, especially in problem cases; the need for a more widespread combined biomedical (BM) and BH approach (i.e., the biopsychosocioeconomic or BSPE model); specific psychological influences (particularly stakeholder appraisals, attitudes, beliefs, and expectations, or AABEs); iatrogenicity (IAG); medically unexplained physical symptoms (MUPS); the dilemma that all participants face in integrating BH concerns into work-related illness and injury (WRII) and work relevant conditions (WRCs);[1] and reasons for current suboptimal practice.

The present state of integration of BM and BH concerns is certainly suboptimal: there is general ignorance (both in terms of not knowing and disregarding) of BH principles in OEM (as well as the converse), an overarching reliance upon AW inactivity and dysfunction rather than function, and poor recognition of the comorbidity of BM and BH factors and the contribution of the latter to the former (i.e., the BPSE approach). Current practice is often adversarial, with a focus on

[1] WRII denotes a condition directly or indirectly caused, exacerbated, or aggravated by work activity. Examples include many musculoskeletal conditions such as sprains and strains, fractures, and acute derangements of the spinal discs, rotator cuff, and knee menisci, as well as occupational behavioral health considerations like untoward effects of excessive job stress. In contrast, WRC indicates a valid WRII complicated by additional preexisting, coincident, or consequent non-work-related influences, including alcohol or opioid dependence and tobacco abuse, fibromyalgia and other nonoccupational chronic pain syndromes, osteoarthritis (OA), and nonoccupational psychological factors (particularly preexisting mood and personality disorders).

G. M. Caruso (✉)
Occupational and Environmental Medicine, Mechanicsburg, PA, USA
e-mail: garson@gmcarusoconsulting.com

P. A. Warren (ed.), *Handbook of Behavioral Health Disability Management*,
https://doi.org/10.1007/978-3-319-89860-5_10

legitimizing BH disability (possibly partially in reaction to rejection by the BM community) instead of focusing on capability, and is thus highly advocagenic and iatrogenic (see Chaps. 5, 6, and 8).

However, the current situation does have many positive elements. OEM in general and workers' compensation (WC) in particular focus on work, which is central to most people's lives. The WC system provides something of a captive audience, with a larger degree of control than group health insurance, and thus a ready-made platform for intervention. Although the multiple stakeholders involved in WC systems (which include the affected worker [AW] and significant others, employer, insurer, clinician and allied health personnel, attorneys, and regulators) often create barriers to effective intervention, they also furnish a strong opportunity for multilateral input with many potentially useful perspectives. There is a growing recognition of the importance of BH factors in OEM, and an expanding research base on how they affect causation and recovery, effective intervention, and cost-utility considerations.

The major focus of this chapter is enhanced treatment and management of BH concerns in OEM and improving the interface between the two disciplines. Based on the psychological and other influences identified in the previous chapter, I identify and discuss many potential improvements in current management, including (1) heightened understanding of these complex elements and their interactions; (2) appreciation of the perspectives of OEM and BH practitioners; (3) adoption of the capacity, limitation, risk, restriction, and tolerance (CLRRT) paradigm; (4) conceptual shifts and applied changes in administrative and clinical practice; (5) increased recognition of potential problem cases; and (6) specific interventions which may contribute to improvement in current practice and outcomes.

10.2 Prevention

There are four recognized levels of prevention in OEM:

- Primary, or deterrence of WRIIs and WRCs before they occur
- Secondary, or early identification and mitigation of WRIIs and WRCs before they cause significant morbidity (i.e., prevention of progression from preclinical to clinical manifestation)
- Tertiary, or amelioration of established WRIIs and WRCs to restore function and minimize complications (i.e., minimization of negative effects once they occur)
- Quaternary, or avoidance or minimization of unnecessary health system interventions (Pandve, 2014), primarily in the form of administrative and clinical IAG

Most mental, emotional, and behavioral disorders start early in life, and many are well established by the time an individual reaches working age (Kessler et al., 2007); this is also true of maladaptive AABEs and the effects of ACEs (Anda, Butchart, Felitti, & Brown, 2010; see in Chap. 8). Thus, primary prevention is largely beyond the scope of the workplace, although a WHO summary report

(WHO, 2004) outlined many societal and some workplace interventions to reduce the risk and impact of mental disorders. Most industrial efforts in primary prevention are focused on the promotion of healthy workplaces, particularly reduction of unnecessary stress (Harder, Wagner, & Rash, 2014a; Chaps. 5, 6, and 8). A Price waterhouse Coopers report on workplace mental health in Australia (PWC, 2014) estimated an average return on investment (ROI) of 2.3 for companies which implement effective changes to improve workplace mental health. The remainder of this chapter addresses secondary through quaternary prevention in OEM where appropriate; all three levels are relevant to avoidance of delayed and failed recovery from WRII and WRCs and the occurrence of unnecessary disability (DFR/UD).

10.3 Enhancement of Understanding

10.3.1 Fragmentation of Knowledge

Given the current lack of widespread understanding and acceptance of the nature, diagnosis, and management BH disorders in the context of OEM, including balanced approaches to causation, IAG, and recognition and care of MUPS, a fundamental need is a cohesive, evidence-based, and usable body of knowledge. Although there is a growing medical literature on BH applications in OEM (and less so on the converse), this information is fragmented and disorganized, and not applicable in organized or effective ways. The situation has been systemically addressed by many notable authors and researchers, including Hadler (2005), Kahn and Langlieb (2003), Loisel et al. (e.g., 2013), Schultz and Gatchel (2005), and Waddell and colleagues in the United Kingdom (e.g., Waddell & Burton, 2006), as well as the present volume. However, particular needs include agreement on a basic core or body of knowledge acceptable and accessible to wide variety/majority of clinicians, more diagnostic precision in both OEM ("chronic sprain") and BH ("major depressive disorder"), and development of administrative and clinical best practices, as well as more widespread management based on those principles. Although all of these improvements will naturally evolve with time, the major influence of BH factors in OEM, and the corresponding real effects on the lives of all stakeholders, makes these changes more urgent.

10.3.2 Perspective: What OEM Needs to Understand About BH

OEM and WC administrators and clinicians need to understand and accept that BH factors, particularly AABEs, are fundamental to human life, influencing predispositions, perceptions, thoughts, and behaviors of all stakeholders in WC (including themselves!) and disability processes, and thus need to be accepted, embraced, and, in many situations, utilized. In contrast to many conditions seen in

OEM (e.g., sprain and strain or fracture), BH disorders are often more complicated in causation, evaluation, and management and often do not have a finite treatment or easily predictable course. Clinical BH is a more subjectively based specialty than many BM concerns, more reliant on individual self-report and less on "objective" measures like imaging studies, increasing the complexity of management. By their very nature, BH disorders are often incompletely resolved even with optimal care and continue to influence the AW in work and life activity.

10.3.3 Perspective: What BH Needs to Understand About OEM

OEM is a "practical" specialty, with an overarching focus on functional restoration from WRII (or WRC) versus simple relief of symptoms (although this is more true in theory than practice). Accurate determination of causation is paramount for claim acceptance and reimbursement, at least in WC cases. There are multiple stakeholders involved which extend beyond the usual boundaries of the basic patient-clinician relationship; the AW can be considered to be at the center of a triangle, the apices of which include employer, insurer, and clinician (with less salient involvement of others such as allied health personnel and attorneys). There is a fairly well-defined regulatory framework (e.g., specified conditions of care, benefits, durations, and processes for claim adjudication) within which all stakeholders must work. Overall, the specialty is based on what may be an excessive emphasis on objective vs. subjective factors (e.g., impairment vs. disability).

10.3.4 The CLRRT Paradigm and Free Will and Personal Responsibility

10.3.4.1 CLRRT Paradigm

As previously noted, optimal function is the overarching goal of both OEM and BH. In both specialties, complete restriction from work activity is usually not required during treatment and recovery from illness or injury (in BH work absence is usually psychiatric emergency, and work may be more beneficial than harmful, unless work factors are a direct contributor to disorder).

Talmage, Melhorn, and Hyman (2011) described five relevant terms in determining an AW's ability to perform a given job description and suggested an ordered process for making return to work determinations. Misunderstanding and misapplication of these concepts underlies a great deal of advocogenicity and iatrogenicity in both OEM and BH (see Chap. 9).

Capacity refers to attributes such as strength, flexibility, and endurance, and cognition and judgment, most often in terms of the affected worker's current ability (Talmage, 2011). Subnormal capacity is described by the clinician in terms of *limitations*, which are activities that the affected worker cannot physically or mentally perform. Physical examples are the inability of a worker with an untreated rotator cuff tear to effectively engage in above-the-shoulder work or an individual that can only exercise to four metabolic equivalents (METs) to perform work frequently requiring six METs of exertion. Behavioral health examples include difficulties with perception, cognition, and decision-making, as well as conforming to constraints of the job situation and interpersonal interaction.

Risk refers to the chance of harm to the affected worker, enterprise, or general public if the affected worker engages in specific work activities. The presence of identifiable risks may necessitate the use of work *restrictions*, which are activities that the affected worker can but should not perform. A common physical example is the prohibition of individuals with uncontrolled seizure disorders from working as aircraft pilots or commercial motor vehicle operators. Behavioral health risk concerns include potential injury to self or others, or physical plant or product, or disruption of normal operations due to compromised attention, perception, or judgment, or aggressive or violent behavior.

Thus, clinicians may describe work limitations (what the AW cannot physically or mentally do), but they impose work restrictions (what the AW should not do, primarily out of safety concerns).

Tolerance is a psychophysiologic concept which describes the affected worker's ability and motivation to sustain work or activity at a given level, particularly in the presence of pain and/or fatigue. Tolerance is in large part dependent upon the rewards available for performing the activity of interest. Tolerance is not an objective or scientifically verifiable concept and is not an appropriate subject for work restrictions or limitations. Clinicians frequently assume activity intolerance, accept inaccurate self-reports by AWs (often contradicted by sub rosa observation), or mistake intolerance due to symptoms as limitations and/or need for protective restrictions; while this is a usually well-intentioned and an ostensibly benign practice, it generally does more harm than good.

10.3.4.2 Free Will and Personal Responsibility

The free will and individual accountability of the AW is a concept which does not get much attention in OEM, but it is critical in optimal management of WRCs and claim resolution. This concept has been most forcefully advanced by Waddell and colleagues (e.g., Waddell & Aylward, 2010), who noted the following:

Some personal characteristics and psychological processes are deeply ingrained or beyond the control of the individual, but conscious choice, motivation and effort still play a central role in sickness and disability. … In practice, choice may be constrained by biological or psychological limitations, by genuine (even if mistaken) perceptions and beliefs, and by social or occupational factors beyond the control of the individual, lack of autonomy and self-esteem. … But, for all the qualifications, most sick and disabled people bear personal responsibility for their actions. Very few have a severe mental illness or disorder that absolves them from responsibility.

For most people with common health problems, decisions about being (un)fit for work, taking sickness absence or claiming benefits are conscious and rational decisions, free choices with full awareness and intent, for which they must take responsibility. Accepting that they have a genuine health problem, most claimants are nevertheless answerable to 'whether it would be unreasonable to expect [me] to seek or be available for work'. The principle of 'reasonableness' is sufficiently broad to allow for the nature and severity of the health condition and for social circumstances. The corollary is that any judgements must be made with understanding and compassion.

The benefit system must then take account of moral hazard. The structures and (dis)incentives of the benefit system influence claimant behaviour, and the present structure sometimes creates 'welfare dependency'. Ideally, social security structures should work with rather than against human nature, work with self-interest, and encourage rather than discourage desired social behaviour. Health care and social security should encourage and support people to help themselves, to move from dependency to fulfilling their potential (Waddell & Ayward, 2010, pp. 21–2).

10.4 Fundamental Conceptual Shifts

10.4.1 Change from Disability to Ability Emphasis

The single most important conceptual shift is a change from emphasis on incapability to capability, particularly a functional restoration approach during recovery from WRII or WRC (Gatchel, McGeary, McGeary, & Lippe, 2014). This is applicable to BH as well as "physical" disorders; work is generally beneficial to mental health (Black, 2008; Waddell & Burton, 2006), and inability to work due to a BH condition should be considered a psychiatric crisis requiring an immediate response (Bilsker, Wiseman, & Gilbert, 2006; Warren, Chaps. 1 and 4), not a routine occurrence. A particular problem is assignment of unnecessary and/or inappropriate work activity proscriptions and/or temporary total disability status, which is a major source of IAG (see Chap. 8). This alteration in approach to AWs also entails much stronger and more widespread consideration and implementation of vocational rehabilitation in WC, STD, LTD, and even SSA cases.

10.4.2 Expansion of Management to Concept of WRCs

There has historically been a reluctance on the part of employers and insurers to include BH concerns in WC claims and instead to maintain a focus on "objective" and "physical" factors; this was and is rational, due to a high potential for unintentional and intentional abuse (and unintended consequences, such as labeling) by claimants and their agents. However, as explored in the previous chapter, a large body of research supports the comorbidity of BM and BH factors in WRCs and psychosocial drivers of DFR/UD. We need to take a more holistic, BPSE view of the AW (see in Chap. 8) in both understanding and managing these conditions, which is likely to be more administratively and clinically effective (and cost-effective as well). In a recent interview, Goldberg (2017) pointed out the following.

The payer community has to be prepared to address head-on psychological issues. And so (psychological issues) either predate the injury or are caused by or complicated by the injury. It's probably the most effective way to treat the patient. The irony is that workers comp carriers have actually been paying for treatment for Anxiety and Major Depressive Disorder and personality disorders and sleep disturbance and insomnia, and catastrophizing all along under the guise of the "physical injury" because the patients who have these conditions either exacerbated by or underlying the injury, or caused secondarily by the injury, they're the ones who are stuck on opioids. I don't think opioids are the right treatment for these conditions. And then these patients end up maybe never getting a true psych diagnosis submitted on the claim form and never get seen by a psychologist or psychiatrist, but they go to surgeons and get operated on inappropriately. They go to pain specialists and get a lot of injections that may or may not help them - often don't help them. So the payers have subsidized the procedural community really well, and they've subsidized the pharmacy community really well, and to what end? And so, if treating physicians are already using antidepressants and antianxiety medications and muscle relaxants to treat in addition to opioids, then actually they're already treating psychological conditions. So to say we're afraid of a tsunami of psych claims is really putting your head into the sand (Goldberg, 2017, p. 13).

It is critically important that BH issues be considered early in the course of a claim, as an integral part of an AW's condition, and not shunted aside or ignored until BM options are exhausted. There is, however, a critical need to find a common ground ("sweet spot") at which effective management for the AW and fair responsibility for payors meet (see Chap. 9).

10.4.3 Adherence to a "First Do No Harm" Mandate

Medical care (especially in WC) is not an inherently benign process (IOM, 2000), and we must temper our natural advocacy for – and desire to "cure" – patients with reasonable and informed practice which does not add to the individual, business, or societal burden of illness. Administrative and clinical IAG and its outgrowth of "type II medical malpractice" were extensively discussed in the prior chapter; specific concerns are further addressed in Sect. 5.1. Harm avoidance includes the concept of hypothesis about, vs. "definitive" diagnosis of, an individual's medical condition, when the latter is uncertain, e.g., using a working impression such as "pain of uncertain etiology" vs. a vague diagnosis like "chronic strain" (Simpkin & Schwartzstein, 2016). More of the same BM method, if it is not working to reduce symptoms and improve function, is not an answer in these claimants, particularly if it is iatrogenic. A more rational approach may include recognition of MUPS/SSD, with a shift in the ultimate goal away from "cure" and toward coping, management, and maximization of residual comfort and function (see Sect. 10.7.10).

10.4.4 Reduction or Elimination of Stigma

The basis of stigma in BH conditions and its contribution to suboptimal care was discussed in Sect. 9.6 of Chap. 9; this stereotyping and the resultant discrimination are a major barrier to more widespread acceptance and treatment of BH disorders (Harder et al., 2014b). A 2015 report by the National Alliance on Mental Illness (NAMI, 2017) outlined the business case for stigma reduction and proposed general organizational interventions.

10.5 Basic Practical Changes

10.5.1 Keeping Inappropriate Patients Out of WC and Disability Systems

As noted above, medical care in general, and within WC systems in particular, is not always a benign process, with a high potential for iatrogenic effects, and claimants should not be admitted to WC systems without clear indications, especially for common health or mental health problems (CHPs or CMHPs)[2] with only a tenuous relationship to work activity (Waddell & Burton, 2004). Current practices are suboptimal, with many individuals undergoing care under WC claims for questionable medical indications (often as a result of medicalization). There are many reasons for this, including claimant AABEs (e.g., erroneous beliefs about WRII and expectations of entitlement), clinician and insurer failure to more carefully consider and forcefully enforce valid causation, early legal representation by claimants, advocogenicity by multiple stakeholders, and the legal and regulatory context (including low thresholds for establishing prima facie medical evidence and imperfections in the subsequent process of evaluation, particularly independent medical examinations [IMEs]). Improvement will require: (1) increase in knowledge of and attention to forensic concerns in causation (e.g., the physics and therefore likelihood of injury) by all stakeholders; (2) stronger mechanisms for recognition and rejection of questionable claims by insurers (including adjuster training in basic medicine and causation and increased involvement of medical professionals, including nurses, physicians, and others);

[2]CHPs are disorders which frequently occur in adult populations; the prototype is probably musculoskeletal (especially low back) pain. CMHPs include anxiety and depressed mood, "stress," and periodic sleep disturbance, all of which may be normal human responses to WRII. See Chap. 8.

(3) increased clinician recognition and involvement, including greater confidence in and willingness to explain rationales for causation decisions to claimant, employer, and insurer; and (4) a more rational legal and regulatory climate in which these stakeholders must function.

10.5.2 Avoidance of IAG

Advocogenicity and iatrogenicity take many forms in current administrative and clinical practice, the latter including both BM and BH conditions (Morgan, 2005; see Chap. 9). A comprehensive discussion of IAG and its avoidance is beyond the scope of this chapter (see, for example, Caruso et al., 2011); however, some opportunities for intervention and reduction in WC systems are listed here.

Administrative Interventions

- Excessive concern with procedural and legal aspects of claims should be avoided. Reasonable due diligence should be applied to legal and technical aspects of cases, but the major priority should be effective and efficient AW recovery from legitimate WRII.
- Unnecessary delays in case management should be eliminated or minimized. Once the legitimacy of a claim is decided, management should be expeditious: decisions on treatment (e.g., medications and therapy) should be prompt, and questions, e.g., with the treating practitioner, should be resolved as soon as possible (Medical Director review and involvement can be helpful in this process).

Clinical Interventions

- The possibility of medicalization of CHPs or CMHPs or nonmedical (e.g., administrative) concerns should be considered and refrained from at the beginning of a claim or as a case evolves (particularly involving new body parts not included in an original illness or injury).
- Clinicians must carefully consider psychosocial aspects of a WRC, e.g., BH factors which may be contributing to complaints and symptoms and suboptimal recovery; they must also avoid assumption of a "psychogenic" cause for symptoms and be cautious about the diagnosis of malingering.
- Inappropriate and excessive advocogenicity, particularly providing long periods of unnecessary work disability, should be avoided.
- Excessive diagnostic investigations, including exhaustive testing and overdiagnosis, may be iatrogenic and should be discouraged. Evidence-based guidelines should be utilized when available, with practitioner override when indicated by clinical judgment. This is also true of treatment, including clinician familiarity with treatment alternatives and judicious use of medications including opioids; interventions should be focused on functional rehabilitation.

10.5.3 Multi-stakeholder Collaboration and Improved Communication

Despite the interdependence of the clinician, employer, insurer, and others in the care of WC claimants, these stakeholders remain functionally separated in the majority of current practice. Waddell (2006) pointed out that all players must be "onside" to maximize management of WC claims, and centrality, or a common focus on the shared goals of recovery and rehabilitation, is one of the five tenets of Colledge & Johnson's (2000) SPICE model. Collaborative, integrated care has been shown to improve multiple treatment outcomes in nonindustrial settings (Watson et al., 2013), and Katon and Seelig (2008) described implementation in industrial situations. Bevan (2015a) reviewed the medical literature showing multiple benefits of early, multi-stakeholder interventions in musculoskeletal disorders, including reduction in sick leave, work productivity losses, health-care and disability benefit costs, risk of permanent work disability and job loss, and development of comorbid mental illness. However, Cullen et al. (2017) concluded that there is still a need for multi-domain, synergistic workplace interventions involving many perspectives and actually mobilizing multiple stakeholders in management of both musculoskeletal and mental health conditions.

Pransky, Shaw, Franche, and Clarke (2004) pointed out that interpersonal communication "… presents a powerful yet largely untapped strategic opportunity to improve outcomes in work disability" (p. 632). Better results in WC claims have been demonstrated with increase in communication between the AW and clinician (Shaw et al. 2011a) and AW and supervisor (Linton, Boersma, Traczyk, Shaw, & Nicholas, 2016) and between the clinician (especially proactively) and both AW and employer (Dasinger, Krause, Thompson, Brand, & Rudolph, 2001; Kosny et al., 2006).

Bruns and Disorbio (2009) emphasized the need for a cooperative, interactive process between physician and psychologist in decision-making for surgery; examples include procedures performed late in the course of chronic pain syndromes, especially those focused on pain relief like implantation of spinal cord stimulators (Campbell, Jamison, & Edwards, 2013). Drewlo (2014) provided an extensive analysis of factors affecting collaboration between primary care physicians and psychologists. Solano, Pirrotta, Ingravalle, and Fayella (2009) described a unique alliance between family physicians and psychologists, working together in the same office, which was well received by patients and promoted a holistic approach to care. Several organizations currently promote efforts to integrate medicine and BH and provide information that can inform collaboration.[3]

[3]The American College of Occupational and Environmental Medicine (ACOEM; http://www.acoem.org/) offers a 1-day seminar for health-care professionals titled "Getting Difficult Cases Unstuck: Strategies for Stalled Recovery and Prolonged Work Disability." Other examples include the Center for Integrated Primary Care of the University of Massachusetts Medical School (https://umassmed.edu/CIPC), the Integrated Behavioral Health Workforce Project of Antioch University (https://www.antioch.edu/new-england/resources/centers-institutes/center-behavioral-health-innovation/), and the American Psychological Association Practice Organization (http://www.apapracticecentral.org/business/collaboration/primary-care.aspx).

10.5.4 Adoption of a Cost-Utility Versus Absolute Cost Approach

Cost of treatment of BH concerns is a major, and legitimate, concern of employers and insurers. Cost offset determinations for these stakeholders (i.e., whether early detection and treatment of medical condition offsets total costs, including medical, indemnity, and productivity, and other costs) are complex (Langlieb, Druss, & Rosenheck, 2003; Langlieb, Stoline, & Sharfstein, 2003). These considerations become even more complicated in the context of WRCs, in which contributing factors are nebulous, industrial causation difficult if not impossible to determine, and outcome benefits uncertain. However, a blanket approach considering only initial costs (e.g., for CBT) is limited, shortsighted, and suboptimal. There is now good research evidence for cost-effectiveness of interventions; for example, Bevan (2015b) found that carefully done early interventions in WC claims can be cost-effective, and cost-utility has been demonstrated for short courses of CBT without (Lamb et al., 2010; Norton, McDonough, Cabral, Shwartz, & Burgess, 2015) and with (Rogerson, Gatchel, & Bierner, 2010) physical therapy. The APA (2017) recently reviewed cost-utility of workplace treatment of BH (including addiction) disorders, citing evidence of benefit in medical care, disability, and productivity costs.

10.6 Early, Late, and Ongoing Recognition of Problem Cases

10.6.1 Use of Associated Predictive Factors

Sears, Blanar, Bowman, Adams, and Silverstein (2013) found that an Injury Severity Score (ISS) calculated from initial *ICD-9* codes predicted work disability and medical costs. Going further, a search for problem cases should begin with First Report of Injury (FROI) and early insurer contact. The latter should be looking for historical elements which may impact the course of a claim, including the following (Schultz et al., 2016; Steenstra et al., 2017):

- Past medical history, e.g., poor baseline health and comorbidities (especially diabetes, medically unexplained syndromic illnesses like fibromyalgia, and overweight)
- Personal factors, e.g., age, prior WC or other insurance claims experience and/or disability, and alcohol, drug, or tobacco use
- BH factors, e.g., preexisting anxiety, bipolar, depressive, personality, or other disorders, and negative attitudes and beliefs about the condition and expectations for recovery
- Workplace factors, e.g., part-time status, job characteristics associated with delayed recovery like high physical demand, low satisfaction, and PI

Based on the natural history of a given disorder (e.g., musculoskeletal sprain and strain), all stakeholders should develop a preliminary expectation regarding appropriate management and recovery trajectory and time course. (Guidelines like the MDGuidelines and ODG may be useful.) Depending upon its quality (which may be highly variable), initial clinician evaluation may provide more useful information in all of these areas and generally will provide clarification of diagnosis (and thus natural history, management, and anticipated outcome).

10.6.2 Screening Instruments

Hill and Fritz (2011) suggested three uses of psychosocial screening in physical therapy treatment, including as prognostic factors, treatment effect modifiers (to provide information about specific therapy), and treatment mediators (linking interventions and outcomes). Both the American College of Occupational and Environmental Medicine (ACOEM; Feinberg, 2011) and the Colorado Division of Workers' Compensation (CDWC, 2012) have provided useful guidelines regarding the use of psychometric testing in occupational medicine, and other resources are available to assist usage in assessing chronic pain and potential for disability (Durand & Hong, 2013; Bruns & Warren, Chap. 6). There is currently much published research on individual screening instruments, but no single tool has been identified that satisfactorily addresses all phases and the full complexity of work disability or accounts for all stakeholder perspectives. In general, the available tools are more accurate for prediction of prolonged absenteeism and disability outcome (Karran et al. 2017), and George (2017) observed that concise assessment of multiple constructs (e.g., with the Orebro Musculoskeletal Pain Questionnaire) had more predictive value. Some findings on specific instruments are as follows:

- Turner et al. (2008) developed a multi-domain model incorporating biological and psychosocial factors as well as environmental influences (including clinician, employer, and family responses and work and economic elements) that predicted the development of chronic and disabling back pain.
- The work of Hill et al. (e.g., 2011) demonstrated the StarTBack tool to be useful for risk stratification in a stepped care approach to managing low back pain.
- Shaw et al. (2011b) reported that a 19-item RTW Self-Efficacy Questionnaire predicted disability outcomes when administered as early as 1–2 weeks after injury.
- Gabel, Melloh, Burkett, Osborne, and Yelland (2012) found that the Orebro Musculoskeletal Pain Questionnaire predicted recovery time to 80% functional status and outcome at 6 months in musculoskeletal injury.
- Bruns and Disorbio (2014) observed that the Battery for Health Improvement 2 (BHI 2) provided particular strengths in assessing pain, the subject's reactions to injury, dysfunctional pain cognitions, and pain-related psychopathology, including affective distress, somatization, and substance abuse, characterological traits.
- The WHODAS 2 (both 12- and 36-item versions) has replaced GAF in *DSM-5* and is currently used by Washington State in their Psychosocial Determinants Influencing Recovery (PDIR) program (L & I, 2016); this instrument may also have a role in assessment of rehabilitation (Federici et al., 2017).

- Newcomb et al. (2016) found that screening for major depressive disorder with the PHQ-9 (with appropriate referral) markedly lowered odds of temporary or permanent work restrictions at 1 year.

Most authors suggest using several measures based on the individual situation, as part of combination of methods, including review of medical records and clinical assessment. All of these tests raise questions of practicality (administration and usefulness in the office setting), appropriate interpretation, clinical relevance, and remuneration, all of which will need to be addressed. Clinicians need to not only use these tools, but learn to apply them to identify AWs in whom psychosocial intervention may be both medically indicated and helpful.[4]

10.6.3 Predictive Modeling

There is currently a great deal of activity focused on data analytics in the WC and disability insurance industries, with many claims of dramatic cost savings in the gray literature, but nearly all of the information is proprietary and organization-specific, with little or no peer-reviewed research. In general, this technique can be used to trigger a higher level of review or intervention or for treatment vs. settlement decisions (Advisen, 2015). Given the lack of available information, it is not clear how or whether predictive modeling translates to better or more efficient care, or more desirable outcomes, including decreased DFR/UD. For example, Hayden et al. (2010) found that most prediction models explain less than 50% of outcome variability, and few had been independently tested.

10.6.4 Use of Estimated Disability Durations to Monitor Cases

These data, e.g., as provided by the MDGuidelines or Official Disability Guidelines (ODG),[5] should be helpful to both administrators and clinicians, but do not appear to have been effectively used to date (Fassier, 2013).[6] It may be possible to use them in a stepped care approach in potentially problematic claims, developing valid risk

[4] In my experience as a WC medical director and disability file reviewer, I have noted that routine office-based psychometric testing is becoming more prevalent. However, more often than not, the test results show up in the medical records as an isolated data point, with rare acknowledgment in impressions and plan, and no application to the claimant or claim. Sullivan (2013) observed that "The assessment of psychosocial risk factors is only worthwhile if there are plans to institute an intervention specifically designed to target these risk factors" (p. 414).

[5] Both of these are subscription services. MDGuidelines are available at https://www.mdguidelines.com/; ODG is available at http://www.worklossdata.com/.

[6] Franklin et al. (2013) suggested that this may be due to the basis of these guidelines on actuarial data rather than evidence-based healing periods. My anecdotal observation is that disability durations are often included in evaluation reports and even clinical progress notes, but rarely utilized in practice.

profiles from initial demographic, diagnosis, historical, and workplace factors; setting thresholds for increased vigilance ("watchful waiting"), change to a different adjuster, or a different "track" within the insurer, as maximum estimated disability duration is exceeded; and setting a threshold for formal psychological screening (e.g., with the Orebro Musculoskeletal Pain Questionnaire, WHODAS, or BHI 2, or perhaps a battery), which might again trip threshold for different management, e.g., referral to preferred provider or even disability prevention specialist.

10.7 Optimal Management

Basic tenets of optimal management include establishment of a therapeutic alliance with the AW (Conboy et al., 2010) and appropriate administrative and clinical advocacy, with avoidance of both medicalization and nocebo effects (see in Chap. 9). Shared decision-making (King & Moulton, 2013) improves patient satisfaction and reduces decisional conflict, although its effects on health outcomes are less clear (Shay & Lafata, 2015). All stakeholders should attempt to engage in some degree of treatment planning, anticipating the likely outcome of a claim (e.g., return to work with or without permanent restrictions, need for vocational rehabilitation, or palliative care with ongoing pain management). Both administrators and clinicians need to spend more time on the details of AW lives and medical histories, although this is challenging in the face of volume of cases, time limitations, and current remuneration. There needs to be serious refinement in medical records, particularly in electronic form (Friedberg et al., 2013). The following subsections describe a generally escalating approach to care for BH concerns in OEM, particularly in DFR/UD.

10.7.1 Recognition of BH Issues in AWs

Recognition and identification of BH concerns in the workplace is the responsibility of all stakeholders, including the AW themselves, family members and significant others, colleagues, employers, insurers, and clinicians. BH influences should not be routinely sought in WC claims, since they will exert significant effects in only a minority of cases. However, given what we don't know about BH disorders in WC and disability medicine, and what we do know about the effects of time delays and management and the suboptimal outcomes in AWs with WRCs, all stakeholders – including those listed above, as well as nurse case managers (NCMs), allied health personnel, and others – have to go beyond routine care and "step up their game" in caring for persons at risk. In general, this will require more (1) knowledge, e.g., of the natural history and course of musculoskeletal disorders (and thus unusually delays), and subtle manifestations of BH issues; (2) awareness, e.g., of risk factors for administrative and medical IAG; (3) diligence, in paying more attention to claims and claimants, and having an increased index of suspicion for potential BH concerns (e.g., as explanations for atypical behavior or change in normal productivity); and (4) energy, to act on what one sees and knows about a given case. As noted above, it is important to consider BH influences earlier rather than later in WRII and to avoid prolonged BM treatment (particularly if it is not effective) without at least contemplating psychosocial factors.

10.7.2 Education of All Stakeholders

Given the current state of knowledge about BH disorders and disability in the workplace, education of all stakeholders is and will remain a priority for the foreseeable future. Employers, insurers, and clinicians all need to be better aware of (and thus more comfortable with) potential BH influences. AWs, and family members and significant others, will rarely be sophisticated about these concerns and will require education – at their own, appropriate level of comprehension – about possible effects and their relevance to a given claim, particularly by occupational physicians (Caruso, 2008; Grove, 2006). Other areas which may need to be addressed include erroneous or maladaptive AABEs (Louw et al., 2017 used the term "de-educate to re-educate" in this regard) and establishment of realistic understanding of a given condition, diagnostics, interventions, and expected outcome (Dasinger et al., 2001). There may be a role for motivational interviewing, particularly in return to work in disabling musculoskeletal conditions (Park, Esmail, Rayani, Norris, & Gross, 2017).

10.7.3 Activation of AWs

Unless a musculoskeletal or other disorder requires immobilization (e.g., in fracture, or postoperatively) or produces activity limitation or a requirement for protective restriction (see Sect. 2.3.4.1), almost any level of activity is preferable to inactivity. The continuum runs from simple self-generated bodily activity like walking; home exercise (with or without clinician or physical therapist instruction); formal, supervised occupational or physical therapy (OT/PT) , with or without work hardening; graded exercise therapy (GET), particularly in syndromic illnesses involving chronic fatigue or fibromyalgia (Clark et al., 2017); volunteerism; and stay at work/return to work (SAW/RTW) in restricted or unrestricted duty. Exercise is strongly recommended as an integral part of mental health promotion, prevention, and management (Min, Lee, & Lee, 2013). Absence from work is detrimental to health (Macdonald & Asanati, 2016), and there are numerous physical and psychological benefits to SAW/RTW (Modini et al., 2016; Waddell & Burton, 2006). Reavley, Ross, Killackey, and Jorm (2012) conducted a Delphi study based on literature review, involving consumer advocates, employer representatives, and occupational and mental health professionals, and developed a set of return to work guidelines primarily focused on employers, and ACOEM has provided an excellent guideline for personal physicians in keeping patients at or returning them to work (Jurisic et al., 2017).

10.7.4 Referral and Use of RTW Coordinator/Case Manager

Pomaki, Franche, Murray, Khushrushahi, and Lampinen (2012) identified three main elements of intervention in preventing disability in workers with CMHPs, including facilitation of both access to clinical treatment and navigation through the disability management system, and workplace-based high intensity psychological intervention. Depending upon the nature and severity of the underlying problem, situation, and availability of resources, AWs with BH problems may be referred to employee assistance programs (EAPs) or directly to BH practitioners with varying levels of training (i.e., masters level clinician or social worker or doctoral level psychologist or psychiatrist). Richmond et al. (2015) found strong evidence for the effectiveness of EAPs in reducing both absenteeism and presenteeism due to depressive symptoms. Although there may be some role for simple therapy by the primary treating provider (Caruso, 2008), most AWs with significant BH issues will likely benefit from diagnosis and treatment by a specialist (Kahn, 2008); this is particularly true in those to require extended pharmacotherapy and psychotherapy (see Sects. 7.4 and 7.5) and in cases of suspected DFR/UD and/or MUPS (Creed, Kroenke, Henningsen, Gudi, & White, 2011). For example, Bostick (2017) found limited effectiveness for psychological interventions in low back pain administered by non-psychologists.

The use of a RTW coordinator or case manager – for workplace assessment, planning for transitional duty, and facilitating communication among stakeholders – may be especially important in cases with complicated BH issues. Successful management is more related to attitudes toward and competencies in job accommodation, interpersonal communication, and conflict resolution than professional designation (Gardner, Pransky, Shaw, Hong, & Loisel, 2010). Effectiveness has been demonstrated by many studies (Hamer, Gandhi, Wong, & Mahomed, 2013; Hanson, Burton, Kendall, Lancaster, & Pilkington, 2006; Rinaldo & Selander, 2016).

10.7.5 Pharmacotherapy

Pharmacotherapy should include guideline-based use of non-opioid and opioid analgesics (including topical agents), antidepressants, muscle relaxants, and neuroleptics. OEM physicians who are licensed to prescribe medications may judiciously use antianxiety agents and antidepressants in selected cases (Caruso, 2008; Kahn, 2008), as long as they are well-versed in the characteristics of the preparations they prescribe and vigilant for untoward effects and appropriate clinical response. There is a role for interventional pain management, again within consideration of guidelines, with clear indications and a functional restoration focus.

10.7.6 The Psychotherapy Continuum: Counseling to Intensive Treatment

There is a continuum of available psychotherapeutic interventions ranging from pure self-help, through intermediate measures comprising counseling by OEM and various levels of BH specialists, structured activity scheduling, training in coping skills, relaxation, stress and distress management, and progressive goal setting (PGAP), to interpersonal psychotherapy, including CBT. The following is a brief summary of treatment options with OEM implications.

- Supportive counseling by primary treating OEM physicians of affected workers with relatively minor psychosocial issues (e.g., less severe adjustment disorders), including problem recognition and affirmation, specific advice, and referral to community resources or company sponsored employee assistance programs (EAPs), may be effective (Langlieb, Druss et al., 2003; Langlieb, Stoline et al., 2003). Such physicians should be trained, capable, provided with enough time, and compensated to employ basic evaluative techniques for detection of risk for prolonged work disability, including but not limited to: (1) administration, interpretation, and communication of results of screening questionnaires to patients; (2) exploration of affected worker AABEs and their effects on work disability risk; (3) delivery of basic therapeutic interventions such as correcting misinformation or reframing issues in the routine counseling of most patients; and (4) recognition of more serious psychopathology, with referrals to (and collaboration with) BH professionals with higher levels of specialized training.
- Adjuvant awareness and cognitive therapies include structured activity scheduling and training in coping skills, relaxation, and stress and distress management (Kendall, Burton, Main, & Watson, 2009). These modalities may be helpful to affected workers in managing symptoms and building self-efficacy in self-management of less severe problems, although they do not address underlying causative factors such as family problems or work conflicts, or significant psychiatric disorders (Kahn, 2003).
- Psychotherapy (cognitive behavioral or interpersonal) is generally reserved for more severe psychological dysfunction which substantially impacts affected worker function or complicates or imposes barriers to recovery from WRCs. In general, cognitive-behavioral approaches may work more quickly for behavioral change, whereas interpersonal approaches are more effective at addressing underlying emotional drivers. Both must be provided by BH professionals who have undergone specific training.

CBT can be done in person, in group, or by telephone or the Internet (Donker et al., 2015), although at this point WC and disability carriers will typically only reimburse for face-to-face encounters. Treatment is typically time limited in nature, in most instances being provided for a period of 12–16 weeks (which may assuage employer and payer concerns of open-ended therapy). The treatment must be individualized and focused on work issues and preferably combined with RTW intervention (Cullen et al., 2017). The Progressive Goal Attainment Program (PGAP) is a standardized 10-week functional maximization program designed to minimize disability from a variety of physical and mental health conditions (Sullivan, Adams, & Ellis, 2013).

There are still a number of practical problems with CBT, including geographic access to live practitioners, quality of the intervention, and lack of a strong functional and occupational focus. However, a recent literature review update for the ACOEM Practice Guidelines (Chronic Pain Chapter) found that a large majority of the quality studies surveyed supported the efficacy of CBT, with improvements in pain and function and reduction in disability (ACOEM, 2017).

Compared to CBT, there is a relative dearth of literature on the effectiveness of interpersonal psychotherapeutic approaches in work disability prevention; however, some studies have suggested both positive and cost-effective outcomes, including a significant decrease in psychotropic medication use and work absenteeism (Beutel, Rasting, Stuhr, Ruger, & Leuzinger-Bohleber, 2004); long-term and persistent reductions in health-care utilization, sick leave, and work disability, with a cost break-even point at approximately 3 years after treatment termination (de Maat, Philipszoon, Schoevers, Dekker, & De Jonghe, 2007); and higher work productivity, with positive effects persisting at 2-year follow-up (Berghout, Zevalkink, & Hakkaart-Van Roijen, 2010). Body-oriented psychotherapy (BOPT), either in interpersonal or group delivery, may be a promising modality (Rohricht, Papadopoulos, & Priebe, 2013).

10.7.7 Workplace Interventions

Facilitation of SAW/RTW may include changes to work environment or equipment (including the use of technical aids), design and organization, and relationships and/or working conditions. Effective workplace interventions include early contact with the worker by employer representatives; meaningful interaction among AWs, employers, and health-care practitioners; ergonomic work site visits; and arrangements for work accommodation, i.e., restricted or transitional work (Carroll, Rick, Pilgrim, Cameron, & Hillage, 2009; Tompa, de Oliveira, Dolinschi, & Irvin, 2008). Cullen et al. (2017) identified three major domains of interventions, including health-focused, service coordination, and work modification, and found the strongest evidence for reduction of lost time in practices involving at least two categories (interestingly, CBT for mental health conditions was not effective unless it involved a work focus). van Vilsteren et al. (2015) found that workplace interventions improved pain and functional status in workers with musculoskeletal disorders and significantly decreased time to first return to work and cumulative duration of sickness absence, and Midtsundstad and Nielsen (2016) reported that workplace interventions were significantly related to reduced disability rates. However, although perceived injustice is one of the strongest predictors of adverse recovery outcomes (see Chap. 9), Sullivan (2016) pointed out that the condition is complex, and effective management strategies are not yet available.

10.7.8 Disability Prevention Specialist and/or Specialty Clinic

As understanding and appreciation of the role of medically unexplained physical symptoms (MUPS) in OEM, particularly in DFR/UD, becomes more widespread, new approaches to evaluation and management will evolve. These very complex problems will likely require a combined approach, merging theory and practice from multiple medical specialties, including (but not limited to) health psychology, OEM, orthopedics, and physiatric (rehabilitation) and psychosomatic medicine. Interestingly, the latter is currently a subspecialty of psychiatry (at least in the United States), but the major influence of BH concerns in musculoskeletal medicine argues for a much larger contribution from other, more "physical" specialties, such as OEM, orthopedics, and physiatry, perhaps merging into a new area of concentration focused on addressing SSDs and similar conditions with a functional restoration approach. Fink, Burton, De Bie, Sollner, & Fritzsche, (2011) analyzed the advantages and disadvantages of current models of care (primarily in Europe) and advocated the need for specialty clinics focused on bodily distress syndromes and "functional" disorders (e.g., chronic fatigue and pain, fibromyalgia, and irritable bowel syndromes), which would provide expertise in managing many conditions with common symptoms; these could certainly include an occupational component to deal with WRCs involving significant SSDs. Rohricht and Elanjithara (2014) reported substantial reductions in somatic symptom levels and service utilization with the use of group BOPT in such a specialty clinic setting.

10.7.9 Interdisciplinary Functional Rehabilitation (IFR)

IFR programs are intensive processes focused on pain reduction and capability restoration in nonmalignant chronic and disabling musculoskeletal disorders, which may involve medical treatment, reeducation, physical reconditioning, psychotherapy, and vocational counseling. The "interdisciplinary"[7] nature comes from

[7] Gatchel et al. (2014) note that *multidisciplinary* programs may also include several different categories of experts, but that *interdisciplinary* programs generally involve a much higher level of focused coordination and integration among the specialties.

the involvement of physicians (including psychiatrists); nurses (including case managers); clinical (health) psychologists; occupational, physical, and recreational therapists; medical social workers; and vocational rehabilitation experts. Delivery can be inpatient or outpatient and usually involves several hours daily, most days of the week, for 3–6 weeks. Stanos (2012) provided a detailed overview of four representative programs in the United States. Obviously, this intervention is expensive, but both clinical effectiveness and cost-utility (showing superiority to usual care) have been documented, with some reservations (Becker, 2012; Kamper et al., 2015). Current problems are similar to those cited above for CBT (see Sect. 10.7.6) and include availability and access, quality, cost, and acceptance by both AWs and insurers (Gatchel et al., 2014). At this point this intervention should probably be reserved for individuals with complex disorders refractory to less involved management, although further cost-utility research may demonstrate benefits occurring earlier in the disability process.

10.7.10 Change from "Cure" to "Coping" Approach

In some cases, the complexity of BH influences on OEM conditions (including MUPS and DFR/UD) will make practical solution under current management systems difficult if not impossible, particularly in those in which the risk of iatrogenic harm is high (e.g., from repeated surgery of uncertain benefit or opioid dependence). In these situations, a change from a "cure" to "coping" focus should be considered. The emphasis in these instances should be the maximization of AW comfort and residual function, with priority placed on work and daily living capabilities rather than symptom relief per se (Buchbinder & Underwood, 2012). This may incorporate approaches and techniques from chronic disease (Cheatle, 2016) and disability (Loisel, 2014) management, with an overarching goal of harm reduction (similar to that taken in management of opioid dependence, e.g., HRC, 2017), and may encompass principles of acceptance and commitment (Hayes, Strosahl, & Wilson, 2012). This management strategy is anathema to the current focus on biomedical cure; may be difficult for AWs, clinicians, and other stakeholders to accept; and requires careful individual utilization in a given AW's situation, but may provide the overall best outcome for all involved parties in terms of quality of life, and resource utilization and cost.

10.8 Barriers to Intervention

There are many potential or actual barriers to implementation of improved care of BH issues in OEM, particularly involving MUPS. All the factors discussed in Sect. 8.6 of Chap. 8, including lack of widespread awareness, general trepidation about psychology, stigma, scientific denialism, inertia, lack of practical interventions and resources, and perceived cost, will remain troublesome, until and unless we make concerted efforts to improve the understanding of all stakeholders, including AWs, and our ability to effectively (and cost-effectively) utilize that knowledge and intervene successfully to improve patient outcomes. Other concerns are as follows:

- Incorporation of BH concerns into musculoskeletal medicine, while necessary and inevitable, will add an unfamiliar, subjective complexity to evaluation and care which will be initially uncomfortable for many stakeholders.
- Medical jurisdiction, or primary specialty responsibility, may create dilemmas in cases with "physical" and BH comorbidity (e.g., orthopedics or psychiatry in SSDs after musculoskeletal injury), particularly those in which the primary condition or conditions requiring treatment or causing impairment is not clear.
- Nonspecific, symptom-based diagnosis will remain problematic (Murray, Toussaint, Althaus, & Löwe, 2016) until clinicians learn to sharpen their focus and administrators insist on such a change.
- As noted in Sect. 8.5 of Chap. 8, the subjective elements of BH may provide new opportunities for erroneous AABEs and fallibility in thinking; errors, frank quackery, and fraud in medical care; and inventive approaches by creative attorneys. Adoption of the concept of MUPS in OEM will pose new challenges in terms of balancing insurer control and AW protection from abuse or suboptimal care.
- Even as knowledge (and acknowledgment) of BH issues grows, the dual and related challenges of implementing evidence (Fassier, 2013) and changing clinician and other stakeholder behavior (Mostofian, Ruban, Simunovic, & Bhandari, 2015) will continue to be difficult, and remuneration for treatment may become complicated.

10.9 Summary

Based on concepts discussed in the Chap. 9, this chapter outlined some of the weaknesses and strengths of the current approach to WRIIs, WRCs, and BH disorders in the workplace. As always, prevention is crucial, and four levels of opportunity were identified. Enhancement of current understanding of these conditions, and the BH and OEM perspectives, is necessary. More widespread application of the capacity, limitation, risk, restriction, and tolerance (CLRRT) approach to impairment and considerations of the role of free will and personal responsibility are important. Proposed conceptual changes included a shift from disability to capability emphasis, elimination of classical dualistic thought and expansion of the concept of WRCs, adherence to "first do no harm," and elimination of stigma. Basic practical changes include keeping inappropriate patients of compensation systems, avoidance of iatrogenicity in all forms, improvement in stakeholder collaboration and communication, and adoption of cost-utility approaches to intervention. Improvement in recognition of problem cases is crucial in all phases of claims, but particularly early on. Areas of management intervention include stakeholder education, encouragement of AW activity, appropriate specialist referral and the use of RTW coordinators (case managers), evidence-based pharmaco- and psychotherapy, and specific workplace interventions. Consideration should be given to the establishment of an integrated clinical disability prevention specialist role, as well as clinics focused on MUPS, the use of interdisciplinary functional rehabilitation in selected cases, and an increased emphasis on coping versus cure in appropriate cases. Multiple barriers to intervention are discussed.

References

ACOEM. American College of Occupational and Environmental Medicine. (2017). ACOEM practice guidelines. Chronic pain chapter. In K. T. Hegmann (Ed.), *Occupational medicine practice guideline* (3rd ed.). Elk Grove Village, IL: American College of Occupational and Environmental Medicine.

Advisen. The power of predictive models in workers' compensation claims handling. November 2015. [http://www.advisenltd.com/wp-content/uploads/2015/10/power-of-predictive-models-workers-comp-claims-handling-paper-2015-10-16.pdf].

Anda, R. F., Butchart, A., Felitti, V. J., & Brown, D. W. (2010). Building a framework for global surveillance of the public health implications of adverse childhood experiences. *American Journal of Preventive Medicine, 39*(1), 93–98. https://doi.org/10.1016/j.amepre.2010.03.015

APA. American Psychiatric Association Foundation. (2017). Center for Workplace Mental Health. *Quantifying the cost of depression* . http://workplacementalhealth.org/Mental-Health-Topics/MajorDepressive Disorder/Quantifying-the-Cost-of-Depression. Accessed on 11 Nov 2017.

Becker, A. (2012). Health economics of interdisciplinary rehabilitation for chronic pain: Does it support or invalidate the outcomes research of these programs? *Current Pain and Headache Reports, 16*, 127–132.

Berghout, C. C., Zevalkink, J., & Hakkaart-Van Roijen, L. (2010). The effects of long-term psychoanalytic treatment on healthcare utilization and work impairment and their associated costs. *Journal of Psychiatric Practice, 16*(4), 209–216.

Beutel, M. E., Rasting, M., Stuhr, U., Ruger, B., & Leuzinger-Bohleber, M. (2004). Assessing the impact of psychoanalysis and long-term psychoanalytic therapies on health care utilization and costs. *Psychotherapeutic Research, 14*(2), 146–160.

Bevan, S. (2015a). *Back to work: Exploring the benefits of early interventions which help people with chronic illness remain in work*. Fit for work Europe. http://www.theworkfoundation.com/wp-content/uploads/2016/11/F152_Economics-of-Early-Intervention-FINAL.pdf. Accessed on 19 Nov 2017.

Bevan, S. (2015b). Economic impact of musculoskeletal disorders (MSDs) on work in Europe. *Best Practice and Research in Clinical Rheumatology, 29*, 356–373.

Bilsker, D., Wiseman, S., & Gilbert, M. (2006). Managing depression -related occupational disability: A pragmatic approach. *Canadian Journal of Psychiatry, 51*, 76–83.

Black, C. (2008). *Working for a healthier tomorrow*. London: The Stationery Office.

Bostick, G. P. (2017). Effectiveness of psychological interventions delivered by non-psychologists on low back pain and disability: A qualitative systematic review. *The Spine Journal, 17*(11), 1722–1728.

Bruns, D., & Disorbio, J. M. (2009). Assessment of biopsychosocial risk factors for medical treatment: a collaborative approach. *Journal of Clinical Psychology in Medical Settings, 16*(2), 127–147. https://doi.org/10.1007/s10880-009-9148-9

Bruns, D., & Disorbio, J. M. (2014). The psychological evaluation of patients with chronic pain: a review of BHI 2 clinical and forensic interpretive considerations. Psychological Injury and Law, 7, 335–61. DOI 10.1007/s12207-014-9206-y.

Buchbinder, R., & Underwood, M. (2012). Prognosis in people with back pain. *Canadian Medical Association Journal, 184*(11), 1229–1230. https://doi.org/10.1503/cmaj.120627

Campbell, C. M., Jamison, R. N., & Edwards, R. R. (2013). Psychological screening/phenotype being as predictors for spinal cord stimulation. *Current Pain and Headache Reports, 17*(1), 307. https://doi.org/10.1007/s11916-012-0307-6

Carroll, C., Rick, J., Pilgrim, H., Cameron, J., & Hillage, J. (2009). Workplace involvement improves return to work rates among employees with back pain on long-term sick leave: A systematic review of the effectiveness and cost-effectiveness of interventions. *Disability and Rehabilitation, 32*(8), 607–621.

Caruso, G. M. (2008). A clinical perspective on workplace depression: Current and future directions. *Journal of Occupational and Environmental Medicine, 50*(4), 501–513.

Caruso, G. M., Barth, R. J., Christian, J., Goertz, M., Letz, G., Weiss, M. S., & Warren, P. A. (Co-Author), Kahn, J. P., Talmage, J. B. (Panel Consultants), & Harris, J. S. (Committee Consultant). (2011). Chapter 5: Cornerstones of disability prevention and management. In K. T. Hegmann (Ed.), *Occupational medicine practice guidelines* (3rd ed.). Elk Grove Village, IL: American College of Occupational and Environmental Medicine.

CDWC. Colorado Division of Workers' Compensation. (2012). *Rule 17, exhibit 9: Chronic pain disorder medical treatment guidelines. Section E.2. Personality/psychological/psychosocial evaluation for pain management*, pp. 14–25. https://www.colorado.gov/pacific/sites/default/files/MTG_Ex9_CPD.pdf. Accessed on 25 Nov 2017.

Cheatle, M. D. (2016). Biopsychosocial approach to assessing and managing patients with chronic pain. *Medical Clinics of North America, 100*(1), 43–53. https://doi.org/10.1016/j.mcna.2015.08.007

Clark, L. V., Pesola, F., Thomas, J. M., Vergara-Williamson, M., Beynon, M., et al. (2017). Guided graded exercise self-help plus specialist medical care versus specialist medical care alone for chronic fatigue syndrome (GETSET): a pragmatic randomised controlled trial. *Lancet, 390*(10092), 363–373. https://doi.org/10.1016/S0140-6736(16)32589-2

Colledge, A. L., & Johnson, H. I. (2000). S.P.I.C.E.–a model for reducing the incidence and costs of occupationally entitled claims. *Occupational Medicine, 15*(4), 695–722, iii.

Conboy, L. A., Macklin, E., Kelley, J., Kokkotou, E., Lembo, A., & Kaptchuk, T. (2010). Which patients improve: characteristics increasing sensitivity to a supportive patient-practitioner relationship. *Social Science & Medicine, 70*(3), 479–484. https://doi.org/10.1016/j.socscimed.2009.10.024

Creed, F., Kroenke, K., Henningsen, P., Gudi, A., & White, P. (2011). Chapter 3: Evidence-based treatment. In F. Creed, P. Henningsen, & P. Fink (Eds.), *Medically unexplained symptoms, somatization, and bodily distress: Developing better clinical services* (pp. 69–96). Cambridge: Cambridge University Press.

Cullen, K. L., Irvin, E., Collie, A., Clay, F., Gensby, U., Jennings, P. A., et al. (2017). Effectiveness of workplace interventions in return-to-work for musculoskeletal, pain-related and mental health conditions: An update of the evidence and messages for practitioners. *Journal of Occupational Rehabilitation*. https://doi.org/10.1007/s10926-016-9690-x

Dasinger, L. K., Krause, N., Thompson, P. J., Brand, R. J., & Rudolph, L. (2001). Doctor proactive communication, return-to-work recommendation, and duration of disability after a workers' compensation low back injury. *Journal of Occupational and Environmental Medicine, 43*(6), 515–525.

de Maat, S., Philipszoon, F., Schoevers, R., Dekker, J., & De Jonghe, F. (2007). Costs and benefits of long-term psychoanalytic therapy: Changes in health care use and work impairment. *Harvard Review of Psychiatry, 15*(6), 289–300.

Donker, T., Blankers, M., Hedman, E., Ljótsson, B., Petrie, K., & Christensen, H. (2015). Economic evaluations of Internet interventions for mental health: a systematic review. *Psychological Medicine, 45*(16), 3357–3376. https://doi.org/10.1017/S0033291715001427

Drewlo, M. (2014). *Factors in optimal collaboration between psychologists and primary health-care physicians* (Unpublished doctoral dissertation). Antioch University, Seattle, Washington. https://aura.antioch.edu/cgi/viewcontent.cgi?referer=https://www.google.com/&httpsredir=1&article=1177&context=etds. Accessed on 30 Nov 2017.

Durand, M.-J., & Hong, Q. N. (2013). Chapter 15: Tools for assessing work disability. In P. Loisel, J. R. Anema, M. Feuerstein, E. MacEachen, G. Pranksy, & K. Costa-Black (Eds.), *Handbook of work disability prevention and management* (pp. 229–251). New York: Springer.

Fassier, J. B. (2013). Chapter 27: Identifying local obstacles and facilitators of implementation. In P. Loisel, J. R. Anema, M. Feuerstein, E. MacEachen, G. Pranksy, & K. Costa-Black (Eds.), *Handbook of work disability prevention and management* (pp. 441–460). New York: Springer.

Federici, S., Bracalenti, M., Meloni, F., & Luciano, J. V. (2017). World Health Organization disability assessment schedule 2.0: An international systematic review. Disability and Rehabilitation, 39(23), 2347–2380. https://doi.org/10.1080/09638288.2016.1223177.

Feinberg, S. D. (Chair) (2011). Chronic pain guideline. In K. T. Hegmann (Ed.), *Occupational medicine practice guidelines* (3rd ed.). Elk Grove, IL: American College of Occupational and Environmental Medicine (ACOEM).

Fink, P., Burton, C., De Bie, J., Sollner, W., & Fritzsche, B. (2011). Chapter 4: Current state of management and organization of care. In F. Creed, P. Henningsen, & P. Fink (Eds.), *Medically unexplained symptoms, somatization, and bodily distress: Developing better clinical services* (pp. 97–123). Cambridge: Cambridge University Press.

Franklin, G. M., Turner, J. A., Wickizer, T. M., Fulton-Kehoe, D., & Mootz, R. D. (2013). Disability prevention. In Gebhart, G. F., & Schmidt, R. F., Eds. Encyclopedia of Pain (Second Edition). Berlin, Heidelberg: Springer-Verlag Berlin Heidelberg, 2013:1006–11.

Friedberg, M. W., Chen, P. G., Van Busum, K. R., Aunon, F. M., Pham, C., Caloyeras, J. P., et al. (2013). *Factors affecting physician professional satisfaction and their implications for patient care, health systems, and health policy*. RAND Corporation Research Report RR-439-AMA. http://www.rand.org/pubs/research_reports/RR439.html. Accessed on 13 May 2017.

Gabel, C. P., Melloh, M., Burkett, B., Osborne, J., & Yelland, M. (2012). The Örebro musculoskeletal screening questionnaire: validation of a modified primary care musculoskeletal screening tool in an acute work injured population. *Manual Therapeutics, 17*(6), 554–565. https://doi.org/10.1016/j.math.2012.05.014

Gardner, B. T., Pransky, G., Shaw, W. S., Hong, Q. N., & Loisel, P. (2010). Researcher perspectives on competencies of return-to-work coordinators. *Disability and Rehabilitation, 32*(1), 72–78.

Gatchel, R. J., McGeary, D. D., McGeary, C. A., & Lippe, B. (2014). Interdisciplinary chronic pain management: past, present, and future. *American Psychologist, 69*(2), 119–130. https://doi.org/10.1037/a0035514

George, S. Z. (2017). Beliefs, behavior, and back pain: Insights into psychologically informed management. *North Carolina Medical Journal, 78*(5), 333–334.

Goldberg, R. (2017). Interview. *Workers Compensation, 3*(3), 12–13.

Grove, B. (2006). Common mental health problems in the workplace: How can occupational physicians help? *Occupational Medicine (London), 56*(5), 391–393. https://doi.org/10.1093/occmed/kql028

Hadler, N. M. (2005). *Occupational musculoskeletal disorders* (3rd ed.). Philadelphia: Lippincott Williams & Wilkins.

Hamer, H., Gandhi, R., Wong, S., & Mahomed, N. N. (2013). Predicting return to work following treatment of chronic pain disorder. *Occupational Medicine, 63*, 253–259.

Hanson, M. A., Burton, K., Kendall, N. A. S., Lancaster, R. J., & Pilkington, A. (2006). *The costs and benefits of active case management and rehabilitation for musculoskeletal disorders* (Research report 493). London: Health and Safety Executive.

Harder, H. G., Wagner, S. L., & Rash, J. (2014a). Chapter 9: Workplace reactions and interactions with mental health. In *Mental illness in the workplace: psychological disability management* (pp. 235–252). Surrey, UK: Gower.

Harder, H. G., Wagner, S. L., & Rash, J. (2014b). *Mental illness in the workplace: Psychological disability management*. Surrey, UK: Gower.

Hayden, J. A., Dunn, K. M., van der Windt, D. A., & Shaw, W. S. (2010). What is the prognosis of back pain? Best Practice and Research Clinincal Rheumatology, 24(2), 167–79. https://doi.org/10.1016/j.berh.2009.12.005.

Hayes, S. C., Strosahl, K. D., & Wilson, K. G. (2012). *Acceptance and commitment therapy: The process and practice of mindful change* (2nd ed.). New York: Guilford Press.

Hill, J. C., & Fritz, J. M. (2011). Psychosocial influences on low back pain, disability, and response to treatment. *Physical Therapy, 91*, 712–721.

Hill, J. C., Whitehurst, D. G. T., Lewis, M., Bryan, S., Dunn, K. M., Foster, N. E., et al. (2011). Comparison of stratified primary care management for low back pain with current best practice (StarTBack): A randomised control trial. *Lancet, 378*, 1560–1571. https://doi.org/10.1016/S0140-6736(11)60937-9

HRC. Harm Reduction Coalition. (2017). *Principles of harm reduction*. http://harmreduction.org/about-us/principles-of-harm-reduction/. Accessed on 29 Nov 2017.

IOM. Institute of Medicine. (2000). *To err is human: Building a safer health system*. Washington, DC: The National Academies Press.

Jurisic, M., Bean, M., Harbaugh, J., Cloeren, M., Hardy, S., Liu, H., Nelson, C., & Christian, J. (2017). The personal physician's role in helping patients with medical conditions stay at work or return to work. Journal of Occupational and Environmental Medicine, 59(6), e125–e131. https://doi.org/10.1097/JOM.0000000000001055.

Kahn, J. P. (2003). Chapter 1: Workplace mental health quality. In J. Khan & A. Langlieb (Eds.), *Mental health and productivity in the workplace* (pp. 3–27). San Francisco: Jossey-Bass (Wiley).

Kahn, J. P. (2008). Diagnosis and referral of workplace depression. *Journal of Occupational and Environmental Medicine, 50*(4), 396–400.

Kahn, J. P., & Langlieb, A., Eds. (2003). Mental health and productivity in the workplace. San Francisco: Jossey-Bass (John Wiley & Sons).

Kamper, S. J., Apeldoorn, A. T., Chiarotto, A., Smeets, R. J. E. M., Ostelo, R. W. J. G., Guzman, J., et al. (2015). Multidisciplinary biopsychosocial rehabilitation for chronic low back pain: Cochrane systematic review and meta-analysis. *British Medical Journal, 350*, h444. https://doi.org/10.1136/bmj.h444

Karran, E. L., Traeger, A. C., McAuley, J. H., Hillier, S. L., Yau, Y. H., & Moseley, G. L. (2017) The value of prognostic screening for patients with low back pain in secondary care. *Journal of Pain*, pii: S1526-5900(17)30022-6. https://doi.org/10.1016/j.jpain.2016.12.020.

Katon, W. J., & Seelig, M. (2008). Population-based care of depression: team care approaches to improving outcomes. *Journal of Occupational and Environmental Medicine, 50*(4), 459–467. https://doi.org/10.1097/JOM.0b013e318168efb7

Kendall, N., Burton, A., Main, C., Watson, P., & on behalf of the Flags Think-Tank. (2009). *Tackling musculoskeletal problems: A guide for the clinic and workplace: Identifying obstacles using the psychosocial flags framework*. London: The Stationery Office.

Kessler, R. C., Amminger, G. P., Aguilar-Gaxiola, S., Alonso, J., Lee, S., & Bedirhan Ustun, T. (2007). Age of onset of mental disorders: A review of recent literature. *Current Opinions in Psychiatry, 20*(4), 359–364.

King, J., & Moulton, B. (2013). Group health's participation in a shared decision-making demonstration yielded lessons, such as role of culture change. *Health Affairs (Millwood), 32*(2), 294–302. https://doi.org/10.1377/hlthaff.2012.1067

Kosny, A., Franche, R. L., Pole, J., Krause, N., Côté, P., & Mustard, C. (2006). Early healthcare provider communication with patients and their workplace following a lost-time claim for an occupational musculoskeletal injury. *Journal of Occupational Rehabilitation, 16*(1), 27–39.

L & I. Washington State Department of Labor & Industries. (2016). *Reducing disability: Psychosocial determinants influencing recovery (PDIR)*. http://www.lni.wa.gov/ClaimsIns/Files/OMD/MedTreat/2016PDIRResourceFinal.pdf. Accessed on 25 Nov 2017.

Lamb, S. E., Hansen, Z., Lall, R., Castelnuovo, E., Withers, E. J., Nichols, V., et al. (2010). Group cognitive behavioural treatment for low-back pain in primary care: A randomised controlled trial and cost-effectiveness analysis. *Lancet, 375*(9718), 916–923. https://doi.org/10.1016/S0140-6736(09)62164-4

Langlieb, A. M., Druss, B. G., & Rosenheck, R. (2003). Chapter 3: Cost-effectiveness, cost containment, and worker productivity. In J. P. Kahn & A. M. Langlieb (Eds.), *Mental health and productivity in the workplace: A handbook for organizations and clinicians* (pp. 48–59). San Francisco: Jossey-Bass.

Langlieb, A. M., Stoline, A. M., & Sharfstein, S. S. (2003). Chapter 2: Mental health care providers and delivery systems. In J. P. Kahn & A. M. Langlieb (Eds.), *Mental health and productivity in the workplace: A handbook for organizations and clinicians* (pp. 28–47). San Francisco: Jossey-Bass.

Linton, S. J., Boersma, K., Traczyk, M., Shaw, W., & Nicholas, M. (2016). Early workplace communication and problem solving to prevent back disability: results of a randomized controlled trial among high-risk workers and their supervisors. *Journal of Occupational Rehabilitation, 26*(2), 150–159. https://doi.org/10.1007/s10926-015-9596-z

Loisel, P. (2014). *The work disability prevention paradigm: Disability prevention and strategies.* Presentation at SEAK National Workers' Compensation and Occupational Medicine Conference, July 22, 2014.

Loisel, P., Anema, J. R., Feuerstein, M., MacEachen, E., Pranksy, G., & Costa-Black, K. (Eds.). (2013). *Handbook of work disability prevention and management* (pp. 59–67). New York: Springer.

Louw, A., Zimney, K., Johnson, E. A., Kraemer, C., Fesler, J., & Burcham, T. (2017). De-educate to re-educate: aging and low back pain. *Aging Clinical and Experimental Research, 29*(6), 1261–1269. https://doi.org/10.1007/s40520-017-0731-x

Macdonald, E. B., & Asanati, K. (2016). Absence from work. *Contemporary Social Science, 11*(1), 30–39.

Midtsundstad, T. I., & Nielsen, R. A. (2016). Do workplace interventions reduce disability rates? *Occupational Medicine, 66*, 691–697.

Min, J.-A., Lee, C.-U., & Lee, C. (2013). Mental health promotion and illness prevention: A challenge for psychiatrists. *Psychiatry Investigation, 10*, 307–316.

Modini, M., Sadhbh, J., Mykletun, A., Christensen, H., Bryant, R. A., Mitchell, P. B., et al. (2016). The mental health benefits of employment: Results of a systematic meta-review. *Australasian Psychiatry, 24*(4), 331–336.

Morgan, R. F. (Ed.). (2005). *The iatrogenics handbook: A critical look at research and practice in the helping professions.* Chico, CA: Morgan Foundation Publishers.

Mostofian, F., Ruban, C., Simunovic, N., & Bhandari, M. (2015). Changing physician behavior: what works? *American Journal of Managed Care, 21*(1), 75–84.

Murray, A. M., Toussaint, A., Althaus, A., & Löwe, B. (2016). The challenge of diagnosing nonspecific, functional, and somatoform disorders: A systematic review of barriers to diagnosis in primary care. *Journal of Psychosomatic Research, 80*, 1–10. https://doi.org/10.1016/j.jpsychores.2015.11.002

NAMI. National Alliance on Mental Health Illness of Massachusetts. (2017). *Bad for business: the business case for overcoming mental illness stigma in the workplace.* http://ceos.namimass.org/wp-content/uploads/2015/03/BAD-FOR-BUSINESS.pdf . Accessed on 12 Nov 2017.

Newcomb, R. D., Steffen, M. W., Breeher, L. E., Sturchio, G. M., Murad, M. H., Wang, Z., & et al. (2016). Screening for major depressive disorder in the occupational health setting. *Occupational Medicine, 66*(5), 390–393. https://doi.org/10.1093/occmed/kqw043

Norton, G., McDonough, C. M., Cabral, H., Shwartz, M., & Burgess, J. F. (2015). Cost-utility of cognitive behavioral therapy for low back pain from the commercial payer perspective. *Spine, 40*(10), 725–733. https://doi.org/10.1097/BRS.0000000000000830

Pandve, H. T. (2014). Quaternary prevention: Need of the hour. *Journal of Family Medicine and Primary Care, 3*(4), 309–310.

Park, J., Esmail, S., Rayani, F., Norris, C. M., & Gross, D. P. (2017). Motivational interviewing for workers with disabling musculoskeletal disorders: Results of a cluster randomized control trial. *Journal of Occupational Rehabilitation*. https://doi.org/10.1007/s10926-017-9712-3

Pomaki, G., Franche, R.-L., Murray, E., Khushrushahi, N., & Lampinen, T. M. (2012). Workplace-based work disability prevention interventions for workers with common health conditions: A review of the literature. *Journal of Occupational Rehabilitation, 22*(2), 182–195.

Pransky, G., Shaw, W., Franche, R. L., & Clarke, A. (2004). Disability prevention and communication among workers, physicians, employers, and insurers–current models and opportunities for improvement. *Disability and Rehabilitation, 26*(11), 625–634.

PWC. Price Waterhouse Cooper. (2014). *Creating a mentally healthy workplace: Return on investment analysis*. https://www.headsup.org.au/docs/default-source/resources/beyondblue_workplaceroi_finalreport_may-2014.pdf?sfvrsn=90e47a4d_6. Accessed on 29 Oct 2017.

Reavley, N. J., Ross, A., Killackey, E. J., & Jorm, A. F. (2012). Development of guidelines to assist organizations to support employees returning to work after an episode of anxiety, depression, or a related disorder: A Delphi consensus study with Australian professionals and consumers. *BMC Psychiatry, 12*, 135.

Richmond, H., Hall, A. M., Copsey, B., Hansen, Z., Williamson, E., Hoxey-Thomas, N., et al. (2015). The effectiveness of cognitive behavioural treatment for non-specific low back pain: a systematic review and meta-analysis. *PLoS One, 10*(8), e0134192. https://doi.org/10.1371/journal.pone.0134192

Rinaldo, U., & Selander, J. (2016). Return to work after vocational rehabilitation for sick-listed workers with long-term back, neck and shoulder problems: A follow-up study of factors involved. *Work, 55*(1), 115–131.

Rogerson, M. D., Gatchel, R. J., & Bierner, S. M. (2010). A cost utility analysis of interdisciplinary early intervention versus treatment as usual for high-risk acute low back pain patients. *Pain Practice, 10*(5), 382–395. https://doi.org/10.1111/j.1533-2500.2009.00344.x

Rohricht, F., & Elanjithara, T. (2014). Management of medically unexplained symptoms: Outcomes of a specialist liaison clinic. *Psychiatric Bulletin, 38*, 102–107.

Rohricht, F., Papadopoulos, N., & Priebe, S. (2013). An exploratory randomized controlled trial of body psychotherapy for patients with chronic depression. *Journal of Affective Disorders, 151*(1), 85–91.

Schultz, I. Z., & Gatchel, R. J. (Eds.). (2005). *Handbook of complex occupational disability claims: Early risk identification, intervention, and prevention*. New York: Springer Science+Business Media.

Sears, J. M., Blanar, L., Bowman, S. M., Adams, D., & Silverstein, B. A. (2013). Predicting work-related disability and medical cost outcomes: estimating injury severity scores from workers' compensation data. *Journal of Occupational Rehabilitation, 23*(1), 19–31. https://doi.org/10.1007/s10926-012-9377-x

Shaw, W. S., Pransky, G., Roter, D. L., Winters, T., Tveito, T. H., & Larson, S. M. (2011a). The effects of patient-provider communication on 3-month recovery from acute low back pain. *Journal of the American Board of Family Medicine, 24*(1), 16–25. https://doi.org/10.3122/jabfm.2011.01.100054

Shaw, W. S., Reme, S. E., Linton, S. J., Huang, Y. H., & Pransky, G. (2011b). Development of the return-to-work self-efficacy (RTWSE-19) questionnaire– psychometric properties and predictive validity. *Scandinavian Journal of Work, Environment, and Health, 37*(2), 109–119. https://doi.org/10.5271/sjweh.3139

Shay, L. A., & Lafata, J. E. (2015). Where is the evidence? A systematic review of shared decision making and patient outcomes. *Medical Decision Making, 35*(1), 114–131. https://doi.org/10.1177/0272989X14551638

Schultz, I. Z., Law, A. K., & Cruikshank, L. C. (2016). Prediction of occupational disability from psychological and neuropsychological evidence in forensic context. International Journal of Law and Psychiatry, 49(Pt B), 183–196. https://doi.org/10.1016/j.ijlp.2016.10.005.

Simpkin, A. L., & Schwartzstein, R. M. (2016). Tolerating uncertainty – the next medical revolution? *New England Journal of Medicine, 375*(18), 1713–1715.

Solano, L., Pirrotta, E., Ingravalle, V., & Fayella, P. (2009). The family physician and the psychologist in the office together: A response to fragmentation. *Mental Health in Family Medicine, 6*, 91–98.

Stanos, S. (2012). Focused review of interdisciplinary pain rehabilitation programs for chronic pain management. *Current Pain Headache Reports, 16*, 147–152. https://doi.org/10.1007/s11916-012-0252-4

Steenstra, I. A., Munhall, C., Irvin, E., Oranye, N., Passmore, S., Van Eerd, D., Mahood, Q., & Hogg-Johnson, S. (2017). Systematic review of prognostic factors for return to work in workers with sub acute and chronic low back pain. Journal of Occupational Rehabilitation 27(3), 369–381. https://doi.org/10.1007/s10926-016-9666-x.

Sullivan, M. J. L. (2013). What is the clinical value of assessing pain-related psychosocial risk factors? Pain Management, 3(6), 413–6. https://doi.org/10.2217/pmt.13.55.

Sullivan, M. J. L. (2016). Introduction to the special issue on justice-related appraisals and recovery outcomes. *Psychological Injury and Law, 9*, 1–5.

Sullivan, M. J. L., Adams, H., & Ellis, T. (2013). A psychosocial risk-targeted intervention to reduce work disability: Development, evolution, and implementation challenges. *Psychological Injury and Law, 6*(3), 250–257. https://doi.org/10.1007/s12207-013-9171-x

Talmage, J. B. (2011). Chapter 6: The occupational medicine perspective on behavioral health concerns. In P. A. Warren (Ed.), *Behavioral health disability: Innovations in prevention and management* (pp. 133–144). New York: Springer.

Talmage, J. B., Melhorn, J. M., & Hyman, M. H. (2011). Chapter 2: How to think about work ability and work restrictions: Risk, capacity, and tolerance. In J. B. Talmage, J. M. Melhorn, & M. H. Hyman (Eds.), *AMA guides to the evaluation of work ability and return to work* (2nd ed., pp. 9–21). Chicago: AMA Press.

Tompa, E., de Oliveira, C., Dolinschi, R., & Irvin, E. (2008). A systematic review of disability management interventions with economic evaluations. *Journal of Occupational Rehabilitation, 18*, 16–26.

Turner, J. A., Franklin, G., Fulton-Kehoe, D., Sheppard, L., Stover, B., Wu, R., et al. (2008). ISSLS prize winner: early predictors of chronic work disability: a prospective, population-based study of workers with back injuries. *Spine, 33*(25), 2809–2818. https://doi.org/10.1097/BRS.0b013e31817df7a7

van Vilsteren, M., van Oostrom, S. H., de Vet, H. C. W., Franche, R. L., Boot, C. R. L., & Anema, J. R. (2015). Workplace interventions to prevent work disability in workers on sick leave (review). *Cochrane Database of Systematic Reviews*, Issue 10. Art. No.: CD006955. https://doi.org/10.1002/14651858.CD006955.pub3.

Waddell, G., & Aylward, M. (2010). *Models of sickness and disability applied to common health problems*. London: Royal Society of Medicine Press.

Waddell, G., & Burton, A. K. (2004). *Concepts of rehabilitation for the management of common health problems*. London: The Stationery Office.

Waddell, G., & Burton, A. K. (2006). *Is work good for your health and well-being?* London: The Stationery Office.

Waddell, G. (2006). Preventing incapacity in people with musculoskeletal disorders. British Medical Bulletin, 77–78, 55–69.

Watson, L. C., Amick, H. R., Gaynes, B. N., Brownley, K. A., Thaker, S., Viswanathan, M., et al. (2013). Practice-based interventions addressing concomitant depression and chronic medical conditions in the primary care setting: a systematic review and meta-analysis. *Journal of Primary Care and Community Health, 4*(4), 294–306. https://doi.org/10.1177/2150131913484040

WHO. World Health Organization. (2004). *Prevention of mental disorders: Effective interventions and policy options. Summary report*. http://www.who.int/mental_health/evidence/en/prevention_of_mental_disorders_sr.pdf. Accessed on 26 Nov 2017.

Chapter 11
Physical Therapy Treatment and the Impact of Behavioral Health Concerns

Jill S. Galper

11.1 Introduction: What Is Physical Therapy?

Physical therapy "is a dynamic profession with an established theoretical and scientific base and widespread clinical applications in the restoration, maintenance and promotion of optimal physical function" (APTA, 2014). Physical therapists (PTs) and physical therapist assistants (PTAs) are involved in the treatment of people with movement dysfunction and pain and also provide services to promote health and wellness in order to prevent injury and the progression of symptoms, impairments, and activity limitations in a person with an illness or injury. The *Guide to Physical Therapist Practice* notes that services are provided to people of all ages who either have conditions impacting "muscular, neuromuscular, cardiovascular, pulmonary and integumentary systems or the negative effects attributable to unique personal and environmental factors as they relate to human performance" (APTA, 2014). In the USA and its territories, the practice of physical therapy is regulated by the state in which the PT and the PTA practice.

PTs and PTAs regularly treat people with musculoskeletal disorders, which are conditions and injuries affecting muscles, bones, and joints that can result in pain, limited mobility and function, and decreased quality of life and productivity. The Executive Summary of the Bone and Joint Initiative notes that these disorders impact people of all ages at a higher incidence than any other medical condition. The prevalence of arthritis is expected to increase to 25% of the adult population by 2030, and the associated economic burden and impact on quality of life will also increase (Lezin & Watkins-Castillo, 2016). It is therefore prudent that PTs and PTAs effectively manage these and other conditions.

J. S. Galper (✉)
VP, Occupational Health Services, Malvern, PA, USA
e-mail: jill.galper@imxmed.com

P. A. Warren (ed.), *Handbook of Behavioral Health Disability Management*,
https://doi.org/10.1007/978-3-319-89860-5_11

A patient's response to physical therapy treatment is impacted by factors associated with the patient, factors associated with the therapist, and the relationship between them. Patient-related factors include the severity and acuity of the injury or illness, comorbid conditions (including pre-existing mental illness), the patient's engagement in treatment, emotional status, and beliefs. Physical therapist-related factors include his/her knowledge, experience, beliefs, and attitudes. Behavioral health concerns impact the patient's adherence to treatment and self-management, participation, and engagement with treatment and recovery of function. These concerns also impact the PT/PTA's beliefs regarding activity, selection of treatment technique, and communication style and content.

The purpose of this chapter is to explore how behavioral health concerns can impact physical therapy treatment, identify tools available to clinicians to identify, evaluate and treat these patients, and discuss how physical therapists can coordinate and collaborate with mental health professionals when psychological factors impact treatment and recovery. While psychological and behavioral health concerns can affect any patient regardless of diagnosis, this chapter will focus on the treatment of patients with musculoskeletal disorders. There has been a significant amount of additional published articles in this area since publication of the first edition of this chapter in 2011, some of which has been included in this current chapter.

11.2 Factors Impacting the PT/PTA

There is evidence that the beliefs and treatment orientation of a healthcare provider affect the patient's beliefs and treatment outcome. Vlaeyen and Linton (2006) wrote that a PT who has fear-avoidance beliefs may counsel his/her patient to stop any activity that hurts and fail to teach the patient to distinguish between hurt and harm. Coudeyre et al. (2006) investigated the fear-avoidance beliefs of general practitioners and showed that elevated scores on the physical activities subscale of the Fear-Avoidance Beliefs Questionnaire were associated with recommendations of bed rest or rest during sick leave and less advice to remain active, in contrast to current guideline recommendations. Darlow et al. (2012) performed a systematic review that included 17 studies from 8 countries in order to explore the relationship between the healthcare provider's attitudes and beliefs and the attitudes, beliefs, clinical management, and outcomes of patients with low back pain. They reported the following conclusions:

- There is strong evidence that healthcare providers' beliefs about back pain are associated with the beliefs of their patients.
- There is moderate evidence that healthcare providers with a biomedical orientation or elevated fear-avoidance beliefs are more likely to advise patients to limit work and physical activities and are less likely to adhere to treatment guidelines.

- There is moderate evidence that healthcare providers' attitudes and beliefs are associated with bed rest and patient education recommendations.

Houben, Gijsen, Peterson, de Jong, and Vlaeyen (2005) reported that physiotherapists' attitudes toward musculoskeletal pain are predictive of the treatment recommendations. Lakke et al. (2015) found that the physical therapist's fear-avoidance beliefs affected lifting results during functional capacity evaluation.

Given the relationship between the clinician and patient's beliefs, PTs and PTAs should be aware of his/her beliefs, attitudes, and biases when treating patients. Nijs, Roussel, and Wilgen (2013) recommend that therapists follow a five-step approach when treating patients with chronic pain. The first step is self-reflection. To assist with this process, the therapist can assess his/her own beliefs by completing some of the same self-report measures used by patients, such as the Pain Catastrophizing Scale, Fear-Avoidance Beliefs Questionnaire, etc. Nijs et al. also suggest that the therapist determine whether he/she is using a biomedical or biopsychosocial orientation in patient management and suggest the therapist use the Pain Attitudes and Beliefs Scale for Physiotherapists to help determine the treatment orientation. Schmidt (2016) suggests that a PT take the Pain Attitudes and Beliefs Scale for Physiotherapists and the Neurophysiology of Pain Questionnaire as part of the self-discovery process.

A biopsychosocial approach has been recommended in treatment guidelines since it is a framework that acknowledges that a combination of biological, psychological, and social factors all play a significant role in the recovery of a patient rather than physical (biological) factors alone and targets these factors in treatment. A biomedical approach may exacerbate a patient's maladaptive beliefs (Domenech, Sánchez-Zuriga, Segura-Ortí, Espejo-Tort, & Lisón, 2011). An interesting investigation of the treatment orientation used by therapists was done by Van Wilgen, Beetsma, Neels, Roussel, and Nijs (2014). The study involved audiotaping physical therapists as they evaluated patients with chronic musculoskeletal pain. The investigators performed a qualitative analysis and concluded that physical therapist assessment was still biomedically oriented. It therefore seems that additional training is indicated for some PTs and PTAs.

11.2.1 PTs and PTAs' Education and Training and Biopsychosocial Orientation

Although physical therapist curricula include class(es) in psychology, educational programs for PTs and PTAs emphasize the science and clinical techniques related to physical function. In their textbook *Psychology in the Physical and Manual Therapies*, Kolt and Andersen (2004) state that practitioners would like more education in psychology in their training program. This continues to be the case, as shown by Sanders, Foster, Bishop, and Ong (2013) who found that while physiotherapists acknowledged the importance of engaging in negotiations with patients about the range of biopsychosocial obstacles to recovery, many therapists felt their skills and training were inadequate to deal effectively with the psychosocial obstacles. Synnott et al. (2015) performed a qualitative meta-synthesis to explore physiotherapists' perceptions about identifying and managing cognitive, psychological, and social factors that may act as barriers to recovery in people with low back pain. In their introduction, the authors noted that while guidelines for low back pain have shifted toward a biopsychosocial management approach, the initial training of physiotherapists is of a more biomedical nature. Following their qualitative systematic review, they concluded:

- Physiotherapists partially recognize cognitive, psychological, and social factors in people with low back pain.
- Physiotherapists expressed a preference for dealing with the more mechanical aspects of low back pain, and some stigmatized the behaviors suggestive of cognitive, psychological, and social contributors to back pain.
- Physiotherapists felt that their initial training was insufficient to provide the skills and confidence needed to address and treat the multidimensional pain presentations found in patients with low back pain.

Parry and Brown (2009) surveyed physiotherapy programs in the UK in regard to how communication is taught as part of formal education. They found that most communication modules were completed before students had practical experience in the clinic. They question whether communication training should be done differently during the physiotherapy education process and discuss how to teach and assess these skills. These investigations clearly point out the need for further training, during both formal PT education and as continuing education for practicing PTs.

Several studies have investigated training programs for practicing PTs. Overmeer, Boersmak, Main, and Linton (2009) investigated whether an evidence-based education and skills development program could be used to train physical therapists in a biopsychosocial-oriented treatment model and evidence-based treatment for musculoskeletal pain. They found that PT's attitudes and beliefs became more biopsychosocially and less biomedically oriented following the program and that attitudes toward pain and activity became consistent with guidelines.

Lonsdale et al. (2017) had mixed results in their cluster randomized controlled trial evaluating the impact of 8 h of communication skills training on patient adherence to home exercise, and pain and perceived function in men and women with low back pain. The intervention was the Communication Style and Exercise Compliance in Physiotherapy. They found that patient-reported adherence improved in the short term but the intervention did not influence the patient's pain, regardless of gender. Murray et al. (2015) reported that physiotherapists who completed the Communications Style and Exercise Compliance in Physiotherapy training provided greater support for their patient's needs in a single assessed session.

Matthews et al. (2015) developed a training program for physiotherapists called Knowledge Exchange and Delivery Support (KEDS) to change physiotherapist behavior relative to communication strategies with back pain patients. This was a pilot study, and the authors found the approach to be feasible and acceptable to physiotherapists.

Finally, Synnott et al. (2016) instituted a cognitive functional training program for physiotherapists and then performed a qualitative investigation through semi-structured interviews. There were 13 physiotherapists from 4 countries involved in the training and subsequent study. The participants described increased understanding of the nature of pain, the role of patient's beliefs, and new appreciation of the therapeutic alliance. Practice changes included use of new assessments, changing communication, and adoption of the functional approach. The PTs described greater awareness of their scope of practice following training and reported increased confidence and job satisfaction as a result of addressing cognitive, psychological, and social factors in their practice.

These investigations show promise in changing PT's attitudes and practice, but further developments are needed in physical therapy curricula and ongoing continuing education programs to help PTs and PTAs confidently apply biopsychosocial principles and current best evidence in daily clinical practice.

11.3 Behavioral Health Factors Affecting the Patient's Recovery

There are physiological, psychological, social, and environmental factors that impact a patient's response to injury or illness and his/her subsequent recovery. Physiological factors include the severity and extent of the injury or illness, past medical and surgical history and comorbid conditions, activity level, and age.

Psychological factors that negatively impact recovery may include pre-existing psychological conditions such as anxiety and depression, or anger or anxiety following injury or illness. Social and environmental factors include job dissatisfaction or work performance issues, stress or conflict in relationships at home and/or work, insufficient social support, and the unavailability of modified work or the ability/willingness of the employer to accommodate the patient's functional limitation(s).

Other factors that have been found to negatively impact recovery include fear-avoidance beliefs (Fritz, George, & Delitto, 2001; George et al., 2011; George, Fritz, & Childs, 2008), pain catastrophizing (Sullivan, Stanishn, Waite, Sullivan, & Tripp, 1998), perceived injustice (Carriere et al., 2015, 2017), poor self-efficacy, negative recovery expectations, and low levels of physical activity at baseline (Ebrahim et al., 2015; Gross & Battié, 2005; Jack, McLean, Moffet, & Gardiner, 2010; Linton & Shaw, 2011; Quicke, Foster, Ogollah, Croft, & Holden, 2016).

These factors may manifest in one of the following behaviors during a physical therapy episode of care: poor attendance or punctuality for scheduled appointments, poor availability for appointments, limited or poor participation in the PT program, poor adherence to self-management including home exercises, a patient's focus on symptoms, a negative or pessimistic outlook, and dependent or passive behavior, where the patient is looking to the therapist to "fix" the problem (Jack et al., 2010). PTs and PTAs need to be aware of these factors since they may impact the patient's recovery and lengthen the episode of care beyond what would be anticipated based on physical considerations and the natural history of the injury or illness. Recognition of these behaviors should result in the PT reevaluating the patient and looking for the presence of psychosocial barriers to recovery. Patients who have these barriers may require different treatment than for patients who do not have these factors. This will be discussed further in Sect. 11.5.

11.4 Identification of Psychosocial Risk Factors During an Episode of Care

Because psychosocial factors and the patient's recovery expectations and beliefs impact recovery, it is important that the PT and PTA are aware of the presence of these factors during treatment, since providing the most appropriate treatment can help decrease both the financial costs and personal burdens associated with delayed recovery. In occupational health, psychological and emotional factors are often represented by the yellow flag concept, representing psychosocial factors-beliefs, behaviors, perceptions, and responses in relation to an injury that impact recovery and return to work (Kendall, Linton, & Main, 1997; Nicholas, Linton, Watson, & Main, 2011). While verbal discussion with the patient and identification of behaviors of poor adherence and/or treatment participation can identify the presence of risk factors, there are a number of validated tools that can provide a more objective indicator of risk and can be used to monitor progress during the treatment episode. A comprehensive review of these various questionnaires is beyond the scope of this chapter. Examples of condition-specific questionnaires include the Oswestry Disability Index (Fairbank, Davies, Couper, & O'Brien, 1980) and Neck Disability Index (Vernon & Mior, 1991).

The therapist can compare the observations he/she made of the patient during evaluation and treatment with what the patient identified on the questionnaire. This can provide useful information regarding the patient's perceptions of ability and function, which the PT monitors during the treatment episode in addition to other objective parameters. Also, the activities identified as limited can be targeted in treatment. Many of the questionnaires have scoring criteria. Significantly elevated scores will clue the therapist to consider that nonphysiologic factors are probably involved. The use of these questionnaires is recommended in physical therapy treatment guidelines (Childs et al., 2008; Delitto et al., 2012).

Nonorganic signs, also called *Waddell's signs*, suggest that there is a psychosocial component to pain (Waddell, McCulloch, & Kummel, 1980). The PT can include assessment of these signs during patient initial evaluation or at any time during treatment. The original list had the following five categories of signs, with a positive result being three or more positive categories. If the PT finds positive results, other questionnaires can be used as discussed below to obtain more information that can help with patient management:

- Tenderness: Superficial and diffuse tenderness and/or nonanatomic tenderness.
- Simulation tests: These are based on movements causing pain, with the tests not actually causing the movement, as with axial loading of the head and simulated trunk rotation.

- Distraction tests: These tests assess the patient's response when attention is distracted from the movement being tested, as with sitting verses supine straight leg raise.
- Regional disturbance: Means regional weakness or sensory changes that do not follow neuroanatomical pathway (regional weakness, cogwheel release, or stocking/glove sensory loss).
- Overreaction: This refers to the patient's response to movement/testing and can be verbal or nonverbal. This category has been controversial as the decision as to what constitutes overreaction is not consistent, so this category can be deleted and a positive finding based on two positive of four categories (Waddell, 2004).

Pain can be monitored through verbal or visual pain scales. Significantly elevated pain ratings that persist beyond the initial injury or illness phase (e.g., pain ratings of 8–10/10 on a pain scale) and discrepancies between the patient's perception and the therapist's observations should be noted and addressed, as will be discussed in Sect. 11.5.

In addition to the condition-specific questionnaires and pain ratings, the patient's fear of activity or (re)injury can be assessed and monitored via questionnaires. The Fear-Avoidance Beliefs Questionnaire (FABQ) (Waddell, Newton, Henderson, Somerville, & Main, 1993) and Tampa Scale of Kinesiophobia (Vlaeyen, Kole-Snijders, Boeren, & van Eek, 1995) can be used to determine whether the patient has fear-avoidance beliefs or fear of (re)injury. Identifying whether a patient has fear-avoidance beliefs or fear of (re)injury is important since evidence suggests that a different treatment approach is recommended for these patients (George, Fritz, Bialosky, & Donald, 2003). In their study, George et al. showed that patients who do not have fear-avoidance beliefs and who were treated with fear-avoidance-based PT had more disability versus those receiving standard physical therapy. Patients with fear-avoidance beliefs who received fear-avoidance-based physical therapy had less disability than those patients receiving standard treatment. The fear-avoidance-based treatment de-emphasized anatomical findings during patient education and used a graded exercise program, which was based on a predetermined quota of exercise intensity, duration, or repetition. This suggests that subclassification of patients with and without psychosocial barriers to treatment is important. The following questionnaires can assist the PT in this assessment.

The FABQ includes 16 statements regarding the nature and presumed cause of the patient's pain and the degree to which the patient believes the pain to preclude physical activity and return to work. The questionnaire has two sections, a physical activities (FABQ-P) section and a work activities (FABQ-W) section. Each section is scored separately. Elevations in the scores on the FABQ-W section have been shown to negatively correlate with return to work in patients with acute low back pain, with scores exceeding 29 predictive of poor outcome (Fritz et al., 2001). A study suggested that scores as low as 20 are correlated with disability as measured by the Oswestry Disability Index (ODI) at 6 months (George et al., 2008). Marchand et al. (2015) found that elevated scores on the FABQ-P subscale at baseline were a negative predictor for improved disability in a population of patients with neck and low back pain. The Tampa Scale of Kinesiophobia (TSK) (Vlaeyen et al., 1995) is a questionnaire that consists of 17 questions that is scored on a four-point Likert scale where higher scores reflect greater fear of movement. It has not been used as frequently as the FABQ in the physical therapy literature but can be used by PTs as an alternative to the FABQ.

Lee et al. (2013) triaged patients to participate in a cognitive behavioral physical therapy approach based on a moderately elevated score of the Örebro Musculoskeletal Pain Questionnaire (OMPQ). The Work-Related Recovery Expectations Questionnaire (ERQ), TSK, ODI, numeric pain rating, and some other tools were used as outcome measures. They investigated the efficacy of an integrated work rehabilitation program that incorporated physical training, a cognitive behavioral approach, and activities related to a participant's job requirements. The participants had non-specific low back pain of less than 12 weeks duration and moderately elevated scores on the Örebro of 106–145 points. The PTs in the intervention group received training in a cognitive behavioral approach. The intervention group received individualized graded activity program, pacing techniques, work conditioning, return to work goal setting, self-management strategies, job analysis, and ergonomic advice. Patients who missed a treatment were phoned. Discharge occurred if the patient was able to return to work, had subjective improvement of 70% or more, or if there was a plateau in progress. Compared with the control group who received usual care of exercise and physical agents, the intervention group made significant improvement in work recovery expectation, pain, self-efficacy, and satisfaction with treatment.

Cairns, Foster, Wright, and Pennington (2003) wrote that distress (a term that represents a composite of psychological distress, depressive symptoms, and depressive mood) associated with low back pain is common and investigated the use of the Distress Risk Assessment Method in conjunction with the Roland-Morris Disability Questionnaire for the management of recurrent low back pain. They found that increased levels of distress markedly increase the risk of poor outcome.

Pain catastrophizing has been associated with delayed recovery and is characterized by the tendency to magnify the threat value of a pain stimulus and to feel helpless in the presence of pain. It affects how people experience pain. The Pain Catastrophizing Scale (PCS) was developed by Sullivan et al. who showed that catastrophizing was associated with disability, with the rumination subscale the strongest predictor of pain and disability (Sullivan et al., 1998).

Sullivan, Scott, and Trost (2012) demonstrated that perceived injustice has a role as a determinant of pain and disability following injury. Perceived injustice and return to work were explored by Carriere et al. (2017) who found that a person's perception of injustice is associated with their expectancies to return to work. Sullivan, Adams, Horan, Mahar, Boland, and Gross (2008) developed and evaluated the psychometric properties of the Injustice Experience Questionnaire (IEQ), which is a 12-item scale developed to measure a person's perceived injustice associated with a musculoskeletal injury. They demonstrated acceptable construct validity of the scale and felt it was a useful complement to psychosocial assessment of people with persistent pain conditions.

Lenz et al. (2016) described the development of a concise multidimensional yellow flag tool that includes both vulnerability and resilience factors called the

Optimal Screening for Prediction of Referral and Outcome (OSPRO-YF). This is intended for use by orthopedic PTs and looks for depressive symptoms, anxiety, anger, fear avoidance, kinesiophobia, catastrophizing, self-efficacy, and pain acceptance.

Wijma, van Wilgen, Meeus, and Nijs (2016) presented a method for PTs to use to perform a clinical biopsychosocial PT assessment of patients with chronic pain. Patients with chronic pain who have central sensitization have pain processes modulated by behavioral, emotional, social, and cognitive factors. Therefore, the authors suggest that the initial exam should take into account both somatic and psychosocial factors. The article discusses how the examination is performed to allow for an interactive and patient-centered process and education. In addition to providing a structure to the evaluation, the article includes a table with a list of helpful questionnaires, which is a helpful resource for PTs and PTAs.

The tools discussed above (as well as others) are available for use by PTs and do not take much time for the patient to complete (generally less than 10 min). It is recommended that PTs use them during the episode of care. Therapists should not use these tools to negatively label or judge their patient but rather should regard them as an additional source of information about the patient that can help guide selection of the appropriate intervention, as will be discussed below.

11.5 Physical Therapy Intervention

11.5.1 The Optimal Treatment Process

Many patients are referred to PTs by a medical practitioner, although all US states and its territories now permit some form of direct access, meaning patients can choose to see a physical therapist without referral. Specific regulations vary by state. All PT intervention begins with an evaluation, which includes medical history, patient interview, examination, diagnosis, and development of treatment goals and a care plan. The plan includes a time frame for treatment and recovery, with outcome measures identified that are monitored during the episode of care. The PT is responsible for coordination and communication with the relevant stakeholders, which may include physicians, nurses, claims adjusters, nurse case managers, and employers. As treatment continues, the patient's response and progress are monitored. The visit frequency and treatment duration depend on a combination of factors including the patient's health status, injury/illness severity, comorbid conditions, and the psychosocial considerations previously discussed. Treatment frequency will decrease as the patient progresses and is better able to self-manage symptoms, exercises, and activities. During the episode of care, all relevant stakeholders should be kept informed of the patient's progress. In cases where the patient has positive self-efficacy and does not have psychosocial or physiological factors that impact recovery, progress is usually steady and parallels soft tissue healing. The patient demonstrates good adherence to treatment recommendations and is a willing active participant in treatment. The patient is discharged when he/she has met the treatment goals (American Physical Therapy Association, 2014).

11.5.2 Therapeutic Alliance

A critical aspect of PT management is the therapeutic alliance (also referred to as the working alliance) between the clinician and patient. The therapeutic alliance has been described as the social connection between therapist and patient. There is a consistent correlation of positive therapeutic alliance and improved pain, disability, and treatment satisfaction in medicine, psychology, and physical rehabilitation (Hall, Ferriera, Maher, Latimer, & Ferriera, 2010; Ferreira et al., 2013; Fuentes et al., 2014) In fact, some authors suggest that the quality of the alliance is more important than the type of treatment in predicting positive therapeutic outcomes (Martin, Garske, & Davis, 2000; Stillwell and Harman, 2017).

The therapeutic alliance in physical therapy has three main components (Ferreira, et al., 2013):

1. Therapist-patient agreement on goals
2. Therapist-patient agreement on interventions
3. The affective bond between the therapist and patient

In more recent physical therapy publications, the therapeutic alliance is most commonly discussed in articles concerning management of patients with delayed recovery or chronic persistent symptoms. However, this working alliance is important in all patient treatment, no matter the stage of recovery, and requires the clinician to adopt a patient-centered approach.

11.5.3 PT for Patients with Delayed Recovery

As treatment continues, the PT may note that the patient's adherence to treatment is not optimal and that recovery is not progressing as anticipated. Reevaluation of the patient is appropriate to ensure nothing was missed during the prior exam. Poor patient adherence in physical therapy may manifest as poor attendance, arriving late for scheduled visits, not following advice, not performing prescribed exercises or activities, and doing more or less than advised (Jack et al., 2010). In cases where there are indicators of delayed recovery, identifying barriers to recovery and communicating with the patient and other stakeholders are important, as continuing with treatment as usual is unlikely to lead to positive results. Assessment of treatment barriers should include PT self-reflection and evaluation of the patient's beliefs, treatment expectations, and psychosocial barriers to recovery as discussed previously.

The importance of good communication and listening skills and patient education is consistent with what patients said was important to them in a qualitative study by Slade, Molloy, and Keating (2009). All patients in that investigation had received treatment of exercise therapy for chronic low back pain by multiple providers. Recurrent themes, within a core theme of partnership, included:

1. Engagement and participation were key exercise ingredients. Patients wanted:
    (a) Mutuality in the process of problem-solving and negotiation to establish goals
    (b) The therapist to ask what he/she thinks
    (c) The therapist to consider the patient's life circumstances and preferences and to consider time availability
    (d) Continuity of care and connection
2. Patients wanted the therapist to listen.
3. Patients wanted to understand the rationale behind why exercise was important.

The findings from Slade et al. (2009) also resonate with the principles of interviewing patients with chronic pain discussed by Diener et al. (2016). They state that:

It could be argued that a skilled interview which embraces and incorporates a biopsychosocial approach may be a key first step of a successful TNE (Therapeutic Neuroscience Education) treatment. (page 357).

The authors also discuss the importance of empathy; the ability to perceive and understand something of the patient's experience of pain, vulnerability, and suffering; and expression of appropriate concern.

Awareness of patient preferences, beliefs, and the therapeutic alliance allows the therapist to use placebo effects and minimize nocebo effects during treatment (Stillwell & Harman, 2017).

Martinez-Cevera, Olteanu, Gil-Martinez, Diaz-Pulido, and Ferrer-Pena (2017) performed a pilot randomized controlled trial of patients with lateral elbow pain (epicondylalgia) in order to investigate the influence of expectations and a specific mobilization technique. They reported statistically significant changes in kinesiophobia and perceived disability in the positive expectations group, demonstrating the use of the placebo effect. This shows the power of patient's beliefs.

Schmidt (2016) states that the process of actively engaging the patient in goal planning, communication, and shared decision-making throughout the treatment process appears to enhance self-efficacy and promote exploration of new challenges and encourages the patient to actively seek solutions to his/her problems.

Goldsmith et al. (2017) demonstrated a relationship between patient satisfaction and patients' sense of being supported by practitioners. The investigation involved interviews of patients who had undergone total knee replacement. Patients felt that "good" PTs had effective communication skills, treated each patient as a person, had time for him/her, and tailored the services, including the number of visits.

The results of the previously completed questionnaires can help direct the discussion of the PT and PTA with his/her patient to obtain more information about a response. In other words, there can be a dialogue or exchange, which can help the clinician better understand the patient's experience and preferences and guide the selection of specific interventions, while the patient feels heard.

11.5.3.1 Graded Activity and Graded Exposure for Patients with Fear-Avoidance Beliefs

Proposed treatment for patients classified as having fear-avoidance beliefs includes education, graded exposure, or graded exercise (Crombez, Eccleston, Vansteenwegen, & Lysens, 2002; George, Bialosky, & Fritz, 2004; Sullivan, Adams, Rhodenizer, & Stanish, 2006; Vlaeyen, de Jong, Geilen, Heuts, & van Breukelen, 2001). Graded exposure involves gradual and progressive exposure to activities the patient identified as being afraid to perform. George et al. developed a questionnaire (the Fear of Daily Activities Questionnaire) to assist in the identification of activities (George, Valencia, Zeppieri, & Robinson, 2009). Blickenstaff and Pearson (2016) stated that graded exposure has demonstrated effectiveness in populations with low to moderate catastrophizing scores but not in patients with high scores. Graded activity involves the use of activity quotas. The patient and therapist agree on a specified amount of exercise the patient will perform daily, and the patient maintains an activity log. The quota is increased weekly by a specified amount. If the patient failed to meet the quota, there is discussion with the patient about what occurred during the week, and the quota amount or activity list may be adjusted.

The use of this graded activity for low back pain patients who do not have fear-avoidance beliefs has been shown to slow recovery (George et al., 2003). It is therefore important for PTs to employ this treatment when appropriate. The state of the current research is such that one approach has not been found to be definitively better than another. A combination of approaches may be helpful, where progressive exposure to a feared activity is part of the weekly activity quota.

11.5.3.2 Exercise Therapy for Patients with Chronic Pain

In the articles reviewed in preparation for this chapter, it was found that while specific recommendations for people with chronic pain may differ in specifics, all share use of actively engaging the patient in progressive exercise and activity and education. Harmon, MacRae, and Vallis (2014) developed a checklist to assist PTs treating patients with chronic low back pain. In their article, patient self-management was reported to be the key. Their checklist is a clinical tool for behavior change they felt is needed because most published articles do not offer detail regarding how to perform and apply the techniques described. They also stressed the importance of the patient being engaged in treatment, which can be accomplished by a patient-focused approach.

Pain neuroscience education (PNE) is an approach to treatment that focuses on education to help the patient reconceptualize the pain process, so hurt and harm can be distinguished (Louw et al., 2016, Louw and Puentedura 2013). This approach encompasses a cognitive behavioral approach. Blickenstaff and Pearson (2016) list the following factors needed for the cognitive approach to have an effect:

1. The patient needs to be dissatisfied with his/her current perceptions about pain in order to be open to a reconceptualization.
2. The new explanation must be intelligible to the patient.
3. The new explanation must be plausible and beneficial to the patient.
4. The new explanation must be shared and confirmed by the direct environment of the patient.
5. Interaction with the PT is necessary. They report that individual education may be more effective than group education.

These authors also make the important point about the need for consistency between healthcare providers in regard to exercise prescription and instruction. Conflicting messages may threaten the patient's sense of safety, which is important in achieving the treatment goals. In my own professional experience, I have found this to be true. When both the treating physician and I encouraged activity and provided similar explanations regarding pain, our patients were more confident and open to activity. In contrast, in cases where a physician told his/her patient that there was significant degeneration of the lumbar spine, and suggested it would only get worse with time, it was much more difficult for the patient to accept that activity was positive. Consistency between PTs and PTAs treating the patient is also important to avoid conflicting messages that may confuse and worry the patient.

A system of cortical reorganization has been developed for patients with chronic pain called *graded motor imagery*. The treatment aims to address the changes that occur in the central nervous system of patients with persistent pain referred to as central sensitization. Central sensitization has been defined as an increased responsiveness of nociceptive neurons in the central nervous system to normative and subthreshold afferent input (Woolf, 2007, Nijs (2015)). This can result in a person perceiving normal movements as painful and threatening. Graded motor imagery is a three-stage treatment that aims to gradually engage cortical motor networks to decrease central sensitization without triggering the protective response of pain. This process was first developed to treat phantom limb pain but has been extended to treat other chronic pain conditions.

The three stages of treatment include left/right discrimination, motor imagery, and mirror therapy. Left/right discrimination involves the patient viewing an image of a body part and deciding whether the image depicts the left or right limb. This treatment addresses the change in the cortex called "smudging" (Butler and Moseley, 2013) that refers to a change in how the body part is represented in the cortex. As the cortical representation of the affected body part normalizes, the patient is able to more quickly discriminate between sides. Motor imagery requires the patient to imagine moving the body part in a very detailed way. Mirror therapy involves the patient placing the affected side inside a mirror box so that body part is unseen and then moving the unaffected side in a mirror that appears as if he/she is moving the affected side. Activities and movements are progressed over treatment (Bowering et al., 2013). This treatment is thought to reconcile motor output and sensory feedback and activate areas in the cortex that are connected with visual processing (Moseley, 2004). Mirror therapy has been used to treat chronic regional pain syndrome, type 1 (CRPS I) (Moseley, 2004). A 2015 Cochrane review (Smart, Wand, & O'Connell, 2016) reported that low-quality trials suggest that graded motor imagery including mirror therapy might be useful for reducing the pain and disability associated with CRPS I after trauma, surgery, or stroke. Rather than using the three components of graded motor imagery sequentially, Louw et al. (2017) investigated the change in shoulder motion following a single session of mirror therapy in patients with shoulder pain with more than a 10 degree difference between sides. The session involved ten repetitions performed slowly, with the patient watching the entire extremity in the mirror while slowly performing movements (average time for ten repetitions was 3 min). They reported a significant increase in shoulder flexion motion following the session with an average improvement of 14.5°. They suggest that mirror therapy may have application for patients without central sensitization and the presence of psychosocial factors. Further study is needed, but these results are interesting.

O'Sullivan, Dankaerts, O'Sullivan, and O'Sullivan (2015) and Bunzli, McEvoy, Dankaerts, O'Sullivan, and O'Sullivan (2016) describe the PT's role as mentor, equipping patients with knowledge and independent problem-solving skills. These authors describe "cognitive functional therapy" as a comprehensive biopsychosocial approach that addresses the mechanisms driving chronic low back pain and associated disability. As with PNE, this approach focuses on reconceptualizing pain as a biopsychosocial problem, functionally retraining maladaptive and feared postures and movement patterns and addressing contributing lifestyle patterns. The approach emphasizes active rehabilitation and incorporates education and mindfulness training underpinned by a strong therapeutic alliance that emphasizes an open and motivational communication style. O'Sullivan et al. investigated cognitive functional therapy in patients with chronic low back pain (2015).Their intervention was done once per week and was gradually reduced to once every 2 weeks. Their intervention had four main stages: cognitive training, functional movement training, functional integration, and physical activity and lifestyle training:

1. Cognitive training involved changing the perception of pain meaning there is tissue damage (through the use of video and discussion) and reviewing radiological tests and talking about the poor correlation of clinical presentation and radiological findings. In addition, there was discussion about pain fluctuations and events (physical, psychological, and social) that occurred during the week. Reflective communication, self-management practices, functional enhancement, and goal orientation continued in the other stages.
2. Functional movement training: A graded exposure model was used, with training based on the specific tasks a patient avoided due to pain or that provoked pain. The exercises were progressed. Pain behaviors during activity were identified and abolished, with practical demonstration by the PT. Videos and mirrors were used to provide feedback and enhance body awareness.

3. Functional integration: The exercises from stage 2 were integrated into daily tasks based on the patient's functional impairments. The movements were practiced with the PT so the patient's confidence increased. If a patient avoided a task, the task was rehearsed, and the patient was encouraged to include them in daily life. The goal was to improve movement capacity and enhance body awareness while reducing avoidance.
4. Physical activity and lifestyle training: Patients were encouraged to perform exercise 3–5 days per week and increased duration up to 20–40 min. No specific form of exercise was prioritized. The emphasis was on performing exercise in a relaxed and mindful manner to facilitate normal movement. Tips on sleep hygiene and stress coping strategies were developed in collaboration with the patient.

O'Sullivan et al. (2015) showed significant reductions in functional disability and pain following treatment and maintained over a 12-month follow-up period. They also found reductions in depression, anxiety, back beliefs, fear of activity, and catastrophizing, while self-efficacy was improved. Bunzli et al. (2016) used the same cognitive functional therapy program and compared and contrasted the patient's perspectives regarding improvement after the program. This was done by in-person interviews. They identified three groups from their analysis: large improvers, small improvers, and unchanged. They identified two themes that encapsulated the key requirements for a successful outcome: (1) changing pain beliefs and (2) achieving independence. A strong therapeutic alliance, development of body awareness, and the experience of control over pain were needed to change pain beliefs in the large improver group. Independence was achieved by the large improvers through self-efficacy, problem-solving skills, decreased fear of pain, and better stress coping. They also found that small improvers had inconsistent self-efficacy and more fear and difficulty coping after the program and believe this group may need more ongoing support.

Beattie, Silfes, and Jordan (2016) proposed a different type of delivery of physical therapy treatment for patients with recurrent low back pain. The treatment emphasized patient education and self-management techniques. They proposed an alternative to the typical short-term PT treatment of 12 sessions within a 4–8 week time frame. Instead, PTs used less frequent sessions over a longer time frame, stressing the therapeutic alliance to develop individualized, patient-preferred approaches for activity-based self-management. This was done to involve the patient in long-term performance of physical activity and education in self-management while providing support, with the goal of impacting the recurrence of low back pain. This approach requires further investigation to determine its efficacy.

There are helpful books available to patients that complement the education and instruction provided by PTs and PTAs during an episode of care. Examples include *Explain Pain* by Moseley and Butler and a number of books by Adriaan Louw covering a variety of topics like headache, back pain, whiplash, and others (Orthopaedic Physical Therapy Products, https://www.optp.com/Neuroscience#.WW4tX4Tyupo).

11.6 Referral and Coordination of Treatment

PTs work as part of a healthcare team. The members of that team will vary, depending on the circumstances and healthcare setting. Frequently, the team will consist of the physician who referred the patient for therapy, the patient, and the therapist (and the therapist's staff involved in treatment). Additional individuals involved in treatment include medical case managers, vocational experts, and medical specialists treating the patient (e.g., physiatrist, orthopedist, neurologist, etc.). Interdisciplinary treatment programs frequently include occupational and recreational therapists, a social worker, and a psychologist. When a patient is referred to a PT for treatment, it is helpful for the physician to identify his/her medical diagnosis and next follow-up appointment. When the injury is work related, and the patient is not able to work, information from the employer regarding the patient's essential job functions and the ability to modify or accommodate work is needed. While this can be provided at least in part by the patient, verifying the information with the employer is important to ensure accuracy of the information. A medical case manager involved with the patient can be a helpful source of information for the therapist.

Coordination and communication are important aspects of PT management. There needs to be good coordination of treatment within the PT facility so the patient receives consistent treatment, education, and instruction. Consistency in staff is helpful and supports the therapeutic alliance. Regular communication between treating clinicians and other stakeholders is also important. Therapists usually send regular progress reports to referring physicians that include current examination results and treatment recommendations. The progress report can include concerns in the event the patient is not making the expected recovery. The PT should also attempt to contact the referral source by phone or email to discuss concerns. When treating patients with chronic symptoms, coordination and communication are vital to ensure a consistent message, and instructions are given to the patient.

In cases where the patient has pre-existing mental health illness that may interfere with his/her ability to participate or engage in treatment, the PT should contact the physician and discuss his findings and concerns. If a patient has psychosocial factors and is not adhering to or participating with treatment or has significantly elevated scores on the Pain Catastrophizing Scale, the physician should be contacted, and referral to a behavioral health specialist should be considered.

One advantage of on-site interdisciplinary treatment programs is that there are regular patient conferences to share information and collaboratively review/modify treatment plans and goals. In an outpatient physical therapy setting, communication between healthcare team members may be more challenging but is equally important to ensure coordination of goals and treatment plans and to obtain helpful information and suggestions to help progress the patient's PT program. The patient should give permission for the PT and behavioral health specialist to communicate about him/her. Discussion can include the treatment barriers and the patient's physical abilities and limitations that may help the behavior health specialist with specific treatment targets and goals.

11.7 Appropriate Documentation of Limitations in Objective Impairment/Functioning

PTs routinely send the referring provider information about his/her patient. This is almost always done after the first visit, and progress reports thereafter are usually timed to coincide with the physician's visit. This requires that the therapist is aware of when the physician's appointment is scheduled. Copies of these reports may also be sent to the medical case manager and in some cases to the insurer. The report should include:

- *Subjective data*
  - The patient's reported symptoms.
  - Results of pain and/or disability questionnaires – the therapist should indicate if the scores meet the criteria for minimal clinical important difference.
- *Objective data*
  - Range of motion, strength, etc. compared with previous findings.
  - Functional abilities – what can the patient do relative to work and home activities?
  - Functional limitations – what work and home activities are limited because of the health condition? Can these limitations be accommodated? The therapist should provide specifics.
- *Assessment (the therapist's interpretation of the data)*
  - Discuss the overall findings and their meaning. When reevaluating the patient, report the areas of improvement. Improvement includes change in both impairment and function. Barriers to improvement should be discussed in detail.
  - Discuss the patient's attendance and participation in therapy.
  - If relevant, provide an assessment about the patient's work ability – either full or modified duty. If the therapist feels that the patient cannot work full time, objective rationale for his/her opinion should be included.
  - Discuss the need for further treatment. The therapist should identify specific short- and long-term goals with time frames. If no further treatment is required, this should be clearly stated.
- *Plan of care*
  - State the overall goals in measurable terms that indicate the predicted level of functional improvement.
  - Make a general statement about the interventions to be used.
  - State the proposed treatment duration and frequency needed to achieve the treatment goals. It is reasonable to decrease treatment frequency during the episode of care, as the patient improves and can do more at home.

Problems frequently noted in documentation include:

- The use of esoteric abbreviations that no one but the therapist understands.
- Illegible handwriting.
- Subjective assessment does not include pain scales or validated disability questionnaires. The inclusion of these tools has been previously discussed and is recommended because it provides a more objective method of documenting the patient's symptoms and perceived function and allows therapist to monitor scores over time.
- Lack of functional data – unfortunately, this information is frequently not assessed as part of the therapy program, even though the patient may be out of work due to a work-related injury. Barriers to including this information include the therapist's inability to perform functional assessment and/or allowing the time to perform the assessment.
- Unclear treatment recommendations – rather than the therapist clearly identifying a recommendation (usually to discontinue therapy), some therapists write something akin to "per physician." It is this author's opinion that this type of recommendation is insufficient. As the functional expert, the therapist should be able to provide recommendations regarding the need for further treatment, work, home abilities, etc. and provide reasonable treatment goals. When therapy is no longer needed, either due to attainment of goals or due to lack of progress, the therapist should clearly indicate this.

PTs and PTAs should refer to and follow the American Physical Therapy Association's Guidelines: Physical Therapy Documentation (APTA-Board of Directors, Documentation Guidelines). This document includes general guidelines; addresses the elements to include in initial evaluation/examinations, reexamination, treatment visits, and discharge/discontinuation summaries; and is a helpful resource for the PT and PTA.

11.8 Treatment Outcomes

Treatment outcomes are the results of implementing a plan of care and are related to the treatment goals that were collaboratively developed by the PT and patient (and possibly family members and other care givers). Treatment outcomes may include the result of self-report tool(s); identified impairments in motion, strength, balance, etc.; activity abilities and limitations; and ability to perform the job (or modified work) or relate to patient education and satisfaction. These outcomes, selected by the PT at the time of the initial evaluation, should be monitored during a treatment episode and may be modified based on the patient's change in status or health condition.

11.9 Summary

While the focus of physical therapy treatment is on management of movement dysfunction, PTs need to establish a therapeutic alliance with their patients and be aware of our own beliefs and treatment biases and the beliefs, fears, biases, and preferences of our patients. In addition, the PT and PTA need to be aware of the psychosocial and environmental factors that can lead to delayed recovery and chronic pain syndromes and have tools to effectively address them early in the treatment process. There are a number of behavioral indicators a patient may exhibit that suggest psychosocial risk factors are present, and a PT should investigate further with one or more of the questionnaires discussed. This will provide information that can be used in treatment planning and serve as an outcome measure of program effectiveness. This chapter has discussed these tools and the need for effective communication, which is critical to effective patient management.

It is an exciting time to practice as a PT as there are state regulations allowing autonomous practice, and research has found some promising interventions to help people with delayed recovery and chronic pain. No specific intervention has been found to be definitively superior to another at this time. A number of interventions have been discussed that are available to the PT/PTA. The PT is therefore charged with considering both the patient's physical and psychosocial factors and preferences and to engage the patient so there is collaboration in treatment planning. While the PT may practice autonomously, coordination and collaboration with other healthcare practitioners and stakeholders are essential, especially when treating patients with chronic pain. Behavioral health specialists can be a valuable resource for the PT when, despite all best efforts, a patient is not engaged in physical therapy treatment. Clinical guidelines, such as the Chronic Pain Guidelines from the American College of Occupational and Environmental Medicine (2017), have recognized the value of both PT and behavioral health interventions when treating people with chronic pain. In the workers compensation area, there continues to be some resistance, at least in parts of the USA, with engaging behavioral health specialists in treatment. Hopefully this resistance will decrease in the near future so the person with chronic pain has access to both the physical and psychological interventions needed to promote optimal recovery.

References

American College of Occupational & Environmental Medicine. (2017). *Chronic pain guideline.* Beverly Farms: OEM Press.

American Physical Therapy Association. (2014). Retrieved June 14, 2017, from http://guidetoptpractice.apta.org/content/1/SEC1.extract. https://doi.org/10.2522/ptguide3.0_1

American Physical Therapy Association Board of Directors. Guidelines: Physical therapy documentation of patient/client management (BOD G03-05-16-41). Available at: http://www.apta.org/uploadedFiles/APTAorg/About_Us/Policies/Practice/DocumentationPatientClientManagement.pdf. Accessed 18 July 17.

Beattie, P. F., Silfes, S. P., & Jordan, M. (2016). The evolving role of physical therapists in the long-term management of chronic low back pain: Longitudinal care using assisted self-management techniques. *Brazilian Journal of Physical Therapy, 20*, 580–591.

Blickenstaff, C., & Pearson, N. (2016). Reconciling movement and exercise with pain neuroscience education: A case for consistent education. *Physiotherapy Theory and Practice, 32*, 396–407.

Bowering, K. J., O'Connell, N. E., Tabor, A., Catley, M. J., Leake, H. B., Moseley, G. L., et al. (2013). The effects of graded motor imagery and its components on chronic pain: A systematic review and meta-analysis. *Journal of Pain, 14*, 3–13.

Bunzli, S., McEvoy, S., Dankaerts, W., O'Sullivan, P., & O'Sullivan, K. (2016). Patient perspectives on participation in cognitive functional therapy for low back pain. *Physical Therapy, 96*, 1397–1407. https://doi.org/10.25522/ptj.20140570

Butler, D., & Moseley, L. (2013). *Explain Pain*. Adelaide: NOI Group Publications.

Cairns, M. C., Foster, N. E., Wright, C. C., & Pennington, D. (2003). Level of distress in a recurrent low back pain population referred for physical therapy. *Spine, 28*(9), 953–959.

Carriere, J. S., Thibault, P., Adams, H., Milioto, M., Ditto, B., & Sullivan, M. J. L. (2015). Expectancies mediate the relationship between perceived injustice and return to work following whiplash injury. *Journal of Pain, 16*, 1280–1287. https://doi.org/10.1016/j.jpain.2015.09.001

Carriere, J. S., Thibault, P., Adams, H., Milioto, M., Ditto, B., & Sullivan, M. J. L. (2017). Expectancies mediate the relationship between perceived injustice and return to work following whiplash injury: A 1-year prospective study. *European Journal of Pain*. https://doi.org/10.1002/ejp.1023. Epub ahead of print.

Childs, J. D., et al. (2008). Neck pain: Clinical practice guidelines linked to the international classification of functioning, disability, and health from the orthopedic section of the american physical therapy association. *Journal of Orthopaedic & Sports Physical Therapy, 38*, A1–A34.

Coudeyre, E., Rannou, F., Tuback, F., Baron, G., Coriat, F., Brin, S., et al. (2006). General Practitioners' fear-avoidance beliefs influence their management of patients with low back pain. *Pain, 124*, 330–337.

Crombez, G., Eccleston, C. V. J. W., Vansteenwegen, D., & Lysens, R. E. P. (2002). Exposure to physical movements in low back pain patients: Restricted effects of generalization. *Health Psychology, 21*, 573–578.

Darlow, B., Fullen, B. M., Dean, S., Hurley, D. A., Baxter, G. D., & Dowell, A. (2012). The association between health care professional attitudes and beliefs and the attitudes and beliefs, clinical management and outcomes of patients with low back pain: A systematic review. *European Journal of Pain, 16*, 3–17.

Delitto, A., et al. (2012). Clinical practice guidelines linked to the international classification of functioning, disability, and health from the orthopaedic section of the american physical therapy association. *Journal of Orthopaedic & Sports Physical Therapy, 42*, A1–A57. https://doi.org/10.2519/jospt.2012.42.4.A1

Diener, L., Kargela, M., & Louw, A. (2016). Listening is therapy: Patient interviewing from a pain science perspective. *Physiotherapy Theory and Practice, 32*(5), 356–367. https://doi.org/10.1080/09593985.2016.1194648

Domenech, J., Sánchez-Zuriga, D., Segura-Ortí, E., Espejo-Tort, B., & Lisón, J. F. (2011). Impact of biomedical and biopsychosocial training sessions on the attitudes, beliefs, and recommendations of health care providers about low back pain: A randomized clinical trial. *Pain, 152*, 2557–2563.

Ebrahim, S., Malachowski, C., Kamal el Din, M., Mulla, S. M., Montoya, L., Bance, S., et al. (2015). Measures of patients' expectations about recovery: A systematic review. *Journal of Occupational Rehabilitation, 25*, 240–255. https://doi.org/10.1007/210926-014-9535-4

Fairbank, J. C. T., Davies, J. B., Couper, J., & O'Brien, J. P. (1980). The Oswestry low-back pain disability questionnaire. *Physiotherapy, 66*, 271–273.

Ferreira, P. H., Ferreira, M. L., Maher, C., Reishauge, K. M., Latimer, J., & Adams, R. D. (2013). The therapeutic alliance between clinicians and patients predicts outcome in chronic low back pain. *Physical Therapy, 93*, 470–478.

Fritz, J. M., George, S. Z., & Delitto, A. (2001). The role of fear-avoidance beliefs in acute low back pain: Relationships with current and future disability and work status. *Pain, 94*, 7–15.

Fuentes, J., Armijo-Olivo, S., Funabashi, M., Miciak, M., Dick, B., Warren, S., et al. (2014). Enhanced therapeutic alliance modulates pain intensity and muscle sensitivity in patients with chronic low back pain: An experimental controlled study. *Physical Therapy, 94*, 477–489.

George, S. Z., Bialosky, J. E., & Fritz, J. M. (2004). Physical therapist management of a patient with acute low back pain and elevated fear-avoidance beliefs. *Physical Therapy, 84*, 538–549.

George, S. Z., Fritz, J. M., Bialosky, J. E., & Donald, D. A. (2003). The effect of a fear-avoidance-based physical therapy intervention for patients with acute low back pain: Results of a randomized clinical trial. *Spine, 28*, 2551–2560.

George, S. Z., Fritz, J. M., & Childs, J. D. (2008). Investigation of elevated fear-avoidance beliefs for patients with low back pain: A secondary analysis involving patients enrolled in physical therapy clinical trials. *The Journal of Orthopaedic and Sports Physical Therapy, 38*, 50–58.

George, S. Z., & Stryker, S. E. (2011). Fear-avoidance beliefs and clinical outcomes for patients seeking outpatient physical therapy for musculoskeletal pain conditions. *Journal of Orthopaedic and Sports Physical Therapy, 41*(4), 249–259. https://doi.org/10.2519/jospt.2011.3488

George, S. Z., Valencia, C., Zeppieri Jr., G., & Robinson, M. E. (2009). Development of a self-report measure of fearful activities for patients with low back pain: The fear of daily activities questionnaire. *Physical Therapy, 89*, 969–979.

Goldsmith, L. S., Suryaprakash, N., Randall, E., Shum, J., McDonald, V., Sawatzky, R., et al. (2017). The importance of informational, clinical and personal support in patient experience with total knee replacement: A qualitative investigation. *BMC Musculoskeletal Disorders, 18*, 127–140. https://doi.org/10.1186/212891-017-1474-8

Gross, D. P., & Battié, M. P. (2005). Work-related recovery expectations and the prognosis of chronic low back pain within a worker's compensation setting. *Journal of Occupational and Environmental Medicine, 47*, 428–433.

Hall, A. M., Ferriera, P. H., Maher, C. G., Latimer, J., & Ferriera, M. L. (2010). The influence of the therapist-patient relationship on treatment outcome in physical rehabilitation: A systematic review. *Physical Therapy, 90*, 1099–1110. https://doi.org/10.2522/pt.20090245

Harmon, K., MacRae, M., & Vallis, M. (2014). The development and testing of a checklist to study behavior change techniques used in a treatment programme for Canadian armed forces members with chronic non-specific low back pain. *Physiotherapy Canada, 66*, 313–321. https://doi.org/10.3138/ptc2013-55BC

Houben, R. M. A., Gijsen, A., Peterson, J., de Jong, P. J., & Vlaeyen, J. W. S. (2005). Do health care providers' attitudes towards back pain predict their treatment recommendations? Differential predictive validity of implicit and explicit attitude measures. *Pain, 114*, 491–498.

Jack, K., McLean, S. M., Moffet, J. K., & Gardiner, E. (2010). Barriers to treatment adherence in physiotherapy outpatient clinics: A systematic review. *Manual Therapy, 15*, 220–228. https://doi.org/10.1016/i.math.2009.12004

Kendall, N., Linton, S., & Main, C. (1997). *Guide to assessing psychosocial yellow flags in acute back pain: Risk factors for long term disability and work loss*. Wellington: ACC.

Kolt, G. S., & Andersen, M. B. (2004). Using psychology in the physical and manual therapies. In G. S. Kolt & M. B. Andersen (Eds.), *Psychology in the physical and manual therapies*. Edinburgh: Churchill Livingstone.

Lakke, S. E., Soer, R., Krijnen, W. P., van der Schans, C. P., Reneman, M. F., & Geertzen, J. H. B. (2015). Influence of physical therapists' kinesiophobic beliefs on lifting capacity in healthy adults. *Physical Therapy, 95*, 1224–1233.

Lee, W.-Y. A., Lee, W.-C. E., Law, S.-W., Lau, W.-K. A., Leung, S.-M., & Sieh, K.-M. (2013). Managing psychosocial contributors in low back pain patients-a randomized controlled trial. *Journal of Orthopaedics, Trauma and Rehabilitation, 17*, 46–51. https://doi.org/10.1016/j.jotr.2012.12.002

Lenz, T. A., Beneciuk, J. M., Bialosky, J. E., Zeppieri Jr., G., Dai, Y., Wu, S. S., et al. (2016). Development of a yellow flag assessment tool for orthopaedic physical therapists: results from the optimal screening for prediction of referral and outcome (OSPRO) cohort. *Journal of Orthopaedic and Sports Physical Therapy, 46*, 327–343. https://doi.org/10.2519/jospt.2016.6487. Epub 2016 Mar 21.

Lezin, N., & Watkins-Castillo, S. (2016). The impact of musculoskeletal disorders on Americans-opportunities for action, executive summary of the burden of musculoskeletal diseases in the United States: Prevalence, societal and economic cost. *Bone and Joint Initiative*. www.boneandjointburden.org. Accessed 14 June 2017.

Linton, S. J., & Shaw, W. S. (2011). Impact of psychosocial factors in the experience of pain. *Physical Therapy, 91*, 700–711.

Lonsdale, C., Hall, A. M., Murray, A., Williams, G. C., McDonough, S. M., Ntoumanis, N., et al. (2017). Patient skills training for practitioners to increase patient adherence to home-based people rotation for chronic low back pain: results of the cluster randomized controlled trial. *Archives of Physical Medicine and Rehabilitation*. https://doi.org/10.1016/j.apmr.2017.02.025

Louw, A., & Puentedura, E. (2013). *Therapeutic neuroscience education: Teaching patients about pain-a guide for clinicians*. OPTP – Orthopaedic physical therapy products.

Louw, A., Puentedura, E. J., & Zimney, K. (2016). Teaching patients about pain. It works, but what should we call it? *Physiotherapy Theory and Practice, 32*(5), 328–331. https://doi.org/10/1080/09593985.2016.1194669.

Louw, A., Puentedura, E. J., Reese, D., Parker, P., Miller, T., & Mintken, P. E. (2017). Immediate effects of mirror therapy in patients with shoulder pain and decreased range of motion. *Archives of Physical Medicine and Rehabilitation*. https://doi.org/10.1016/j.apmr.2017.03.031. [Epub ahead of print].

Marchand, G. H., Myhre, K., Leivseth, G., Sandvik, L., Lau, B., Bautz-Holter, E., et al. (2015). Change in pain, disability and influence of fear-avoidance in a work-focused intervention on neck and back pain: A randomized controlled trial. *BMC Musculoskeletal Disorders, 16*, 1–11. https://doi.org/10.1186/s12891-015-0553-y

Martin, D. J., Garske, J. P., & Davis, M. K. (2000). Relation of therapeutic alliance with outcome and other variables: A meta-analytic review. *Journal of Counseling and Clinical Psychology, 68*, 438–450.

Martinez-Cevera, F. V., Olteanu, T. E., Gil-Martinez, A. G., Diaz-Pulido, B., & Ferrer-Pena, R. (2017). Influence of expectations plus mobilization with movement in patients with lateral epicondylalgia: a pilot randomized controlled trial. *Journal of Rehabilitation*. https://doi.org/10.12965/jer.1732848.424

Matthews, J., Hall, A. M., Hernon, M., Murray, A., Jackson, B., Taylor, I., et al. (2015). Brief report on the development of a theoretically-grounded intervention to promote patient autonomy and self-management of physiotherapy patients: Face validity and feasibility of implementation. *Biomedcentral Health Services Research, 15*, 260. https://doi.org/10.1186/s12913-015-0921-1

Moseley, G. L. (2004). Graded motor imagery is effective for long-standing complex regional pain syndrome: A randomized controlled trial. *Pain, 108*, 192–198.

Murray, A., Hall, A. M., Williams, G. C., McDonough, S. M., Ntoumanis, N., Taylor, I. M., et al. (2015). Effect of self-determination theory-based communication skills training program on physiotherapists' psychological support for their patients with chronic low back pain: A randomized controlled trial. *Archives of Physical Medicine and Rehabilitation, 96*, 809–816.

Nicholas, M. K., Linton, S. J., Watson, P. J., & Main, C. J. (2011). "Decade of the flags" working group-early identification and management of psychological risk factors ("yellow flags") in patients with low back pain a reappraisal. *Physical Therapy, 91*, 737–753.

Nijs, J., Roussel, N., & Wilgen, C. P. (2013). Thinking beyond muscles and joints: Therapists' and patients' attitudes and beliefs regarding chronic musculoskeletal pain are key to applying effective treatment. *Manual Therapy, 18*, 96–102.

Nijs, J., Van Houdenhove, B., & Oostendorp, R. A. (2015). Recognition of central sensitization in patients with musculoskeletal pain: Application of pain neurophysiology in manual therapy practice. *Manual Therapy, 15*, 135–141.

O'Sullivan, K., Dankaerts, W., O'Sullivan, L., & O'Sullivan, P. B. (2015). Cognitive functional therapy for disabling nonspecific chronic low back pain: Multiple case-cohort study. *Physical Therapy, 95*, 1478–1488.

Overmeer, T., Boersmak, K., Main, C. J., & Linton, S. J. (2009). Do physical therapists change their beliefs, attitudes, knowledge, skills and behavior after a biopsychosocially oriented university course? *Journal of Evaluation in Clinical Practice, 15*, 724–732.
Parry, R. H., & Brown, K. (2009). Teaching and learning communication skills and physiotherapy: What is done and how is it done? *Physiotherapy, 95*, 294–301.
Quicke, J. G., Foster, N. E., Ogollah, R. O., Croft, P. R., & Holden, M. A. (2017). The relationship between attitudes, beliefs and physical activity in older adults with knee pain: secondary analysis of a randomized controlled trial. *Arthritis Care and Research*. https://doi.org/10.1002/acr.23104. (accepted 9/27/2016).
Sanders, T., Foster, N. E., Bishop, A., & Ong, B. N. (2013). Biopsychosocial care and the physiotherapy encounter: Physiotherapists' accounts of back pain consultations. *BMC Musculoskeletal Disorders, 14*, 65. http://www.biomedcentral.com/1471-1-2474/14/65
Schmidt, S. G. (2016). Recognizing potential barriers to setting and achieving effective rehabilitation goals for patients with persistent pain. *Physiotherapy Theory and Practice, 32*, 415–426.
Slade, S. C., Molloy, E., & Keating, J. L. (2009). Listen to me, tell me: A qualitative study of partnership in care for people with non-specific chronic low back pain. *Clinical Rehabilitation, 23*, 270–280.
Smart, K. M., Wand, B. M., & O'Connell, N. E. (2016). Physiotherapy for pain and disability in adults with complex regional pain syndrome (CRPS) types I and II. *Cochraine Database Systematic Review, 2*.
Stilwell, P., & Harman, K. (2017). Contemporary biopsychosocial exercise prescription for chronic low back pain: Questioning core stability programs and considering context. *Journal of Canadian Chiropractic Association, 61*, 6–17.
Sullivan, M. J., Adams, H., Rhodenizer, T., & Stanish, W. D. (2006). A psychosocial risk factor-targeted intervention for the prevention of chronic pain and disability following whiplash injury. *Physical Therapy, 86*, 8–18.
Sullivan, M. J., Stanishn, W., Waite, H., Sullivan, M., & Tripp, D. A. (1998). Catastrophizing, pain and disability in patients with soft-tisse injuries. *Pain, 77*, 253–260.
Sullivan, M. J. L., Adams, H., Horan, S., Mahar, D., Boland, D., & Gross, R. (2008). The role of perceived injustice in the experience of chronic pain and disability: Scale development and validation. *Journal of Occupational Rehabilitation, 18*, 249–261.
Sullivan, M. J. L., Scott, W., & Trost, Z. (2012). Perceived injustice: A risk factor for problematic pain outcomes. *Clinical Journal of Pain, 28*, 383–488.
Synnott, A., O'Keefe, M., Bunzli, S., Dankerts, W., O'Sullivan, P., & O'Sullivan, K. (2015). Physiotherapists Ms. statement ties were feel unprepared to treat people with low back pain and psychosocial factors that influence recovery: A systematic review. *Journal of Physiotherapy, 61*, 68–75.
Synnott, A., O'Keefe, M., Bunzli, S., Dankerts, W., O'Sullivan, P., Robinson, K., et al. (2016). Physiotherapists report improved understanding of and attitude toward the cognitive, psychological and social dimensions of chronic low back pain after cognitive functional training. *Journal of Physiotherapy, 62*, 215–221.
Van Wilgen, P., Beetsma, A., Neels, H., Roussel, N., & Nijs, J. (2014). Physical therapists should integrate illness perceptions in their assessment in patients with chronic musculoskeletal pain: A qualitative analysis. *Manual Therapy, 19*, 229–234.
Vernon, H., & Mior, S. (1991). The neck disability index: A study of reliability and validity. *Journal of Manipulative and Physiological Therapeutics, 14*, 409–415.
Vlaeyen, J. W., de Jong, J., Geilen, M., Heuts, P. H., & van Breukelen, G. (2001). Graded exposure in vivo in the treatment of pain-related fear: A replicated single-case experimental design in four patients with chronic low back pain. *Behaviour Research and Therapy, 39*, 151–166.
Vlaeyen, J. W., Kole-Snijders, A. M., Boeren, R. G., & van Eek, H. (1995). Fear of movement/(re) injury in chronic low back pain and its relation to behavioral performance. *Pain, 62*(3), 363–372.
Vlaeyen, J. W., & Linton, S. J. (2006). Are we fear-avoidant? *Pain, 124*, 240–241.
Waddell, G. (2004). *Back pain revolution*. London: Churchill Livingstone.

Waddell, G., McCulloch, J. A., & Kummel, E. (1980). Nonorganic physical signs in low-back pain. *Spine, 5*, 117–125.

Waddell, G., Newton, M., Henderson, I., Somerville, D., & Main, C. J. (1993). A fear-avoidance beliefs questionnaire (FABQ) and the role of fear-avoidance beliefs in chronic low back pain and disability. *Pain, 52*, 157–168.

Wijma, A. J., van Wilgen, C. P., Meeus, M., & Nijs, J. (2016). Clinical biopsychosocial physiotherapy assessment of patients with chronic pain: The first step in pain neuroscience education. *Physiotherapy Theory and Practice, 32*, 368–384.

Woolf, C. J. (2007). Central sensitization: Uncovering the relation between pain and plasticity. *Anesthesiology, 106*(4), 864–867.

Chapter 12
Employee Assistance Programs and Behavioral Health Disability

David Weis

12.1 Overview/History of EAPs in the United States

The history of EAPs in the United States dates back to the early 1940s (Masi, 2011). It was at this time that there was a scattered growth of alcoholism programs in major industrial firms, including Dupont, Eastman Kodak, and Kemper Insurance. Despite the growing interest in alcoholism assistance programs, many of them did not succeed for a number of reasons. The programs at that time seemed to lack an emphasis on productivity/cost-effectiveness and therefore took on a moral tone that alienated business people. Additionally, there was a social stigma attached to alcoholism as well as a denial about the extent of the problems that alcoholism created.

Another factor that contributed to the initial lack of success with EAP programs was that workplace supervisors were tasked with screening for alcoholism. This put supervisors in a precarious position in that they are typically individuals who have not received professional graduate training pertaining to the assessment of mental health and substance abuse conditions. Employers usually want their management team to avoid getting involved in personal issues with employees. Employers want their managers to monitor for job performance only and leave it up to the EAP professional to weigh in on how/if the personal issues impact job performance. Additionally, EAPs have received the requisite professional training and are skilled at screening for alcoholism. If the alcohol screen produces a positive score, then, the individual is typically referred for a more formal assessment.

The current EAP referral process includes both supervisory and employee referrals. For example, an employee may be experiencing symptoms that could be Major Depressive Disorder (MDD) with no workplace issues. That employee could then seek EAP services for further screening of these symptoms. The EAP can help to screen for psychological conditions, provide counseling related to problems that

D. Weis (✉)
TEAM Corporation, Roseville, MN, USA
e-mail: dweis@team-mn.com

P. A. Warren (ed.), *Handbook of Behavioral Health Disability Management*,
https://doi.org/10.1007/978-3-319-89860-5_12

may be contributory for these symptoms, or even to have the EAP refer the individual for additional long-term psychological treatment. The supervisory referral process is still necessary when the employee's workplace performance is impacted. The referral process is discussed in greater detail later in this chapter.

As EAPs continue to develop, there is growing concern among EAP professionals regarding that companies were calling themselves EAPs, but offering minimal or shoddy services. This resulted in a lack of standardization of EAP services that were being offered to employers and employees.

Roman and Blum (1988) noted that the paucity of standardization led to a conceptual framework for the delivery of EAP services. This framework resulted in the core for eight components essential to EAP program development and delivery. This framework is what is referred to as the EAP core technology. This signaled the advance at the first attempt at empirically determining what does an EAP actually do. Below are the eight core technologies:

1. Consultation and training to the work organization leadership (managers, supervisors, and union officials) seeking to manage troubled employees, enhance the work environment, and improve employee job performance. This core technology addresses the need for the EAP to provide consultation to managers around the management of behaviors in the workplace. This particular core component requires the workplace supervisor to reach out to the EAP with questions about workplace performance. This removes the supervisor from inappropriately serving as a lay counselor and allows the supervisor to focus on performance vs. having to try and understand the "why" behind deteriorating workplace performance.
2. Active promotion of the availability of EAP services to employees, their family members, and the work organization. A core function of a well-integrated EAP is the ability to be able to actively promote the program to employees and their dependents. This must be a coordinated effort between the designated company EAP supervisor or designated professional and the EAP provider. Generally speaking, the better the EAP program is promoted within the workplace, the better utilization will be because employees will be familiar with the benefit if/when they need it.
3. Confidential and timely problem identification/assessment services for employees with personal concerns that may affect job performance. This core component reflects on the importance of the confidential nature of EAP that is important in order for employees to feel comfortable with the service without fear that private information will somehow get back to their supervisor or human resources. Confidentiality is one of the most critical requirements for an EAP to be effective.
4. Use of constructive confrontation, motivation, and short-term interventions with employees to address problems that affect job performance. The value of this core function is the EAP focus on providing short-term intervention vs. the long-term care model that is evident with non-EAP providers. Care models for EAP

have always been on short-term intervention as a way to enable the employee to return to optimal level of functioning in the workplace.

5. Referral of employees for diagnosis, treatment, and assistance, as well as case monitoring and follow-up services. By design, EAPs do not operate under a medical model. In the medical model, a person receives either medical or mental health assessment, a diagnosis is given, and a treatment plan is developed. Moreover, the individual receives a bill for the treatment services received.

   In the EAP service model, an EAP professional completes an assessment for current problem areas. If problematic issues are identified, then they are assessed for their impact on the employee's functioning in the workplace. If the employee requires longer-term treatment, the EAP professional refers the employee for that treatment. Generally speaking, longer-term care is covered by the employee's health insurance. The critical piece under this core function is that the EAP provider does not disengage from the EAP process at that point. Instead, the EAP provider facilitates the referral to the provider and, then, follows up with the employee to ensure that the referral is effective. Most importantly, it is critical for the EAP professional to assess the employee is improving in functioning. There will be further discussion on the outcome variables with EAP later in this chapter.

6. Assisting work organizations in establishing and maintaining effective relations with treatment and other service providers and in managing provider contracts. In this core component, the EAP works to establish a "preferred provider network" where they can refer employees for specific treatment once the EAP completes the initial assessment. Navigating the behavioral healthcare delivery system can be complicated. An effective EAP establishes relationships with treatment providers and helps vet these providers so that employees are getting the right care at the right time with the right provider.

   Some behavioral health conditions require long-term treatment, and this is where the EAPs provide long-term follow-up by reaching out after the individual has returned to the workplace. By doing so, the EAP ensures that the employee is continuing to function in the workplace without continued problems. This type of follow-up typically occurs with employees with substance abuse conditions.

   Another facet of this core is that EAP providers develop (i.e., either internally or via a vendor) a broad network of EAP affiliates who agree to provide EAP services on behalf of the EAP. This allows EAPs to provide contracted services with multistate employers or with international employers. Recent trends in the provision of EAP services are the development of EAP networks across countries. The difficulty with international EAP work is that the western application of EAP does not often translate to other countries and EAPs are then left to try and develop relationships with providers that are indigenous to that culture.

7. Consultation to work organizations to encourage availability of and employee access to health benefits covering medical and behavioral health problems including, but not limited to, alcoholism, drug abuse, and emotional disorders.

EAPs often assist employers as they make decisions regarding the coverage of behavioral healthcare insurance.

8. Evaluation of the effects of EAP services on work organizations and individual job performance. This particular core will be discussed later in this chapter as it relates to methodology used to evaluate EAP effectiveness.

The application of the above EAP core technology provides greater standardization to EAP service delivery and implementation. The usage of the EAP core technology has been especially important as EAPs have moved from an internal EAP delivery model (the EAP was "internal" to the organization) to an external delivery model where both EAP staff and affiliates (i.e., "external" providers) deliver the service. When EAP staff and EAP affiliates share in the delivery of service, there is greater opportunity for variance in the quality of care. The standardization of the EAP core components served to rectify this.

It is also essential to note that the EAP counseling is not the same as traditional outpatient psychotherapy. This is because EAP work is focused on the issues as they relate to return-to-work and a wellness model. EAP affiliates may employ a medical model which focuses on pathology or a biopsychosocial model which evaluates the physical and psychological conditions as well as psychosocial issues to provide a more comprehensive treatment.

12.2 The Employee Assistance Program Role

There are several ways that the EAP can assist the employer/employee in the provision of EAP services.

First, EAPs provide reasonable suspicion training for employers regarding substance abuse. This training is most often presented to managers and supervisors to facilitate making decisions about whether to seek and when to refer an employee to the EAP. The ideal is that the employee seeks EAP on his or her own, but that may not occur when an alcohol abuse or dependence pattern is present. Usually the employee is "leveraged" into treatment by a spouse or employer after either failing a drug or alcohol test at work. This leveraging refers to an external motivation (i.e., the threat of a spouse leaving the employee or the employee being terminated) as the motivator for seeking treatment. The leveraging can also occur within a "supervisory referral." This will be discussed in more detail later in this chapter.

Once the employee is referred, the EAP professional conducts a thorough assessment. In the example above, the EAP professional must determine if the employee requires further professional treatment, such as with substance abuse conditions. If so, the EAP will refer the employee for substance abuse treatment outside of the EAP as formal substance abuse treatment. Substance abuse treatment is not provided under the short-term EAP model as substance abuse treatment is delivered over the course of days/weeks/months.

12.2.1 What Is the Current Status of the EAP Field?

There are several observations worth noting as to the current status of the field. There are a number of environment drivers that impact the positioning and sustainability of EAPs and behavioral health (Sharar & Pompe, 2014). One of the issues is the lack of consistent utilization of EAP services. On average, there are 4.5 members who used the EAP for counseling per year per every 100 covered employees (Attridge, Cahill, Granberry, & Herlihy, 2013). This seems to suggest that while there are a large number of individuals with a mental health diagnosis, very few actually seek treatment. Why is this so? What are the barriers to treatment? Historically, individuals have not generally sought EAP services due to the stigma attached to seeking treatment. Mental health treatment was perceived as a "weakness" that could be countered by "pulling yourself up by your bootstraps and moving on." With the increased publicity available around seeking treatment (i.e., many celebrities identifying that they have mental health conditions), it has become commonplace to seek services in this day and age. It should be noted that there are some identifiable barriers that can prevent getting treatment; there is a lack of mental health providers available to provide services (Sheparis & Walsh, 2017). There may also be socioeconomic factors that inhibit seeking treatment such as cost and difficulty getting to providers in remote areas (Sheparis & Walsh, 2017).

Another driver is that historically EAPs are not effective at demonstrating their value to both the purchaser and the public. There are a few reasons why this is so. One is that historically EAPs have not actively published studies that to demonstrate EAP efficacy. This is changing in that recently the Employee Assistance Professional Association (EAPA) has created a research foundation that seeks to begin to study EAP effectiveness and to support this research with proposals for funding (Sharar & Pompe, 2008).

Another reason why EAPs have lacked outcome studies is that their methodological quality is generally weak and doesn't incorporate stronger research design into evaluating EAP workplace interventions (Sharar & Pompe, 2008).

Additionally, employers generally prefer the data that the EAP gathers regarding its employees to be evaluated internally as opposed to data that may be collected/analyzed from other sources (i.e., multi-employer groups) and thereby not unique to the purchasers specific workforce. The reason for this is that employers want to see data that are unique to their employee and not extrapolated from a large database. Many employers who purchase EAP services appreciate the use of data as it relates to employee utilization of EAP services. Moreover, employers tend to want to keep these data "in-house" versus having its data synthesized into a data set pertaining to multiple employers.

The pricing of EAP services is one of the most important drivers to threaten the utility of EAPs. The old axiom "you get what you pay for" is certainly true in the EAP field. EAPs are now considered a business commodity. On one hand, this is a positive development since employers are recognizing the value of EAPs. However, regional EAPs have now found themselves in a "pricing war" with large national vendors who sell EAP services at a vastly reduced price. Frequently, employers' decision to purchase of EAP services is based on price alone and without understanding that low-cost EAP services are not necessarily synonymous with high-quality EAP services. Consequently, when these types of decisions are made on cost alone, it negatively impacts on the overall quality of EAP services provided. Many regional EAPs have a distinct advantage over nationally based EAPs in that they are more aware of the underlying issues that employers and employees are experiencing in that region. Moreover, regional services are better situated to customize EAP services to address those needs in a more expedient manner. One of the frequent complaints from employers who have been surveyed about EAP services is that they discover after contracting with a large EAP vendor that the purchased services cannot be customized, and so EAP services do not necessarily meet their requirements as defined in their request for proposal (Employee Assistance Professional Association, 2005).

The last driver that impacts EAP viability is that the EAPs have not incorporated technology into the delivery of its services. Technology should not be just another method to drive efficiency, cut costs, or "do more with less" (Sharar & Pompe, 2008). Instead, technology offers increased expediency in providing EAP services, such as with offering virtual EAP services.

However, the delivery of EAP with technology is not without its problems. EAPs must ensure they have fully vetted through due diligence all potential legal and ethical issues of virtual care before any such services are offered. For example, many large EAPs are now offering telephonic services as a means of controlling costs. The business case for providing services is that EAPs can utilize a call center located anywhere that employs staff counselors to deliver EAP services. This service model may be more cost effective since the EAP staff provides set telephonic services. This results in fixed EAP costs since there are only limited EAP services that are provided. When EAPs contract with different affiliates, the costs can vary widely due to regional pricing differences or differences in what services are contracted.

Telephonic therapy has also been evaluated in more than 30 research studies and is being used successfully with certain cases such as anxiety disorders, MDD, panic disorders, and trauma-related disorders (Attridge, 2017). However, there are several factors that must be considered when evaluating the implementation of a telephonic counseling model with EAPs. Generally speaking, telephonic counseling is viewed as a viable alternative to face-to-face counseling in that it is more convenient for employees, it protects the anonymity of the employee, and it is less expensive to deliver than traditional face-to-face counseling.

There are several points to consider in the implementation of telephonic services within an EAP. First, it is essential to complete due diligence to determine whether there are specific limitations to the implementation of a telephonic EAP model. A potential shortcoming with the delivery of EAP telephonic services is that the EAP professional may be licensed in a different state from where the employee resides. This is an important concern as State licensures laws can vary considerably from State to State. Moreover, some States have specific limitations in how many hours a licensed professional may provide EAP services in that State. For example, the

State of Ohio limits psychologists to 10 h. Thus, licensure portability issues may significantly limit the number of telephonic services that an EAP may offer to employees in different states.

A second consideration is whether telephonic EAP services are comparable to traditional face-to-face EAP services. However, most research has only analyzed the traditional EAP model of face-to-face services between the client and EAP counselor. Most of the studies conducted to date have not directly compared in-person versus telephonic EAP services using randomized controlled trials that are required in strong research design (Sharar, Popovits, & Donahue, 2010). Thus, it is not clear if one method is better for service delivery than the other.

Additionally, concern around virtual intervention and how it relates the issue of client confidentiality is particularly important. One of the legal requirements regarding patient or employee care relates to confidentiality. Both State and federal laws exist that specifically delineate what information must be kept confidential.

Confidentiality is a crucial component of any EAP. There are a couple of caveats to the confidentiality that are mentioned regarding EAP services. EAP providers have certain regulatory considerations (i.e., legal/ethical and licensure) that may affect the clinical course for an employee.

If the EAP provider suspects that there may be elder/child abuse, the provider has both legal and ethical obligation to report that to the appropriate authorities (Employee Assistance Professional Association, 2017a, 2017b). The EAP provider must clearly note the EAP itself does not conduct an investigation into the allegation, but is just required to report it (Employee Assistance Professional Association, 2017a, 2017b).

If an EAP client is determined to have active suicidal ideation, then, the EAP provider has both a legal and ethical responsibility to ensure that the client is referred for psychiatric assessment immediately. This is accomplished by the EAP professional calling a local psychiatric hospital and initiating the employee's transfer to the psychiatric facility or local emergency department. Lastly, if an EAP client is determined to be actively homicidal, the EAP provider has a duty to warn and protect the individual or individuals who may be in danger. In addition, the EAP professional must call the local police department to advise them of this danger. In this instance, the EAP professional specifically notes that she/he must breach confidentiality because of potential harm to others. Moreover, the EAP must comprehensively document what the client noted and what steps were taken to warn the potential victim, as well as noting the police department involvement.

Another concern regarding confidentiality pertains to data breaches, such as those making regular headlines nationally recently. This begs the question of whether virtual EAP services can truly maintain both a secure means to provide those services as well as to make an absolute guarantee to maintain confidentiality.

Moreover, the use of telephone and tablet apps is being offered as another potential method of communication with employers and employees. Since apps can be vulnerable to potential hacking, the usage of these apps must be vetted with the same due diligence and care as when evaluating the usage of telephonic modes for EAP service delivery. Moreover, because so many business utilize web-based business applications, many employers have a similar expectation for EAPs to do so as well. The quandary exists in how EAPs can develop secure web-based platforms for service delivery. Any new EAP service platform must meets the legal standards regarding confidentiality, while enhancing availability to its services. This point is especially salient as EAP profit margins are slim. It is only when EAPs address these concerns that they can remain a sustainable benefit for employer groups.

It should be noted that there has been resistance to the increased use of technology in the EAP field. Part of this resistance is due to the fact that the EAP field, in general, needs to address the future reduction of younger EAP clinicians into EAPs in the future (2017 EAPA National Conference, Interview with Dr. Paul Roman). Currently, many EAPs professionals currently have not been exposed to technology, therefore reluctant, or may not even know how to go about implementing a technology platform.

12.2.2 Accessing EAP Services

The mission of any effective EAP is to identify and help employees with personal problems to receive proper assessment/referral. Realistically, this is not always the case as sometimes employees do not believe they need EAP services. For example, if an employee has a substance abuse issue, the employee's denial of the issue creates a personal resistance to accept that a problem exists and that there is need to address it. However, this is also true for other concerns such as behavioral health conditions that impact the workplace.

12.3 Types of EAP Referrals

12.3.1 Informal or "Friendly" Referral

The ideal method for which employees can access this benefit is the voluntary referral. In is this type of referral the employee/dependent calls the EAP on their own accord. They have either heard about the EAP from their HR/Benefits department, have seen EAP promotional, and/or are aware of the benefit via a co-worker, or in some cases, a supervisor has made them aware of the benefit.

When a supervisor has made the employee aware of the benefit, this is called a "friendly referral." In this case, there are no job performance concerns, and the supervisor is merely demonstrating concern for the employee by reminding them of the free and confidential service. In fact, supervisors are generally the "hands and feet" of a well-integrated EAP as they are on the frontlines and tend to know more about an employee's personal life by virtue of working with the individual. Moreover, when a supervisor makes a friendly referral, it removes the workplace supervisor from the faux-counselor role and allows the supervisor to focus on the employee's work/job performance. With this type of referral, nothing is ever released back to the employer unless the employee consents to it. Because there are no job performance indicators, documentation can be kept to a minimum, and there are no other stakeholders involved in the referral.

12.3.2 *Supervisory Referral*

A supervisory referral is generally not a mandatory referral to the EAP. However, the supervisor may indicate that EAP involvement is strongly encouraged. Yet, the referral itself is still voluntary. That is, the employee can decide whether to comply with the referral. With this type of referral, management consultation is essential. Management consultation involves EAP interacting with management around if, when, and how to refer "troubled" or marginally performing employees to the EAP. The purpose of the management consultation is to help supervisors take the most appropriate action when dealing with troubled or impaired employees and resolve negative situations in a respectable and accountable manner. During a consultation, there are several objectives that EAP professionals address:

- Help the supervisor sort out objective job performance issues from personal feelings and actions.
- Consider whether or not the employee's behavior is symptomatic of a personal problem.
- Support the supervisor in dealing with his or her own feelings of frustration regarding the employee.
- Assist in determining if the employee is a good candidate for a formal referral to the EAP or possibly needs a drug test or medical evaluation. This is discussed further in the section pertaining to substance abuse.
- Register the consultation in our database so the EAP can track the employee follow-through.
- Provide clarification to the referring supervisor regarding appropriate next steps after the employee has been formally referred to the EAP.

12.3.2.1 Responsibility of the EAP with Friendly or Voluntary Supervisory Referrals

With friendly and voluntary supervisor referrals, the EAP has certain professional responsibilities that must be addressed. EAP professionals must:

- Ensure that an accurate and comprehensive assessment is conducted to facilitate the most appropriate intervention for the employee. This assessment includes a gathering of current symptomology and its impact on the workplace; a review of medical history including any relevant psychiatric history; psychosocial issues/

stressors that impact on the employee's current situation; medical history, including noting what type of other professionals are involved with the employee's care (e.g., primary care physician, occupational medicine, etc.); prescribed medications; usage of street drugs or inappropriate utilization of prescribed medications; and types of treatments that the employee is receiving. In addition, a comprehensive EAP assessment the EAP professional must also evaluate whether the person has active suicidal or homicidal thinking.

- Obtain the appropriate signed releases from the employee to update the employer of compliance with the referral. In some instance, this type of referral is not considered a mandatory referral, so an employee may elect to not authorize communications with the employer under this type of referral. If a release of information is signed by the employee, the only information that can be released to the employer is the information pertaining to the referral. No other clinical information is shared. If the employee refuses to sign the release, no information is released.

The EAP provides case management services until either the employee completes all requirements of the referral. This case management function includes following up with the employee and the treatment provider to ensure that the employee is satisfied with the referral and engaging in treatment. If the employee does not comply with the referral, all EAP services are terminated. If the employee does not complete the referral, then it is up to the employer if/how the employer will address that with the employee in the context of their work performance.

12.4 Fitness for Duty (FFD) Referral

The role of the EAP in regard to the FFD referral is to assist the employer in assessing the employee's behavior and arranging for an independent FFD assessment with the most appropriate provider. This type of EAP referral is a mandatory referral. In other words, the employee must comply with the referral. The type of professional to complete the FFD is determined by the clinical issues that are occurring. Moreover the FFD professional must assess whether these issues impact on the person's ability to work.

EAP serves as the "navigator" to ensure the assessment is comprehensive and that the results of the FFD make a determination around the employee's ability to return to work. If the employee is able to return to work, then a plan to return to work is made by the FFD and EAP professionals. If the employee is not able to return to work, the FFD addresses what type of intervention or treatment needs to take place in order for employee to regain functioning to return to the workplace.

The FFD referral presents a unique challenge for the EAP provider. Historically, FFD referrals revolved around employees who abused substances and impaired workplace performance. These types of referrals arose out of the occupational workplace services programs mentioned earlier in this chapter. For example, an employee may show up to work, smelling of alcohol. The supervisor may decide to refer the employee to the EAP for a chemical dependency evaluation. Upon completion of the chemical dependency evaluation, the EAP provider may refer the employee to a treatment program for more intensive professional care. As EAPs have become more sophisticated, coupled with employers becoming more concerned about impairment in the workplace, FFD referrals now not only include drugs/alcohol assessment but now also include the screening for psychiatric and neurological disorders.

There are a number of stakeholders that are involved in the FFD referral process. Some of the stakeholders include occupational medicine, workplace security, the professionals providing treatment to the employee, specialists (e.g., pain, psychology, psychiatry, neurology, etc.), supervisor, employer, workers compensation, disability professionals (if a workplace injury has occurred), union, etc.

There are also different aspects that must be considered pertaining to the initiation of the FFD process. For example, what role will the EAP take to coordinate communication between the stakeholders? In some instances, the EAP professional will need to meet with the employer to fully understand what the employer's policy and procedures are as it relates to the referral. For example, what happens if the employee does not follow up with the referral? Will the employee be terminated? What if the employee does not complete the entire treatment episode (the reason for the referral)? The employer will need to address these questions, and most often this is done via their policy.

An additional aspect that the EAP must discuss is what needs to happen for the employee to return to work. For example, will the employer allow the employee to receive treatment and continue to work? Does the employee have to have a clear drug screen in order to return to work? Most EAPs serve to coordinate and address these issues so that it is clear to all parties what must occur for the employee to return to work. It is important for the savvy EAP professional to must not only provide and receive information from all involved parties, but a treatment summary and other pertinent data must be made part of the EAP records as well to document what took place. By going through the EAP, any treatment records are kept separately from an employee's routine medical records. By doing so, this provides another layer of protection for confidentiality.

It helps to visualize this process since it can be complex. Moreover, there are different professionals who become involved at specific times during the EAP FFD process.

The algorithm below in Fig. 12.1 is a conceptual overview the flow of the fitness for duty process. The model below was developed and applied with a large regional healthcare provider (Weis, 2014). The model was developed by the author as a framework for how EAP would interact with the different stakeholders involved in the FFD evaluative process. It also depicts the different elements of EAP involvement in the FFD referral process.

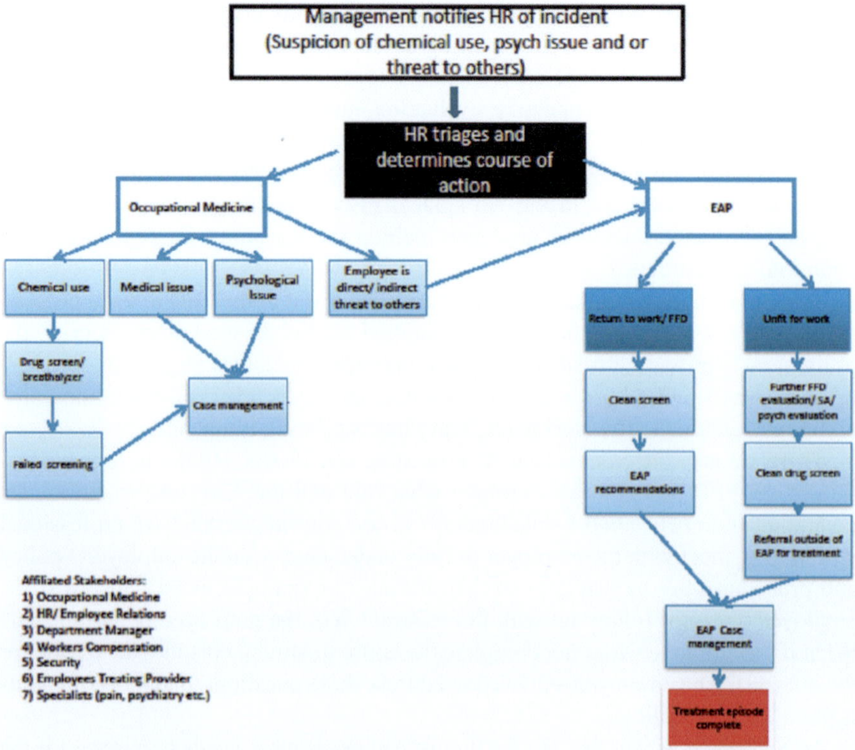

Fig. 12.1 Weis EAP fitness for duty model

12.4.1 Responsibility of the Employer for Mandatory Employee Referrals

The employer has responsibilities to complete as part of the EAP FFD process as well. When the employer makes a mandatory EAP referral, the employer must do the following:

Continue to monitor the employee's performance even after the referral. In other words, the employer has a burden to follow-up with the employee referred under the fitness for duty scenario. This is an area in which many employers tend to skip over; this follow-up is critical in that it ties the reason for referral to the employee's expected workplace compliance. This follow-up process can reduce the employer's liability regarding the employee claiming that no notification was given by the employer pertaining to workplace behavior.

A second responsibility that the employer must do is to update the EAP with any new developments with the employee's job performance so that the EAP can address accordingly. Generally, the EAP professional will maintain ongoing communication with the employer to determine if the employee is satisfactorily maintaining job performance, after the EAP FFD process is completed. It is important for the employer to remember that the actual fitness for duty evaluation is actually a snapshot of a "moment in time" for evaluating that employee.

Typically, the FFD evaluator determines whether the employee is able to return to work after thoroughly evaluating the individual. A critical step is for the employer to continue to assess the employee's job performance and to keep reaching out to the EAP to complete the FFD process, to ensure the employee's successful reintegration back into the workplace.

Lastly, the employer must determine what will happen if the employee is non-compliant with the FFD referral. Typically, the employer will have very specific policies and procedures associated with a FFD referral. There may be times that an employer does not have a specific workplace policy that will drive a FFD referral. In that case, it is the role of the EAP as a consultant to refer the employer to their legal counsel. Typically, once this occurs, the EAP no longer provides consultation to the employer.

12.4.2 Responsibility of the EAP for FFD Referrals

The EAP must complete an initial assessment of employee in order to evaluate whether there are potential concerns that require additional comprehensive FFD assessment. This type of evaluation can either be conducted by the EAP or arranged through an affiliate provider. There is some dissension among EAPs about whether or not the EAP should be involved in this type of referral. It is my opinion that, at the very least, EAPs need to play a role in assisting employers with these types of referrals due to the complicating factors involved in workplace behavioral health risk management.

A discussion of the role of the EAP in FFD referrals will be now be explored further. EAPs act as intermediaries to:

1. Arrange for a comprehensive forensic assessment of the employee by a provider that has expertise in conducting forensic evaluations. The EAP and forensic evaluator determine what, if any, other professionals need to be a part of the evaluation. For example, if the employer has concern about the cognitive ability of the employee, a neuropsychological evaluation may be warranted. The EAP professional is responsible for ensuring that the evaluator has all of the documentation necessary to conduct the fitness for duty evaluation.
2. If there are substance abuse concerns with the employee, a thorough chemical health assessment must be completed. It is prudent that every FFD forensic evaluation should minimally include either a psychiatric and/or psychological evaluation or a battery of standardized psychological testing that are administered specific to the noted concerns. This level of testing provides a standardized, objective assessment of potential psychological and medical conditions that may impede the employee's functioning in the workplace.

3. Once a referral is made to an FFD professional, that professional must determine if the employee has any objectively identified psychological or medical conditions that impact on workplace functioning. If one or more condition is identified, then, the FFD professional must determine if the employee's condition(s) impact on the employee's ability to complete workplace duties safely. If the employee cannot safely work, then, the FFD professional must detail what types of treatments or interventions are required to facilitate the employee's return to work.

12.4.3 Additional Consideration Regarding FFD Referrals

It is imperative that the employer has specified workplace policies. This is frequently lacking in workplaces. These workplace policies determine what actions and role the employer takes when making a FFD referral.

Employers frequently look to EAPs to assist them in developing policy and procedure for fitness for duty concerns. Many EAPs (especially external models) do not have the required training or skills to provide this type of assistance to employers. This is because there are differences in State and federal laws pertaining to the workplace which adds considerable complexity to policy development. Moreover, external EAPs typically do not have that level of integration and consequently may not know how communication and processes flow within the organization.

Historically, internal EAPs have been more involved in workplace policy development because they have a greater level of integration within the company.

It is essential for employers to have set workplace policies because these also delineate the extent to which the EAP will be involved. Depending on the employer's policy and procedure under this referral, the EAP may not be initially involved when an employer wants an FFD completed. Typically, the role of the EAP under this type of referral is to act as a case manager facilitating communication between the forensic evaluator and the employer.

For example, the forensic evaluator will provide the return to work status regarding the employee to the EAP professional. The EAP professional then becomes the custodian of the record in order to protect the employee from having their records accessible from human resources (HR), safety, or other stakeholders that do not need to have that level of detail. If forensic evaluator indicates that the employee is able to return to work, the EAP will inform the employer, and the employee is released back to work. If the forensic evaluator indicates that the employee cannot to return to work, the EAP will inform the employer that the employee is not released to return to work. The forensic evaluator will then recommend what treatment or intervention(s) that need to take place in order for the employee to return to work. It is then up to the EAP to facilitate a referral to an appropriate provider and then to ensure that the employee complies with the treatment recommendation(s).

It is important to know that forensic evaluator does not provide any type of treatment. The reason is that a forensic evaluator cannot simultaneously be in a treating and forensic role. This is considered unethical behavior by many professions. Moreover, it greatly reduces the professional's ability to remain unbiased. Thus, the forensic evaluator conducts a thorough assessment (psychiatric, psychological, substance abuse) and then will make a determination for return to work based on the results of the comprehensive assessment. If the forensic evaluator determines that the employee cannot return to work, it may be necessary for the employee to take a leave of absence. This may be covered under short-term and long-term disability or even the Family Medical Leave Act (FMLA).

12.5 EAP and Behavioral Health Disability

EAPS can play an integral role regarding behavioral health disability. There are a number of reasons why the involvement of the EAP is essential. First, the EAP is often the "go to" professional organization that employers use regarding employees with workplace productivity concerns. Employers look to a well-integrated EAP to be their "eyes and ears" in assisting employees with behavioral health issues. Historically, employers have done a relatively good job of mining data related to medical conditions and their impact on work. However, when the employer is asked about how they address workplace behavioral health conditions, they have more difficulty defining if/how to intervene with their employees around these issues. If an employee accessed EAP services preventatively through self-referral, this may serve to reduce the severity of a psychological condition later. Another reason why EAP are in a key position to address workplace behavioral health conditions is that EAPs focus on the need to return the employee to work as effectively and efficiently as possible. The EAP is not concerned with the healthcare reimbursement structure for their services as EAP is often a "pre-purchased" benefit and the EAP is paid whether the employees use it or not. Finally, EAPs have access to employer benefit information that is helpful if the EAPs have to refer the employee for longer term care that is covered by the employee's workplace health plan. The axiom that is used in some EAP settings is: "the right care, at the right time, with the right provider." Employers appreciate this focus. EAPs are frequently in a unique position to help employees navigate a complex behavioral healthcare delivery system. The current medical healthcare delivery system can be difficult to navigate and the behavioral health system is even more so. Because of specific training, most EAP professionals understand the nuances of facilitating referrals that make for effective behavioral health treatment.

12.5.1 *EAP and Workplace Mental Health Risk Management*

Before the programmatic aspects of an EAP program are explored, it is important to examine how EAPs can better manage the behavioral health risks in the workplaces they serve.

Most EAPs must take a comprehensive approach in addressing workplace mental health concerns. Consequently, EAPs must identify:

12.5.2 *Risk Prevalence*

The American Psychological Association (APA, 2014) reported that of the 3068 adults who completed their Stress in America survey, three in four adults in the study experienced at least one symptom related to stress in the past month. The top sources of stress were money, work, the economy, family, and personal health. Because of their potential to assess/intervene early, EAPs have much to offer here in terms of identifying who is at risk and then either providing short-term counseling or referring employees to the proper treatment provider.

In the US National Random Sample Epidemiological Interview Data (2012), full-time workers were much more likely to have experienced a behavioral health disorder in the past 12 months with 20% of workers experiencing clinical levels of a behavioral health disorder (Karg et al., 2017). This demonstrates a key role that EAPs can play in identifying and referring to treatment if the employee cannot be treated within the contracted EAP model by the employer.

12.6 Secondary Effects of Mental Health Disorders on Other Disability Factors

Undiagnosed mental health conditions can negatively impact on the treatment that is obtained. For example, an employee receives treatment for newly diagnosed diabetes. While the initial diagnosis is diabetes, and that drives the treatment that the employee receives, empirical research has consistently demonstrated that comorbid psychological conditions frequently occur as well. Without appropriate identification of the underlying psychological condition, the treatment for the diabetes may not be successful. Anxiety disorders and MDD occur frequently with individuals who have been diagnosed with diabetes. Consequently, it is imperative that *both* physical and psychological conditions are identified as soon as possible for optimal treatment outcomes (Attridge Consulting, Inc., 2017).

Yet, the paradox is that in spite of high prevalence, most of the employees that need treatment do not get it. There are a number of reasons why those who need it most do not get it including social stigma, lack of physician assessment and diagnosis of psychological conditions, and lack of or inappropriate treatment, such as with the use of psychotropic medication only. Therefore, either a self-referral or supervisory referral to an EAP can be the first step in identifying a potential psychological condition and obtaining appropriate treatment.

12.7 Workplace Costs Related to Mental Health

According to Substance Abuse and Mental Health Services (SAMSHA) (2014), the prevalence for adults experiencing a mental illness in any given year is 43.6 million (18.1%). The prevalence rate for adults with a substance use disorder is 20.2 million (8.4%). Interestingly, 7.9 million adults in a given year will experience both a mental illness and substance use disorder. It is difficult to deny the impact of these conditions in the workplace as they are the most common among employees (Partnership for Workplace Mental Health, 2016). Additionally, employers are recognizing that employees have comorbid behavioral health and medical conditions that cost 2–3 times more in medical costs than just those with medical conditions alone (Milliman, 2017).

As employers have evaluated the costs related to healthcare (both behavioral and medical) in the workplace, they have realized that it is not just the cost to treat the condition(s) themselves but also the indirect cost of the condition(s) to the workplace in lost productivity and absenteeism. There are two conclusions from the Partnership for Mental Health (2016) study: more workers are absent from work because of stress and anxiety than because of physical illness injury; more days of work loss and work impairment are caused by mental illness than many other chronic conditions such as diabetes, asthma, and arthritis. If the data for Major Depressive Disorder (MDD) alone are examined, employees with Major Depressive Disorder report productivity levels at 70% of their peak performance (Partnership for Mental Health, 2016). An additional consideration related to the workplace is the costs related to disability. Of note, MDD is the leading cause of disability for people 15–44 years of age in the United States (Partnership for Mental Health, 2016). Approximately 80% of persons with MDD reported some level of functional impairment (Partnership for Mental Health, 2016). Given that major depressive disorder is a treatable condition with many new treatment options available, this seems to be a point where EAPs can begin to impact the consequences of this condition. Over the course of my career as an EAP professional, I have worked with stakeholders within employer groups to target outreach to both employees and providers related to high-risk conditions. One pilot project that I initiated involved developing a "depression toolkit" for primary care physicians (PCPs) to use in conjunction with the behavioral health managed care carve-out with a large employer in the Midwest. As the EAP provider, we developed a full campaign to help reduce the stigma of MDD in the workplace, gave providers a "tool" to help them screen for Major Depressive Disorder in the PCP setting, and gave providers access to free number they could call to consult with a psychiatrist with questions related to initiating medication for the employee as well. All of the materials used in the campaign promoted the EAP as a referral source for the PCP in the event the provider thought the employee could benefit from psychotherapy, while the PCP treated the biological basis of the Major Depressive Disorder if indicated. This resulted in a spike in EAP referrals from treating PCPs for the treatment of Major Depressive Disorder. This was an innovative yet fairly simple way, for the EAP to address Major Depressive Disorder with this large employer group in the Midwest.

12.8 Absenteeism: Demonstration of Return on Investment (ROI) with EAP Services

It is estimated that MDD costs US workplaces $23 billion dollars annually (Gallup Report, 2017). For many years, EAPs have focused on lowered absenteeism as a return on investment (ROI) that employers obtain when they invest in EAP services. However, absenteeism is just one measure that EAP professionals can demonstrate this ROI. A new and promising measurement tool for evaluating other measures as well of EAP effectiveness is the Workplace Outcome Suite (WOS) (Sharar, Pompe, & Lennox, 2012). This instrument is specifically designed for EAPs and is short with just 25 total items and 5 scales. Moreover, the WOS has been psychometrically tested and validated. Thus, this means the WOS has been found to accurately measure workplace issues easily (Lennox, Sharer, et al. 2010). The Workplace Outcome Suites five scales that are at the heart of the workplace issues that EAP address: absenteeism, presenteeism, work engagement, life satisfaction, and workplace distress. Because of this, many EAPs routinely utilize the WOS as part of their workplace and employee assessments. In a pooled study of 20 EAPs, Sharar and Pompe (2014) found that change in work absenteeism dropped from 13.28 days of missed work without EAP involvement to 7.49 days of missed work 90 days after EAP intervention. The WOS is the best empirically supported instrument to date and has demonstrated a 43.6% improvement in workplace absenteeism with EAP intervention (Sharar & Pompe, 2014).

12.8.1 Risk Prevention: EAP Assistance in Integration of Employer Services

Employers have accepted the reality that workplace behavioral health issues are not going away and the employers need to not only "mine" their workplace data to discover the drivers of their increased healthcare costs, but they must embrace EAPs and other professionals who develop proactive, evidenced-based approaches to address the costs. This is an area where EAP positively impact the bottom line for employers because EAPs' unique position in working with both employers and employees regularly. Consequently, EAP professionals are able to assist employees in navigating the very complicated healthcare system. Moreover, EAPs offer specific services regarding employee workplace productivity, such as health risk screenings, smoking cessation, stress management, as well as physical fitness, nutrition, and weight loss. As employers better understand how mental health greatly impacts on the workplace, there has been increased willingness to integrate mental health services in EAP services to promote better employee health and safety.

12.9 Risk Identification: EAP Usage of Screening Tools

There are a number of evidenced-based screening tools used by EAPs to assess for potential psychological conditions. It is important to note that a positive screening tool score does not necessarily mean that a person conclusively has a psychological condition (Jensen-Doss, A., & Hawley, K.M., 2011). This is because screening tools do not go through the same validation and standardization processes such as those with psychological tests. A positive screening score on one of several screening tools such as those used by EAP professionals indicates the person requires further evaluation and potentially a referral to a mental health professional.

12.9.1 Michigan Alcohol Screening Tool (MAST)

The MAST is one of the most widely used screening tools to assess for potential alcohol abuse. It is a 25-item questionnaire that is designed to provide a rapid assessment of lifetime alcohol problems (Selzer, 1971). The MAST takes about 8 min to administer and 5 min to score and interpret. A shortcoming of the MAST is that it assesses for lifetime alcohol problems and does not screen for acute alcohol issues. However, it is still a reasonable tool to use when assessing for alcohol-related problems.

The EAP professional utilizing the MAST needs to be mindful that just like other assessment tools, this should be used in tandem with other assessment tools and a thorough clinical interview. There are some clinicians in the alcohol/drug addiction field who will also conduct a collaborative interview with other persons in the client's support system who can provide helpful information in formulating a treatment plan. There is some debate among professionals as to how helpful the collateral interview is in that there may be a lack of transparency on the part of the interviewee. This is particularly true especially if the client is the primary breadwinner, and reporting problems with substance abuse may result in a referral for substance abuse treatment.

Another consideration pertaining to the usage of collateral interviews may result in a lack of transparency around problems with substance abuse if there is abuse within the family system. While collateral interviews can certainly be helpful, it is not necessarily something an EAP professional completes if there is a workplace performance issue related to the employee.

12.9.2 Physician Health Questionnaire (PHQ-9)

The PHQ-9 is a brief assessment tool used to screen for severity of major depressive disorder (MDD) over time. It consists of nine questions that ask a patient to self-report degree of symptomology on a Likert scale ranging from 0 to 5 with 0 being "not at all" and 5 being "nearly every day." The higher the score is, the more likely the person is endorsing symptoms of MDD.

12.9.3 Beck Major Depressive Disorder Inventory (BDI)

This assessment tool consists of a 21-question multiple-choice self-report inventory. It is one of the most widely used psychometric tests used for measuring the severity of depressive symptoms (Beck, 1972). The assessment tool is also based on a Likert-type scale that looks at severity on a scale from 0 to 3. "0" indicates little feelings of sadness and "3" indicates sadness that is intolerable. While the BDI is used in a variety of settings, it was designed for research settings, originally. Moreover, it does not have any validity indices so that there is no means to ascertain whether the person is over- or under-reporting symptoms.

Much like the MAST, there are some limitations in using the PHQ-9 and BDI alike in that because both are self-report tools. Moreover, responses may be exaggerated or minimized by the person completing the questionnaire. Bowling (2005) also found that the client's response may change when the PHQ-9 is given in EAP settings. In addition, because these questionnaires are completed in a clinical setting, social expectations have shown to elicit a different response compared to administration via a postal survey (Bowling, 2005).

Despite the limitations of the discussed screening tools, they provide EAP professionals with a means to further assess for potential psychological and substance abuse issues. If a positive screen is determined, the EAP must then evaluate whether the issue can be ethically and legally addressed in an EAP settings. This is because there are limitations with the short treatment model of the EAP. Moreover, for some psychological conditions, the person may require more intensive, evidence-based treatment than an EAP can provide.

A well-integrated EAP is most effective when it receives referrals (either self or supervisory) early on in when an employee's personal struggles occur. However, the EAP may become involved at an acute stage to assist the employee in either (a) providing short-term intervention via the EAP or (b) referring the employee into their insurance benefit for longer-term treatment. Despite this effective EAP model, some employees may not comply with a referral until the problem becomes more severe. For this reason, many employers are becoming proactive in addressing these types of workplace concerns more frequently.

12.9.4 Risk Reduction: Types of Effective Treatment for Employees with Mental Health Conditions

There are numerous evidence-based practices that are more rigorously evaluated and demonstrated to be effective (Attridge, 2017). The most common treatment modality is psychotherapy, such as with cognitive behavioral therapy (CBT) or with psychotropic medication. Typically, CBT focuses on maladaptive thought patterns that impact decisions. The goal of this approach is to facilitate the individual to choosing more adaptive ways to thinking about personal and workplace concerns. The prescribing of psychotropic medication involves the utilization of medications that are specifically for the treatment of psychological conditions. Additional modalities that have demonstrated to be effective include exercise, adequate sleep hygiene, stress interventions, nutrition counseling, and mindfulness meditation (Partnership for Workplace Mental Health, 2016).

12.10 Workplace Costs Related to Substance Abuse

As stated earlier, the addiction field is really where EAP began. It is commonly accepted that alcohol and drug use among employees and their family members can be an expensive problem for business and industry (National Council on Alcoholism and Drug Dependence, 2017). The impact on alcohol/drugs often focuses on four areas: premature deaths/fatal accidents, injuries/accident rates, absenteeism/extra sick leave, and loss of production. Historically, the focus of research has primarily been on alcohol and illicit drug use (e.g., marijuana and cocaine), but that has changed with the recent introduction of opioids into the United States today.

From the employer perspective, there is much more focus on the costs of prescriptions being written for conditions like chronic pain vs. illicit use. Many employees who use these prescription medications are now addicted to them. Given that opioids are euphoric and reduce a person's ability to focus, their usage in employees is a very real workplace issue. Thus, many employers want to address these potential addiction issues with EAP assistance.

Because employees with alcohol abuse issues at risk for 2.7 times are more likely to have workplace injuries than those without these concerns, it provides a great fit for EAP to provide employer/employee education as well as screening of these concerns for employees (National Council on Alcoholism and Drug Dependence, 2017).

Moreover, the cost of alcohol and drug abuse in the workplace accounts for 70 + % of costs associated for workplace productivity in those that abuse substances (Cognichoice, 2016). In addition, 24% of workers report drinking during the workday at least once in the past year (Cognichoice, 2016). Thus, it quickly becomes clear that substance abuse and the impact on workplace productivity is a considerable concern.

Typically, an employee who is identified as having a substance abuse issue in an EAP is referred outside for more intensive treatment. At that point, the employee's insurance generally covers the treatment expense. On average, addictions treatment costs $1583 per patient, with a corresponding $11,487 return in benefits to society. Most of the benefits come from reduced crime and increased employment earnings (Cognichoice, 2016).

12.10.1 Treatment Options

There are several treatment options available for employees that need treatment for an alcohol addiction. The levels of care for addiction range from standard outpatient treatment (weekly psychotherapy that is specific to substance abuse) progressing to intensive outpatient therapy (a combination of individual and group psychotherapy) to a residential treatment facility where an employee will spend several days to weeks receiving intensive treatment.

The primary focus of the EAP with employees who abuse substances is to determine which type of professional provides the most appropriate treatment. In addition, an EAP also provides a referral to substance abuse treatment facilities. The treatment goal is to guide the employee back to sobriety. However, if the employee does elapse, it is ideal that the EAP professional already has a relationship with the employee to quickly intervene and to streamline the referral process to the most appropriate provider.

12.10.2 Evaluating the Workplace Effectiveness of EAP Interventions

Despite the popularity and prevalence of EAPs, and the historical emphasis on how EAP can improve work performance, there has been very little rigorous evaluation of the workplace effects of EAP counseling (Sharar et al., 2012). It is apparent that EAP has clearly made a mark with US employers. What has been lacking is that measures of the effectiveness of EAP service have not routinely captured whether EAP providers achieve results that are relevant to workplace effectiveness. It is this type of data that is most meaningful to stakeholders such as HR, employee benefits, and occupational health and safety.

The typical measures of EAP often focus on process metrics such as utilization rates, presenting problems, and demographics, but fail to demonstrate the program's effectiveness in obtaining a positive outcome in the workplace. Therefore, in the future, EAP providers must recognize that employers are concerned about absenteeism and presenteeism, higher levels of work engagement, and reduced levels of stress at work and provide measures that obtain this information. The measures that EAP has used historically have fallen short in demonstrating the actual effect of obtaining a positive effect in the workplace. What follows are some of the measures that have been used to evaluate EAP effectiveness:

1. *Measures of client satisfaction.* Many EAP counselors are typically rated highly by clients that have experienced little or no change in their work environment. Anecdotally, the return rate for client satisfaction was around 20% which is quite low (Sharar et al., 2012).
2. *Case studies or testimonials.* First-hand, positive anecdotal accounts of an employee's personal experience with EAP are valuable but since they are subjective perceptions are therefore imprecise. Moreover, case studies or testimonials do provide any standardized, quantifiable, or reliable outcome data. This means that they have limited value to document the effectiveness of EAP services.
3. *Utilization rates.* A "high" utilization rate reflects a common perception that the EAP must be successful, but it, in reality, only indicates the extent to which employees use the EAP. Utilization rates do not provide any objective data regarding whether the EAP had a positive workplace impact.
4. *Other published studies.* While a step in the right direction, the number of published studies is quite small, outdated, and not easy to find (Attridge & Wallace, 2010). This means that the majority of EAP research currently does not meet the high-quality standards for research, such as RCTs, and replication in a number of EAP settings as well as a variety of EAP clients.

12.11 Models of Return to Work

There is no single framework for conceptualizing return to work and accommodations for mental health disability. However, there are a number of principles and processes that can be utilized to address the return to work process. Many of the models that will be discussed below employ a multi-causal focus that evaluates individual and work factors.

12.11.1 Process Models

The return to work (RTW) process is not a straightforward path. Many issues can arise along the process. However, the RTW process addresses identifying the individual issues that negatively impact on the employee's return to work.

One way to look at this approach is to look at the individual characteristics of the worker who is absent from work. The process model examines age, sex, and personal dimensions linked to physical and mental health, particularly the person's psychiatric history. The process model holds that obtaining the psychiatric history of the worker is a critical step in the initial assessment as a positive history may be an indication of mitigating factors. Consequently, it is essential to explore this further with the individual to ascertain what treatment has worked and what didn't. Moreover, the savvy EAP professional will ascertain types of treatment as well as any potential compliance issues with treatment.

An additional factor to consider is the psychosocial environment at work. This looks at structural dimensions (i.e., the workplace rules and policies regarding "what to do," "how to do it," and "how much time" is needed to perform a given task) as well as the human dimensions of work (i.e., communication between superiors, subordinates, and colleagues).

When the EAP professional utilizes this approach, then the issues that contribute to a delay in returning to work are identified. For example, how will the employees' co-workers interact with him/her if they come back to work with a limited duty restriction? What if the employee returns to work but is not able to keep up with demands of the work environment (Human Solutions Report, 2017)? If the EAP is involved in the case from the outset, you can see how they could play a critical role in the success of the employee returning to work.

12.11.2 Phase Model

This phase model views the return to work process as a process of time. The phase model emphasizes the usage of time to allow workers to return to work at a pace that allows employees to readapt to the workplace environment. The phase model notes that this process helps employees stay at work once they return. An important variable in this model is considering the time factor of when to return to work and what coordinated outreach needs to occur to facilitate an effective RTW. Medical management, as well as the timing of interventions, is critical to increase the probability of a successful RTW (Roelen et al., 2012). This study found that in order to maximize the RTW probability in the first months after being off, it is important to reach out to the employee within the first 2–3 weeks after RTW (Roelen et al., 2012). The discussion of the four phases in this model follows:

(a) *Being off work (and receiving treatment).* This is typically the phase that occurs at the beginning of the time-off episode where the employee is actively engaged in treatment with providers. It typically would coincide with the acute phase of the precipitating event that has led to time off.
(b) *Work reintegration (coming back into the workplace)*. The employee is still engaged in treatment, but the process of gradually return to the workplace has begun. It may involve a return to work meeting with the employer/supervisor to

determine what needs to occur when the employee returns. It may also be a time to review any restrictions around returning to work. This phase really establishes the "path" for a successful return to work.

(c) *Work maintenance (avoiding a relapse).* Once the employee has returned to work, usually the EAP professional monitors the employee's functioning in the workplace. If problematic issues are identified, the EAP professional advocates to address these issues so that they can be addressed. The EAP can advocate for the employee, the employer, or both.

(d) *Work improvement and career advancement.* The EAP professional can continue to work with the employee or employer to facilitate the employee's sustained success as well as assisting the employee in working toward job promotions (Human Solutions Report, 2017).

12.12 Work Outcomes

Review of treatment outcomes has ascertained that the treatment of any impairment in functioning is essential to regaining work productivity (Lelliott et al., 2008). For example, the usage of psychotropic medication is essential to treat the brain chemistry component of MDD. However, psychotropic medications alone are insufficient to fully treat MDD. Instead, the empirical research consistently indicates that the combination of medication and specific psychological treatment, such as cognitive behavioral therapy, are superior to regaining functioning (Lelliott et al., 2008). Moreover, psychosocial issues, which are not valid conditions, but personal preferences, beliefs, and expectations, play a role in recovery as well (Warren, 2011). Thus, any BH treatment must parse valid psychological conditions from psychosocial issues since psychosocial issues are under voluntary control. That is, the individual can learn to control behaviors to make behavioral changes in the workplace. Second, while some psychotropic medication side effects can interfere with the ability to perform work duties (i.e., disturbed sleep and impaired concentration), these are frequently managed by sufficient follow-up with the prescribing psychiatrist to minimize the impact of side effects on functioning.

12.12.1 Innovations in EAP Involvement with Primary Care

EAPs have begun to collaborate with the primary care professionals (PCPs) assessment skills to screen for psychological conditions (Attridge, 2017). In addition, collaborative care models emphasize participation of physicians and mental health professionals (i.e., such as those found in the EAP treatment models) in the assessment and treatment of all types of disability concerns, including psychological conditions. As a consequence, there is now an emphasis on the return to work as part of the treatment process. Currently, EAPs play a role in educating PCPs on the interaction between employee functioning and workplace performance. Frequently, outpatient treatment in the primary care settings focus exclusively on symptom reduction without really understanding the need to return employees to work as part of treatment outcomes. This lack of understanding creates an opportunity for EAPs to interact with PCPs to develop return to work goals.

Additional education/training for treating professionals must also address the lack of screening for psychosocial issues that are present when the employee obtains treatment. This can be a difficult gap to bridge in to a capitated model where the provider is reimbursed a select amount for a certain population vs. billing a fee for a particular service.

One type of change that can be made easily is to collaborate with the PCP's nursing staff. This enhances communication regarding the return to work goal for the employee. This is where EAPs can foster a true collaborative relationship in regard to preventative work.

Additionally, collaborative care models currently focus on improving accessibility of mental healthcare in primary care settings, increase case-specific communication between different treatment providers seeing the employee, and promote greater treatment continuity and follow-up care. The collaborative effort increases the likelihood that the employee can return to work utilizing best clinical practices. Some examples of work-focused interventions include collaborative disability case management, early contact with the absent worker from the supervisor, ongoing communication with the absent employee, and an agreed-upon rehabilitation plan including work tasks as well as flexibility in creating work accommodations and return-to-work arrangements. Adherence to these tasks ensures the quality of the provided treatment is monitored and delivered in such a way that return to work is the treatment outcome goal.

12.13 Future Trends in EAP Services

EAPs have a long history of supporting employees and organizations in a variety of ways. The role of the EAP in supporting worker mental health and job performance is already a key component to the overall success of thousands of organizations. A recent industry survey by Chestnut Global Partners (2017) ascertained that participants identified their top needs for the EAP industry as (1) increased EAP utilization rates, (2) the production of measurable outcomes that improve the perceived value of EAP by purchasers, and (3) improved collaboration/case management and coordination of care. These innovations are now discussed below.

12.13.1 Factors That Increase EAP Utilization

As employers and employees alike become more aware of EAP programs, the utilization of EAP services has steadily increased. EAP utilization is one measure of EAP effectiveness. The employer generally likes to see higher utilization rates as that typically indicate their employees and their dependents are aware of the benefit and are using it. However, high utilization does not speak to the effectiveness of the EAP professional or the provided EAP services. Over the years, EAPs have touted EAP utilization as the prime measure of EAP effectiveness. However, the utilization of EAP services does not speak to the efficacy of the EAP services. To that end, EAP professionals must expand the measurement of EAP effectiveness beyond utilization. With the development of tools, like the WOS, future EAP research can better examine EAP effectiveness.

12.13.2 Measurable Outcomes

The short-term model of EAP counseling has demonstrated effectiveness in helping employees return to optimal levels of functioning in the workplace by addressing specific workplace performance issues (Sharar et al., 2012). However, most of the studies to date remain unpublished, due to employer proprietary restrictions on its employee data, or are simply not shared with the purchaser. However, EAPs can now incorporate the Workplace Outcome Suite (WOS) into all assessments and begin to evaluate treatment efficacy internally. This allows EAPs to determine EAP effectiveness prior to intervention and at the end of the intervention related to the five dimensions described earlier.

12.13.3 Improved Collaboration/Case Management and Coordination of Care

EAP professionals can better differentiate themselves from other providers by enhanced collaboration as well as through the case management and coordination of care. As stated earlier in this chapter, case management is a core technology for EAP that has been somewhat lost in recent years. EAP professionals have a great opportunity to interface with multiple providers and serve as the "link" to fully ensuring that care is well-coordinated. Because EAP is a pre-purchased product by an employer (i.e., the EAP gets paid whether employees use the program or not), the EAP professional does not have financial pressures that prevent him/her from taking additional time to reach out to other professionals such as with a PCP or private practitioner.

12.14 Summary

EAPs have long been available. However, more recently employers and employees alike are beginning to tap into EAP services. EAP provide a variety of services through consultation, assessment, education, collaboration, and case management.

Many of the issues that relate to employees are related to psychological and substance abuse conditions. EAPs provide excellent and quick assessment for these types of concerns. Moreover, EAP professionals can facilitate the referral for longer-term treatment when it becomes clear that psychological and substance abuse conditions are more severe than what can be addressed in the EAP setting.

Future trends for growth in the field include the increase use of technology, legislative and business challenges affecting the workplace, greater recognition of the role of mental health in productivity and organizational health, and positioning issues for EAP as a commodity versus a profession. EAP providers need to learn to move from a position of reacting to employer requests to becoming seen as a consultant or advisor. EAPs must continue to strive to have a "seat at the table" with C-suite/HR/benefits staff to assist in offering EAP services (i.e., their call center capability, reporting and infrastructure, as well as their behavioral health screening expertise). Employers are keenly aware of the costs to their health plan that are medical in nature and have now come to realize that most medical complications (i.e., obesity, heart disease, and diabetes) now also have comorbid behavioral health problems (e.g., Major Depressive Disorders or one of the anxiety disorders). This serves as an opportunity for EAPs to blend their services with employer initiatives.

In terms of business product life cycle, it's time for service innovation in the EAP field. However, innovation does not have to mean ripping out the core, but redefining, adding, or integrating features. As stated earlier, EAPs must think "outside the box" to find ways to identify what they are really good at (i.e., behavioral health assessment) and work with employer groups to show them our value in how we can take our expertise and align in with their organizational goals to enhance access to care, provide greater quality of care, and possibly even reduce costs by ensuring that employees have access to the right care, at the right time, with the right provider.

EAPs need to continue to find innovative, cutting-edge ways to integrate with both providers and other vendors that employer's contract with such as disability and workers' compensation in order to address the potential for behavioral health disability in an expedient manner. This helps employers and employees alike to remain healthy and productive.

References

American Psychological Association. (2014). *Stress in America: paying with our health.* Retrieved September 7, 2017, https://www.apa.org/news/press/releases/stress/2014/stress-report.pdf.

Attridge Consulting Inc. (2017). *Evidence-based workplace mental health risk management: Implications for EAP.* Plenary presentation at the annual institute of the Employee Assistance Society of North America, Atlanta, GA. July 7, 2017, http://hdl.handle.net/10713/6571.

Attridge, M., Cahill, T., Granberry, S., & Herlihy, P. (2013). National behavioral consortium industry profile of external eap vendors. *Journal of Workplace Behavioral Health, Volume, 28*(4), 251–324.

Attridge, M., & Wallace, S. (2010). *Able-minded: return to work accommodations for disability leave and mental disorders.* Vancouver, BC, Canada. Retrieved August 14, 2017, http://archivehshsl.umaryland.edu/handle/10713/3834. Accessed 14 Aug 2017.

Beck, A. T. (1972). *Major depressive disorder: Causes and treatment*. Philadelphia: University of Pennsylvania Press. 0-8122-1032-8.

Bowling, A. (2005). Mode of questionnaire administration can have serious effects in data quality. *Journal of Public Health, 27*(3), 281–291.

Chestnut Global Partners. (2017). Future trends report. An analysis of what is occurring in the fields of employee assistance, organizational health and workplace productivity industries. Retrieved July 28, 2017, http://www.chestnut.globalpartners.com/2017/9/18.

Cognichoice. (2016). 10 Sobering facts on the business costs of addiction in 2016. Retrieved September 7, 2017, http://www.cognichoice.com/2016/02/13. 10-sobering.

Employee Assistance Professional Association. (2005). Retrieved July 7, 2017, https://metroeap.com/wp-content/uploads/2015/08/EAP-buyers-guide.pdf.

Employee Assistance Professional Association. (2017a). Ethical Issues and Codes, Retrieved December 5, 2017, https://www.eapassn.org/about/about-employee-assistance/ethical-issues-and-codes.

Employee Assistance Professional Association. (2017b). National conference keynote session titled: wrestling with EAP core technology: origins and future implications for the profession. Interview with Greg DeLapp & Dr. Paul Roman.

Gallup Report. (2017). *Major depressive disorder costs U.S. workplaces $23 billion in absenteeism.* Retrieved July 10, 2017, http://www.gallup.com/poll/163619/Major Depressive Disorder-costs-workplaces-bllions-absenteeism.aspx.

Human Solutions Report. (2017). *Annual report: able-minded return to work and accommodations for workers on disability leave for mental disorders*. Retrieved August 13, 2017, https://archive.hshsl.umaryland.edu/handle/10713/3834.

Jensen-Doss, A., & Hawley, K. M. (2011). Understanding clinicians' diagnostic practices: Attitudes toward the utility of diagnosis and standardized diagnostic tools. *Administration and Policy in Mental Health Services Research, 38*(6), 476–485. https://doi.org/10.1007/s10488-011-0334-3

Karg, R. S., Bose, J., Batts, K. R., Forman-Hoffman, V. L., Liao, D., Hirsch, E., Pemberton, M. R., Colpe, L. J., & Hedden, S. L. (2017). Past year mental disorders among adults in the United States: Results from the 2008–2012 mental health surveillance study. CBHSQ Data Review. SAMSHA. Retrieved June 22, 2017, https://www.samhsa.gov/data/...N2MentalDis.../NSDUH-DR-N2MentalDis-2014.htm.

Lelliott, P., Boradman, J., Harvey, S., Henderson, M., Knapp, M., & Tulloch, S. (2008). Mental health and work: A report for the national director for work and health. London: Royal College of Psychiatrists. Retrieved October 11, 2017, http://www.rcpsych.ac.uk/clinicalservicesstandards/crupublications/2008.aspx.

Masi, D. (2011). Definition and history of employee assistance programs in correct Understanding and application of EAP necessary for all entities that implement measures for mental health. Kabushiki Kaisha Roudou, Tokyo, Japan, June 2011. Retrieved 11 Aug 2017.

Milliman Medical Index. (2017). Retrieved October 28, 2017, www.milliman.com/uploadedFiles/insight/Periodicals/mmi/pdfs/2014-mmi.pdf.

National Council on Alcoholism and Drug Dependence. Drugs and alcohol in the workplace (2017). Retrieved September 20, 2017, https://www.ncadd.org/aboutaddiction/update'drugsandalcoholintheworkplace.

Partnership for Workplace Mental Health. (2016). Taking on mental health in the workplace: programs that make a difference. Retrieved October 30, 2017, dmec.org/wp-content/.../Taking-on-Mental-Health-in-the-Workplace_5.20.16.pdf.

Roelen, C., Norder, G., Koopmans, P., Van Rhenen, W., Van der Klink, & Bultmann, U. (2012). Employees sick-listed with mental disorders: Who returns to work and when? *Journal of Occupational Rehabilitation, 22*(3), 409–417. https://doi.org/10.1007/s10926-012-9363-3

Roman, P., & Blum, T. C. (1988). Reaffirmation of the core technology for employee assistance programs. *The ALMACAN, 19*(8), 17–22.

Selzer, M. L. (1971). The Michigan alcoholism screening test (MAST): The quest for a new diagnostic instrument. *American Journal of Psychiatry, 127*, 1653–1658.

Sharar, D., & Pompe, J. (2008). Preparing for the challenges of research. *Journal of Employee Assistance, 38*(2), 7–9.

Sharar, D., & Pompe, J., (2014). *How recent innovations in technology and analytics can transform the EAP industry*. Presented at the Northern IL EAPA 36th annual conference.

Sharar, D., Pompe, J., & Lennox, R. (2012). Evaluating the workplace effects of eap counseling. *Journal of Health and Productivity, 6*(12), 5–14.

Sharar, D., Popovits, R., & Donahue, E. (2010). Telephone counseling in employee assistance programs: Is it effective? Is it legal? *Journal of Compensation and Benefits, 26*(1), 1–4.

Sheparis, C., & Walsh, F. (2017). The fragility of freedom, counseling today. *60*(4), 46–50.

Substance Abuse and Mental Health Services Administration (SAMSHA). (2014). Behavioral health trends in the United States: results from the 2014 national survey on drug use and health. Retrieved October 30, 2017, https://www.samhsa.gov/data/sites/default/files/NSDUH-FRR1-2014/NSDUH-FRR1-2014.pdf

Warren, P. A. (2011). *Behavioral health disability: Innovations in prevention and management*. New York: Springer Science+Business Media, LLC.

Weis, D. (2014). *Fitness for duty evaluation EAP algorithm*. Unpublished work.

Chapter 13
Case Management and Behavioral Health Disability

J. David Hubbard, Pamela A. Warren, and Robert M. Aurbach

13.1 Epidemiological and Prevalence of Psychological and Behavioral Health Concerns

Behavioral health disability claims have been reported more frequently over the past several decades (Warren, 2009). This has led professionals to question whether there is an actual increase in actual behavioral health disorders or if there are other issues that are driving this increase (American Medical Association (AMA), 2008; Canadian Medical Association, 1997; CDC, 2009; Gatchel & Schultz, 2005; Melhorn & Ackerman, 2008).

13.2 Comorbid Behavioral Health and Physical Concerns

Empirical research has ascertained that approximately two-thirds of individuals who utilize a high level of medical care were found to have some type of true psychiatric disorder that met the *Diagnostic and Statistical Manual-5* (American Psychiatric Association (ApA), 2013; Von Korf, 1992). Twenty-three percent of these individuals were diagnosed with major depressive disorder. Another 22% of these individuals had a diagnosis of some type of anxiety disorder, while yet another 20% had a diagnosis of Somatization Disorder. Importantly, this type of high

J. David Hubbard
Genex Services, Inc, Plano, TX, USA

P. A. Warren (✉)
Carle Physician Group and University of Illinois Medical School, Department of Psychiatry, Monticello, IL, USA

R. M. Aurbach
Uncommon Approach, Melbourne, VIC, Australia

P. A. Warren (ed.), *Handbook of Behavioral Health Disability Management*,
https://doi.org/10.1007/978-3-319-89860-5_13

utilization of medical care continued throughout these individuals' lives. This finding was later supported by Harter, Baumeister, Reuter, et al. (2007) who determined that the most common behavioral health diagnoses were those related to the depressive, anxiety, and somatoform disorders spectrum.

Importantly, behavioral health concerns tend to have a high comorbidity with physical concerns. The empirical literature has consistently demonstrated that many physical concerns, such as chronic pain, musculoskeletal, cardiac, stroke, obesity, diabetes, as well as different types of injuries have a great deal of concurrent psychological concerns (Dewa & Lin, 2000; Harter et al., 2007; Kessler, Merikangas, & Wang, 2007; Kroenke, 2003; Laitinen-Krispijn & Bijl, 2000; Linton, 1993; Merikangas, Ames, Cui, et al., 2007; Ormel, Petukhova, Chatterji, et al., 2008; Roy-Byrne, Davidson, Kessler, et al., 2008). The prevalence rates for comorbid behavioral health disorders are quite high, averaging 42.2% for individuals with physical concerns. Thus, the empirical research has demonstrated the importance of appropriate evaluation and diagnosis of potential behavioral health concerns when treating an individual for a physical issue (Adler, 2007; Disability Management Employer Coalition, 2009; Evans, Charney, Lewis, et al., 2005; Gatchel & Gardea, 1999; Gatchel, Peng, Peters, Fuchs, & Turk, 2007; Goetzel, Long, Ozminkowski, et al., 2004; Heidel, Klachefsky, McDowell, et al., 2007; Jorm, Angermeyer, & Katschnig, 2000; Katon, Kleinman, & Rosen, 1982; Kavan, 2009; Kessler, Demler, Frank, et al., 2005; Kessler & Wang, 2008; Krause, Frank, Dasinger, Sullivan, & Sinclair, 2001; Langlieb & Kahn, 2005; Lee, Tsang, Breslau, et al., 2009; Leopold, 2003; Lerner, Allaire, & Reisine, 2005; Reggers & Ansseau, 1999; Seedat, Scott, Angermeyer, et al., 2009; Suehs, Argo, Bendele, et al., 2008; Waehrer, Leigh, Cassady, & Miller, 2004).

13.3 Defining Disability in the Behavioral Health Context

While the prevailing view among professionals is that disability is primarily a physical issue, the greater prevalence of behavioral health concerns in the majority of disability claims is typically overlooked. Dr. Brundtland, the former Director General of the World Health Organization (World Health Organization, 2004), noted in 2001 that mental health disorders account for 30% of all years lived with disability (YALY) on a global basis. Specifically, major depressive disorder was reported to be the fourth leading cause of disability. Moreover, it was projected that major depressive disorder would be the second leading cause of disability by 2020. Moreover, within the USA, a similar trend can be observed in the number of individual filing for behavioral health disability with the Social Security Administration (SSA, 17).

Because of the lack of clarity in the definition of disability, case management (case manager) professionals tend to rely on subjective information for "evidence" of disability rather than relying on objective data of functional impairment in the disability determination process. Thus, from the initiation of the claim, the stage is set for adversarial process between the treating professional, case manager, and insurer (Hadjistavropoulos & Bieling, 2001; Talmage, 2007). While it is unrealistic to expect all treating professionals to be fluent in the multiple definitions of disability, it is essential that all treating professionals understand the basic requirements for the objective evaluation and documentation when an individual files a disability claim. Unfortunately, there is a current lack of professional training for all professionals in understanding the difference between disability and impairment, appropriate evaluation, and evidence-based treatment to facilitate an individual's return to work (ACOEM, 2006).

It is essential for case managers to recall that impairment in functioning pertains directly to the actual functioning of the individual across multiple physical, emotional, and cognitive domains. Importantly, case managers should focus on the specific, standardized measures of functioning in each of these systems. This provides a means for case management professionals to discuss specific deficits and how these deficits relate to the individual's ability to perform a workplace duty.

This provides a framework in which the case manager can request information from a treating professional such that he or she can understand and be able to provide the precise information requested (ACOEM, 2006; Warren, 2005, 2009).

In case management, there is misperception about how impairment in functioning relates to behavioral health concerns. This general lack of understanding of the nuances of impairment in functioning is shared not only by the treating professionals but also by the majority of case managers who are involved only on the healthcare side of case management.

Case management involves a wide range of professional knowledge, functions, and responsibilities. Unfortunately, the claimant's work status may not always be a consideration by the case manager. For example, when the case manager is involved on the healthcare side in non-integrated case management, the focus is often more toward reducing healthcare utilization and cost containment. This type of stance may not always be compatible with optimal treatment and return to work efforts. Moreover, it tends to promote an overly simplistic case management style in which important and often complex behavioral health disability decisions are made in regard to reducing the number of professional visits with the treating professional and minimizing the cost of care. Reduction of healthcare utilization and costs are not the sole motivating factors in the case management process. Often, treating professionals are unaware of how a good case manager, with a thorough understanding of both the case manager and behavioral health treatment process, can actually help the treating professional better navigate the behavioral health disability process and reduce the time taken for the documentation process (Powell & Tahan, 2007).

13.3.1 Types of Disability Benefits

It is important to note there are multiple types of disability benefits that an individual may receive.[1] Each type of disability has its own definition as well as required criteria and documentation that must be submitted to receive disability benefits. It is

[1] Behavioral health disability in the contexts of workers' compensation and personal injury law is discussed in detail elsewhere in this volume and will not be discussed here.

also possible that the claimant may be applying for benefits under two or more programs. This is commonly seen when an individual applies for short-term or long-term disability benefits and simultaneously applies for Social Security Disability Insurance. The processes may be similar but will demand different application forms and potentially different clinical documentation. Thus, there are issues related to standardization of definitions and requirements across each type of disability. Each type of disability has its own type case managers who manage dis- ability claims. This can result in multiple case managers involved in a claimant's disability claim. Alternatively, different case managers may interact with one case in a sequential fashion. Frequently, commercial and private insurers have clauses that limit behavioral health disability to specific periods of time. A typical period is 2 years. After this period of time, the claimant is not typically longer eligible to receive further disability benefits from the private insurer, based on common insurance practices. A claimant may either file for private disability or simultaneously file for public disability benefits, such as Social Security Administration (SSDI) disability insurance. Moreover, a claimant may also file for workers' compensation (WC) disability benefits if the claimant and treating professional believe the workplace caused the purported impairment.[2] If the reported behavioral health concern is not work related, then the claimant (if covered at the time the disability occurred) may file for short-term (STD) or long-term (LTD) disability benefits from commercial disability insurer. Typically, STD and LTD insurance benefits are paid either in part or in whole by the employer (Powell & Tahan, 2007).

In STD or LTD, the types of disability are usually broken into two separate categories. These are often termed "own occupation" ("own occ") or "any occupation" ("any occ"). "Own occupation" refers to the claimant's ability to perform the essential tasks of one's own occupation or job. "Any occupation" refers to the inability to perform any type of gainful employment. STD/LTD contracts may further refine this to mean unable to perform the usual tasks of any gainful occupation for which the claimant is reasonably suited by training, education, or experience sufficiently to procure and retain employment (Powell & Tahan, 2007).

In many ways, "any occupation" is similar to the criteria for Social Security Disability Insurance (SSDI). The primary difference is that under SSDI, it is permissible for an individual to have limited employment under a "trial work period" and/or "extended period of eligibility" as defined below.

Trial work period: The trial work period allows a claimant to test one's ability to work for at least 9 months. During the trial work period, the claimant will receive their full social security benefits regardless of how much they are earning as long as they report their work activity and continue to have a disabling impairment. In 2009, a trial work month is any month in which the total earnings are $700 or more or, if self-employed, earn more than $700 (after expenses) or spend more than 80 h in one's own business. The trial work period continues until the claimant has worked 9 months within a 60-month period.

Extended period of eligibility: After the trial work period, the claimant has 36 months during which he or she can work and still receive benefits for any month if the earnings are not

[2] Statute of limitation issues may complicate workers' compensation claims initiated after mental health disability coverage periods have run out.

"substantial." In 2009, earnings of $980 or more ($1,640 if one is blind) are considered substantial. No new application or disability decision is needed for the claimant to receive a social security disability benefit during this period (Social Security Administration, 2004, 2017).

The STD/LTD "any occupation" criteria may not provide for limited or part-time employment and require the claimant to be totally disabled. Many STD policies related to "own occupation" do, however, have provisions that permit part-time or limited duty and do not require the claimant to be "totally disabled" even from one's own occupation. There are hybrid forms of STD/LTD policies which provide that if the claimant is not able to perform the essential tasks of one's work, the claimant is considered to be "totally disabled." Under such a policy, the claimant is generally not permitted to be employed in any other capacity during the time the individual is on disability.

Unless the STD/LTD plan provides rehabilitation incentives or alternative duty programs, the benefits are likely to act as a disincentive for the individual to request accommodations or to request transferring into another position at the workplace. Another concern is that the claimant continues to receive benefits for being disabled from one's usual occupation. This creates a dilemma for the claimant in that one of the primary incentives to return to work is minimized or eliminated altogether. This is especially true in the case where the individual's employment has been terminated, such as when the disability has exceeded the Family Medical Leave Act (FMLA) period. In such a case, should the individual wait until his or her STD/LTD "own occupation" benefits terminate before seeking other employment, the individual may become unemployable due to the gap in work history, loss of job-related skills, and mental attitude. At such a point, the individual and/or treating professional may begin to view the STD or LTD as unemployment insurance and the claimant may become strongly entrenched in the disability role (Hadjistavropoulos & Bieling, 2001).

Unfortunately, many treating professionals continue to see the claimant on a periodic basis only. At these visits, the claimant will typically note continued symptoms. A common response of many treating professionals is to rubberstamp the claimant's disability to leave without the benefit of referring the claimant for psychological evaluation and evidence-based treatment to better address both true psychological concerns and psychosocial issues. True psychological concerns are not under the claimant's voluntary control.[3]

13.3.2 Issues that Arise with Disability Benefits and Objective Evidence of Impairment

A particular problem arises when the claimant experiences a serious illness or injury that will permanently prevent return to work within one's own occupation (Bruns & Disorbio, 2005; Dersh, Gatchel, Polatin, & Mayer, 2002; Gatchel, 2004). Except for

[3] Moreover, true psychological concerns can cause impairment in functioning and require professional treatment to ameliorate. On the other hand, psychosocial concerns are issues that are likely to occur with most people in life. Examples of psychosocial concerns are job dissatisfaction, workplace conflict, and work performance issues, to name a few (Warren, 2013a, 2013b).

certain cases of disability, such as workers' compensation, where the claimant may be required to accept light or alternative work, such requirements do not apply to the majority of STD/LTD disability policies. Moreover, if the individual has applied and has received SSDI benefits, there is no mechanism in place to facilitate the individual's return to the workplace.

It is common for the claimant to develop strong affiliation with a disability role and to not attempt activities of daily living, let alone returning to work. In the field of psychology, this is called "learned helplessness" (Bandura, 1986; Chang & Sanna, 2007; Peterson, Maier, & Seligman, 1993). If and when the disability policy definition changes to "any occupation" (which often occurs in the transition from STD to LTD) and if the claimant is capable of lighter or alternative work, he or she often experiences a "loss of face" resulting from the expectation that they will return to a role that they believe is impossible for them. The claimant, who was previously viewed as being totally disabled, is now faced with a change in disability definition that requires treating professionals, case managers, and the claimant to consider the prospect of other work (ACOEM, 2008; AMA, 2008). Because the claimant is highly likely to have become entrenched in the disability role, it is particularly difficult for the claimant to consider transition back to the workplace (Anssea, Dierick, Buntinkx, et al., 2004; Aylward & Lonsdale 1995, Aylward, 2001; Bigos et al., 1991; Bigos & Battie, 1991; Brundtland, 2001; Waddell, 2006; Waddell & Burton, 2001; Waddell & Burton, 2004; Waddell, Burton, & Aylward, 2007; Waddell et al., 2008a; Waddell et al., 2008b; Waddell, Burton, & Main, 2003; Waddell, Newton, Henderson, Somerville, & Main, 1993).

In many instances, the treating professional and claimant are unfamiliar with the nuances of disability benefit structures (Warren & Hubbard, 2007). For example, an individual may be denied additional disability benefits after a certain period of time has passed or if the claimant is not receiving regular professional treatment. In addition, there is a misconception among the majority of professionals and claimants that behavioral health concerns are permanent in nature and thus require long, open-ended leave from the workplace. Empirical research has consistently demonstrated that the majority of psychological concerns respond quickly to treatment that has been shown empirically to be effective (Warren, 2005). Thus, while the claimant may continue to experience some symptoms, it is imperative for the treating professional and the case manager alike to not assume that they are evidence of impairment (American Psychiatric Association (ApA) (2006a), American Psychiatric Association (ApA) (2006b), American Psychiatric Foundation, Partnership for Workplace Mental Health (2005)). The American Psychiatric Foundation (2005) has noted that an individual can receive treatment and work simultaneously and stressed the points that the majority of individuals with mental health concerns are able to return to the workplace and that extended workplace leave is the exception, not the norm. The common failure to recognize this capacity to work while receiving treatment can lead to iatrogenic disability.

13.3.3 Family Medical Leave Act

Under the Family Medical Leave Act (FMLA), an employee is eligible for job protection for up to 12 weeks of unpaid leave per year when either the employee or a family member suffers from a "serious health condition." The year is frequently interpreted to be a rolling year so that if the individual has taken 12 weeks off in

One year, then another 52 weeks of work must be accrued before the individual is eligible to take an additional 12 weeks of FLMA off. The condition must either prevent the worker from performing his or her job or require the worker to care for a family member. There are three different ways in which FMLA leave can be utilized:

1. *Continuous FMLA leave*: an example is when an employee is absent for more than three consecutive business days and has been treated by a doctor.
2. *Intermittent FMLA leave*: in this instance, the employee is taking time off in separate blocks due to a serious health condition that qualifies for FMLA. Intermittent leave can be in hourly, daily, or weekly increments. Intermittent FMLA is often taken when an employee needs ongoing treatment for one's physical or behavioral health concern.
3. *Reduced schedule FMLA leave*: an employee needs to reduce the number of hours one works per day or per week, often to care for a family member, to reduce stress, or to facilitate reconditioning by easing the employee back into the workplace.

When an employee has used up his or her FMLA, he or she loses the FMLA job protection, which can result in the loss of the individual's work position.

FMLA is not a type of disability insurance. While this may seem self-evident, it is frequently confused by treating professionals with some type of insurance. Alternatively, treating professionals may believe that it affords the employee unlimited leave from the work and protects the employee's job indefinitely. This is an issue to which all case managers should be aware so that they can help educate the treating professional, address appropriate workplace leave absences, and assist the return to work process more effectively.

13.4 Case Management Roles and Requirements in the Context of Treatment

The American Psychiatric Foundation, a branch of the American Psychiatric Association, has taken a role in raising consciousness about the issue of disability by defining the inability to work as a "crisis." Moreover, it has been noted that most treating professionals do not provide intensive care that is comparable to a mental health crisis. Typically, when a person is said to be unable to work, it means that the individual is truly unable to care for one's self on an independent basis. This is because many work activities are similar in nature to personal life activities. Consequently, if a person is truly unable to function at work, it is highly probable that the person cannot function in other life activities as well. For severe mental health concerns, inpatient hospitalization is the most effective means of quickly stabilizing the individual and ensuring the person's safety (Warren, 2005). However, as noted earlier, many treating professionals simply see the claimant on a nonurgent and non-emergent basis (AMA, 2008; Melhorn & Ackerman, 2008; Oyebode, Cantley, & Schroeder, 2008; Talmage & Melhorn, 2005).

13.4.1 General Problems Arising Within the Behavioral Health Claims Process

The relationships between case characteristics, adequacy of care, and claim outcome were examined by Hamm, Reiss, Paul, and Bursztajn (2007). They found that only 22% of behavioral health disability cases had comprehensive psychological evaluations, while 48% of these claims had superficial evaluation and 30% of individuals who had filed a behavioral health disability claim had no evaluation of the reported concerns. This is troubling because it means that the majority of behavioral health disability claims are submitted without the individual being evaluated in a comprehensive manner to even determine whether any type of objective impairment exists before filing for a disability claim (Hamm et al., 2007).

When professional treatment was evaluated in regard to adequacy of care, an alarmingly low 11% of individuals had received appropriate professional care that was sufficient to help the person regain functioning. This is in contrast to 67% of claimants who had received superficial care and the remaining 22% had received no professional treatment at all. Moreover, it was determined that when behavioral health claims related to a physical injury, the claims related to psychosocial stressors were more often to have undergone a superficial diagnostic evaluation and treatment. In general, those behavioral health claims with superficial treatment were less likely to have their claim granted (19.3%) than those with adequate treatment (36.8%) (Hamm et al., 2007). Thus, when the case manager is reviewing a claim, it is important to ask whether the superficial treatment is reflective of the actual severity of the symptoms or reflective of inadequate treatment.

The quality of the documentation submitted to substantiate the claim is typically quite poor; the documentation that is submitted by the claimant is usually highly subjective and demonstrates a pattern of poor communication of the underlying issues with the treating professional. Documentation generated by treating professionals frequently lacks a Diagnostic-IV-TR diagnosis and objective data to support both the diagnosis noted and the reported impairment (Barth, 2005, 2006; Melhorn & Ackerman, 2008; Schultz & Gatchel, 2005). Diagnoses are rarely confirmed, or ruled out, with objective, standardized psychological testing. There is also a pattern of poor collaboration with other treating professionals involved in the claimant's care.

Outside of the workers' compensation claims, healthcare providers typically lack education and training in the assessment and documentation necessary for the evaluation and adjudication of behavioral health disability claims.

Warren and Hubbard (2008a) completed a study regarding behavioral health claims with a large insurer that confirmed these issues were commonplace and that they directly impacted on the claim outcome. Specifically, claims that had even one of the problems noted were more likely to result in extended workplace absence.

13.4.2 *The Impact of Poor Documentation on Disability Claims*

While it may appear self-evident that sufficient documentation is required to make a sound decision regarding the approval or denial of a behavioral health disability, claim, it is quite common for the case manager to receive incomplete or poor documentation. An example of this includes when a treating professional reports a nonexistent diagnosis, such as "stress-related depression." All clinical diagnoses provided by the treating professional must be in the form of an actual *DSM-5* (or current version). Failure to comply with this requirement leads to non-standardized terminology being utilized. Thus, this leads to confusion about the diagnosis and raises doubt about the accuracy of the treating professional's diagnosis and proposed treatment of the claimant.[4] Moreover, the precise criteria for a nonexistent "diagnosis" are unclear to the case manager and treating professionals alike (Talmage, 2007; Warren, 2009). Other examples of poor documentation are:

1. The treating professional not completing all of the forms sent by the claimant and/or case manager
2. The treating professional refusing to release treatment records, even with the appropriate signed release by the claimant[5]

[4]Although the majority of physicians are members of the American Medical Association, rarely does a physician follow the AMA's Guides to the Evaluation of Permanent Impairment (6th edition, 2008). The Guides provide professional instruction to other professionals as well who profess to evaluate and treatment individuals with impairment in functioning. Chapter 5 provides detailed information regarding the appropriate evaluation of individuals with behavioral health disability concerns. Case managers should obtain training in the appropriate utilization of the methods discussed in the Guides. By doing so, this will help the case manager to better understand the fundamentals of appropriate professional evaluation of impairment in functioning.

[5]Although a signed release is not technically required under the federal Health Insurance Portability and Accountability Act (HIPAA, 1996), other state mental health laws may supercede the HIPAA law. Most behavioral health professionals are instructed by their professional organizations to follow the more restrictive law in order to provide protection to their patients/clients. Thus, although the case manager may send a signed release, the treating professional may not honor the insurer's release. This leaves the case manager in the difficult situation of trying to obtain information from the treating professional to make an initial decision regarding the behavioral health disability claim.

3. The treating professional sending incomplete records (which has the same result of not sending the records at all)
4. The treating professional conducting psychological testing that is either not specific to the claimant's reported impairment or reporting invalid testing[6]

In this latter case, since a case manager is not typically trained in objective psychological testing, the case manager is left in the position of attempting to decide whether the psychological testing is an appropriate evidence. Many times, due to the lack of training, case managers simply accept the psychological testing, valid or not, as "proof" of documentation for the claimant's reported impairment.

It is common for the claimant to receive similar treatment with a primary care physician, a master's level therapist or psychologist, as well as a psychiatrist. It is therefore essential to obtain copies of medical records from all providers involved in the claimant's treatment.

In an unpublished study conducted by Warren and Hubbard (2008a), tools were developed by Hubbard and Warren specific to behavioral health disability claims. This allowed for uniform comparison of information being provided by the claimant and each of the healthcare providers. The tools completed by the healthcare provider(s) and claimants frequently demonstrated a remarkable inconsistency in information provided. This ultimately brings into question the issue of claim credibility regarding the submitted documentation.

13.4.3 Standardized Psychological Testing

Unlike physical illness or injury disability claims, behavioral health claims tend to rely on primarily the claimant's subjective claims of symptoms and impairment. Moreover, the treating professional tends to provide a diagnosis without any objective evidence or data as "proof" of "disability". Claims involving physical illness or injury have pathology which can be objectively determined and/or measured by imaging studies, lab results, or even physical examination. Standardized psychological testing provides a more objective means to confirm or rule out and validate the diagnosis, psychopathology, and severity. Behavioral health claims are virtually the only area of disability in which objective testing and examination is not routinely required.

The issue of appropriate psychological testing and its application in the case manager process warrant further discussion. The appropriate testing procedures regarding test administration and interpretation are under the direct auspices of the American Psychological Association (APA). All individuals who utilize psychological tests are required to follow the appropriate testing standards as addressed by the APA and other professional organizations (American Educational Research Association, the American Psychological Association, and the National Council on

[6] Testing that cannot be utilized for specific reasons related to the testing process.

Measurement in Education, 2014). A particular problem in the case management process for behavioral health disability claims is either the absence of objective, standardized psychological testing or the reporting of invalid test results that were reported by the treating professional as being valid (AMA, 2008; Barth, 2005; Warren, 2013a, 2013b).

The need for objective, standardized testing is taught to psychologists during doctoral graduate training. However, a licensed clinical psychological counselor or a licensed clinical social worker is unlikely to have received extensive psycho- logical test training required in the disability assessment process as part of their master's degree training. Specifically, many master's level professionals cannot complete the necessary objective, standardized testing, such as in the case of neuropsychological or intelligence testing (Warren, 2013a, 2013b). Thus, this means these types of treating professionals are limited in the types of documentation and depth of testing that they can provide to a case manager.

Generally speaking, the case manager should look for objective testing that is specific to the reported concern. Typically, a savvy case manager will work with a clinical psychologist trained in disability management to review the submitted testing to ascertain whether the testing (1) is valid and thus can be utilized as documentation, (2) confirms or rules out the reported psychological diagnosis, and (3) utilizes at least two or more objective psychological tests specific to the reported concern (American Medical Association, 2008). Failure to conduct these reviews eliminates the possibility of the case manager exercising independent judgment.

A major concern with the failure to test appropriately is that many individuals had not received the intensive treatment consistent with the diagnosis and severity of symptoms that would have been disclosed had they been properly tested (American Psychiatric Foundation, 2005b; McGlynn, Asch, Adams, et al., 2003; Seelig & Katon, 2008; Wang, Berglund, & Kessler, 2000; Warren, 2005). It is quite possible that an individual does have true psychopathology, resulting in substantial functional impairment, but is receiving only minimal treatment. It is also possible that an individual's concerns are not as severe, and the treatment is at an excessive level for the concern. However, in either instance, the treating professional has not provided the necessary documentation for the case manager to form a judgment (Hamm et al., 2007).

13.4.4 Subjective Information

Another common issue is the utilization of the claimant's subjective information as a substitution for the necessary objective documentation. Although all treating professionals rely, at least initially, on the individual's self-report of symptoms and concerns, the actual treatment process must include a more objective approach that confirms or rules out the perceived issues.

Moreover, the treating professional must utilize objective tools, such as blood tests, CT/MRI scans, and objective, standardized psychological testing to fully evaluate an individual. The empirical literature has demonstrated that treating professionals, as a whole, are not immune to bias in the evaluation process. Furthermore, clinical observation alone is insufficient to confirm or rule out a behavioral health disorder that causes impairment. When the treating professional has simply listed the claimant's concerns, but has not objectively evaluated them, the case manager should be alerted to request additional information in the case management process (Barth, 2005; Melhorn & Ackerman, 2008; Short, Goetzel, Pei, et al., 2009).

The most appropriate means in which to make a diagnosis is based on the diagnostic criteria in the *DSM-5* (ApA, 2013). The multiaxial diagnosis model was removed in the *DSM-5*.

13.4.5 Assessment of the Behavioral Health Disability Claim

Case managers are often placed in the role of making a judgment about whether a claim for disability based on behavioral health concerns should be accepted by the benefit payer. The role of the case manager is not to form or interpose an independent clinical judgment concerning the claimant, but to determine whether the claim is properly substantiated and documented in the first instance, and properly treated if the claim is accepted.

In the typical behavioral health disability claims process, the individual initiates the claim by noting that s/he cannot work in one's current job. Usually, each insurer has its own forms that must be utilized. The individual will use these forms and sign a release so that the insurer may request treatment records. Once records are received, they are reviewed to ascertain whether sufficient objective documentation has been submitted to support the claim (Warren & Hubbard, 2008b). A common misconception is that once the documentation has been submitted, the evidence is sufficient because a treating professional has said that an individual is unable to work (ACOEM, 2006; Melhorn & Ackerman, 2008; Schultz & Gatchel, 2005). However, because of the wide variance in care, a careful review of all documentation must be completed by the case manager.

Moreover, if the case manager is receiving a claim, and a non-specific diagnosis such as "depression" is noted, this represents another yellow flag since depression is simply a symptom and not an actual clinical diagnosis, such as Major Depressive Disorder (MDD) (Warren, 2009; Warren & Hubbard, 2008b).

13.4.6 Assessment of the Treatment Being Provided

When the treating professional is a primary care physician who has provided all care to date, this is a significant yellow flag since primary care physicians typically prescribe medication and are likely to see the individual about every 4–6 weeks (Kroenke, Spitzer, Williams, et al., 1994; Oyebode et al., 2008; Pransky, Shaw,

Franche, & Clarke, 2004; Seelig & Katon, 2008; Teutsch, 2003; Waddell & Burton, 2007). This type of care is not consistent with a health crisis. If this type of documentation is submitted, it is essential for a case manager to contact the primary care physician to ask for additional information. The contact should not be adversarial in nature, but rather coming from the direction of wanting to educate both the claimant and the primary care physician any necessary remedial steps to help provide the appropriate documentation for the claim decision-making process.

Case managers can use best practice standards or treatment guidelines as a tool to evaluate treatment plans.8 Many of these have undergone extensive peer evaluation of empirical research as well as reviewed by other professional organizations to provide an external peer evaluation of the guidelines. However, it is important for a case manager to become familiar with the characteristics of strong practice guidelines and not simply use a guideline in an indiscriminate manner. Bruns, Mueller, and Warren (2010) noted that when a guideline is mandated in some states, the user of the guideline must be aware of the limitations of the guideline whether making clinical, case manager, or legal decisions.

For those behavioral health claims that do not resolve as anticipated, it will be important for the case manager to periodically reevaluate the continuing claim. In these instances, the case manager will need to request and review additional copies of treatment records from the treating professional(s). Careful attention should be paid to whether the individual is experiencing any improvement from the last review. This is especially important in behavioral health claims because the majority of these concerns have evidence-based treatments that help the individual return to the previous level of functioning quickly. Consequently, the fact that an individual is not improving after a significant number of weeks of treatment should raise a yellow flag for closer evaluation (Warren & Hubbard, 2008b).

The following are basic tips for case managers to utilize in the case assessment process:

1. Objective, standardized testing must be performed in strict accordance with the testing manual for each test. Moreover, the testing professional must follow the current American Psychological Association's testing standards. These testing standards are called "The Standards for Educational and Psychological Testing." A testing professional may not deviate from the prescribed administration for each test. If this is done, then the validity of the testing is compromised, or in some cases invalidated completely (APA, 2014).
2. No single objective psychological test can provide a comprehensive assessment of an individual's reported concerns (AMA, 2008; Warren, 2013a, 2013b).
3. It is essential that the case manager understands the difference between subjective screening tools and objective standardized testing. Thus, the case manager is better able to discern those screening tools that are only subjective and are not appropriate for documentation of impairment in functioning.
4. Many psychological reports used by testing professionals are computer generated in that the professional simply uses the scores from the computerized report. In some instances, the computerized program attempts to interpret the testing

results even if they are invalid. Thus, it is important for the testing professional to report that the testing results are, in fact, valid.

5. Many tests have validity indices or base rates. Most case managers do not have the professional training to evaluate these validity indices and should work with a clinical psychologist who is trained in disability management for assistance in making sense of the submitted documentation.
6. When the case manager plans to send psychological tests results out for an independent review by a clinical psychologist, it is essential that the testing professional has provided copies of all the raw data for the independent reviewing psychologist to analyze. When the claimant has signed a release, both master's level professionals and psychologists may release the raw test data and copies of the answer sheets to an independent reviewing psychologist. This independent reviewing psychologist is most typically a clinical or neuropsychologist.

13.4.7 Psychosocial Concerns Versus True Psychological Disorders

Warren and Hubbard (2008a) found that a high level of job dissatisfaction (88%) was associated with behavioral health claims. While it can certainly be understood how one may dislike a job, this does not necessarily mean that a person cannot perform the job. Instead, this is typically noted as a psychosocial concern in the empirical research (Drukteinis, 1997; Lelliott, Tulloch, Boardman, et al., 2008; Melhorn & Ackerman, 2008; Waddell, 2005; Waddell, Burton, & Aylward, 2008a, 2008b; Warren, 2013a, 2013b; Warren & Hubbard, 2007, 2008a, 2008b). Another common psychosocial issue that arises is that of workplace conflict. Warren and Hubbard (2008a) found that many behavioral health claimants (81%) reported workplace conflict as a primary reason for filing the disability claim. Unfortunately, the majority of treating professionals did not ask about the workplace conflict and did not note this in their documentation. Other common psychosocial concerns that occur in behavioral health disability claims are the claimant noting (1) excessive workload, (2) a lack of balance between work and home life, and (3) issues related to childcare. Thus, the case manager should be aware of psychosocial concerns noted and be aware of the possibility of medicalization of those concerns.[7]

In the research examining behavioral health disability claims, Warren and Hubbard (2008a) explored the occurrence of psychosocial issues and objectively determined psychological concerns. There was a pattern of poor communication between the treating professional and the claimant regarding specific issues, such as job dissatisfaction and workplace conflict. In 72% of the examined claims, there was typically no objective psychological testing completed to support the reported concern. The concern with this statistic is that the treating professional typically had

[7] See Sect. 13.4.12.

been conducting treatment for at least 1 month before the claim was filed. This time frame is typically adequate treating professional to conduct objective, standardized psychological testing. Moreover, in those instances where objective psychological testing was completed, 94% of testing results reported by the treating professional were invalid. Consequently, the issues in appropriately differentiating between a true psychological concern and a psychosocial issue are often exacerbated by poor quality documentation. When psychosocial concerns exist,10[8] these can be discerned from objective *DSM-5* diagnoses with the usage of psychological testing.

Warren and Hubbard (2008a) developed a set of tools to quickly gather information specific to behavioral health concerns that can allow a case manager to identify potential psychosocial concerns that may be underlying issues related to the reported claim. One set of tools was specific to the claimant, while the other set was directed to the claimant's treating professional(s). The tools are typically utilized at the claim initiation, as well as follow-up tools to gather accruing documentation over the life of the claim. The tools allow a case manager to evaluate the comprehensiveness of the treating professional's evaluation of the claimant, pinpoint the claimant's report of psychosocial issues, document types of medication prescribed, evaluate treatment compliance, and examine the consistency of the treatment plans. Of equal importance, the tools provide an opportunity for the case manager to examine medication compliance as well and identify medications prescribed by all treating professionals. Specifically, the tools served to identify those behavioral health claims that were likely to have a high probability of a variety of issues that extended the life of the claim for extremely lengthy periods of time. The tools are designed to assist the case manager in working with the claimant and the treating professional.

13.4.8 Utilizing the Expectation of Consistency in Objective Impairment and Functioning

Sufficient and appropriate documentation is typically a problem with behavioral health disability claims (Barth, 2005; Ertel, Koenen, & Berkman, 2008; Melhorn & Ackerman, 2008; Warren & Hubbard, 2008b). A common problem is that many professionals take what the claimant says at face value without benefit of verifying the information through other sources, such as workplace evaluations or even in direct contact with the claimant's human resource department (Short et al., 2009). Without this type of verification, the results of the evaluation and development of a

[8] With behavioral health disability claims, when a psychosocial concern arising from work is the primary catalyst for filing for disability, it is important to recognize that this represents a belief by the claimant that s/he must be completely satisfied with one's job or that one will never experience any workplace conflict. With changes within the workplace, it is highly likely that one will experience job dissatisfaction or conflict at some time during one's employment (ACOEM, 2006). Instead, it is the claimant's coping style that comes into play in these situations. Coping style is shaped by a number of aspects, for example, childhood upbringing, stress management techniques, social support, and one's personality.

treatment plan are jeopardized. Reliance on the claimant's subjective report alone is inherently risky. Frequently, the claimant will report an inability to continue a situation at work that is inconsistent with behavior in other aspects of life.[9]

Typically, limitations in functioning occur consistently, regardless of the setting. Evidence of this type of inconsistency is a yellow flag to a case manager for further investigation and may require obtaining additional information from both the claimant and the treating professional(s).

13.4.9 *Patient Compliance Issues Within the Behavioral Health Disability*

The prevalence of noncompliance with treatment ordered by the treating professional has been found to range from 20% to 50% in a review of the empirical literature. The issue of noncompliance is critical for both the treatment and case management processes (Becker & Maiman, 1975; DiMatteo, Lepper, & Croghan, 2000; Jensen, Albertsen, Borg, & Nabe-Nielsen, 2009; Warren, 2013a, 2013b). There are several forms that noncompliance might take: (1) outright refusal to follow treatment recommendations; (2) agreeing to follow the treatment plan in consultation with the treating professional, but outside of the treatment milieu, not following the treatment plan; (3) following parts of the treatment plan, but not the entire treatment plan; (4) repeatedly canceling appointments and so, the person is receiving sporadic care; and (5) not taking medication as prescribed.

Noncompliance is a serious issue that negatively impacts on treatment outcome. It is almost always under the individual's voluntary control as well. Some exceptions

[9]An example of contradictory information that Warren and Hubbard (2008a) noted was when a claimant who was a customer service representative was diagnosed with Major Depressive Disorder. The treating professional noted that the claimant was not able to perform her job due to an inability to concentrate and interact with the customers or to respond to their requests for assistance in resolving concerns. The claimant was described as being unable to cope with a full day's work and could not manage many activities of daily living, such as traveling in a car, paying bills, or preparing meals, among some of the noted limitations. When the submitted documentation was examined, it was found that the claimant was a single mother with children less than 10 years of age. One child needed to have prescribed medications given at specific times. It was the claimant's responsibility to ensure this occurred. Of significance, the claimant was completely responsible for caring for herself and her children on a daily basis. The treating professional reported that the claimant was unable to concentrate sufficiently to answer customer calls and unable to complete most activities of daily living. Clearly, this is at odds with what the claimant was actually doing. She was able to care for herself as well as her children, including ensuring that prescribed medication was taken at appropriate times by her child. Moreover, the treating professional also went on to note that the claimant was able to drive a vehicle. The inherent problem with the treating professional's assertion is that driving is an activity that requires complex functioning across multiple cognitive domains, including sustained concentration and attention, visuospatial skills, and short- and long-term memory. Consequently, because driving a vehicle requires similar cognitive skills to those in the workplace, it is unlikely that the claimant was not able to function in the work setting with lesser demands, but could function in driving a car, which takes multiple cognitive skills.

to this are when an individual has had a serious mental health concern, such as a psychotic break or with a head injury in which memory is impaired. With valid behavioral health impairment, there are several instances of noncompliance that can result in poor treatment outcomes. Examples include failure to engage in an exercise program with major depressive disorder (since physical activity has been found to be an important variable in the improvement of that condition) and failure to take medication as prescribed. Noncompliance is not an evidence of objective impairment in most cases, but rather a decision to not follow a recommended course of action. Thus, noncompliance is a yellow flag pertaining to a potential psychosocial issue.[10]

The issues of primary and secondary gain are also usually involved when noncompliance occurs in some form. Primary gain occurs when the person experience a positive internal motivation. It is usually not a conscious. It usually allows the person to save face or to avoid a negative situation. For example, a person may develop physical symptoms without any identifiable physical causes, such as in the case of conversion disorder. Conversion disorder is an extreme instance where the person may develop physical symptoms such as stroke-like symptoms, after a hospital visit to a relative who had heart surgery. In this case, the internalized emotions coupled with the stressor produce the physical symptoms (Warren, 2013a, 2013b).

In the case of secondary gain, the behavior is usually linked to an external motivator, such as (1) avoiding an unpleasant task or situation; (2) receiving attention and sympathy from others regarding the physical concerns; (3) receiving monetary benefits because of the physical issues, such as with a lawsuit or with disability benefits; and (4) identification with a "sick or disabled" role. The person may or may not be aware of the motivation. However, when a person is consciously producing or exaggerating symptoms for personal gain, then the person is malingering.[11] If secondary gain is suspected, then the issues of noncompliance and possible malingering should be considered as separate issues, and the case manager should not indulge any assumptions.

Regardless of the reason for noncompliance, the case manager must evaluate whether the claimant is complying with the prescribed treatment. One way to do this is to compare treatment records with the claimant's reports regarding medications

---

[10]When the claimant is out of work and additional factor may create noncompliance, the claimant may no longer have insurance to provide the recommended care. If the claimant wished to have insurance after one's employment terminates, one must obtain it for oneself. Such insurance is typically covered by the Consolidated Omnibus Budget Reconciliation Act (COBRA, 1985). COBRA had allowed employed people and their families to opt to continue to receive group health benefits that are provided by their current group plan. This is typically for a limited period of time (18 months). The costs associated with COBRA are quite high. For example, those who are qualified are usually required to pay the entire healthcare premium to 102% of the cost of the plan. This can result in another form of noncompliance due to the claimant's inability to pay for ongoing treatment, diagnostic procedures, and medications. However, with the institution of the American Recovery and Reinvestment Act of 2009 (ARRA), an individual who is eligible for assistance will pay only 35% of the premium needed to obtain COBRA coverage. Thus, this change should help to ameliorate some of the financial burden and serve to remove one barrier to noncompliance.

[11]See discussion of malingering in Sect. 13.4.10.

prescribed and how the medication is being taken. To further complicate the case management process, the case manager must complete this evaluation process for each treating professional who is treating the claimant. It is especially important with psychotropic medication for the claimant to fully follow the prescription directions to help restore the claimant's health to the previous level of functioning. Consequently, the case manager should pay close attention to medication compliance in the behavioral health disability claims process.

13.4.10 Symptom Exaggeration and Malingering

Although many professionals believe they possess the professional ability to discern if the claimant is exaggerating symptoms[12] or malingering, this has not been supported in the empirical literature (Iverson, 2003, 2007). Instead, the empirical research has consistently demonstrated that the majority of professionals are simply not able to reliably differentiate between a claimant who is exaggerating or malingering and one who is not. The AMA (2008) and others (Aronoff, Mandel, Genovese, et al., 2007; Iverson, 2007; Wiley, 1998) have indicated that all professionals must evaluate for symptom exaggeration and malingering as a normal part of the evaluation process. With behavioral health concerns, this is typically done with the employment of standardized objective psychological tests in addition to other medical tests, such as blood assays. Furthermore, there are specific objective psychological tests to evaluate both types of symptom exaggeration or malingering issues. Without the benefit of objective psychological testing, the case manager is left to "eyeball" the claim and to make basic case management decisions based on subjective information versus objective data about the veracity of the claimant's self-reported symptoms (Warren & Hubbard, 2008b).

It is important to note that symptom exaggeration, although a component of malingering, is not sufficient alone as "proof" that an individual is malingering. A person can exaggerate one's symptoms in situations where she or he believes the treating professional is not taking a concern seriously. However, if the symptoms are related to an actual valid physical concern, then the individual is not malingering. In addition, a person can exaggerate one's symptoms without being aware of the action. The key distinction between symptom exaggeration and malingering is that the person who malingers is conscious of one's actions.[13] Malingering is

[12] Also sometimes referred to as "symptom magnification."

[13] The *DSM-5* (ApA, 2013) noted malingering as "the intentional production of false or grossly exaggerated physical or psychological symptoms, motivated by external incentives such as avoiding military duty, avoiding work, obtaining financial compensation, evading criminal prosecution, or obtaining drugs." Moreover, there are four specific criteria that must be met before malingering is reported by the professional. Aronoff et al. (2007) completed an extensive meta-analysis and found specific behaviors and concerns associated with malingering. In general, the more of these that were identified, the more the potential for malingering is raised. In addition, Iverson (Iverson, 2003, 2007) reported additional factors that serve as catalysts for symptom exaggeration and malingering.

fraudulent in nature. It is useful to note that malingering has been found to occur at a higher prevalence rate in disability situations. The empirical research has noted the malingering prevalence rate to range from 30% to 40% in many disability cases for pain, emotional, and/or cognitive symptoms. These rates of malingering occur in those seeking disability benefits and in litigation cases (Mittenberg, Patton, Canyock, & Condit, 2002). Thus, the treating professional must routinely evaluate whether symptom exaggeration or malingering is occurring. Unfortunately, Warren and Hubbard (2008b) ascertained that this rarely occurs with behavioral health disability claims.

13.4.11 Collaboration Among Treating Professionals

When several treating professionals are providing treatment to the claimant, it is imperative for each of them to collaborate to ensure continuity of care. In addition, this affords the treating professionals the opportunity to discuss the specific diagnosis that each has made in regard to the claimant. Unfortunately, this does not occur as regular part of the treatment process. As a consequence, it is common to see conflicts of diagnosis in the file review process. Diagnosis plays an important role in selecting the treatment that is implemented. Therefore, if there are different diagnoses, it raises significant concern about the consistency, and therefore the appropriateness of the selected treatments being provided that may contribute the potential detriment of the claimant (Warren & Hubbard, 2007).

Warren and Hubbard found that the diagnosis provided differed frequently among treating professionals and that the majority of treating professionals did not collaborate with each other (95%).

13.4.12 Medicalization of Psychosocial Issues

It is important for the case manager to consider the possibility of a psychosocial concern being the primary issue. In many instances, the treating professional has used the information provided by the claimant to make a decision regarding a potential behavioral health diagnosis. However, if the claimant notes issues such as job dissatisfaction, conflict with one's coworkers, or simply "stress," then it increases the probability that the underlying concern is a psychosocial issue rather than a true mental health disorder. Typically, psychosocial concerns do not meet the *DSM-5* criteria for an actual psychological disorder. When psychosocial concerns are noted as the primary catalyst for the claimant filing for disability, the case manager should take steps to carefully evaluate the treating professional's records to ascertain how this is addressed. If the psychosocial concerns are noted as the reason for the claimant's reported concerns, this is known as "medicalization" (Dworkin, 2001; Melhorn & Ackerman, 2008; Waddell, 2005; Warren, 2009; Warren & Hubbard, 2008b).

To fully evaluate the behavioral health disability claim, it is necessary to obtain documentation from all treating professionals who have treated the claimant. The documentation obtained from the treating professional should then be compared to the documentation submitted by the claimant with special attention to psychosocial issues that are reported. This process allows the case manager to ascertain whether there are discrepancies between what the claimant is reporting in the disability claim, what the claimant has discussed with the treating professional, and what the treating professional has noted to be the primary clinical concerns and addressed in the treatment plan and the anticipated return to work date (Warren, 2009; Warren & Hubbard, 2008b).

13.5 The Return to Work Case Management Process in the Context of Behavioral Health

Waddell and Burton (2006a, 2006b) explored the relationship between working and health. They concluded that the activity of work is strongly associated with good physical and mental health. Moreover, they noted that working is therapeutic, and it literally reverses the negative health effects associated with unemployment. The one proviso that they noted is that the quality of work, as well as being safe when working, is essential. Their final finding was that the beneficial effects of work far outweigh the risks of work and the even greater effects of extensive unemployment and/or workplace absence.

Empirical research has found that those who do not work experience a 50% risk of dying in the next 10–17 years after unemployment begins. Moreover, the quality of life regarding physical, emotional, and financial health declines sharply (Gerdtham & Johannesson, 2003; Jin, Shah, & Svoboda, 1995).

The longer an individual is off of work, it becomes more unlikely that s/he will ever successfully return to work (ACOEM, 2006). Within as little as 12 weeks, the chances of success- fully returning to work may be reduced to as little as 50%. The longer an individual is off of work, it becomes more unlikely that she/he will ever successfully return to work relationships with coworkers, who may have been absorbing the work not being performed by the disabled individual while off work. This has the potential for creating strained work relationships when the employee returns to the workplace. The individual who was once a member of the team may perceive oneself or the team may perceive her or him as now being an outsider. The individual also can lose job skills or missing out on changes in the workplace. In some cases, significant changes may be instituted even in a relatively short absence from the workplace. This may result in the need for the employee to undergo retraining to be able to complete workplace duties once more (ACOEM, 2006; Waddell & Burton, 2006a, 2006b). Frequently, the individual experiences a sense of anxiety in returning to the workplace. The American Psychiatric Foundation (2005b) noted that this is not at all unusual, but the norm. This anxiety itself is not a sign that the individual cannot work, but simply a part of the return to work process.

Warren and Hubbard found that treating professionals did not consider return to work at a level consistent with its importance for the overall well-being of the claimant. Eighty-one percent of treating professionals did not address the return to work issue with the claimant. Thus, most claimants did not understand that return to work was an expected treatment goal. Moreover, 81% of treating professionals did not address the workplace accommodation issue with employers. Interestingly, the majority of behavioral health claimants felt that they could return to work with an accommodation. However, if this is not addressed by the treating professional and discussed with the employer, the likelihood for a meaningful discussion, as well as the opportunity for assisting the claimant back to work, is lost.

13.5.1 Workplace Accommodations and Return to Work Planning

In regard to behavioral health concerns, although an individual may be unable to fully return to work for one's own occupation, it is quite common that the individual can either return to work with temporarily reduced work expectations or return to work in another position. Both of these examples are types of workplace accommodations that should be explored by both the treating professional and the case manager. This requires that the case manager be supplied with and utilize objective information from the treating professional(s). When case managers make decisions without sufficient input from the treating professional, they are seen as advancing an agenda other than the claimant's welfare, and this fosters distrust. These issues arise across the case management spectrum, including the behavioral health disability management process (Pransky et al., 2004; Talmage, 2007; Talmage & Melhorn, 2005; Warren & Hubbard, 2007, 2008a, 2008b).

Workplace accommodations, particularly with regard to behavioral health concerns, must be addressed as part of the return to work process. Often, the viewpoint among treating professionals is that this is somehow unsympathetic, harsh, and employer-oriented. The failure to provide the employee with behavioral health concerns with appropriate accommodations leaves him or her more vulnerable to being placed on open-ended disability leave, to his or her long-term detriment.

It is important to recognize that there are gaps in communication between treating professionals and case managers. A necessary component of the case management process is to adequately address time away from work in a comprehensive manner, including addressing the return to work process as an integral part of the claimant's treatment plan. Consequently, it is important that both types of professionals understand the usual communication issues and strive to overcome them to accomplish the com- mon goal of helping the claimant obtain adequate assistance and restore the claimant's previous level of functioning (Pransky et al., 2004; Warren & Hubbard, 2007, 2008b).

13.5.2 Appropriate Roles for the Case Manager

Case managers can help to educate treating professionals regarding insurance policy limitations, an issue about which treating professionals are often unaware. Moreover, case managers can and should provide information to treating professional about the empirically documented problems with long-term workplace absence, particularly related to behavioral health concerns. Unfortunately, most treating professionals are not taught about disability management, federal and states laws regarding disability, or even, appropriate return to work strategies (AMA, 2008; Melhorn & Ackerman, 2008; Warren, 2005, 2009). Instead, most medical and graduate school programs overemphasize treatment alone.

There are other areas in which the case manager can assist in obtaining the best result for the claimant. The issue of professional liability is of great concern in the current environment. There is a mind-set among many treating professionals to err on the side of lengthy workplace absences than to open oneself to the potential of inadvertent harm to the claimant. This is particularly true when treating professional has provided professional care to an individual with behavioral health concerns (ACOEM, 2006; AMA, 2008; APF, 2005; Dasinger, Krause, Thompson, Brand, & Rudolph, 2001). Zinn (1996) revealed that 56% of treating professionals report having limited confidence and knowledge in their ability to determine whether an individual was disabled. More disturbing, the same percentage of treating professionals was willing to exaggerate clinical data to "help" an individual who the treating professional thought was "deserving" of receiving disability benefits.[14] Proactive case management, with a heavy emphasis on education, claimant advocacy, appropriate workplace leave, and objective documentation of impairment with a treatment goal of returning to work are essential to addressing this issue. The case manager must also emphasize to the treating professional how the case manager can simplify the process, providing additional benefit to the treating professional and the claimant and how the treating professional can help in this interactive process (Warren & Hubbard, 2008b).

[14] Talmage and Melhorn (2005) wrote a book for physicians regarding the RTW process. They noted three primary constructs in looking at an individual's ability to work. These constructs are:

1. *Risk*: This is defined as the potential of harm to the individual or others, if the individual engages in a type of specific work.
2. *Capacity*: This is in regard to the physical, mental, and psychological ability to perform the specific tasks of the job.
3. *Tolerance*: This is noted to be the individual's ability to tolerate the specific activity, such as work.

Another professional role in case management is to work with the employer to discuss appropriate workplace accommodations that can be made to assist in the return to work process (Powell & Tahan, 2007). Frequently, employers take an all-or-none stance that either the claimant returns fully to work or does not return at all (ACOEM, 2006). There are many problems with this approach:

1. The employer may be in breach of the current ADA Amendments Act of 2008 (that afford new protections to the employee that are much farther reaching than the previous version of the ADA law).
2. The all-or-nothing position may be counterproductive for the employer. It is often more cost-efficient for the employer to allow the employee to return part-time or on accommodations than to incur the administrative costs of replacing the worker and training a replacement. Workplace accommodations may also reduce overall disability costs by eliminating needless disability caused by prolonged work absence. Additionally, these accommodations are helpful in keeping the employee engaged in the workplace when an eventual return to work is anticipated currently in workplace duties.
3. Specific to behavioral health concerns, employers are frequently in the dark regarding what are appropriate accommodations as well as how long should these accommodations should exist.

The Disability Management Employers Coalition (DMEC) survey (2016) of employers found that most understand that behavioral health concerns exist, but do not feel confident in developing behavioral health workplace disability policies or in making accommodations. Thus, the case manager has the opportunity to discuss appropriate workplace accommodations with the employer and assist them in understanding that the employee may still be receiving treatment but is, nonetheless, still able to work.

13.6 Strategies to Address Weaknesses Occurring in the Behavioral Health Disability Case Management Process

In case management, precise and accurate information is the most critical component. In some contexts, such as the STD/LTD case management process, the case manager does not have the ability to attend the claimant's appointments treating professional. In other contexts, the case manager may be prevented by statutory or regulatory prohibitions from engaging in direct, hands-on, information gathering or simply may not have a caseload allowing for that intensive level of involvement. This potentially creates a gap in the available information, with effects that are potentially detrimental to the case manager's role and the claimant's outcome. In such instances, needed information is usually gathered over the phone or from the office notes. A primary problem with this approach is the case manager's need to obtain information in a timely manner from a source (the treating professional) who has a crowded clinical schedule does not allow for long chats with the case manager. In this situation, the treating professional often views the case manager as a nuisance. An alternative to this approach is to provide the treating professional with a concise list of questions that address the issues pertinent to the claims decision process. If possible, the case manager should try to frame the questions in a yes/no or checkbox answer format to minimize writing by the treating professional. This speeds up the process for the treating professional and also reduces the likelihood of the case manager needing to interpret a treating professional's handwritten comments. Without the necessary documentation from the treating professional, the case manager will eventually need to take some kind of action. This is likely to result in a claim denial due to insufficient documentation to support the claim (Powell & Tahan, 2007).

In the behavioral health process, the STD/LTD case management process is hindered by both state and federal laws regarding confidentiality (Gold & Metzner, 2006; HIPAA, 1996).[15] All states in the USA have privacy laws regarding mental health treatment as well as confidentiality requirements applying to anyone who may seek to obtain mental health information regarding another person. Because of the perceived stigma in the USA regarding mental health treatment, most individuals do not wish others to know of given diagnoses or received treatment. Releases signed by claimants, when available, are not always honored by treating professionals, who are often concerned with avoiding any approbation or liability attached to improper release of information. This leaves the case manager in the position of needing to tell the treating professional that the behavioral health disability claim will be denied absent the necessary documentation. At this point, the case manager is viewed as an adversary who is only concerned about the insurer and not the claimant. An option in this situation is to discuss with the claimant that the treating professional is unwilling to provide the required information. By doing so, the claimant can then request the treating professional to comply. It is an unfortunate circumstance that most treating professionals do not understand the crucial nature that their documentation plays in assisting both the claimant and the case manager.

It was previously noted there are specific issues that occur uniquely within the case manager process applicable to behavioral health claims. Unfortunately, as discussed, most case managers do not have specific training regarding behavioral health issues and yet it is the case manager's responsibility to sort through issues related to the claimant's care and documentation. Many case managers learn on the job about how to address these concerns. While such training is considered the norm for many such positions, it does not provide the in-depth understanding and knowledge of complex behavioral health and comorbid concerns. Thus, a beginning case manager's training is only as good as the training of the more experienced case manager from whom she/he has learned.

[15] While HIPPA technically does not cover workers' compensation claims, treating professionals routinely demand HIPPA compliance measures to ensure that they limit their liability exposure.

It is common to see case managers take a simplistic view of behavioral health disability claims. Moreover, behavioral health comorbidity with physical concerns is typically not addressed, even though empirical research has consistently demonstrated a strong relationship between serious or chronic physical concerns and behavioral health diagnoses. Consequently, all case managers should be aware of limitations in training and take steps to remedy this. There are a number of avenues to address this:

1. Reviewing current empirical literature regarding best practice standards
2. Attending professional conferences in training regarding behavioral health disability issues which are addressed
3. Seeking consultation with a clinical psychologist or psychiatrist trained in disability management to receive individualized instruction regarding evidence-based strategies to be applicable to the circumstances of the case

Case managers should also use disability guidelines that are available commercially.[16]

Each set of guidelines is developed by the specific company or organization. One such organization, ACOEM utilizes professional multidisciplinary panels of experts to review empirical research. The guidelines are then sent for external review to different experts and organizations to ensure independent accuracy of the guidelines and the recommendations made. Moreover, many states legally mandate the usage of certain guidelines. Thus, case managers should be aware of current laws in the state(s) where they work. The usage of professional guidelines permits behavioral health disability claims to be expedited, minimizing delays in starting the disability benefits and minimize the need to obtain copies of the medical records and the associated costs.

It should be noted that disability guidelines are not meant to represent an absolute prescription for the duration of a disability nor the only acceptable plan of treatment. Instead, most of the guidelines usually provide multiple "critical points." This provides the case manager and claims adjusting personnel with an indication of expected costs and treatment modalities used for a given diagnosis, and/or for the recovery period and anticipated return to work date. Depending upon an insurance carrier's internal policies and procedures, these "critical points" may be used to signal when to refer the claim on to the case manager or for a physician review should the claim exceed the anticipated resolution time frame. It is essential to keep in mind that disability and treatment guidelines are also only as good as the empirical research on which they are based. Case managers who use professional guidelines

[16]There are several available guidelines. The most commonly used are the case manager process of the Work Loss Data Institute's (2008) Official Disability Guidelines (ODGs), the Reed Group's (2009) Medical Disability Advisor (MDA) and MDguidelines which are complementary, the American Medical Association's Guides to the Evaluation of Permanent Impairment, 6th edition (2008), and the American College of Occupational and Environmental Medicine's (ACOEM, 2008) Practice Guidelines.

are well advised to become educated about the evidence criteria utilized and to never over-rely on the guideline as an absolute decision-making instrument.

The case manager should also pay close attention to whether the treating professional has discussed return to work directly with the claimant. Frequently, treating professionals do not discuss the process of return to work as a part of the treatment plan. The American Psychiatric Foundation (2005b) has noted that "The belief or policy that one must be fully recovered before returning to work is iatrogenic and inappropriate except in rare, safety-sensitive occupations. Even in these situations, accommodations often make clinical sense for early phases of return to work" (Dasinger et al., 2001). ACOEM (2006) ascertained that a treating professional's discussion and encouragement of a return to work within 1 month after an acute illness or injury were associated with a higher return of work rate. After 1 month, however, momentum is lost, and the interaction of physical, psychological, and psychosocial issues come into play, typically resulting in longer workplace absences.

The case manager also has a critical role in communicating with the employer about the claimant's return to work. Aside from the workers' compensation disability realm, few employers strive to encourage a quick return to work and, in many cases, lack a formal behavioral health return to work policy. The employer may, at times, actually act as an impediment in the return to work process. One reason is that an employer may fear the returning employee, who is not fully recovered, may be disruptive to business. Consequently, the case manager can educate the employer regarding the benefits of facilitating the claimant's return to work. Without the case manager's intervention, the claimant frequently faces daunting barriers to returning to the job. Moreover, many employers simply do not know the types of accommodations that could be made for a claimant with a behavioral health concern. A superior case manager can help the employer address requests for accommodations and help create a win–win scenario for treating professionals, claimants, and employers alike.

13.7 Conclusion

The case management process for behavioral health concerns is a system that has several distinct functions. The basic case management process involves getting information from the claimant and from the treating professional. This information is central to making a well-formed decision regarding the acceptance of the claim, the appropriateness and coordination of treatment, and the planning for return to work and job accommodations. The case manager is responsible for:

1. Ensuring that all critical information is obtained and that it is objective and valid for the purposes intended
2. Monitoring to ensure that the treatment plan is developed appropriately to the severity of the presenting behavioral health concern
3. Facilitating collaboration among all treating professionals
4. Ensuring that a return to work planning has occurred, that accommodations have been considered, and that date has been set, when appropriate

In addition, a superior case manager is skilled in both educating and treating professionals regarding potential insurance issues as well as deficits in the documentation, treatment plan, and return to work planning processes.

In this regard, the case manager is rather like the coach of a baseball team: The coach is not on the field hitting, throwing, and catching. The coach works toward getting the most out of all the players on the team by working together and making sure that they have a winning attitude. The coach collects useful information about team members and the challenges they face and provides them with needed resources. Most importantly, the coach makes sure the right player is doing the job that one is best suited to do to accomplish the overall goal. With the baseball coach, the goal is winning the game. With the case manager, the goal is the claimant's return to a full and productive life, to the greatest extent possible.

References

Adler, H. M. (2007). Toward a biopsychosocial understanding of the patient-physician relationship: An emerging dialogue. *Journal of General Internal Medicine, 22*, 280–285.

American College of Occupational and Environmental Medicine. (2004). *Stress-related conditions* (pp. 387–405). Beverly Farms, MA: American College of Occupational and Environmental Medicine press, OEM Press.

American College of Occupational and Environmental Medicine. (2008). *Occupational medicine practice guidelines: Evaluation and management of common health problems and functional recovery in workers* (3rd ed.). OEM Health Information Press.

American College of Occupational and Environmental Medicine's Stay at Work and Return to Work Committee, Christian, J., Martin, D., Brown, D., Colledge, A., Gean, C., et al. (2006). ACOEM practice guideline for preventing needless work disability by helping people stay employed. *American College of Occupational and Environmental Medicine, Journal of Occupational & Environmental Medicine, 2006.*

American Educational Research Association, the American Psychological Association, and the National Council on Measurement in Education. (2014). *Standards for educational and psychological testing*. Washington, DC: American Educational Research Association, the American Psychological Association, and the National Council on Measurement in Education.

American Medical Association. (2008). *Guides to the evaluation of permanent impairment* (6th ed.). Chicago: American Medical Association.

American Psychiatric Association. (2006a). *Practice guideline for the Compendium of Practice Guidelines: 2006: Treatment of patients With major depressive disorder*. In *Compendium of Practice Guidelines: 2006* (2nd ed.). Arlington, VA: American Psychiatric Association 2006.

American Psychiatric Association. (2006). *Psychiatric evaluation of adults: A quick reference guide, based on practice guidelines for the psychiatric evaluation of adults* (2nd ed.). Washington, DC: American Psychiatric Association.

American Psychiatric Association. (2013). *Diagnostic and statistical manual on mental disorders (DSM-5)* (5th ed.). Washington, DC: American Psychiatric Association Press.

American Psychiatric Association: American Psychiatric Foundation's Partnership for Workplace Mental Health. (2005). *Assessing and treating psychiatric occupational disability*. American Psychiatric Foundation.

American Psychiatric Foundation, Partnership for Workplace Mental Health. (2005). *Assessing and treating psychiatric occupational disability, executive report*. Washington, DC: American Psychiatric Association.

American Recovery and Reinvestment Act of 2009 (ARRA), Pub. L. No. 111-5.

Anssea, M., Dierick, M., Buntinkx, F., et al. (2004). High prevalence of mental disorders in primary care. *Journal of Affective Disorders, 78*(1), 49–55.

Aronoff, G. M., Mandel, S., Genovese, E., et al. (2007). Evaluating malingering in contested injury or illness. *Pain Practice, 7*(2), 178–204.

Aylward, M. (2001). *Psychological injury: Understanding and supporting*. The Stationary Office, London: Department of Social Security.

Aylward, M., & Lonsdale, S. (1995). Disability and its assessment: Controlling access to, and exit from disability and incapacity benefits. Springer-Verlag: Foundation of International Studies on Social Security publications.

Bandura, A. (1986). Fearful expectations and avoidant actions as coeffects of perceived self- inefficacy. *American Psychologist, 41*(12), 1389–1391.

Barth, R. J. (2005). *A physician's guide to return to work*. Chicago: American Medical Association Press.

Barth, R. J. (2006). *Undiagnosed mental illness as the cause of general medical disability claims*. Chicago: The American Medical Association Guides News Letter, American Medical Association.

Becker, M. H., & Maiman, L. A. (1975). Sociobehavioural determinants of compliance with health and medical care recommendations. *Medical Care, 13*, 10–24.

Bigos, S. J., & Battie, M. C. (1991). A prospective study of work perceptions and psychosocial factors affecting the report of back injury. *Spine, 16*(1), 1–6.

Bigos, S. J., Battie, M. C., Spengler, D. M., Fisher, L. D., Fordyce, W. E., Hansson, T., et al. (1991). Industrial back pain complaints: A broader perspective. *Orthopaedic Clinics of North America, 22*(2), 273–282.

Brundtland, G. H. (2001). Director-general world health organization at a council for mental health seminar. *Norway on*, (11 December 2001).

Bruns, D., & Disorbio, J. M. (2005). Chronic pain and biopsychosocial disorders. *Practical Pain Management, 5*(7), 2–9.

Bruns, D., Mueller, K., & Warren, P. (2010). The development of biopsychosocial laws governing treatment of pain and injury. *Psychological Injury and the Law, 3*, 169–181.

Canadian Medical Association. (1997). The physician's role in helping patients return to work after an illness or injury. *Canadian Medical Association, 156*(5), 680A–680F.

Centers for Disease Control: Prevalence of disabilities and associated health conditions among adults – United States, 1999, 2005. Retrieved August 12, 2009., from http://www.cdc.gov/mmwr/preview/mmwrhtml/mm5007a3.htm

Chang, E. C., & Sanna, L. J. (2007). Affectivity and psychological adjustment across two adult generations: Does pessimistic explanatory style still matter? *Personality and Individual Differences, 43*(5), 1149–1159.

Disability Management Employer Coalition. (2016). *DMEC 2016 employer behavioral risk survey*. San Diego: Disability Management Employer Coalition.

Consolidated Omnibus Budget Reconciliation Act of 1985 (P.L. 99-272, 100 Stat. 82).

Dasinger, L., Krause, N., Thompson, P., Brand, R., & Rudolph, L. (2001). Doctor proactive communication, return-to-work recommendation, and duration of disability after a workers' compensation low back injury. *Journal of Occupational and Environmental Medicine, 43*(6), 515–525.

Dersh, J., Gatchel, R. J., Polatin, P., & Mayer, T. (2002). Prevalence of psychiatric disorders in patients with chronic work-related musculoskeletal pain disability. *Journal of Occupational Environmental Medicine, 44*, 459–469.

Dewa, C., & Lin, E. (2000). Chronic physical illness, psychiatric disorder and disability in the workplace. *Social Science & Medicine, 51*, 41–50.

DiMatteo, M. R., Lepper, H. S., & Croghan, T. W. (2000). Depression is a risk factor for non-com- pliance with medical treatment: Meta-analysis of the effects of anxiety and depression on patient adherence. *Archive of Internal Medicine, 160*, 2101–2107.

Disability Management Employer Coalition (DMEC). (2009). *Tools of the trade: A compilation of programs and processes for the absence, disability, health and productivity professional*. San Diego: Disability Management Employer Coalition.

Drukteinis, A. M. (1997). Personnel issues in workers' compensation claims. *American Journal of Forensic Psychiatry, 18*, 3–23.

Dworkin, R. W. (2001). The medicalization of unhappiness. The Hudson Institute, from http://www. hudson.org/index.cfm?fuseaction=publication_details&id=911. Accessed 1 Oct 2009.

Ertel, K. A., Koenen, K. C., & Berkman, L. F. (2008). Incorporating home demands into models of job strain: Findings from the work, family, and health network. *Journal of Occupational and Environmental Medicine, 50*, 1244–1252.

Evans, D. L., Charney, D. S., Lewis, L., et al. (2005). Mood disorders in the medically ill: Scientific review and recommendations. *Biological Psychiatry, 58*, 175–189.

Gatchel, R. J. (2004). Comorbidity of chronic mental and physical health conditions: The biopsychosocial perspective. *American Psychologist, 59*, 792–805.

Gatchel, R. J., & Gardea, M. A. (1999). Psychosocial issues: Their importance in predicting disability, response to treatment, and search for compensation. *Neurologic Clinics, 17*(1), 149–166.

Gatchel, R. J., Peng, Y. B., Peters, M. L., Fuchs, P. N., & Turk, D. C. (2007). The biopsychosocial approach to chronic pain: Scientific advances and future directions. *Psychological Bulletin, 133*(4), 581–624.

Gerdtham, U. G., & Johannesson, M. (2003). A note on the effect of unemployment on mortality. *Journal of Health Economics, 22*, 505–518.

Goetzel, R. Z., Long, S. R., Ozminkowski, R. J., et al. (2004). Health, absence, disability, and presenteeism cost estimates of certain physical and mental health conditions affecting U.S. employers. *Journal of Occupational & Environmental Medicine, 46*(4), 398–412.

Gold, L. H., & Metzner, J. L. (2006). Psychiatric employment evaluations and the health insurance portability and accountability act. *American Journal of Psychiatry, 163*, 1878–1882.

Hadjistavropoulos, T., & Bieling, P. (2001). File review consultation in the adjudication of mental health and chronic pain disability claims. *Consulting Psychology Journal: Practice and Research, 53*(1), 52–63.

Hamm, R. M., Reiss, D. M., Paul, R. K., & Bursztajn, H. J. (2007). Knocking at the wrong door: Insured workers' inadequate psychiatric care and workers' compensation claims. *International Journal of Law and Psychiatry, 30*(4–5), 416–426.

Harter, M., Baumeister, H., Reuter, K., et al. (2007). Increased 12-month prevalence rates of mental disorders in patients with chronic somatic diseases. *Psychotherapy and Psychosomatics, 76*(6), 354–360.

Heidel, S., Klachefsky, M., McDowell, D., et al. (2007). *Assessing and treating psychiatric occupational disability: New behavioral health functional assessment tools facilitate return to work [electronic version] (report from the Partnership for Workplace Mental Health)*. Arlington, VA: American Psychiatric Foundation.

Iverson, G. L. (2003). Detecting malingering in civil forensic evaluations. In A. M. Horton & L. C. Hartlage (Eds.), *Handbook of forensic neuropsychology* (pp. 137–177). New York: Springer.

Iverson, G. L. (2007). Identifying exaggeration and malingering. *Pain Practice, 7*(2), 94–102.

Jensen, J. N., Albertsen, K., Borg, V., & Nabe-Nielsen, K. (2009). The predictive effect of fear a-voidance beliefs on low back pain among newly qualified healthcare workers with and without previous low back pain: A prospective cohort study. *Musculoskeletal Disorder, 10*, 117. From http://www.biomedcentral.com/1471-2474/10/117

Jin, R. L., Shah, C. P., & Svoboda, T. J. (1995). The impact of unemployment on health: A review of the evidence. *Canadian Medical Association Journal, 153*(5), 529–540.

Jorm, A. F., Angermeyer, M., & Katschnig, H. (2000). Public knowledge of and attitudes to mental disorders: A limiting factor in the optimal use of treatment services. In G. Andrews & S. Henderson (Eds.), *Unmet need in psychiatry* (pp. 399–413). Cambridge, MA: Cambridge University Press.

Katon, W., Kleinman, A., & Rosen, G. (1982). Depression and somatization: A review. Part I. *American Journal of Medicine, 72*, 127–135.
Kavan, M. G. (2009). Generalized anxiety disorder: Practical assessment and management. *American Academy of Family Physicians, 79*(9), 785–791.
Kessler, R. C., Demler, O., Frank, R. G., et al. (2005). Prevalence and treatment of mental disorders, 1990 to 2003. *The New England Journal of Medicine, 352*(24), 2515–2523.
Kessler, R. C., Merikangas, K. R., & Wang, P. S. (2007). Prevalence, comorbidity, and service utilization for mood disorders in the United States at the beginning of the twenty-first century. *Annual Review of Clinical Psychology, 3*, 3137–3158.
Kessler, R. C., & Wang, P. S. (2008). The descriptive epidemiology of commonly occurring mental disorders in the United States. *Annual Review of Public Health, 29*, 115–129.
Krause, N., Frank, J. W., Dasinger, L. K., Sullivan, T. J., & Sinclair, S. J. (2001). Determinants of duration of disability and return-to-work after work-related injury and illness: Challenges for future research. *American Journal of Industrial Medicine, 40*(4), 464–484.
Kroenke, K. (2003). Patients presenting with somatic complaints: Epidemiology, psychiatric comorbidity and management. *International Journal of Methods Psychiatric Research, 12*, 34–43.
Kroenke, K., Spitzer, R. L., Williams, J. B. W. M., et al. (1994). Physical symptoms in primary care: Predictors of psychiatric disorders and functional impairment. *Archives of Family Medicine, 3*, 774–779.
Laitinen-Krispijn, S., & Bijl, R. V. (2000). Mental disorders and employee sickness absence: The NEMESIS study. *Social Psychiatry and Psychiatric Epidemiology, 35*, 71–77.
Langlieb, A. M., & Kahn, J. P. (2005). How much does quality mental health care profit employers? *Journal of Occupational & Environmental Medicine, 47*(11), 1099–1109.
Lee, S., Tsang, A., Breslau, J., et al. (2009). Mental disorders and termination of education in high-income and low- and middle-income countries: Epidemiological study. *The British Journal of Psychiatry, 194*(5), 411–417.
Lelliott, P., Tulloch, S., Boardman, J., et al. (2008). Mental health and work. The Royal College of psychiatrists commissioned by the cross government health work and Well-being Programme. From http://www.workingforhealth.gov.uk/documents/mental-health-and- work.pdf.
Leopold, R. S. (2003). *A year in the life of a million workers*. Metropolitan Life Insurance Company.
Lerner, D., Allaire, S. H., & Reisine, S. T. (2005). Work disability resulting from chronic health conditions. *Journal of Occupational & Environmental Medicine, 47*(3), 253–264.
Linton, S. J. (1993). A controlled study of the effects of an early intervention on acute musculoskeletal pain problems. *Pain, 54*(3), 353–359.
McGlynn, E. A., Asch, S. M., Adams, J., et al. (2003). The quality of health care delivered to adults in the United States. *Journal of New England, Medicine, 348*, 2635–2645.
Melhorn, J. M., & Ackerman, W. E. (Eds.). (2008). *Guides to the evaluation of disease and injury causation*. Chicago: American Medical Association.
Merikangas, K. R., Ames, M., Cui, L., et al. (2007). The impact of comorbidity of mental and physical conditions on role disability in the US adult household population. *Archives of General Psychiatry, 64*(10), 1180–1188.
Mittenberg, W., Patton, C., Canyock, E. M., & Condit, D. C. (2002). Base rates of malingering and symptom exaggeration. *Journal of Clinical Experimental Neuropsychology, 24*, 1094–1102.
Ormel, J., Petukhova, M., Chatterji, S., et al. (2008). Disability and treatment of specific mental and physical disorders across the world. *British Journal of Psychiatry, 192*, 368–375.
Oyebode, T. O., Cantley, L., & Schroeder, M. (2008). Impairment and disability evaluation: The role of the family physician. *American Family Physician, 77*(12), 1655–1666.
Peterson, C., Maier, S. F., & Seligman, M. E. P. (1993). *Learned helplessness: A theory for the age of personal control* (p. 359). New York: Oxford University Press. xi.
Powell, S. K., & Tahan, H. A. (2007). *Case manager's core curriculum for case management* (2nd ed.). Philadelphia: Lippincott Williams & Wilkins.

Pransky, G. S., Shaw, W. S., Franche, R. L., & Clarke, A. (2004). Disability prevention and communication among workers, physicians, employers, and insurers: Current models and opportunities for improvement. *Disability & Rehabilitation, 26*(11), 625–634.

Reed Group. (2009). Medical disability advisor. 6th ed. Retrieved June 10, 2009, from http://www.medicaldisabilityadvisor.com/

Reggers, J., & Ansseau, M. (1999). Lifetime prevalence of DSM-1V psychiatric disorders in the Liège study: Preliminary results. Abstracts of the VIII Congress of the International Federation of Psychiatric Epidemiology.

Roy-Byrne, P. P., Davidson, K., Kessler, R. C., et al. (2008). Anxiety disorders and comorbid medical illness. *General Hospital Psychiatry, 30*(3), 208–225.

Schultz, I. Z., & Gatchel, R. J. (Eds.). (2005). *Handbook of complex occupational disability claims*. New York: Springer Publishing.

Seedat, S., Scott, K. M., Angermeyer, M. C., et al. (2009). Cross-national associations between gender and mental disorders in the World Health Organization world mental health surveys. *Archives of General Psychiatry, 66*(7), 785–795.

Seelig, M. D., & Katon, W. (2008). Gaps in depression care: Why primary care physicians should hone their depression screening, diagnosis, and management skills. *Journal of American College of Occupational and Environmental Medicine, 50*(4), 451–458.

Short, M. E., Goetzel, R. Z., Pei, X., et al. (2009). How accurate are self-reports? Analysis of self-reported health care utilization and absence when compared with administrative data. *Journal of Occupational & Environmental Medicine, 51*(7), 786–787.

Social Security Administration (2007). Disability evaluation under social security listing of impairments. Social Security Administration, pub. No. 64–039.

Social Security Administration. (2017). Research, statistics, & policy analysis annual statistical report on the social security disability insurance program, 2007. Baltimore: Social Security Administration.

Social Security Administration Office of Disability Programs (2004). Understanding social Security's disability programs: Mental impairments, SSA Pub. No. 64–086.

Suehs, B., Argo, T. R., Bendele, S. D., et al. (2008). Texas medication algorithm project procedural manual, major depressive disorder algorithms. *Texas Department of State Health Services*, 1–71.

Talmage, J. B. (2007). Failure to communicate: How terminology and forms confuse the work ability/disability evaluation process. *Journal of Insurance Medicine, 39*, 192–198.

Talmage, J. B., & Melhorn, J. M. (2005). Working with common psychiatric problems. In *A physician's guide to return to work* (pp. 305–319). Chicago: American Medical Association Press.

Teutsch, C. (2003). Patient-doctor communication. *Medical Clinics of North America, 87*, 1115–1145.

The Health Insurance Portability and Accountability Act of 1996 (HIPAA), Pub. Law No. 104–191 (1996).

The World Health Organization. (2004). The world health Report. Changing history. (p. 2004). Geneva: The World Health Organization.

Von Korf, M. (1992). Disability and depression among high utilizers of health care. *Archive of General Psychiatry, 49*, 91–99.

Waddell, G. (2005). Yellow flags: Psychosocial risk factors for chronic pain and disability. In M. Szpalski & R. Gunzburg (Eds.), *The failed spine* (pp. 151–156). Philadelphia: Lippincott, Williams & Wilkins. 2005, Chap 17.

Waddell, G. (2006). Preventing incapacity for work in people with musculoskeletal disorders. *British Medical Bulletin, 77*(1), 55–69.

Waddell, G., & Burton, A. K. (2001). Occupational health guidelines for the management of low back pain at work: Evidence review. The Royal College of Physicians. The Faculty of Occupational Medicine. *Journal of Occupational Medicine, 51*, 124–135.

Waddell, G., & Burton, A. K. (2004). *Concepts of rehabilitation for the management of common health problems*. London: The Stationery Office.

Waddell, G., & Burton, A. K. (2006a). Is work good for your health and well-being? (Monograph) The Stationery Office, London

Waddell, G., & Burton, A. K. (2006b). Is work good for your health and well-being? *Occupational Health Review, 24*, 30–31.

Waddell, G., & Burton A. K. (2007). *Advising patients about work. (An evidence-based approach for general practitioners and other healthcare professionals.)* The Stationery Office, London 2007.

Waddell, G., Burton, A. K., & Aylward, M. (2007). Work and common health problems. *Journal of Insurance Medicine, 39*, 109–120.

Waddell, G., Burton, A. K., & Aylward, M. (2008a). A biopsychosocial model of sickness and disability. *The Guides Newsletter*. Chicago, American Medical Association, May/June: 1–13.

Waddell, G., Burton, A. K., & Aylward, M. (2008b). *A biopsychosocial model of sickness and disability*. In R. J. Barth & D. Randolph (Eds.), *Psychosocial Aspects of Disability. Proceedings of EUMASS/AADEP conference, Dublin 2006* (p. 2008). Chicago: American Medical Association.

Waddell, G., Burton, A. K., & Kendall, N. (2008). *Vocational rehabilitation: What works, for whom, and when?* The Stationery Office, London: Commissioned by the Vocational Rehabilitation Task Group and the Industrial Injury Advisory Council. 2008.

Waddell, G., Burton, A. K., & Main, C. J. (2003). *Screening to identify people at risk of long-term incapacity for work: A conceptual and scientific review*. London: The Royal Society of Medicine Press.

Waddell, G., Newton, M., Henderson, I., Somerville, D., & Main, C. J. (1993). A fear-avoidance beliefs questionnaire (FABQ) and the role of fear-avoidance beliefs in chronic low back pain and disability. *Pain, 52*, 157–168.

Waehrer, G., Leigh, J. P., Cassady, D., & Miller, T. R. (2004). Costs of Occupational Injury and Illness across States. *Journal of Occupational & Environmental Medicine, 46*(10), 1084–1095.

Wang, P. S., Berglund, P., & Kessler, R. C. (2000). Recent care of common mental disorders in the United States: Prevalence and conformance with evidence-based recommendations. *Journal of General Internal Medicine, 15*(5), 284–292.

Warren, P. A. (2005). *The management of workplace mental health issues and appropriate disability prevention strategies*. San Diego, CA: Work Loss Data Institute.

Warren, P. A. (2013a). Those who hesitate are lost: The case for setting behavioral health treatment and disability standards, part I. *Psychological Injury and Law, 6*(3), 183–195.

Warren, P. A. (2013b). Those who hesitate are lost: The case for setting behavioral health treatment and disability standards, part I. *Psychological Injury and Law, 6*(3), 196–207.

Warren, P. A., & Hubbard, J. D. (2007). The disability claims process and determining mental health diagnoses versus workplace dissatisfaction. *American Academy of Disability Evaluating Physicians, 5*(2), 13–24.

Warren, P. A., & Hubbard, J. D. (2008a). *Psychosocial issues related to behavioral health disability claims*. Fort Dearborn Insurance Company.

Warren, P. A., & Hubbard, J. D. (2008b). I claim, you claim: How to ensure proper claims management. *Case in Point Journal, August/September*, 32–36.

Warren, P. A. (2009). Behavioral Health as a Causation Issue in Workers' Compensation and Disability Claims. *IAIABC Journal, 46*(2), 17–56.

Wiley, S. D. (1998). Deception and detection in psychiatric diagnosis. *Psychiatric Clinics of North America, 21*(4), 869–893.

Work Loss Data Institute. (2008). *Official Disability Guidelines*. Encinitas, CA: Work Loss Data Institute.

Zinn, W. (1996). Physician perspectives on the ethical aspects of disability determination. *Journal of General Internal Medicine, 11*(9), 525–532.

Chapter 14
Managing Behavioral Health in Private Disability Insurance

Les Kertay

14.1 Understanding Private Disability Benefit Systems

Understanding the similarities and differences between DI and other health and income protection coverages, in historical context, can help behavioral health providers work with the system in a way that promotes the best possible outcome for patients. By clarifying unfamiliar and sometimes idiosyncratic terminology and outlining the generic process of disability determination under DI contracts, behavioral health providers will understand better what is expected.

14.1.1 Distinguishing Private Disability from Other Coverages

Private DI systems differ from other forms of illness and injury compensation, some of which are covered elsewhere in this volume, as well as from health insurance. These compensation systems have different goals, different rules and regulations, and often different terminologies. Unfortunately, conflating them can lead to confusion for practicing behavioral health professionals and, ultimately, to poor outcomes for patients.

Insurance is designed to manage risk. Individuals buy coverage, or have it provided by employers, to manage personal risk. A certain portion of our income is used to buy insurance, as a hedge against a catastrophic loss which is beyond our personal means. Home insurance mitigates the risk of losing a house to fire or some other events. Health, dental, disability, or other coverage is a hedge against medical losses that we cannot personally absorb.

L. Kertay (✉)
Dr. Les Kertay & Associates, LLC, Chattanooga, TN, USA
e-mail: les@drleskertay.com

P. A. Warren (ed.), *Handbook of Behavioral Health Disability Management*,
https://doi.org/10.1007/978-3-319-89860-5_14

On the other side of this equation is the insurer, whose role is to provide a promise of support to mitigate losses, in exchange for premiums paid. The insurer manages risk by balancing the odds of paying claims against the premiums collected. Tools for managing risk include raising and lowering premiums, changing contractual definitions, defining limits and scope, etc. For both insurer and insured, the specifics of risk management vary depending on the type of insurance.

For example, health insurance is designed to provide payment for treatment. This is familiar territory for practicing clinicians, who have been trained to diagnose and treat. The health insurer agrees to pay for certain treatments, based on defined criteria for medical necessity, for specified conditions, within state and federal regulations, in exchange for a specified premium. The insurer's risk is managed by limiting the panel that can provide treatment; by negotiating rates; by limiting the treatments for which payment will be made, based on best available evidence; and by setting deductibles, copay amounts, and premiums. From the treating provider's perspective, the most important of these is *managed care*, meaning that the insurer will try to control what treatments are provided, over what period of time, for what amounts. Treating providers tend to perceive these conditions, which are the insurer's means of managing risk, as intruding on clinical judgment, and it is a major source of strain between health insurers and treating clinicians.

Similarly, workers' compensation (WC) carriers cover treatment for medical impairments, with specifications related to whether the condition is work related as defined by statute and whether the treatment is found reasonable and medically necessary for that work-related condition. The potential conflict with treating clinicians is similar to that encountered with health insurers but now additionally complicated by the question of work-relatedness. This can lead to situations in which even clinically appropriate treatment is not covered by the WC payer, because the condition is deemed not related to an injury in the workplace.

Private DI policies typically do not manage risk by controlling treatment. Instead, it is the definition of disability in the contract that determines what is covered and what is not. To complicate matters more, each DI company may have a different definition of disability, and each company may have multiple contracts, each with a variation on the general definition. The insurer manages risk by defining the terms for evaluating whether or not the individual is precluded from performing important work-related duties, as a result of an injury or illness. This is a world foreign to many health providers, with unfamiliar terminology, processes, and requirements. For the behavioral health practitioner, there are additional complications because of the nature of the conditions we treat. A patient may be diagnosed with a behavioral health condition, may be symptomatic and need treatment, and may have some functional limitations, but nevertheless not be found disabled under the contract. This can be confusing and frustrating for both the patient and his or her treating provider.

14.1.2 The History and Purpose of Private Disability Systems

Providing compensation and care for those who became injured or ill is not new. Four millennia ago, the Law of Ur provided rules for compensating specific injuries. Only a little more recently, the 1750 BC Code of Hammurabi employed a similar scheme. Many ancient cultures developed laws that provided set rewards for the loss of function related to specific injuries. Beginning with the feudal systems of the Middle Ages, these codified systems were replaced with the benevolence or caprice of the local lord (Guyton, 1999) and later those of industrial owners and employers.

Recognized by many as the precursor to modern disability insurance coverage, in 1848, the Railway Passengers' Assurance Company of London sold the first accident insurance as part of the price of a train ticket. The coverage expanded to losses experienced from any accident in 1852, and in 1863, James Batterson founded the Travelers Insurance Company, bringing to the US coverage for accidents while traveling. Seventeen years later, the St. Lawrence Life Association began issuing policies that combined coverage for accidents and illnesses, forming for the first time a comprehensive policy covering the same types of conditions as in modern disability insurance policies. The policies had liberal definitions, affordable for the carriers because claim incidence was low – it not being thought seemly to file a claim unless there was truly an incapacitating condition – and the number of policies continued to grow. However, when the world's economies collapsed in the 1930s, liberal policy definitions combined with grave economic circumstances to greatly increase incidence, and many insurers left the marketplace to stem losses, reducing the number of policies dramatically (Lynch, 2001).

Companies began offering policies again after World War II, but this time with tighter definitions of what qualified for disability. Alongside these employer-provided policies, individuals, often professionals such as attorneys or physicians, became a market for high-end policies which were expensive compared to the employer-provided policies, but with rich benefits and relatively liberal definitions. Over time, with each major economic downturn, companies made efforts to tighten definitions to mitigate coverage risks (Lynch, 2001). When the dot.com bubble burst in the early 2000s, individual disability policies were significantly narrowed, and beginning with the bursting of the housing bubble and the economic collapse of 2008, the trend began to shift from employer-provided coverage to voluntary benefits.

In parallel, public coverage for disability was developed, eventually enacted as the Social Security Disability Insurance (SSDI) program. That program, too, adjusted definitions of disability over time, sometimes swinging from definitions that were too broad, leading to excessive claims costs at the federal level, to definitions that were too narrow, depriving the most vulnerable populations of coverage. Inadequate funding and perceived abuse of the system are perennial topics of discussion (Berkowitz, 2000). With respect to behavioral health diagnoses, changes to the SSDI program were implemented at the beginning of 2017. Those changes include a requirement that psychiatric conditions cited as the basis of a claim for disability benefits be "medically documented" for at least 2 years, and the diagnostic categories were updated to mirror the *DSM-5* (SSA, 2017b).

Throughout this history, the *stated* goal of disability coverage has remained a noble effort: to protect the income of individuals and families who are, or become, unable to work as a result of a nonoccupational injury or illness. The *perceived* goal, accelerated by the inception of SSDI in 1956, is arguably less noble: having paid for coverage, either directly or indirectly, individuals sometimes perceive collecting benefits under disability coverage as a right, rather than a last-ditch backstop. The balance between disability income protection under rare circumstances on the one hand, and as entitlement on the other hand, informs much of the difficulty in understanding, and working with, the private disability system.

14.1.3 Defining Terms

To effectively work with behavioral health conditions in the context of disability insurance, it is helpful to understand the unfamiliar and sometimes confusing terminology employed. The following definitions are idealized and may differ slightly depending on specific contractual conditions but give general guidance. They are organized into two sections: terms related to clinical judgment and terms related to administrative determinations (Kertay, 2016).

14.1.3.1 Terms Primarily Related to Clinical Judgment

Impairment is a "significant deviation, loss, or loss of use of any body structure or function in an individual with a health condition, disorder, or disease" (AMA, 2011). Medical impairment is measurable, with loss of function defined as inability to, or difficulty with, performing activities of daily living (ADLs), instrumental activities of daily living (IADLs), or other important tasks. Note that "work" is not considered an ADL or IADL; an individual may not be able to dress independently, for example, once dressed might nevertheless be able to work. Also, it is important to bear in mind that impairment is measurable; an individual might have a symptom such as anxiety, but not be medically impaired because they are still capable of performing all important functional activities (Table 14.1).

Limitation is tied to the capacity to perform a function (see 14.4.2). In the context of disability, a functional limitation is something that an individual is unable to do, without regard to motivation. That is, a limitation is something that cannot be done, no matter how hard the individual tries. Typically, it is both specific and measurable (AMA, 2011). In major depressive disorder, for example, psychomotor retardation, if present, is not a limitation, but an individual with severe psychomotor retardation might be functionally limited in the ability to perform rapid

Table 14.1 Listing of ADLs and IADLs

ADL function	**Independent**	**Needs help**	**Dependent**	**Cannot do**
Bathing				
Dressing				
Grooming				
Mouth care				
Toileting				
Transferring				
Walking				
Climbing stairs				
Eating				
IADL function	**Independent**	**Needs help**	**Dependent**	**Cannot do**
Shopping				
Cooking				
Managing medications				
Using the phone				
Looking up information				
Doing housework				
Doing laundry				
Driving/using public transport				
Managing finances				
Computer use				

hand movements, such as sorting on a fast-moving conveyor belt or rapid typing. Symptoms are not limitations, but they may contribute to the development of limitations.

Restriction is tied to risk associated with actual harm, to self or others, from performing an action (see 14.4.1). Whereas a limitation is something an individual *cannot* do as the result of a medical impairment, a restriction is intended to prevent something the individual *should not* do. Medically necessary restrictions from activities are assigned when doing a particular task is likely to lead to specific, actual harm. In a seizure disorder, for example, individuals are often restricted from driving, because a seizure while driving is likely to lead to an accident. As with limitations, an increase in symptoms is not, in itself, reason for restricting activity. For example, an individual with a social anxiety disorder will be anxious around others, but need not be restricted; in fact, the anxiety will not improve unless they are exposed to circumstances that trigger anxiety, but with a new set of skills (exposure and response prevention).

Maximum medical improvement (MMI) is more frequently encountered in WC than in private disability, because it refers to a plateau in clinical progress that triggers an impairment rating connected with a work-related condition. An individual is at MMI when she/he has made as much progress as is likely. It is not necessary to be fully cured, or asymptomatic, to be at MMI. It is simply that further progress is unlikely (AMA, 2011). This can be a frustrating concept for providers, who want their patients to be cured. In terms of private disability, the applicability is that an individual doesn't need to be cured of a psychiatric condition to return to work; what's needed is that she/he be at a baseline level consistent with the ability to perform occupational duties.

14.1.3.2 Terms Primarily Related to Administrative Determinations

Occupational duties, or *essential duties*, are those tasks that are central to doing a job. A job duty can be deemed *essential* for a number of reasons. A job duty is essential if the job exists to perform that function. For example, a pilot's job is to fly planes, so the ability to fly is an essential duty. A job duty might also be essential if only a few people can perform it or if the function is so highly specialized that employees are hired specifically because of their expertise (Eskay-Auerbach, 2016).

In disability determinations, the inability to perform one or more essential job duties is typically part of the definition of disability. Health providers can be confused by this. For example, an individual may be restricted from driving, which makes it impossible to get to work without a ride, or public transportation. But unless the job itself requires driving, it is not an essential duty. Similarly, a patient might have severe agoraphobia that makes it difficult, or impossible, to leave home, or risks harm if she/he does so. But if the individual works from home, that impairment may not be relevant to the occupation.

Occupation will be contractually defined but is typically the general class of work that the individual performs, whereas *job* is the nature of the role that is performed for a specific employer. Nursing, for example, is an occupation, within which there are multiple possible jobs. Nursing shares a set of broad skills and functional requirements, such as the ability to effectively apply a body of medical knowledge to patient care. Within the occupation, nurses may have a variety of jobs, such as a floor nurse, a nurse in a physician's office, a reviewer of medical records, etc. Whether the policy pays for the individual's ability to perform a particular *job*, or any of the jobs within the broader *occupation*, will depend on the specific contract under which benefits are being paid.

Accommodation in the context of disability insurance is a modification of the workplace or the way in which tasks are ordinarily performed, so that an employee can work (US EEOC, 2010). Examples might include ramps and other modifications to allow the use of a wheelchair, a sit-stand workstation that allows change in position, or the use of speech recognition software for someone who has lost the ability to type. Defining what is a "reasonable" accommodation under the law is beyond the scope of this chapter. However, the important point is for treating providers to consider whether there is a modification that would allow an individual who has an impairment and is functionally limited in some ways, nevertheless, to work. In the arena of behavioral health, for example, accommodations might be the ability to work from home and with flexible hours. For an individual with a bipolar disorder and who is judged temporarily restricted from overstimulating environments due to risk of exacerbated mania, such an accommodation can make the difference between working and not.

Residual functional capacity (RFC) "describes what an individual is able to do, despite functional limitations resulting from a medically determinable impairment(s) and impairment-related symptoms (SSA, 2017a, 2017b)." This is an administrative determination that relies on medical evidence provided by treating or evaluating clinicians. Although RFC most often is related to SSDI and public disability systems, it is a useful concept for clinicians to keep in mind when making clinical determinations related to the ability to work. Often, it is as important, or more important, to consider what a patient *can* do, than to consider what they cannot.

Disability has a medical meaning, but when it comes to private disability, it refers to an administrative determination made by a claims professional who evaluates medical and vocational information and applies it to a contractual definition. If the individual's circumstances meet the contractually specified definition of disability, then and only then are they considered disabled under the policy.

Among the confusions this causes for clinicians is that disability is a term used differently in different legal circumstances. For example, under the Americans with Disabilities Act (ADA, 1990), *disability* refers to a condition that impacts an individual's function, but with which they could work, if provided an accommodation. That definition was expanded considerably under the ADA Amendments Act of 2008 (ADA 2008), allowing even more behavioral health conditions to qualify for consideration of accommodations. Under the ADA, in other words, an individual might claim a disability because they want the right to request an accommodation, so they *can* work, as compared to a private disability policy, under which an individual claims disability because they believe they *cannot* work and want benefits paid as a result. The same word is used, for two opposite purposes.

Another confusion is that it is possible for a clinician to believe his or her patient is unable to work due to an impairing condition and she/he might have functional limitations and/or restrictions, but still not be disabled under the policy definition. This can occur, for example, when an individual is deemed unable to work around the public due to a behavioral health condition, but they may be denied benefits if working around the public is not part of their occupation or job.

14.1.4 Making Disability Determinations

As noted above, evaluating impairment is a clinical judgment, but determining disability is administrative. Typically, a claims professional is responsible for assembling the information related to the claim and determining if the totality of the information gathered matches the contractual definition of disability. Each claim is unique, and circumstances are never exactly the same. In addition, there will be nuanced differences between the claim determination processes that apply to short-term disability (typically the first 3–6 months) or long-term disability. Roughly speaking, the generic sequence of steps is as follows:

1. *Determine eligibility*: The claims manager determines that the claimant is eligible for coverage. This requires ensuring that the claimant had a valid policy in

effect at the time they left work due to illness or injury, either by paying individual premiums or through the employer.

2. *Pre-ex*: There may be other contractual issues that impact eligibility. One common issue occurs when there is a "preexisting" clause in the contract and the claimant leaves work soon after becoming eligible. These clauses vary widely, but a common one is that if the claimant leaves work within the first 12 months of becoming eligible, then information is sought to determine if the claimant received treatment for the same condition, or set of symptoms, in the "look-back" period, typically 3 months prior to becoming eligible. If so, the claimant may not receive benefits even if she/he is profoundly impaired.
3. *Obtain information about the claimant's activities*: The claims manager will interview the claimant and inquire about what the claimant reports she/he is able to do, or has trouble doing, and why the claimant feels she/he is unable to work.
4. *Obtain medical information*: The claims manager will obtain from the claimant, or request directly from the treating providers, medical records for the time period surrounding the claim. In addition, the claims manager will ensure that there is a treating provider certifying that, in the provider's opinion, the claimant has functional limitations and/or medically necessary restrictions.
5. *Obtain vocational information*: The claims manager will evaluate the essential occupational duties of the claimant's employment at the time of the illness or injury. As noted above in the definitions of 14.1.3.2, whether the essential duties relate to job or occupation will be determined by the contract. A job description from the employer is usually the starting point for this evaluation, but if there is ambiguity or more detail is needed, a vocational professional may be asked to provide clarification.
6. *Evaluate the medical information*: If the medical information supports functional limitations or activity restrictions that would obviously preclude the essential duties of the job or occupation, the claims manager can make a determination to pay the claim. This may happen, for example, if the claimant is hospitalized with catastrophic injuries that clearly prevent any occupational duties. If the circumstances are less certain, the claims manager may ask a healthcare professional – a nurse, a physician, or a behavioral health specialist such as a licensed professional counselor (LPC), licensed clinical social worker (LCSW), or licensed psychologist (LP) – to evaluate and interpret the medical information, with respect to what office visit notes say, or don't say, about functional impairment. When the medical information involves psychological or neuropsychological testing, psychologists with appropriate training are asked to review those data. These health professionals may be internal to the insurer, as employees or contractors, or may be contracted through a vendor.
7. *Evaluate the vocational information*: Once the claims manager has a clear understanding of the occupational requirements and of the medical impairment with associated functional limitations and medically necessary activity restrictions, she/he will compare the two sets of data. If there is clinical evidence that is consistent with the conclusion that one or more occupational duties are precluded, the claim is likely to be valid and payable. If no essential occupational duties are

Table 14.2 Idealized claim evaluation process

	Activities	Impairment	Duties
Claim	Claimant statement	Attending physician statement	Job description
Validation	Interviews, field visit, surveillance, social media searches	Clinical and medical evaluation of evidence presented, independent records review, independent evaluations	Occupational analysis, employer contacts, accommodations analysis
	Can't do what?	*Because of what?*	*With what impact?*

Eskay-Auerbach & Kertay (2016)

precluded, then the claim is likely not payable. If the claims manager is uncertain, this is another area in which a vocational expert may assist in evaluating the claimant's functional abilities against the occupational requirements.

8. *Form a conclusion about benefits*: Assuming the claimant is eligible (steps 1 and 2), the claims manager will evaluate the information obtained in steps 3–7 and determine if the available information meets the definition of disability.

The generic claims process is pictured in Table 14.2. The broad question that the claims manager needs to answer is "what can the claimant not do, based on what medical cause, and what are the implications for performing occupational duties?" Put more succinctly, "can't do what, because of what, and with what impact?"

There are several points in this process that can confuse health providers and that can seem to run counter to clinical reasoning. For example, with respect to pre-ex, the claimant/patient may be profoundly impaired and obviously unable to work, but the claim may not be payable because the claimant is not eligible due to pre-ex. The principle is similar to all insurance products: an individual can't go out and buy a policy to cover the loss of his or her home, after the house burns down. The policy must be in place before the loss.

Another area of confusion for providers can occur when the claims manager, and/or the medical advisors who evaluate the information provided, does not accept the treating provider's point of view. This may happen for a variety of reasons. It may be that the documentation provided is insufficient in depth and detail to clearly support the provider's opinion. It may be that the provider has information that isn't in the record. Or it is possible that the claims manager, or the consulting health providers, has information that is not available to the attending; sometimes the claimant presents one set of data to one provider and different information to another, and the information is contradictory.

Finally, at times the occupational information that is available to the claims professional may contradict what the patient tells his or her provider. For example, the patient may tell the provider that she/he spends 80% of the time interacting with the public, but the occupational data or the job description describes this as a minor duty. In that case, even if the patient is deemed unable to interact effectively with the public, the essential occupational duties might not be impacted.

Many of these issues can be remedied by better understanding the disability determination process and by understanding what the insurer needs in order to make the best possible determination. Remedying any deficiencies in the provider's interaction with claims staff is addressed in the remainder of this chapter.

14.2 The Challenge of Behavioral Health Conditions in Private Disability

The claims manager's job is relatively straightforward when the claimant describes daily activities consistent with what is expected, when medical findings demonstrating functional limitations are clear-cut and there are well-established best practices to guide reasonable activity restrictions, and when limitations and restrictions can be compared to well-defined requirements to perform important occupational duties. Often, with straightforward physical conditions that cause temporary impairment, and in the absence of complications, this straightforward decision-making occurs easily and promptly, and the system works as it was designed. Income protection benefits are provided for the necessary convalescence and recovery period, and support continues until the claimant is able to return to work.

Medical conditions are defined by both *signs,* which are the measurable findings that health providers see, and *symptoms*, which are what the patient experiences. A patient presents to his or her physician with symptoms of knee pain. The doctor observes swelling, joint crepitus, restricted range of motion, and internal damage on imaging. When the findings are severe enough, chronic, and do not respond to conservative treatment, surgery may be performed, followed by a generally known period of rehabilitation and recovery. If the ability to bend, stoop, climb, or walk long distances are an essential part of the job, the claims manager can determine with reasonable certainty that benefits will be paid for the period of time the claimant is unable to perform those activities (limitations), or should not yet perform them for risk of reinjury (restrictions).

14.2.1 Claimant Reports in Behavioral Health Conditions

Behavioral health conditions, however, often do not provide such a clear-cut picture. One problem is the degree to which the symptoms of a behavioral health disorder impact an individual's *perceived* ability to accomplish certain tasks, which may not reflect his or her *actual* functional capacity. For example, one of the common characteristics of a major depressive disorder is decreased motivation and loss of pleasure or interest in activities previously enjoyed. When a claimant tells the claims manager that she/he doesn't really feel like doing anything and doesn't leave the house, is the claimant experiencing a symptom of MDD or expressing job dissatisfaction and a choice not to go to work? How does a claims manager evaluate the difference? How does the clinician?

Moreover, even if the claims manager decides to conduct surveillance or have someone conduct a home visit, how does she/he evaluate what the claimant does? If the claimant doesn't come out of the house during the period of surveillance or looks disheveled and withdrawn during a case manager visit, is that because the claimant doesn't *want* to leave the bedroom or because she/he is *unable* to leave?

14.2.2 Clinician Reports and Diagnoses in Behavioral Health Conditions

Similarly, in behavioral health the diagnosis of a clinical impairment – the condition(s) causing functional loss – relies on symptoms, with limited measurable signs. There is, for example, no blood test that reliably characterizes a major depressive episode. Psychiatric diagnoses often have poor reliability (Aboraya, Rankin, France, El-Missiry, & John, 2006, Frances A, Freedman et al., 2013, Matuszack & Plasecki, 2012), a problem made worse with the introduction of the 5th Edition of the *Diagnostic and Statistical Manual* of the American Psychiatric Association (*DSM-5*) (APA, 2013; Frances, 2013) and complicated by the simultaneous use in the USA of both the *DSM-5* and the *ICD-10*, which relies on the older categories of the *DSM-IV*.[1] Too often, practicing clinicians fail to apply rigor to making behavioral diagnoses, perhaps stretching the definition of criterion A of Post-Traumatic Stress Disorder (PTSD) to include upsetting events such as job harassment or diagnosing Bipolar Disorder II when one of the cluster B personality disorders would be more accurate.

Even having rigorously established a diagnosis, how does the clinician determine the degree to which the patient is *unable* to concentrate, for example, as compared to the degree to which the patient's amotivation leads him or her to give insufficient effort? More to the point in the disability process, how does the

[1] The *ICD-10* (WHO, 1992) is the *International Statistical Classification of Diseases and Health Related Problems, 10th Revision*. It was endorsed in 1990 by the Forty-third World Health Assembly and began to come into use by member states in 1994 (WHO, 2017). When it was adopted in the USA in 2016, it created a conflict between most health insurers, which require *ICD-10* codes for billing, and behavioral health providers who use the *DSM-5*, because the *ICD-10* uses the classification scheme of the *DSM-IV*. Moreover, the *ICD-10* has its own definitions and criteria, outlined in *The ICD-10 Classification of Mental and Behavioural Disorders* (WHO, 1993), which parallel but do not exactly match *DSM-IV* criteria. The confusion generated by these conflicting sets of diagnostic criteria adds to lack of clarity in diagnosis and complicates discussions of diagnostic and treatment guidelines; the discrepancies may or may not be resolved by the release of the *ICD-11*, which is due in 2019 (WHO, 2017). For the treating professional providing a diagnosis in the DI system, the best guidance is to clarify which diagnostic criteria are being used and how the patient's symptoms meet those criteria.

claims manager understand the difference? Finally, what clinical data can the treating professional provide in order to facilitate the most accurate claim determination?

14.2.3 Occupational Duties and Behavioral Health

A significant deficiency in making claim determinations related to behavioral health conditions is that there is a paucity of information that correlates cognitive and emotional capacities with job requirements. One common resource still used by vocational experts, the Dictionary of Occupational Titles (DOT), was first published in 1938 and last updated in 1999 (Miller, Cain, Roos, & Roos, 1980; US DOL, 1991). The DOT is silent on emotional, mental, or behavioral job requirements, instead categorizing only the essential physical demands of occupations. The Occupational Information Network (O-NET, 2017) was intended to replace the DOT and has more to say about broad levels of skill needed for occupations but still lacks specificity for particular determinations. Finally, employer job descriptions can be used but are notoriously inadequate to the task of specifying measurable mental demands.

The net result is that clinicians often rely on what their patient tells them about the job, which may or may not be accurate. Especially when the patient has psychological symptoms, or has anxiety about returning to work, self-described job requirements are likely to be distorted. For the claims manager, she/he must rely on experience or on the best assessment of a vocational professional, who faces the same challenges as the rest of the profession.

14.2.4 The Role of Professional Clinical Resources Internal to the Insurer

Claims managers have expertise and training in understanding contracts and the intricacies of the regulatory requirements for making claim determinations. However, they typically do not have the same depth of medical knowledge as the clinicians providing them information, and they may not know what questions they should be asking. As a result, private insurers will often employ, or contract with, professional resources – nurses, counselors, social workers, physicians, and/or psychologists – to help them interpret the clinical data supplied by treating providers.

Although the independence of these internal resources has been the subject of controversy (Hadjistavropoulos, 1999; Hadjistavropoulos & Bieling, 2001; MacLeod, LaChapelle, Hadjistravropoulos, & Pfeifer, 2001), and sometimes litigation (Metropolitan, 2008), their ideal role is straightforward: evaluate the medical information submitted by treating providers, including office visit notes, test results,[2] and completed forms; determine the extent to which they are consistent internally and with the severity of the claimed impairment; and interpret the information in a way that non-clinicians can understand. Sometimes, when the provider's notes are unclear, when additional detail is needed, or if the internal clinician interprets the data differently, a phone call with the treating provider is made. In addition to evaluating and interpreting clinical data from treating providers, internal clinical resources may also help educate claims manager, help formulate questions for independent evaluations, and make recommendations about potential return-to-work plans with or without accommodations.

There is ongoing debate about the presumed bias of internal resources and the presumption that the treating provider knows the patient best and is therefore in the best position to judge the patient's condition and functional ability. Balanced against that perspective is the potential ethical conflict of the treating provider who also finds him−/herself in a forensic role by providing information in support of a disability claim (Greenberg & Shuman, 1997; Greenberg & Shuman, 2007). It is also true that the internal clinician often has access to medical records the treating provider may not have and has the time to review the totality of the records in detail. This chapter will not resolve the debate, but it is fair to say that the ideal role of the internal reviewer is to help facilitate accurate understanding of medical information and through that interpretation help achieve the best outcome for the claimant, whether that outcome is prompt payment for a well-supported impairment or the conclusion that the claimant can, and should, return to work.

14.3 The Functional Impact of Behavioral Health Is Multifaceted

When those involved in disability claims operate from a purely biomedical perspective, many of the nuances of the claimant's condition may be missed, complicating claims management. Behavior impacts claims on multiple levels: psychiatric disorders; psychological symptoms that fall short of a diagnosable condition; psychosocial factors that are neither conditions nor symptoms, but which act as barriers to function; and behavioral overlays that represent motivation, disability beliefs, and other similar factors. One of the strengths of behavioral health providers on the whole, within the private disability context, is that they are well-educated in the

[2] Although office notes and other information may be reviewed by other behavioral health providers, when formal psychological or neuropsychological test results are part of the record, these results are normally reviewed by appropriately trained psychologists. If the psychologist providing the testing has a question about this, she/he should verify that the review will be conducted by an appropriate professional.

ability to distinguish these impacts and to offer viable assistance to the patient in efforts to regain functioning.[3]

14.3.1 *The Biopsychosocial Perspective*

Disability, as defined in this chapter, is a prototypically biopsychosocial phenomenon. The biopsychosocial nature of impairment and disability is discussed in more detail elsewhere in this volume (see Chap. 5) and in depth in other works (Caruso, 2013; Loisel & Anema, 2014). To reiterate, many factors will contribute to the decision to apply for disability benefits, and many will impact the duration of the claim. The patient's attitude toward work and disability (Berecki-Gisolf, Clay, Collie, & McClure, 2012; Berglind & Gerner, 2005; Cole, Mondloch, & Hogg-Johnson, 2002; Franche & Krause, 2002; Laisne, Lecomte, & Corbiere, 2012), the provider's attitude toward disability (Dasinger, Krause, Thompson, Brand, & Rudolph, 2001; Franche & Krause, 2002), other provider-related factors (Englund, Tibblin, & Svarsudd, 2000; Pransky, Katz, Benjamin, & Himmelstein, 2002; Rainville, Pransky, Indahl, & Mayer, 2005), the patient's perception of workplace support (Caruso, 2013; Foreman, Murphy, & Swerissen, 2006; Franche & Krause, 2002; Young et al., 2005), and the availability of compensation while away from work (Franche & Krause, 2002, Young et al., 2005) are all predictive of absence duration. Additional factors include studies related to characteristics of the patient's experience at work, including perceived injustice (Scott & Sullivan, 2012, Sullivan, Scott, & Trost, 2012. Sullivan, Yakobov, Scott, & Tait, 2014), catastrophizing (Besen, Gaines, Linton, & Shaw, 2017; Moore, Thibault, Adams, & Sullivan, 2016; Quartana, Campbell, & Edwards, 2009) fear avoidance (Grotle, Vollestad, Velerod, & Brox, 2004; Moore et al., 2016) and disability beliefs (Caruso, 2013, Loisel & Anema, 2014). At times, malingering and/or symptom exaggeration has an impact as well (Gill, Green, Flaro, & Pucci, 2007; Young, 2015).

It is important to remember that by far the majority of individuals who leave work with an illness or injury receive disability benefits for a period of recovery time and then return to work. When recovery is unnecessarily and unreasonably delayed, it is more often than not because there are psychosocial factors that are

[3]The author of this chapter writes with the assumption that disability is best understood as a biopsychosocial phenomenon, and not as one that is purely biomedical. In the author's experience, DI carriers, and insurers in other systems such as WC, are gradually moving to adopt the biopsychosocial perspective in managing claims, particularly those with a behavioral health component. That said, in adjudicating DI claims, the claims manager must make a clear determination regarding eligibility for benefits based on the contract. Because that black-and-white decision does not automatically lend itself to a biopsychosocial perspective, there is a tendency to rely more on biomedical reasoning. It is important for treating and evaluating behavioral providers to provide information that is detailed, clearly understandable, and oriented toward function. In essence, the behavioral health provider can help build the bridge between biopsychosocial and biomedical perspectives.

contributing and creating barriers to return to work. Behavioral health providers are in a unique position to understand, and mitigate, unnecessarily prolonged disability durations.

14.3.2 Layers of Impact

It is critically important to differentiate the impact of psychiatric condition, psychological symptoms, and psychosocial factors as they impact on a claim for benefits under a private disability contract. Claims systems are beginning to understand the importance of psychosocial factors as they impact incidence and duration and are looking for ways to mitigate barriers to work. Unfortunately, confusion about the different ways in which psychological and social factors impact claims and the interventions appropriate to each interfere with effective claim determination and management.

14.3.2.1 Behavioral Health Conditions

Behavioral health conditions are diagnosable syndromes, each with distinct diagnostic criteria that must be met, that can be identified and treated, and more often than not will resolve with effective, evidenced-informed treatment. As noted throughout this chapter, a diagnosis does not mean the patient has a significant impairment in day-to-day functioning. By definition, psychiatric diagnoses cause distress and/or functional impairment, but distress does not mean that the individual has reduced functioning, and a functional impairment may not be significant enough to interfere with daily tasks, including work. From the perspective of the private disability benefit systems, however, a diagnosed condition is a necessary, but not sufficient requirement for determining disability.

It is important to generate a clear and accurate diagnosis and to effectively document it. Good documentation will specify how the diagnostic criteria are met, provide reliable observations that support the asserted severity, and will specify the method by which the diagnosis was derived, e.g., structured interview, testing and behavioral observations, etc. Well-documented clinical observations, findings from formal mental status examination, and/or test results are needed to supplement the patient's self-report. In addition, it is important to state which diagnostic scheme is being used, whether *DSM-5* or *ICD-10*. Documentation that fails to provide clearly delineated diagnostic criteria, or that stretches the definitions of those criteria, will complicate the evaluation of the information and will delay the adjudication of the claim. Unfortunately, such inadequate documentation is common, and low inter-rater reliability in *DSM-5* diagnostic categories is one of the major sources of its criticism (Frances, 2013; Wakefield, 2016).

Although a properly documented psychiatric diagnosis does not translate automatically into disability, determining its functional impact will be clearer because the condition is well defined. Psychiatric conditions may be the primary cause for a disability claim, or it may be co-occurring as a separate condition. It also may impact the claim as a comorbidity that aggravates the severity of another condition or complicates recovery. Whether alone or in combination with other conditions, psychiatric condition will be evaluated for functional impact and the degree to which the impairment meets the contractual definition of disability.

14.3.2.2 Psychological Symptoms

Psychological symptoms are often substituted for carefully documented diagnoses in medical records. It is common to see "depression" and "anxiety" noted in medical records from primary care providers, for example, and it is not uncommon to see symptoms such as these substituted for specific diagnostic categories in some mental health records. Symptoms such as these should be documented, and psychological symptoms can color the perception of physical conditions; pain perception, for example, is increased when an individual feels depressed (Dickens, McGowen, & Dale, 2003; Thompson, Correll, Gallop, Vancampfort, & Stubbs, 2016; Woo, 2010), and anxiety is known to exacerbate the experience of pain (Theunissen, Peters, Bruce, Gramke, & Marcos, 2012; Woo, 2010).

However, absent the careful documentation of a psychiatric diagnosis, reported psychological symptoms cannot be correlated with specific functional impairment, and it will be impossible to evaluate the extent to which the individual is functionally limited or requires clinically necessary activity restrictions. It is possible the "depression" is a psychiatric condition that has been inadequately specified, or it may be that the symptoms are present as a variation of mood, but without an underlying diagnosis. Absent a clarified diagnosis, symptoms are symptoms, and may not be considered the basis of a documented disability under the terms of the contract.

14.3.2.3 Psychosocial Factors that Impact Disability Claims

"Psychosocial factors" are those life stressors that get in the way of normal daily activities, without rising to the level of a particular psychological symptom and without equating to a diagnosed psychiatric condition. Poor economic circumstances, family conflict, educational deficits, workplace conflicts, and changing workplace demands are all conditions that can interfere with an individual's ability to cope. Some, including a growing body of research involving adverse childhood experiences (ACE), can be predictive of poor claim outcome and delayed recovery (Schussler-Fiorenza et al., 2016). Unresolved, psychosocial stressors can decrease motivation for work and/or create barriers that interfere with functional recovery and return to work. Psychosocial factors are not impairing conditions, but they are important considerations when it comes to understanding the totality of a claim and managing to a better outcome.

14.3.2.4 Behavioral Overlay

A fourth layer of impact is behavioral overlay. Individuals who experience chronic health conditions can become frustrated and can come to believe that it is necessary to exaggerate in order to be taken seriously. Others may be irritable and argumentative, either in response to circumstances or as a personality characteristic. Still others may deliberately exaggerate or manufacture symptoms, either in order to play a sick role, as in factitious disorder, or for monetary gain, as in malingering. The important point is that these behavioral factors may complicate the evaluation of claims or may impeded recovery, but they are not conditions that lead to impairment and are not the source of functional limitations or clinically necessary activity restrictions.

14.3.2.5 Different Layers Require Different Interventions

The differing layers of impact play different roles in claim determination, claim duration, and claim outcomes, and they require different interventions. Psychiatric conditions, for example, are known to respond effectively to medications, evidence-based psychotherapies, or a combination. Vague psychological symptoms, on the other hand, may respond to psychiatric and/or psychological interventions, but the outcomes are less certain because the conditions are less clear. Psychosocial factors that act as barriers to work do not require behavioral health intervention; instead, they will respond to interventions designed to facilitate problem-solving and increased coping support (see the flags methodologies, for example, as developed in the UK; Kendall, Burton, Main, & Watson, 2009). Behavioral overlays require interviewing skills from the claims managers and require strong enough communication skills to navigate sometimes difficult emotions. The claims managers are not clinicians, typically, and have varying degrees of training in the requisite skills that require to navigate these relationships. Behavioral overlays also may require methods such as testing or surveillance to address deliberate exaggeration or falsification. The main point is that they should not be confused with behavioral health conditions requiring treatment. When providers are clear about these distinctions, documentation improves, and patients are more likely to have claims adjudicated promptly and fairly. When claims insurers are clear about the distinctions, there will be less confusion about what to expect in documentation, and it will be easier to define what interventions are appropriate.

14.4 Determining Work-Relevant Behavioral Health Impairments

Clinicians typically are trained to determine the nature of a behavioral health condition and then to treat that condition in such a way that symptoms are reduced and the patient feels better. However, a further analysis is required to determine whether a patient who files a disability claim is functionally impaired with respect to occupational duties. This additional level of analysis, the impairment evaluation, is not usually taught in either medical training or the training of psychologists and other psychotherapy providers. The risk, capacity, and tolerance model presented here is a consistent, valid approach for specifying functional abilities (Hyman, 2016; Talmage, Melhorn, & Hyman, 2011).

14.4.1 Risk: Determining Clinically Necessary Restrictions

Risk refers to the chance of direct harm to the patient, or to others, as a result of a health condition, if the patient engages in certain activities. Activity restrictions are based on this risk of harm and define what the patient *should not do*, in order to avoid or minimize *actual harm* that might be caused. Note that exacerbated symptoms are not in themselves the appropriate basis of activity restrictions, unless those symptoms correlate with underlying harm, or are themselves harmful.

In physical medicine, a classic example of appropriate restrictions based on determining risk are seizure precautions. A patient with an incompletely controlled seizure disorder is assigned activity restrictions designed to minimize harm in the event of a seizure. Those restrictions typically include working at heights, operating heavy or fast-moving machinery, driving, and other activities where a sudden seizure could result in injury. These restrictions apply regardless of whether the activity occurred at work or outside it.

Ideally, restrictions are based on quantitative research that demonstrates the statistical likelihood of harm arising from a specific activity, but these specifications are often not available. As an alternative, consensus guidelines can be used to assign risk and associated activity restrictions. For example, the American College of Cardiology provides guidelines for participation in competitive sports (Morantz, 2005), and there are developing guidelines for return-to-play determinations related to sports-related concussions (Harmon et al., 2013).

Absent either statistical guidance or consensus documents, activity restrictions can be assigned based on clinical reasonableness. For example, behavioral health practitioners might reasonably restrict a patient in the midst of a severe major depressive episode, who is demonstrating extreme psychomotor retardation, from operating safety-sensitive machinery or when rapid decision-making is required. Here too, activity restrictions that are clinically necessary would logically apply regardless of circumstances; i.e., it is not clinically reasonable to restrict a patient from operating machinery at work due to psychomotor retardation but to leave driving unrestricted.

In behavioral health conditions, risk is often more difficult to define than it is in physical conditions. Since risk implies actual harm, and since behavioral health conditions are most often diagnosed by reported symptoms, providers may assume that exacerbated symptoms mean harm to the patient. However, consider, for example, an anxiety disorder. We know that exposure to an anxiety-provoking stimulus will increase symptoms, but not only is exposure not harmful, it is necessary in order to improve the underlying condition. Careful analysis of potential underlying harm is required.

Within the context of disability determinations, activity restrictions should be based on the risk of actual harm, they should define specific activities, and they should be characterized with respect to any modifications or accommodations that can mitigate the risk. The focus is on performing activities, rather than on resolving symptoms, and those activities need to be specifically defined. "No work" is not a useful activity restriction in the context of disability determination, since it is neither specific nor consistent across circumstances. "No work" also only very rarely is in the best interests of patients; being at work, with or without accommodations, conveys benefits for both physical and psychological health (Kertay, Eskay-Auerbach, & Hyman, 2016; Waddell & Burton, 2006).

14.4.2 Capacity: Determining Functional Limitations

Whereas risk focuses on what a patient *should not* do, capacity focuses on what a patient *can* or *cannot* do. Functional limitations are activities that the patient is unable to perform, regardless of desire or motivation. These limitations are typically measurable in some objective way, based on history, observation, and formal assessment.

In behavioral health conditions, cognitive functions such as concentration, attention, memory, and planning ability can be measured by screening such as a formal MSE or through more extensive neurocognitive testing. Emotional capacities, such as the ability to effectively communicate needs and relating effectively to coworkers and customers, can be assessed through therapy interactions and through testing. Importantly, clinical data is required to support a functional limitation. A positive screening measure, such as an abnormal MSE finding, a positive screen using a PHQ-9 (Kroenke, Spitzer, & Williams, 2001) or one of the many brief, self-report measures of depression, anxiety, or trauma, is an indication that more comprehensive assessment is needed to confirm or rule out functional limitations associated with a behavioral condition.

Functional limitations may or may not correlate with perceived ability. Just as assigning activity restrictions should be based on determining risk of actual harm rather than solely on increased symptoms, so symptoms do not always define a functional limitation. For example, individuals diagnosed with a major depressive disorder may, when the condition is active, describe themselves as having poor memory or as having trouble concentrating. Often, however, the patient's subjective description will be worse than performance measured on testing. Limitations are defined as the actual inability to perform certain functions, not on perceived difficulty.

Documenting functional limitations through formal MSE, behavioral observations, and episodically repeated testing will be helpful in the disability determination process, whereas documenting only symptom report will be less helpful. In documenting, the behavioral health clinician should ask themselves, what can the patient do and not do, objectively, rather than relying only on what the patient describes. Similarly, relying solely on the clinician's own opinion based on prior experience will not be sufficient to describe why *this* patient, at *this time*, is functionally unable to perform certain activities.

14.4.3 Tolerance: Choice, Motivation, and Other Factors

Having evaluated risk of harm and assigning appropriate activity restrictions, and having specified capacity by determining objectively demonstrable functional limitations, what remains to be considered is tolerance. Tolerance is more closely aligned with the patient's self-assessment and their symptoms. Tolerance is primarily a psychological state that represents the perceived ability to comfortably perform certain activities. Symptoms such as fatigue, pain, and/or motivation are all features of tolerance, rather than objectively measurable functional limitations, or conditions requiring clinically necessary activity restrictions. In other words, the patient may have the *ability* to perform a specific task or set of work-related tasks, and there may be no *harm* in doing so, but she/he may be uncomfortable to the point of a perceived decrease in ability.

For example, a patient who has had a well-documented mild traumatic brain injury (mTBI, or concussion) may report subjective symptoms beyond the point at which testing demonstrates a return to baseline functioning. Such symptoms are not functional limitations nor do they require activity restrictions. Instead, they may derive from hypersensitivity to remembered incapacities, as a result of intense self-monitoring, or they may result from anxiety related to returning to normal functioning in the environment in which the injury occurred.

As another example, the individual with a diagnosed panic disorder that first occurred in the workplace may continue to feel anxious about returning to work, even after the panic attacks are well-controlled. Objectively, the individual is able to perform work duties (no limitations), and there is no actual harm to the individual when returning to the workplace (no restrictions), but symptoms of anxiety may make the return subjectively uncomfortable.

A useful question for the provider to ask himself or herself in this context is, "If my patient wanted to return to work, would I let them?" If the answer is "yes," then two things are clear: the patient is capable of performing occupational duties, and there is no clinically necessary reason to restrict them from doing so. The issue, then, is one of tolerance and can be documented as such and can also become the focus of discussion with the patient. If the answer, on the other hand, is "no," then it should clarify the issues that objectively prevent the patient from returning, and documenting the associated clinical findings will be extremely helpful in the disability determination process.

14.4.4 Using Documented Behavioral Impairment in Disability Determination

Impairment evaluation relies on a systematic application of evidence that is relevant to function. The behavioral health clinician must determine, and document, clinical data that support statements of functional limitations and clinically necessary restrictions. For the claims manager to effectively utilize clinical data in determining disability, an independent examiner or the treating provider must document features that are consistently associated with changes in the ability to perform work-related tasks. Utilizing the risk, capacity, and tolerance model outlined above will help focus the documentation. Some additional factors that are relevant to a disability determination include:

- *Documented symptom severity*: are the reported symptoms described in detail sufficient to determine their likely impact on functional abilities?
- *Behavioral observations*: what behaviors does the patient/claimant demonstrate that are consistent with the reported symptoms and demonstrate functional changes? For example, in a patient who reports severe anxiety that is perceived to interfere with concentration, do office visit notes document wandering attention, thought derailment, difficulty focusing on the topic of discussion, etc.? Clearly documenting behavioral observations can help bridge symptom report and functional impairment.
- *Formal mental status examinations (MSE)*: many electronic medical record (EMR) systems automatically generate a template for mental status examination, and the MSE should be a standard part of every office visit with a patient that is claiming disability. Well-documented MSE findings can help corroborate functional impairment associated with a behavioral health condition and can also document change over time.
- *Formal risk assessments*: like the MSE, formally documenting a formal risk assessment in each session helps establish symptom severity and can help determine the need for activity restrictions designed to minimize risk.
- *Treatment intensity*: because being out of work has such negative health consequences (Waddell & Burton, 2006), a high degree of treatment intensity is expected; i.e., a behavioral health condition that impedes work capacity should be considered a clinical emergency. Treatment intensity may vary for a number of reasons, but in general more frequent treatment would be expected in an acutely impairing episode than would be expected in a mild-to-moderate and/or

stable condition. Documented consideration of higher levels of treatment intensity, such as inpatient, intensive outpatient, or partial hospitalization programs, speaks to the perceived severity of the condition and to the need for a degree of treatment inconsistent with work-concurrent treatment.

- *Documented focus on functional restoration*: when office notes reflect discussions with the patient about functional status, performance of ADLs, and return to work, the notes will be more helpful in assessing work-relevant impairment.
- *Consistency analysis*: consistency among the above-noted factors, across time, across providers, and across circumstances is an important part of evaluating functional impairment related to a behavioral health condition. Consistency strengthens the evidence for degree of impairment, while inconsistency undermines it. For example, when a patient is driving, using a computer extensively at home, and is otherwise able to engage in complex cognitive activity, that is inconsistent with a patient who is said to be unable to concentrate enough to use the computer at work. Similarly, it is inconsistent for a patient who is noted in a narrative report or on a disability form to be severely functionally limited, to be noted in contemporaneous office visit notes to be improving, participating in complex activities at home or in non-work organizations. Inconsistency will undermine the credibility of a claim of occupation-precluding behavioral health impairment.

14.5 Communicating Effectively in the Context of Private Disability

A presumption of this chapter, and underlying much of the book, is that it is in the patient's best interests to remain as functional as possible, for as long as possible. That includes the ability to work, which is a key component of an individual's financial well-being, physical and mental health, and sense of purpose. In short, having the patient enter the workforce despite a disability, stay at work if they are working, or return to work if they are out is the best outcome for the individual, the healthcare system, the employer, and the disability insurer. If it is necessary for the patient to be out of work, then the key is to document and communicate with all stakeholders in such a way that insurers can pay appropriate benefits promptly, with the eventual goal of returning the individual to work as quickly and safely as possible. Communications that facilitate these outcomes are the focus of this section.

14.5.1 Communicating with Patients

Behavioral health providers, along with primary care physicians, are on the front lines of claims within the private disability system. Patients will turn to their providers if they are sick, or injured, and believe they are unable to work. Their reaction typically will be in reverse order from the evaluation of impairment outlined above.

Table 14.3 The risk-capacity-tolerance inversion

Provider	Patient
Risk: *Is it safe for Joe to work?* Will performing necessary work activities cause harm to joe or to others?	**Tolerance:** *I'm too tired to work* Symptoms are perceived to prevent work, not just to make it uncomfortable
Capacity: *What can't Joe do?* What is it that joe cannot do despite being motivated to do so?	**Capacity:** *I just can't stay awake to work* Symptoms become impossible barriers
Tolerance: *What symptoms might be exacerbated by working?* What experiential barriers might exist?	**Risk:** *If I go to work tired, I could get really hurt!* Fear of (re)injury means I shouldn't work

Table 14.3 shows the inversion of priorities when patients and their providers evaluate the ability to work. For the provider, objective evaluation of risk and capacity is primary. For the patient, symptom reduction is primary.

Early interactions with health providers may make the difference between staying at work, or at most taking a leave for only as long as is needed, and an unnecessarily extended workplace absence that can have profound negative consequences for mental and physical health, financial well-being, and prospects for long-term employment. Naturally, a careful evaluation of medical impairment is the first priority. If there is genuine, clearly established risk of harm and/or functional incapacity to perform work duties, careful documentation will help ensure that appropriate available benefits are paid. Even more importantly, a safe, effective plan to help the patient return to full functioning, including but not limited to work, will be based on the best possible understanding of the patient's condition.

However, if the result of an impairment evaluation is that there is no clinical reason for the patient to be out of work, then the provider's job is to reassure the patient and encourage maximum functioning while offering appropriate treatment. As Dowrick, Ring, Humphris, and Salmon (2004) pointed out, not all reassurances are the same, and not all are helpful. Patients want first of all to be heard and taken seriously. Reassurance that acknowledges and validates the patient's experience, explains symptoms in a way that the patient can connect to experience, and helps the patient understand how to cope will be both the most helpful and also the most likely to have a positive impact. With behavioral health conditions or behavioral symptoms that impact physical complaints, a critical component of effective communication will be for the patient to feel the provider believes their symptoms are real while offering a believable alternative that allows for shared decision-making and does not evoke defensiveness (Salmon, 2006).

Finally, it may be helpful to address the time it takes to communicate about disability. Although not a primary problem for behavioral providers, most of whom have longer sessions than the average medical appointment, there is a frequently expressed sentiment that "it takes too long" to talk with patients about return to work. With respect to the claim determination process and encouraging patients to return to work, it is less the amount of time spent discussing work than it is about the content of the discussion. When a patient complains about anxiety related to work, for example, a clinician may be inclined to simply take the patient's word for conditions in the workplace, because to discuss it takes longer. But it takes the same amount of time to encourage a patient to learn new coping skills as it does to fill out paperwork in support of disability. In the long run, the time invested in helping a patient remain as functional as possible is time well spent, in terms of both patient outcomes and in terms of effective communication within the private DI system.

14.5.2 Communicating with Insurers

Communicating with insurers of all sorts is part of the business of being a health provider, albeit one that can seem a necessary evil and can feel adversarial. Insurers can require additional paperwork, for which the provider will likely not be paid. In private disability, the insurer will often require some form of attending physician's statement (APS), a behavioral health questionnaire (BHQ), or a form for functional capacity assessment (FCA). These forms may ask questions in terms that are unfamiliar (see 14.1.3 above), and may not have been part of the clinician's training. Moreover, once those forms are submitted, the insurer may question the provider's opinion. At times the communication can feel adversarial.

It will be helpful for the behavioral health provider to understand that the claims manager with whom they will communicate is the ultimate decision-maker regarding the patient's benefits under the contract. The clinician will have behavioral expertise that is critical to the claims manager's determination, while the claims manager will have expertise in interpreting the contract that ultimately determines whether benefits are payable or not. The first principle of communicating with the insurer is to provide information necessary to understand the severity of a health condition and its functional impact, in a form that will be best understood by a well-educated lay person (as opposed to another clinician). For the clinician, it may seem that the clinical data speaks for itself and that the clinician's opinion should be sufficient. For the claims manager, however, that clinical interpretation only matters as it informs an interpretation of the contract. Providing information that is clear, that concisely summarizes the clinical opinion in plain language, and that is based on a concrete understanding of how the patient's condition does or does not impact the ability to function in daily life will be the most helpful.

A word about privacy protection is in order, as it pertains to communication with the insurer. Behavioral health providers will almost always be "covered entities" under the Health Insurance Portability and Accountability Act (HIPAA) and so much follow the rules set out under HIPAA, as interpreted by the Department of Health and Human Services (HHS, 2013). In addition, behavioral health providers will have a code of ethics with which they much comply as professionals.

However, disability insurers are usually *not* covered entities under HIPAA, unless they also have a medical insurance component, and they are not subject to the same ethics codes but rather to general business ethics. For the insurer, the main goal is to obtain sufficient information to validate the functional implications of a claimed disabling impairment. Typically, that will mean that contemporaneous office visit notes are more helpful than narratives, because they provide more data, in a longitudinal context. Insurers will also typically ask for test results, which will be interpreted by internal or contracted psychologists.

For the provider, the main goal may be to protect his or her patient's privacy, and insurer requests may seem intrusive. Some providers may take the position that they cannot, or should not, release patient records, citing HIPAA, state law, or professional ethics. However, if the patient has signed a release and is asking the provider's help in providing information in support of obtaining benefits, those arguments create an unnecessary barrier. The most useful approach will be to ensure the signed release is valid and to keep psychotherapy notes, as defined under HIPAA, separate from the medical record to be released. If the medical record contains the basic elements required for reimbursement under health insurance rules, including information about treatment, evaluation, risk assessment, mental status, and treatment plan, that will almost always be sufficient for the insurer; session content is not the critical information. This will be particularly true if the record references functional evaluation and treatment includes a focus on returning the patient to work, if possible.

14.5.3 Communicating with Employers

Behavioral health providers are not often involved in discussions with employers, and it can be argued that it is not the clinician's job to help the employer engage in returning the patient to work (Denne, Kettner, & Ben-Shalom, 2015). However, clinician involvement with the employer can have a positive impact on return-to-work outcomes (Bensen, Young, & Shaw, 2015; Franche et al., 2005 & Young et al., 2005), and the availability of modified work is a strong predictor of disability duration (Fransen et al., 2002; Fulton-Kehoe et al., 2008; Pransky, Verman, Okurowski, & Webster, 2006 & Turner et al., 2008). Communicating with the employer can help the behavioral health provider better understand the work duties of the patient's occupation, and can help reduce the stigma associated with behavioral health conditions. With this understanding, the provider can help smooth the patient's return to work, as well as reduce the patient's anxiety about the transition back into the workplace.

A question with which behavioral health providers may not be familiar is the concept of a work accommodation. As noted in 14.1.3.2, an accommodation is a change to the workplace, or to the way in which a main duty is performed, that would allow an individual to work effectively. Since we have argued that being in the workforce is the most desirable outcome, whenever possible, an earlier return to work with an accommodation is better than further delay. Table 14.4 shows some common functional impairments that might be associated with a behavioral health condition, or with behavioral symptoms, and suggested workplace accommodations that might allow the patient to work.

Table 14.4 Behavioral limitations and potential accommodations

Functional capacity	Measure	Potential accommodation
Maintain concentration and attention	Mental status examination, formal testing of executive functions, working memory, and processing speed	Frequent breaks, self-paced work, moving work space to a less distracting area, work from home, self-prompting software
Ability to follow instructions	Mental status examination, formal "homework," behavioral observations	Prompts and job aids, self-prompting software, frequent reminders, real-time feedback
Think critically	Mental status examination, formal testing of problem-solving, interpretation of proverbs, observed difficulties navigating daily problems	Additional time to complete tasks, checks and balances for critical decisions, clearly outlined limits on decision-making authority
Make decisions independently	Observed problems navigating daily problems, documented overreliance on reassurance from others	Checks and balances for critical decisions, clear limits on decision-making authority, graduated transition back to work
Engage with the public	Observe interactions with office staff, self-monitoring notebook, documenting non-work activities that involve being in public	Gradually reintroduce public-facing duties, temporary accommodation to limit exposure, temporary work from home in a nonpublic-facing role
Engage with coworkers	Observe interactions with office staff and others, documenting interactions	Graduated exposure, temporarily assigning a non-team role
Work independently	Ability to manage ADLs and IADLs alone, driving self to appointments, completing household tasks independently	Temporary additional supervision or assigning a "work partner"
Recall important information	Formal mental status examination, memory testing, monitoring homework assignments or other important information over time	Notebooks and logs, job aids, detailed list of activity steps
Learn complex tasks	Formal mental status examination, memory testing, learning new behaviors assigned in therapy	Detailed outlines of procedures, behaviorally anchored performance measures, reminders
Adapt to changing circumstances	Observe interactions with others, monitor responses to schedule changes or changes in the office, document interactions with others at home	Temporarily assign more routine work, clearly outlines expectations and tasks
Multitask, or rapid shifting of focus	Formal mental status examination, executive function testing, observed/described interactions at home	Temporarily assign more routine work, allow additional time to complete tasks, work from home

Finally, disability insurers may have support available for the claimant who is motivated to return to work, but who may not be able to return to the same occupation. Depending on the contract, vocational rehabilitation and/or retraining benefits may be available. Support for assistive devices is also sometimes available. By connecting with the employer, on behalf of the patient, it may be possible to bridge the gap between the patient's abilities and the employer's needs and to involve the insurer in the return-to-work effort.

14.5.4 Filling out Forms

The most common form encountered in connection with private disability coverage is an attending physician's statement (APS) or its equivalent (see Fig. 14.1). The key information for the disability insurer will be diagnosis, findings that support the diagnosis, symptoms, limitations, restrictions, and the expectations for when restrictions can be lifted. Potential accommodations, if requested, will also be important.

The guidance provided in this chapter will be helpful in completing the form effectively, for the patient and for the insurer. It is most helpful to be clear about the

Patient name	Date of birth	Identifying number
Primary diagnosis	Secondary diagnosis	
Objective findings (signs)		
Subjective findings (symptoms)		
Diagnostic testing completed		
Current treatment		
Other providers		
Limitations		
Restrictions		
Date restrictions began	Date restrictions are expected to end	
Name	Degree	Specialty
Address		Phone
Signature		Date

Fig. 14.1 Attending physician's statement (idealized)

distinction between symptoms, which are the patient's report, and signs, which are test results, behavioral observations, or other data that support the clinician's diagnosis and assessment of function. Sections on limitations and restrictions will be best completed by following the guidance provided in 14.2.3 and by asking yourself the main question, "If my patient wanted to work, would I let him/her?" If the answer is no, that will guide your assessment of what the patient *cannot do* (limitations) and/or what the patient *should not* do (restrictions). Issues of tolerance are best entered under symptoms, and not as a restriction.

The insurer may also request a supplemental form, sometimes referred to as a behavioral health questionnaire (BHQ), or a similar title. These forms will have additional questions specific to behavioral health conditions and will ask more functionally oriented questions. The principles for completing them remain the same. The most helpful information, both for the insurer's ability to adjudicate the claim and for the patient whose claim is being evaluated, will be (a) clearly described in plain language; (b) supported by behavioral observations, with limited assumptions about internal experience or motivation; and (c) focused more on functional capacity than on symptoms. If a question is unclear, ask for clarification or indicate the issue, rather than trying to guess what the insurer wants to know. If the answer is unknown, or outside the practitioner's expertise, "I don't know" is a more helpful response than guessing.

14.6 Disability Management and Evidence-Informed Behavioral Health Practices

There is an accumulating body of evidence to support the proposition that behavioral health treatment that is (a) timely, (b) evidence-informed, and (c) culturally appropriate can help improve productivity, help individuals stay at work, reduce the duration of workplace absence, and help ensure a successful and sustained return to work (Beales et al., 2017; Blank, Peters, Pickvance, Wilford, & McDonald, 2008; Dewa, Thompson, & Jacobs, 2011; Harnois & Gabriel, 2000). Insurers across disability benefit systems are recognizing gradually that support for behavioral care may help obtain better outcomes.

Clearly, if the primary condition causing functional impairment is a diagnosed psychiatric condition, appropriate treatment for that condition will contribute to recovery, both of mental health and of function. However, the value of behavioral care is not limited to treatment for psychopathology. The longer a claim extends, the more that psychological symptoms, psychosocial barriers, and behavioral overlays contribute to claim duration (Shaw, Pransky, & Winters, 2009). As a result, time-limited interventions geared toward functional restoration can be helpful in reducing claim durations by facilitating return to work. Examples include work-oriented cognitive behavioral therapy (Devente, Kamphuls, Emmelkamp, & Blonk, 2008; Lagerveld, Blonk, Brenninkmeijer, Wijngaards-de, & Schaufell, 2012; Reme,

Grasdal, Lovvik, Lie, & Overland, 2015) and applications designed specifically to facilitate functional recovery, such as Progressive Goal Attainment Program (PGAP; Adams, Ellis, Stanish, & Sullivan, 2007, Rafferty, Murphy, O'Shea, Newell, & McGuire, 2013, Sullivan et al., 2005, Sullivan, Adams, Rhodenizer, & Stanish, 2006, Sullivan & Simon, 2012,) .

The application of these programs remains in its early stages, and evidence is accumulating slowly. At the same time, there is limited knowledge among behavioral health providers about their role in the private disability system. Behavioral clinicians have a great deal to contribute to better work-related outcomes, both by applying appropriate best practices in caring for patients who file, or are considering filing, disability claims, and also by understanding the importance of work for mental health.

14.7 Summary and Conclusions: What the Disability Insurer Needs from Behavioral Health Providers

Misunderstanding the goals, language, and processes of the disability determination process can lead to an unnecessarily adversarial relationship between treating clinicians and the insurer and can lead to confusion for the evaluating clinician performing an independent examination. Treating behavioral health clinicians, despite training in psychological and/or neuropsychological assessment, rarely have training in evaluating patients with respect to daily function and how functional capacities relate to work. At the same time, claims managers have a limited understanding of the clinical issues encountered daily by treating providers. Effectively navigating communication between these different perspectives is an important part of ensuring the best outcomes for patients who are also claimants. What follows is a summary of the general guidance in this chapter for the behavioral health clinician, intended to help generate information that will assist the claims manager to best adjudicate the claim (Eskay-Auerbach & Kertay, 2016):

1. Decide whether your involvement in the disability claim is in your patient's best interests. "Advocacy" is often taken to mean that it is the treating provider's job to help the patient obtain benefits. As we have seen elsewhere in this volume, obtaining benefits may or may not be in the patient's best interests from a clinical perspective. True advocacy is helping a patient get what she/he needs, which is very often that she/he should stay at work, or return to work, as quickly as is possible.
2. Decide whether you have the requisite skills to evaluate the patient's functional capacities with respect to work. If so, providing clear, accurate, and timely information to the insurer is the best way to quickly and accurately resolve the claim.
3. Understand the distinction between a clinical evaluation of impairment, for which supporting data is supplied, and a disability determination, which is an administrative decision and based on contractual definitions in addition to clinical perspectives.

4. Generate a clear and accurate diagnosis. Functional limitations and clinically necessary restrictions occur in the context of an impairment, and an impairment is based on a clear clinical diagnosis. Good documentation will specify how the diagnostic criteria are met, will provide reliable observations that support the asserted severity, and will specify the method by which the diagnosis was derived, e.g., structured interview, testing and behavioral observations, etc. Well-documented clinical observations, findings from formal mental status examination, and/or test results are needed to supplement the patient's self-report. In addition, it is important to state which diagnostic scheme is being used, whether *DSM-5* or *ICD-10*. Documentation that fails to provide clearly delineated diagnostic criteria, or that stretches the definitions of those criteria, will complicate the evaluation of the information and will delay the adjudication of the claim.
5. Assess the functional impact of the impairing condition. Having established the diagnosis clearly, the next step is to determine the functional impact of the signs and symptoms documented. Specifically, what can the patient do, and not do, with respect to day-to-day activities. Ask yourself, "if this patient wanted to work, would I let them?" If the answer is affirmative, then clearly the patient is not functionally limited from doing job-related activities, and there is no reason to clinically restrict them from occupational duties. If the answer is negative, be sure that you have documented the reasons, as clearly as possible.
6. Support all conclusions with evidence, and apply evidence-based or evidence-informed practices. When guidelines are available, with respect to functional capacities and/or activity restrictions, follow them, and provide the reference. When guidelines are not available, as often can be the case with mental health conditions, you will have to rely on clinical experience and the best available data. Most importantly, provide the rationale for your conclusions.
7. Communicate clearly and precisely, with an eye toward describing function. One of the errors often seen in office notes occurs when clinicians describe patient reports as if they were observed first hand. Use precise language about the sources of your information. For example, there is a difference between "the patient has trouble sleeping" and "the patient reported they have trouble sleeping," or perhaps "the patient's wife informed that the patient says he has trouble sleeping."

References

Aboraya, A., Rankin, E., France, C., El-Missiry, A., & John, C. (2006). The reliability of psychiatric diagnosis revisited. *Psychiatry (Edgmont), 3*(1), 41–50.

ADA Amendments Act of 2008. 42 U.S.C. 12101.

Adams, H., Ellis, T., Stanish, W. D., & Sullivan, M. J. L. (2007). Psychosocial factors related to return to work following rehabilitation of whiplash injuries. *Journal of Occupational Rehabilitation, 17*(2), 305–315.

American Medical Association. (2011). *Guides to the evaluation of permanent impairment* (6th ed.). Chicago: American Medical Association.

American Psychiatric Association. (2013). *Diagnostic and statistical manual of mental disorders* (5th ed.). Washington, DC: American Psychiatric Publishing.

Americans with Disabilities Act of 1990. 42 U.S.C. 12101.

Beales, D., Kyaw-Myint, S., Smith, A., O'Sullivan, P., Pransky, G., Linton, S., et al. (2017). Work productivity loss in young workers is substantial and is associated with spinal pain and mental health conditions. *Journal of Occupational and Environmental Medicine, 59*(3), 237–245.

Bensen, E., Young, A. E., & Shaw, W. S. (2015). Returning to work following low back pain: Towards a model of individual psychosocial factors. *Journal of Occupational Rehabilitation, 25*, 25–27.

Berecki-Gisolf, J., Clay, F. J., Collie, A., & McClure, R. J. (2012). Predictors of sustained return to work after work-related injury or disease: Insights from workers' compensation claims records. *Journal of Occupational Rehabilitation, 34*(5), 355–382.

Berglind, H., & Gerner, U. (2005). Motivation and return to work among the long-term sick-listed: An action theory perspective. *Disability and Rehabilitation, 24*, 719–726.

Berkowitz, E. D. (2000). *Statement before the subcommittee on Social Security of the Committee on Ways and Means,* July 13, 2000. http://www.ssa.gov/history/edberkdib.html. Accessed 27 October 2017.

Besen, E., Gaines, B., Linton, S. J., & Shaw, W. S. (2017). The role of pain catastrophizing as a mediator in the work disability process following acute low back pain. *Journal of Applied Behavioral Research, 22*(1), e12085.

Blank, L., Peters, J., Pickvance, S., Wilford, J., & McDonald, E. (2008). A systematic review of the factors which predict return to work for people suffering episodes of poor mental health. *Journal of Occupational Rehabilitation, 18*(1), 27–34.

Caruso, G. M. (2013). Biopsychosocial considerations in unnecessary work disability. *Psychological Injury & the Law, 6*, 164–182.

Cole, D. C., Mondloch, M. V., & Hogg-Johnson, S. (2002). Listening to injured workers: How recovery expectations determine outcomes – A prospective study. *Canadian Medical Association Journal, 166*, 749–754.

Dasinger, L. K., Krause, N., Thompson, P. J., Brand, R. J., & Rudolph, L. (2001). Doctor proactive communication, return to work recommendation, and duration of disability after a workers' compensation low-back injury. *Journal of Occupational & Environmental Medicine, 43*, 515–525.

Denne, J., Kettner, G., & Ben-Shalom, Y. (2015). Final report: The role of the physician in the return-to-work process following disability onset. *Mathematica Center for Studying Disability Policy.* https://www.dol.gov/odep/topics/pdf/RTW_Role%20of%20Physician_2015-03.pdf. Accessed 12 Nov 2017.

Devente, W., Kamphuls, J. D., Emmelkamp, P. M., & Blonk, R. W. (2008). Individual and group cognitive-behavioral treatment for work-related stress complaints and sickness absence: A randomized controlled trial. *Journal of Occupational Health Psychology, 13*(3), 214–231.

Dewa, C. S., Thompson, A. H., & Jacobs, P. (2011). The association of treatment of depressive episodes and work productivity. *Canadian Journal of Psychiatry, 56*(12), 743–750.

Dickens, C., McGowen, L., & Dale, S. (2003). Impact of depression on experimental pain perception: A systematic review of the literature with meta-analysis. *Psychosomatic Medicine, 65*(3), 369–375.

Dowrick, C. F., Ring, A., Humphris, G. M., & Salmon, P. (2004). Normalisation of unexplained symptoms by general practitioners: A functional typology. *British Journal of General Practitioners, 54*, 165–170.

Englund, L., Tibblin, G., & Svarsudd, K. (2000). Variations in sick-listing practice among male and female physicians of different specialties based on case vignettes. *Scandinavian Journal of Primary Health Care, 18*, 48–52.

Eskay-Auerbach, M. (2016). Physician certification for family medical leave. In L. Kertay, M. Eskay-Aurbach, & M. H. Hyman (Eds.), *The AMA guides to navigating disability benefit systems*. Chicago: American Medical Association.

Eskay-Auerbach, M., & Kertay, L. (2016). The health care professional and private disability insurance claims. In L. Kertay, M. Eskay-Aurbach, & M. H. Hyman (Eds.), *The AMA guides to navigating disability benefit systems*. Chicago: American Medical Association.

Foreman, P., Murphy, G., & Swerissen, H. (2006). *Barriers and facilitators to return to work: A literature review*. Latrobe University, Melbourne: Australian Institute for Primary Care.

Frances, A. (2013). *Saving normal: An insider's revolt against out-of-control psychiatric diagnosis, DSM-5, big pharma, and the medicalization of ordinary life*. New York: Harper Collins.
Franche, R. L., Cullen, K., Clarke, J., Irvin, E., Sinclair, S., & Frank, J. (2005). Workplace-based return-to-work interventions: A systematic review of the quantitative literature. *Journal of Occupational Rehabilitation, 15*(4), 607–631.
Franche, R. L., & Krause, N. (2002). Readiness for return-to-work following injury or illness: Conceptualizing the interpersonal impact of health care, workplace, and insurance factors. *Journal of Occupational Rehabilitation, 12*, 233–256.
Fransen, M., Woodward, M., Norton, R., Coggan, C., Dawe, M., & Sheridan, N. (2002). Risk factors associated with the transition from acute to chronic occupational back pain. *Spine, 27*(1), 92–98.
Freedman, R., Lewis, D. A., Michels, R., Pine, D. S., Schultz, S. K., Tamminga, C. A., et al. (2013). The initial field trials of DSM-5: New blooms and old thorns. *The American Journal of Psychiatry, 170*(1), 1–5.
Fulton-Kehoe, D., Stover, B. D., Turner, J. A., Sheppard, L., Gluck, J. V., Wickizer, T. M., & Franklin, G. M. (2008). Development of a brief questionnaire to predict long-term disability. *Journal of Occupational & Environmental Medicine, 50*(9), 1042–1052.
Gill, D., Green, P., Flaro, L., & Pucci, T. (2007). The role of effort testing in independent medical examinations. *Medico-Legal Journal, 75*(2), 64–71.
Greenberg, S., & Shuman, D. W. (2007). When worlds collide: Therapeutic and forensic roles. *Professional Psychology: Research & Practice, 38*, 129–132.
Greenberg, S. A., & Shuman, D. W. (1997). Irreconcilable conflict between therapeutic and forensic roles. *Professional Psychology: Research & Practice, 28*(1), 50–57.
Grotle, M., Vollestad, N. K., Velerod, M. B., & Brox, J. I. (2004). Fear-avoidance beliefs and distress in relation to disability in acute and chronic low back pain. *Pain, 112*(3), 343–352.
Guyton, G. P. (1999). A brief history of worker's compensation. *The Iowa Orthopaedic Journal, 19*, 106–110.
Hadjistavropoulos, T. (1999). Chronic pain on trial: The influence of litigation and compensation on chronic pain syndromes. In A. R. Block, E. F. Kremer, & E. Fernandez (Eds.), *Handbook of pain syndromes: Biopsychosocial perspectives*. Mahwah, NJ: Lawrence Erlbaum Associates.
Hadjistavropoulos, T., & Bieling, P. (2001). File review consultation in the adjudication of mental health and chronic pain disability claims. *Consulting Psychology Journal: Practice & Research, 53*(1), 52–63.
Harmon, K. G., Drezner, J. A., Gammons, M., Guskiewicz, K. M., Halstead, M., Herring, S. A., et al. (2013). American medical society for sports medicine position statement: Concussion in sport. *British Journal of Sports Medicine, 47*(1), 15–26.
Harnois, G., & Gabriel, P. (2000). Mental health and work: Impact, issues, and good practices. Geneva: Mental Health Policy & Service Development, Department of Mental Health & Substance Dependence, World Health Organization. http://www.who.int/mental_health/media/en/712.pdf. Accessed 17 November 2017.
Health and Human Services. (2013). Modifications to the HIPAA privacy, security, enforcement, and breach notification rules under the health information technology for economic and clinical health act and the genetic information nondiscrimination act; other modifications to the HIPAA rules. 45 CFR Parts 160 & 164.
Hyman, M. H. (2016). Work ability and return to work. In L. Kertay, M. Eskay-Aurbach, & M. H. Hyman (Eds.), *The AMA guides to navigating disability benefit systems*. Chicago: American Medical Association.
Kendall, N. A. S., Burton, A. K., Main, C. J., & Watson, P. (2009). *Tackling musculoskeletal problems: A guide for clinic and workplace*. London: The Stationery Office.
Kertay, L. (2016). The health care professional's role in disability benefit systems. In L. Kertay, M. Eskay-Aurbach, & M. H. Hyman (Eds.), *The AMA guides to navigating disability benefit systems*. Chicago: American Medical Association.
Kertay, L., Eskay-Auerbach, M., & Hyman, M. H. (2016). Introduction. In L. Kertay, M. Eskay-Aurbach, & M. Hyman (Eds.), *The AMA guides to navigating disability benefit systems*. Chicago: American Medical Association.

Kroenke, K., Spitzer, R. L., & Williams, J. B. (2001). The PHQ-9: Validity of a brief depression severity measure. *Journal of General Internal Medicine, 16*(9), 606–613.

Lagerveld, S. E., Blonk, R. W., Brenninkmeijer, V., Wijngaards-de, M. L., & Schaufell, W. B. (2012). Work-focused treatment of common mental disorders and return to work: A comparative outcome study. *Journal of Occupational Health Psychology, 17*(2), 220–234.

Laisne, F., Lecomte, C., & Corbiere, M. (2012). Biopsychosocial predictors of prognosis in musculoskeletal disorders: A systematic review of the literature. *Disability & Rehabilitation, 34*(5), 355–382.

Loisel, P., & Anema, J. R. (2014). *Handbook of work disability: Prevention and management.* New York: Springer.

Lynch, K. M. (2001). *Essentials of disability income insurance* (3rd ed.). Bryn Mar, PA: American College Press.

MacLeod, F. K., LaChapelle, D. L., Hadjistravropoulos, T., & Pfeifer, J. E. (2001). The effect of disability claimant's coping styles on judgments of pain, disability, and compensation: A vignette study. *Rehabilitation Psychology, 46*, 417–435.

Matuszack, J., & Plasecki, M. (2012). Inter-rater reliability in psychiatric diagnosis. *Psychiatric Times, 29*(10).

Metropolitan Life Ins. Co. v. Glenn, 554 US 105. (2008). https://supreme.justia.com/cases/federal/us/554/105/. Accessed 30 Oct 2017.

Miller, A. R., Cain, D. J., Roos, P. S., & Roos, P. A. (1980). *Work, jobs, and occupations: A critical review of the dictionary of occupational titles. Final report to the US Department of Labor from the committee on occupational classification and analysis*. Washington, DC: National Academy Press.

Moore, E., Thibault, P., Adams, H., & Sullivan, M. J. L. (2016). Catastrophizing and pain-related fear predict failure to maintain treatment gains following participation in a pain management program. *Pain Reports, 1*(2), e567.

Morantz, C. A. (2005). ACC statement on preparticipation cardiovascular screening for competitive athletes. *American Family Physician, 72*(3), 523–527.

Pransky, G., Katz, J. N., Benjamin, K., & Himmelstein, J. (2002). Improving the physician role in evaluating work ability and managing disability. *Disability & Rehabilitation, 24*, 867–874.

Pransky, G. S., Verman, S. K., Okurowski, L., & Webster, B. (2006). Length of disability prognosis in acute occupational low back pain: Development and testing of a practical approach. *Spine, 31*(6), 690–697.

Quartana, P. J., Campbell, C. M., & Edwards, R. R. (2009). Pain catastrophizing: A critical review. *Expert Review of Neurotherapeutics, 9*(5), 745–758.

Rafferty, M. N., Murphy, A. W., O'Shea, E., Newell, J., & McGuire, B. E. (2013). Effectiveness of a cognitive behavioural therapy-based rehabilitation programme (progressive goal attainment program) for patients who are work-disabled due to back pain: Study protocol for a multicentre randomised controlled trial. *Trials, 14*, 290.

Rainville, J., Pransky, G., Indahl, A., & Mayer, E. K. (2005). The physician as advisor for patients with musculoskeletal complaints. *Spine, 30*, 2579–2584.

Reme, S. E., Grasdal, A. L., Lovvik, C., Lie, S. A., & Overland, S. (2015). Work-focused cognitive-behavioural therapy and individual job support to increase work participation in common mental disorders: A randomised controlled multicentre trial. *Occupational & Environmental Medicine, 72*, 745–752.

Salmon, P. (2006). Explaining unexplained symptoms: The role of beliefs in clinical management. In P. W. Halligan & M. Aylward (Eds.), *The power of belief: Psychosocial influence on illness, disability, and medicine*. New York: Oxford University Press.

Schussler-Fiorenza, R. S. M., Eslinger, J. G., Zimmerman, L., Scaccia, J., Lai, B. S., Lewis, C., & Allsic, E. (2016). Adverse childhood experiences, support, and the perception of ability to work in adults with disability. *PLoS One, 11*(7), e0157726.

Scott, W., & Sullivan, M. (2012). Perceived injustice moderates the relationship between pain and depressive symptoms among individuals with persistent musculoskeletal pain. *Pain Research & Management, 17*(5), 335–340.

Shaw, W. S., Pransky, G., & Winters, T. (2009). The back disability risk questionnaire for work-related, acute back pain: Prediction of unresolved problems at 3-month follow-up. *Journal of Occupational and Environmental Medicine, 51*(2), 185–194.

Social Security Administration. (2017a). Residual functional assessment: Introduction: Programs Operations Manual System (POMS). https://secure.ssa.gov/poms.nsf/lnx/0424510001. Accessed 29 Oct 2017.

Social Security Administration. (2017b). *Disability evaluation under Social Security: Mental disorders – adult*. https://www.ssa.gov/disability/professionals/bluebook/12.00-MentalDisorders-Adult.htm. Accessed 25 Nov 2017.

Sullivan, M. J., Adams, H., Rhodenizer, T., & Stanish, W. D. (2006). A psychosocial factor-targeted intervention for the prevention of chronic pain and disability following whiplash injury. *Physical Therapy, 86*(1), 8–18.

Sullivan, M. J., Scott, W., & Trost, Z. (2012). Perceived injustice as a risk factor for problematic pain outcomes. *The Clinical Journal of Pain, 28*(6), 484–488.

Sullivan, M. J., Yakobov, E., Scott, W., & Tait, R. (2014). Perceived injustice and adverse recovery outcomes. *Psychological Injury & the Law, 7*(3), 325–334.

Sullivan, M. J. L., & Simon, G. (2012). A telephonic intervention for promoting occupational re-integration in work-disabled individuals with musculoskeletal pain. *Translational Behavioral Medicine, 2*(2), 149–158.

Sullivan, M. J. L., Ward, L. C., Tripp, D., French, D. J., Adams, H., & Stanish, W. D. (2005). Secondary prevention of work disability: Community-based psychosocial intervention for musculoskeletal disorders. *Journal of Occupational Rehabilitation, 15*(3), 377–392.

Talmage, J. B., Melhorn, J. M., & Hyman, M. (2011). How to think about work ability and work restrictions: Risk, capacity, and tolerance. In J. B. Talmage, J. M. Melhorn, & M. H. Hyman (Eds.), *AMA guides to the evaluation of work ability and return to work*. Chicago: American Medical Association.

Theunissen, M., Peters, M. L., Bruce, J., Gramke, H. F., & Marcos, M. A. (2012). Preoperative anxiety and catastrophizing: A systematic review and meta-analysis of the association with chronic post-surgical pain. *The Clinical Journal of Pain, 28*(9), 819–841.

Thompson, T., Correll, C. U., Gallop, K., Vancampfort, D., & Stubbs, B. (2016). Is pain perception altered in people with depression? A systematic review and meta-analysis of experimental pain research. *The Journal of Pain, 17*(12), 1257–1272.

Turner, J. A., Franklin, G., Fulton-Kehoe, D., Sheppard, L., Stover, B., Wu, R., et al. (2008). ISSLS prize winner: Early predictors of chronic work disability: A prospective, population-based study of workers with back injuries. *Spine, 33*(25), 2809–2818.

US Department of Labor. (1991). *Dictionary of occupational titles* (4th ed.). Washington, DC: US Department of Labor.

US Department of Labor. (2017). O*NET online, https://www.onetonline.org. Accessed 28 Oct 2017.

US Equal Employment Opportunity Commission. (2010). EEOC policy on reasonable accommodations. http://www.eeoc.gov/eeoc/internal/reasonable_accommodation.cfm#1. Accessed 29 Oct 2017.

Waddell, G., & Burton, A. K. (2006). *Is work good for your health and Well-being?* London: The Stationery Office.

Wakefield, J. C. (2016). Diagnostic issues and controversies in the DSM-5: Return of the false positives problem. *Annual Review of Clinical Psychology, 12*, 105–132.

Woo, A. K. M. (2010). Depression and anxiety in pain. *Reviews in Pain, 4*(1), 8–12.

Word Health Organization, WHO. (1993). The ICD-10 classification of mental and behavioural disorders. http://www.who.int/classifications/icd/en/bluebook.pdf?ua=1. Accessed 25 Nov 2017.

World Health Organization, WHO. (1992). *International statistical classification of diseases and related health problems, tenth revision*. Geneva, Switzerland: World Health Organization.

World Health Organization, WHO. (2017). International standard. http://www.who.int/classifications/icd/en/. Accessed 25 Nov 2017.

Young, A. E., Wasiak, R., Roessler, R. T., McPherson, K. M., Anema, J. R., & van Poppel, M. N. M. (2005). Return-to-work outcomes following work disability: Stakeholders motivations, interests, and concerns. *Journal of Occupational Rehabilitation, 15*, 542–556.

Young, G. (2015). Malingering in forensic disability-related assessments: Prevalence 15 ± 15%. *Psychological Injury & the Law, 8*(3), 188–199.

Chapter 15
The Legal System and Behavioral Health

Robert M. Aurbach

15.1 Causes of Action and Their Prevalence

It is beyond the scope of this chapter to examine the practices and causes of action available in all jurisdictions and under all laws. Rather, the purpose of this chapter is to acquaint the reader with general concerns that arise more or less frequently. Of necessity, individual variations in practice are excluded from this discussion, and no criticism of any individual's legal practice or of any specific class of practitioners is intended or implied.

The prevalence of behavioral concerns in our system of legally based dispute resolution (henceforth, "the legal system") is not well known. One of the reasons for this lack of information is the diversity of contexts in which the person experiencing behavioral health concerns can interact with the legal system. Any dispute submitted to legal resolution involves the claimant and defendant in a bewildering maze of unfamiliar rules and demands, the subjugation of control of various aspects of one's life to external authority, and the stress of having a matter of great personal concern winding, sometimes interminably, through a system that is opaque to him or her. These more general impacts of the legal system will be dealt with elsewhere in this analysis.

At the same time, some issues within the legal system focus directly on the behavioral health challenges of the litigant. A basic tenant of American law is that there must be a case or controversy over which the court-like entity has jurisdiction for the legal system to be invoked. The shorthand term for the recognized case or controversy is "cause of action." The causes of action in which behavioral health issues are most likely to be in issue include workers' compensation claims and enforcement of rights both under the Americans with Disabilities Act (ADAAA) (as amended) and under federal and state laws against violation of civil rights, in tort claims of various types, and in the enforcement of disability insurance provisions

R. M. Aurbach (✉)
Uncommon Approach, Inc, Melbourne, VIC, Australia
e-mail: Rob@uncommonapproach.com

P. A. Warren (ed.), *Handbook of Behavioral Health Disability Management*,
https://doi.org/10.1007/978-3-319-89860-5_15

and claims for Social Security Disability Insurance (SSDI). There are also several factors affecting our knowledge of the prevalence of behavioral health claims that cut across most or all of the various causes of action and affect many of such claims.

15.1.1 Workers' Compensation

Workers' compensation is the generic name given for the 53 state and territorial programs that provide medical treatment and indemnity benefits to workers covered under the provisions of the specific law for injuries and occupational illnesses occurring in the course and scope of work.

In addition, the Federal government has a general program for governmental employees and several specific programs for specialty populations. The SSDI program covers long-term disability. Some sovereign tribal entities have adopted their own tribal workers' compensation provisions.

Each of the statutory schemes in these jurisdictions is different and provides different benefits and procedures for the perfection of rights. The differences include very significant variation in the extent to which claims are brought to the attention of a centralized record keeper and variations in the manner in which centralized records of claims made in the system are recorded. There is no central collector of standardized workers' compensation statistical data; although several organizations do research across many or all jurisdictions to an extent, no research quantifying the prevalence of behavioral health concerns across all jurisdictions has been published.

Moreover, the extent to which behavioral health concerns are compensable under the various workers' compensation laws varies widely. Some states allow claims for workers' compensation based solely upon the behavioral impacts experienced in the workplace; some states limit claims based upon behavioral concerns to those that are resultant from a sudden, discernable trauma or the direct or indirect result of physical trauma; and some states purport to ban such claims altogether. In this environment, many behavioral health concerns are not separately reported from the physical injury to which the claim is attached. These reporting difficulties are further compounded by the development of mental health concerns arising as a secondary result of prosecuting a claim through the system. There is no state or territory that measures the prevalence or extent of these iatrogenic secondary psychological claims, although they are undoubtedly a major contributor to claim costs (Aurbach, 2015). Accordingly, the prevalence behavioral health concerns in workers' compensation can only be estimated (Warren, 2009).

15.1.2 Americans with Disabilities Amendments Act of 2008

The ADAAA provides protection against employment discrimination for persons with physical and mental limitations or challenges. The ADAAA requires covered entities, including certain private employers, to provide reasonable accommodations to the known physical or mental limitations of an otherwise qualified individual with a disability who is an applicant or employee, unless such covered entity can demonstrate that the accommodation would impose an undue hardship, pursuant to U.S.C. 12112(b)(5) (A).Two crucial issues under the law are the definition of disability and the concept of "essential functions" of the job. Section U.S.C. 12102(2) provides that covered worker is disabled under the act if one has a physical or mental impairment that substantially limits one or more of the major life activities of an individual, have a record of such impairment, or are regarded as having such impairment. A worker with a disability who can perform the essential functions of his or her job is disabled under the act and entitled to its protections. Under the definitions in the original act, workers with behavioral health concerns were seldom afforded protection because of failure to qualify as a protected disabled person.

The ADA was amended in 2008 (Public Law 110-325, effective January 1, 2009), and the amendments appear to have greatly expanded the effective definition of disability with respect to behavioral concerns. The definition of disability itself remained unchanged, but the effects of mitigating measures (except for vision correction lens) are not to be considered when determining the extent of interference with the major functions of everyday life. Under the new amendments, virtually any condition that can interfere with work and is subject to control with medication, treatment, or assistive technology is likely to be covered, including common behavioral health concerns. The definition of major functions of everyday life has been expanded to cover bodily functions. Episodic conditions or conditions in remission are to be considered active.

The ADAAA appears to have given significant additional range of protection for behavioral health concerns ranging from depressive disorders, anxiety disorders and trauma-related disorders, neurodevelopmental disorders, and attention deficit/hyperactivity disorders, at least where there is sufficient proof on the record. It should be noted, however, that there were not many appellate cases reported during the first 5 years under the amendments despite an apparent increase in ADAAA claims (Goldberg, 2013).

15.1.3 Civil Rights Enforcement Under 42 U.S.C. 1983 and Under State Civil Rights Laws

After the Civil War, Congress passed remedial legislation intended to keep the states from perpetuating the discrimination against persons of color. The complaining person must prove two critical issues: a "person" subjected the aggrieved party to acts "under color of state law" and the acts deprived the aggrieved person of rights, privileges, or immunities guaranteed under federal law or the US Constitution. The state itself is not a "person" within the meaning of the section, and the requirement for action "under color of state law" refers to an action taken in the context of the authorized duties of the accused. Thus, if state law authorizes law enforcement officers to conduct traffic stops of suspected violators, the officer is a person acting under the cover of state law when he makes such traffic stops. If the reason for stopping a person is related to, say, the ethnicity of the person stopped, rather than to the driving behavior, the claim under Section 1983 may be complete.

Certain groups are afforded a heightened standard of judicial protection. These groups are called "suspect classifications," and claims of actions against such groups may go forward with a lower standard of evidence of discriminatory intent. Persons with behavioral health concerns are not considered a "suspect classification" under the law. As a result, successful claims under Section 1983 for discrimination based upon the aggrieved person's behavioral health have been rare. The effects of the alleged discrimination in causing or exacerbating behavioral conditions are sometimes offered as an element of harm for which monetary compensation is sought. Many states have a parallel remedy under state law, subject to similar limitations. Some states have specific anti-discrimination laws pertaining to people with behavioral health concerns.

The impact of behavioral health concerns in claims under the various federal and state anti-discrimination laws is not accurately documented for a variety of reasons, including, but not limited to, the differences in record-keeping protocols that make combining the data from such records difficult and the lack of detail surrounding the nature and source of damages alleged present in statistical summaries of such claims.

15.1.4 Psychological Torts

There are a number of causes of action for the redress of personal injuries, and they are generically referred to as "torts." Several of them pertain to injuries to the behavioral health of the aggrieved person, and collectively they may be described as psychological torts. An essential feature of traditional tort law is the notion of fault. An act must be intentionally done, or done negligently, in violation of a duty to avoid harm, to be actionable (at least in the absence of some special "no-fault" statutory provision). Of necessity, these claims are difficult to prove, and of varying degrees of success, because of the inherently hidden nature of the harm. Even with a competent diagnosis, some jurors tend to discount behavioral health injuries either because of perceived lack of objectivity associated with them or because of a tendency to separate emotionally from the possibility that they could similarly be harmed.

15.1.4.1 Intentional Infliction of Emotional Distress

Intentional infliction of emotional distress is a cause of action utilized for the redress of intentional psychological harm. The harm complained of is a change in the behavioral health status of the plaintiff. Therefore, the plaintiff is subject to examination with regard to both current and past behavioral health. Since the cause of action is predicated on an adverse change of condition, the cause of action forces the plaintiff to prove that he or she has been the victim of wrongdoing and that, as a result, his or her behavioral health has suffered.

The change in behavioral health status is relatively hard to prove, and the cause of action requires the plaintiff to attach the public stigma of behavioral health concerns to themselves in a public manner. Given these concerns, juries do not generally respond well to these actions. They are not commonly asserted as stand-alone grounds for recovery.

15.1.4.2 Hostile Working Environment (Sexual Harassment)

Sexual harassment lawsuits may proceed under one or more of three available theories. The case might allege that the plaintiff was actually subjected to unwanted physical contact, that he or she was given or offered benefits in exchange for sexual concessions or threatened with adverse consequences if such concessions were refused, or that he or she was subjected to a hostile working environment that contained unwanted sexual content. The nature of this last theory for claiming sexual harassment places the behavioral health of the claimant into issue in the case, as the unwanted nature of the content must be proven, as well as any harm for which damages are sought.

These lawsuits are reasonably common, and some of the successful ones have been highly visible. Persons subject to sexual harassment are readily seen as "victims" for whom much of the stigma of public assertion of behavioral health concerns may be diminished.

15.1.4.3 Post-traumatic Stress Disorder and Other Psychological Claims Rising from Traumatic Events

When a traumatic event causes damage, psychological injuries are often claimed as an element of the damages. The claims themselves are based upon the negligence or intentional act that caused the damage, such as an assault or a failure to maintain proper control of an automobile. An element of any tort action is that it caused damage and the size of the damage award is based, at least in part, on the extent of the damages that are proven. Accordingly, a change in the plaintiff's behavioral status is often alleged as part of the damages in the case. The assertion of that element of damages places the plaintiff's psychological state in issue in the lawsuit, subjecting him or her to examination, testimony, and cross-examination concerning both prior and present behavioral health concerns. Post-traumatic stress disorder is a common example of this element of damages. The diagnosis, which was originally developed to describe the effects of the incredible brutality and stress of warfare, has been (often inappropriately) generalized by enterprising plaintiff attorneys (and sympathetic mental health practitioners) to apply to the emotional aftermath of almost any unpleasant experience. It should be noted that the negative effects of "medicalization" of the claim upon the claimant (see Sect. 15.5, below) are sometimes inadvertently caused by the desire to find a diagnosis to support an enhanced claim for damages. Tort claims are most often filed in at the state court level where record keeping is not detailed and often is only generally tabulated as to the nature of the claim. Detailed central tabulation at the state level is rare, and multistate tabulation of records is hampered by inconsistent record-keeping formats. Details such as the elements of damage asserted are often not available for study absent specific examination of individual files. Moreover, when a jury awards damages, it often does not specify the specific harm for which the damages were awarded. Accordingly, little is known about the prevalence of the assertion of these elements of damages, or about the success associated with such assertions, except in connection with local studies in a specific jurisdiction.

15.1.5 Disability and Health Insurance Claims

Insurance for disability has at least two incarnations: some states, such as California, have mandatory short-term employer-based disability insurance programs for most workers. The majority of states do not have such programs, and disability insurance is available as a private purchase insurance option or as part of an employee benefit program. In most instances, insurance-based disability programs contain provisions for the settlement of disputes outside of a traditional legal framework. Provisions requiring arbitration, or other alternative dispute mechanisms, are common in disability insurance contracts.

Health insurance has similar dynamics, with most health insurance available on a private purchase or employee benefit basis. Public-based health insurance options are more prevalent among the states but often cover specific populations, rather than the broad spectrum of workers in general. Use of mandatory alternative dispute resolution procedures is quite frequently a feature of such insurance contracts.

In this context, disputes concerning care for behavioral health concerns seldom find their way into the formal court system. Rather, disputes over whether the insurer has met the obligations of the insurance contract in good faith are sometimes asserted as a cause of action in state courts. The behavioral health concerns of the plaintiff sometimes find their way into such lawsuits as elements of the damages alleged, but for the reasons stated above in connection with psychological torts, the prevalence of such allegations is not well documented across broad populations.

The SSDI system also has a captive dispute resolution protocol involving its own specialized judges and criteria for proof. Importantly, the criterion for receipt of benefits is proof of the inability to do any kind of work. Thus, in this context, the claimant must consider himself or herself completely disabled to get benefits and model a lifestyle consistent with that expectation. SSDI reports that 34.8% of its claims are for behavioral health concerns, but additional claims present a combination of physical and behavioral reasons for disability (Annual Statistical Report on the Social Security Disability Insurance Program, 2015; Warren, 2009).

15.1.6 General Considerations Concerning Reporting of the Prevalence of Behavioral Health Claims

There are several reasons to believe that behavioral health claims are significantly underreported (Warren, 2009). These include the stigma attached to behavioral health claims and the tendency for them to be swept up in general privacy protection requirements, the concentration of the legal system of the documentation of physical ailments, and the failure to properly diagnose and document elements of harm that are based on behavioral health issues.

15.1.6.1 Stigma

Notwithstanding the remedies outlined above for redress of discriminatory treatment of persons with behavioral health concerns, stigmatization of such persons is widespread. Responses vary from overt discrimination to social disadvantage, and the subtle value judgments of persons with such challenges are even imbedded in our language. We have no lack of derogatory terms for people with behavioral health challenges. "Crazy," "whacko," and "nut case" are not complementary terms when used to describe a person. "Special" takes on a whole different meaning in the phrase "special education." Thus, we are taught from a young age that such challenges are shameful and should be hidden from view. Emphasis is placed in privacy policies, especially those concerning health records, to especially safeguard records concerning behavioral health issues. Service groups such as the Black Dog Foundation and beyondblue in Australia and the Anxiety and Depression Association of America and the Depression and Bipolar Support Alliance in the United States have focused upon overcoming this stigma by encouraging persons with depressive disorders to come forward and seek help. Most recently, the British royal family has been publically involved in such initiatives. These phenomena evidence the degree to which behavioral health concerns are regarded as something which has been hidden from public view. As a result, it is reasonable to assume that some percentage of the affected population self-selects avoidance of any activity that could "label" them and therefore that the reported prevalence of such claims is artificially suppressed.

15.1.6.2 Concentration on Physical Ailments

The legal system operates on the presumption that the complaining party has the burden of proving the harm claimed. That proof must be made to skeptical claims examiners or to a judge or jury with no personal stake in the outcome. In that context, the natural tendency is to seek and concentrate upon elements of claims or damages that are objectively verifiable and demonstrable. Subjective claims concerning conditions that have no obvious physical manifestations are simply harder to prove, since they require the person or group delegated the authority to determine facts in the dispute to accept the word of an expert or the assertion of an interested party. As a result, there is a natural tendency for advocates in the system to focus first on the objectively demonstrable harms and damages and to throw additional issues in for whatever they are worth. In the traditional assessment of the value of a tort claim, for instance, the presumptive measure of damages is some multiple of "actual" damages (medical expense, lost wages, property damages) and "special" damages (including most behavioral harms such as depressive or anxiety disorders arising from the physical harm) that may or may not be included in the calculation. As a result, especially given the stigmatization associated with such claims and the tendency for assertion of such damages to generally place the behavioral health of the claimant into issue in the case, assertion of such claims is likely artificially suppressed or is often hidden as a secondary element of damages. In addition, treating physicians often do not look for behavioral harm resulting from a physical injury (American Medical Association, 2008a, 2008b) and therefore often miss them when they are present, due to lack of training or awareness, time pressures, or lack of a behavioral baseline from which differences can be noticed.

15.1.6.3 Failure to Diagnose Behavioral Health Concerns

Since advocates tend to focus on physical harms and claimants have a tendency to minimize or keep secret behavioral health concerns, symptoms are often not brought to the attention of the examining health-care providers. The health-care provider diagnoses and treats the conditions brought to his or her attention and may or may not delve into behavioral health issues. Even if the health-care provider who is treating the claimant for his or her physical symptoms both notices and understands the significance of presenting signs or symptoms of behavioral health issues, they are often inadequately equipped, by training and experience, to diagnose or treat such conditions. Referral to an appropriate mental health specialist is an extra step, for which there is little reinforcement. As a result, behavioral health concerns often go undiagnosed, further suppressing the reported prevalence of such issues in the legal system.

15.2 What Works, and What Does Not Work, in Legal Representation of Persons with Behavioral Health Concerns

The legal system is a complex and unintuitive dispute resolution mechanism. Navigation of the intricacies of that system is possible for the persons who do not have legal representation, but such litigants are often at a substantial disadvantage in utilizing (and defending against) the procedural and evidentiary requirements of a lawsuit and in understanding the development of the law with respect to their particular cause of action and its requirements.

To understand the impact of the legal system on participants with behavioral health challenges, it is necessary to closely examine the roles played by the advocates upon whom they rely for guidance through the unfamiliar processes of the legal system. The lawyer for the claimant (plaintiff) in an action has a substantially different role than the lawyer for the person or entity against whom the claim is filed (defendant). Understanding those roles and the underlying economic motivations is crucial to understanding the impact of participation in the system. It is also helpful to understand the issues that are created by the health-care professionals upon which either side relies.

15.2.1 Plaintiff's Lawyers

There are two distinct varieties of plaintiff's lawyers, operating under different economic models and therefore subject to differing sets of motivations. The private plaintiff's lawyer is generally compensated by the plaintiff, either out of the plaintiff's resources or (most often) out of the proceeds of the recovery from the case.

The public attorney is paid a salary by an entity for which he or she works and provides services to the plaintiff without expecting compensation from the plaintiff. Regardless of the role and source of compensation, the role of the plaintiff's lawyer is to win the case before him. The lawsuit is, to the plaintiff's attorney, a classic "zero-sum" game where one party wins and the other loses.

15.2.1.1 The Private Plaintiff's Attorney

The private plaintiff's attorney is most often compensated on the basis of a "contingent fee" arrangement whereby the attorney invests his or her time in the perfection of the case without compensation, in exchange for a contractual right to a percentage of the proceeds of the claim. The percentage of the ultimate recovery can vary widely, but most often is between 25 and 33% of the award of damages to the plaintiff. This arrangement creates two motivations: the attorney is unlikely to accept cases on this basis that are unlikely to generate a substantial award (and thus a substantial fee) either because the case is unlikely to be successful or because the case has too little at stake by way of economic outcome to generate a fee that will compensate the attorney at the rate they desire. The calculation of the assessment of the case is complex and subject to both economic and noneconomic influences. A case that "develops the law" in a new and untested direction might be accepted if the potential for the eventual outcome is high enough or if the attorney particularly believes in the direction of development for which he or she is advocating.

Private plaintiff's attorneys may also accept cases on the basis of payment at a predetermined hourly rate. The rates charged by attorneys vary quite widely, depending on the market in which they operate, their experience, and overhead. Typically, a claimant is asked to deposit a "retainer" in such cases, against which the attorney draws periodically at the specified hourly rate. If the retainer is depleted, the plaintiff is usually required to deposit further funds before the attorney invests additional time in the case.

The private plaintiff's attorney is often caught between two paradigms. On the one hand, he or she often feels that they are advocates for the disadvantaged and the champion of the little person. On the other hand, the economics of practice, particularly under contingent fee arrangements, require them to reduce all claims to monetary value, prioritize their representation choices based on the potential size of the award, and focus their resources on the maximization of that award.

The economics of practice under contingent fee arrangements also dictate that a percentage of cases will fail to generate fees or will generate fees that are insufficient to adequately compensate the attorney for the time invested. This creates a motivation to keep the volume of open cases large enough to generate an income stream and to file all cases under every conceivable legal theory that is available or that can be imagined as an extension of existing law. The long pendency of lawsuits exacerbates the tendency to keep high volumes of cases presenting multiple theories of relief. It is not unusual for a case to persist for over a year from the initial filing of the complaint that initiates it until judgment after trial that resolves it, and this period can be substantially extended by appellate proceedings. The long resolution times combined with the economics of contingent fee practice also create a substantial pressure to settle pending lawsuits by agreement, and the urge to settle sometimes puts the attorney into a conflict of interest situation with the client who wants his or her "day in court."

In cases of certain rights violation allegations, and many cases involving workers' compensation, the defendant may be required to pay some or all of the claimant's attorney fees, subject to order of the court adjudicating the case.

15.2.1.2 The Public Plaintiff's Attorney

There are public advocacy organizations that employ attorneys to provide free representation to qualifying individuals. Most often, cases that have the potential to generate a fee through a monetary award to the plaintiff are excluded from these services upon the presumption that a private plaintiff's attorney can be found to provide representation. Where the remedy sought is the enforcement of a right, or the development of the law in a particular direction, the public plaintiff's attorney may become involved.

Since the public plaintiff's attorney is paid a fixed (and often comparatively low) salary, there is no motivation to maximize the monetary value of the claim. Rather the motivation comes from the choice to represent the population and the political, philosophical, and social agenda of the employing organization. Cases are sometimes determined to be worthy by the organization, and plaintiffs are then recruited to allow the organization to go forward and seek development of the law in a particular direction. The concerns of the particular litigants in such cases are not necessarily the attorney's primary focus.

Public plaintiff's attorneys are often regarded as possessing inferior skills, based upon perceptions of their chosen role. This is often inaccurate, as these attorneys often develop superior knowledge and skills in a focused area of law and possess strong internal motivation. It is also true that public plaintiff's law is used as a training ground for inexperienced attorneys, who eventually move on to more lucrative practice.

15.2.2 The Defense Attorney

Defense attorneys also come in various incarnations. Private defense attorneys may be employed to defend an insurer who is potentially liable for damages on the claim or by the defendant directly. Governmental attorneys defend public agencies from claims against those entities. In either case, the defense attorney may be directly employed by the client or may work for a private firm of attorneys representing the client. The defense role is also to win the case brought to them. Since contracted attorneys are in a purely reactive mode, responding to claims that have already been asserted, they are in a modified zero-sum game. Reduction of a liability below the expected level may be considered a "win" since the attorney had no choice concerning the acceptance of the claim and entered the case too late to have free reign to defend as he or she sees fit. In-house counsel sometimes has the opportunity to avoid claims by proactive intervention.

15.2.2.1 Defense Attorneys Who Are Compensated According to Contract

Defense attorneys who contract with insurers, private entities or persons, or governmental agencies for defense of claims against them are usually compensated on the basis of an agreed hourly rate (although a flat rate per case defended is occasionally utilized). The motivation set for such attorneys is a balance of efficiency in claims resolution (to please the client) and a desire to aggressively defend the claim (to accumulate the greatest number of billable hours). The defense attorney is not in primary control of the overall approach to litigation, however. The employing entity most often decides the litigation approach either on a case-by-case basis, or as an overall policy, and finds an attorney who will acquiesce in the strategy. Depending on the willingness of the paying entity to fund aggressive litigation, the behavior of the contractual defense attorney may range from a desire to quickly settle every claim to an aggressive procedural and substantive defense. Strategy in such aggressive defenses includes tactics designed to delay resolution of the claim and "starve out" the claimant and procedural manipulations designed to sap the litigation resources of the plaintiff through multiplication of expensive preliminary procedures such as extensive discovery and motions practice. These tactics are successful when the willingness of the plaintiff and his or her advocate to invest further time and energy is impacted. The ultimate goal of this "scorched earth" defense is to encourage the plaintiff to give up the claim or force settlement at a fraction of the value of the claim.

15.2.2.2 Salaried Defense Attorneys

The salaried defense attorney, whether working for a governmental agency or as in-house counsel for either the defendant directly or for one's insurer, is less motivated by the economic ramifications of practice and more by the management of risk for their employer. Typically, such defense counsels are motivated to minimize the damages in particular cases, as an overall measure of their effectiveness. In-house (noninsurance) and governmental defense attorneys may also take action within their organization to prevent similar claims from arising in the future. However, when given direction to do so, salaried defense attorneys are also capable of utilizing the considerable resources of their organizations to engage in aggressive defense practices.

15.2.3 Treating Professionals

Both the plaintiff and defense bars rely on behavioral health professionals in making their cases between more attractive and saleable in court. When there is a relationship between a court advocate and a health-care professional that is habitual in nature, it is likely that economic motivations influence both, although that influence may not be recognized at a conscious level. The advocate is searching for an opinion that suits the needs of the theory of the case. The health-care provider gets a referral for an evaluation and potentially for treatment after the lawsuit. If the opinion does not match the needs of the attorney, then the health-care provider does not get more referrals. Even without conscious intent, the defense bar and plaintiff's bar develop, over time, their stables of "reliable" health-care providers, and the health-care providers tend to nurture that relationship. Even where the relationship is entirely innocent of opinion influence, the tendency for attorneys to choose health-care providers with known tendencies friendly to their position is common. Bias in determining the individual's psychiatric disability status can result (Harding, 2004).

15.2.4 What Works, and Does Not Work, in the Legal System?

It is important to understand that, despite popular misconceptions, the legal system in the United States is not designed to necessarily produce a just result but rather is designed as a decision generation engine. At the end of the day, when the legal system is done with a claim, there will be a decision. The parties may or may not find it satisfying, but there will be finality, and there are extensive rules designed to preclude re-litigation of the same issue after the legal system has processed it completely. This production of finality is one of the chief functional successes of the legal system.

Access to attorneys for representation is generally not a significant problem, but there are notable exceptions in particular circumstances. There is no national shortage of attorneys, and as evidenced by lawyer advertisements, there is competition among attorneys for clients. Most fee-generating cases can be matched with an attorney hungry enough to take them on, albeit not always the most experienced attorney for the case at hand.

However, plaintiffs with certain classes of cases that will not generate a fee commensurate with the work involved in perfecting the claim may experience difficulty in finding representation. This phenomenon is particularly evident with respect to workers' compensation claims where the benefit in issue is limited to treatment for medical or behavioral concerns. In such cases, the usual measure of compensation is a percentage of the benefit obtained by the services of the attorney. If the value of the benefit sought is sufficiently low and the difficulty in perfecting the right is sufficiently high, the plaintiff's attorney is unlikely to accept the case. Defense lawyers know this and discourage representation by threatening aggressive defense that will require a substantial investment of time to overcome. The result is that some workers' compensation clients seeking treatment only for medical or behavioral concerns (or seeking only modest levels of other benefits) are effectively denied representation by the structure of the system. Some states have developed public advocacy attorney organizations to manage this phenomenon. The phenomenon is also present in other claims where there is a contingent fee arrangement and the potential damages (and therefore the attorney's fee) are relatively low.

Public advocacy attorneys, and encouragement of representation on a pro bono basis by bar organizations, are widespread and available to qualifying individuals with appropriate claims. Representation on this basis may not be as available in rural areas, although the special needs of disadvantaged populations are a particular emphasis of many public advocacy organizations. As noted earlier, the representation of individuals may sometimes be compromised by the overall social, philosophical, or political agenda of the organization.

Contingent fee arrangements allow plaintiffs to pursue claims without the necessity of placing large sums of money on retainer for their attorney, when such resources are often not available. This allows claims to be freely brought. The consequences of such fee arrangements include crowding of the courts, "strike suits," and subsidization of dubious claims by claimants with more conventional claims. Success in litigation generates fees, and therefore claimant's attorneys are encouraged to pursue the reduction of claims to an economic value through the legal process, often to the exclusion of other remedies. This creates expectations in the public (fed by lawyer advertisements) that perceived wrongs are a potential source of monetary awards. The courts then experience demand for their dispute resolution services based upon the expectations of the public, and long delays are the result, as demand outstrips judicial resources. While some courts have resorted to alternative dispute resolution techniques to manage their caseload, delay in litigation resolution remains a problem.

The ultimate extension of this trend is the "strike suit." A claim of dubious merit may be filed with the knowledge that the cost of defending the claim exceeds the value of a small settlement to make the claim "go away." While there are court rules designed to control this behavior, most judges are former practicing attorneys, and some are reluctant to enforce the intent of such rules, whether by reference to their own former practices or because of continuing relationships with the attorneys against whom such enforcement would fall.

As a practical matter, contingent fees usually compensate attorneys at a level that is disproportionately high for the effort expended. This is regarded as justified because of the risk of failure of the claim and the resultant risk that the attorney will be uncompensated for his or her efforts. As a practical matter, the practice results in systemic subsidization of dubious claims, and efforts to extend the law, by claimants that have routine claims that will generate fees without any substantial risk of uncompensated work. It also results in a lack of willingness to take on anything but routine low-risk claims by some attorneys, potentially affecting access for people with unique circumstances.

On the defense side, privately contracted defense attorneys get paid to defend claims and not to find solutions for problems or prevent their recurrence. The image of a "junkyard dog" is given grudging admiration as a model for behavior. The task of managing risk exposure and return to work efforts is most often delegated to other personnel.

In general, the legal system stops when the claim is resolved. There is no follow-up to see if the litigants have resolved their issues and moved on with their lives. While economic provision for future medical care is made in workers' compensation cases and some tort cases, litigants are often left to seek resources for the resolution of their behavioral health concerns on their own. The advocate for the claimant has no systemic motivation to assist him or her after the claim is completed, depriving the claimant of what may have been their only support system during the lengthy pendency of the litigation. Planning for functional adaptation and treatment after the dispute is resolved is often lacking. Once the projected future costs of functional recovery are reduced to a monetary figure and an award is made, the claimant is most frequently left to his or her own devices with regard to actually obtaining services.

Some practices in the legal system overcompensate for harm. The doctrine of "punitive (or exemplary) damages" allows a litigant with actual damages to seek an additional award in many tort (but not workers' compensation) cases. This award is not designed to compensate the claimant but rather to punish the defendant for wrongdoing and/or serve as an exemplar for others to avoid the behavior that formed the basis for the complaint. Punitive damages exacerbate the tendency for the system to cast the claimant in the role of "victim" and encourage "legalization" of the claim. They are also quite popular with attorneys who work on a contingent fee basis, as the attorney gets their percentage of these awards.

The process of litigation is itself highly stressful on the litigants. The claim is submitted to a dispute resolution forum that has its own (often counterintuitive) rules that require professional help to navigate. The claimant's personal behavioral health may be placed in issue, depending on the nature of the claim, and his or her privacy invaded. Loss of a sense of personal control is frequently experienced, as is enhanced focusing on the wrong suffered or condition experienced. The process is long, invasive, and uncertain in outcome. The stress of litigation can exacerbate the harm that gave rise to the claim or create new behavioral concerns. These facts are sometimes used by the defense as part of a strategy to discourage claimants from pursuing their rights.

15.3 Determining Current Behavioral Functioning in the Legal System

The determination of harm in the legal system arises from a simpler time when the issues presented were less complex. The legal system, with its reliance on prior precedent for future guidance, has been slow to adapt to the demands of more complex case presentations. This weakness of the system in its adaptation is particularly evident with respect to behavioral health concerns. As behavioral health effects have gained recognition as elements of damage, the issue of correctly assessing the mental aspects of the harm from the physical or other elements of damages has become difficult. So too has the issue of causation, where the ability to attribute the onset of behavioral health concerns to a specified event is critical to the establishment of the requirement that the event complained of caused the harm for which damages are sought. This issue of causation particularly applies to tort and workers' compensation cases. Thus, the determination of the level of current behavioral functioning and the determination of the causal connection between prior events and the current behavioral health status are issues of importance in the legal system, even though the current status of scientifically based determination of behavioral health functioning sometimes cannot keep pace (Melhorn and Ackerman 2008). This can lead to further complication of the already complicated relationship between lawyers and behavioral health practitioners discussed earlier in Sect. 15.2.3 and result in more unpredictability and variation in diagnosis and impairment rating than would be desirable.

15.3.1 The Legal Standard of Proof Concerning Scientific Evidence

For testimony concerning the degree of harm, or the causal link between the acts giving rise to the legal claim and the harm, to be considered by the entity in the legal system that will decide the facts (the judge or the jury, depending on the cause of action, the tactical choices of the parties, and the requirements of applicable statutes), the testimony must be determined to be reliable. The general rule of law is that reliable evidence will (with exceptions not usually relevant here) be considered in the determination of the case, and unreliable evidence will not. In general, for evidence of a scientific nature to be considered ("admissible"), the reliability of the evidence is determined by a rule of evidence.

With respect to scientific evidence, the Circuit Court of Appeals for the District of Columbia announced, in 1923, a standard of evidence still used in some states in a case that has become known as the *Frye* opinion (Frye v. United States, 293 F. 1013 (CADC, 1923). In that opinion, the court announced a standard for reliability of scientific evidence that was based upon the general acceptance of the basis of the scientific testimony in the particular field of scientific inquiry. This standard is conservative when it comes to the acceptance of new or novel theories, definitions, or (importantly for behavioral concerns) diagnoses. If a new behavioral diagnosis is not "generally accepted" in the behavioral health community, it cannot form the underlying basis of testimony that a particular claimant does or does not suffer from it.

In 1993, the US Supreme Court announced a new standard and overruled the *Frye* case. In *Daubert v. Merrell Dow* (henceforth, *Daubert*), the court rejected the inflexibility of the *Frye* test in favor of an independent judicial assessment of the reliability of the evidence. Factors to be considered by the court reviewing scientific evidence reliability include the degree to which the scientific theory has been empirically tested, the extent to which it has been peer reviewed and published, and the qualifications and professional stature of the witness presenting the testimony. Because of the procedural footing of the case, it did not become binding on the states, and at present, approximately one third of the states still follow the *Frye* standard, one third follow *Daubert*, and the remainder have developed their own standard or a hybrid between *Frye* and *Daubert*. Thus, the legal standard for admissibility of scientific evidence, and therefore the admissibility of testimony that a particular person has a particular behavioral health concern, is subject to state-by-state variation and uncertainty.

This is particularly true when a plaintiff is attempting to "extend" the law by establishing that a novel, or newly discovered or described, behavioral health concern is an appropriate basis for an award of damages. Testimony about the objective existence of the "new" behavioral health concern can become the principle litigated issue in some cases. The plaintiff in such a setting may be subjected to unusual systemic pressures to internalize the purported diagnosis.

In the context of this uncertainty, the presence on the *Diagnostic and Statistical Manual-5* (American Psychiatric Association, 2013) presents complications not present with respect to prior editions. Presence of a diagnosis in the *DSM-5* (APA, 2013) was almost always accepted as sufficient under that *Frye* or *Daubert* standards for establishing the definition of a behavioral health. The same cannot be confidently said at this time with respect to *DSM-5*. There is substantial professional disagreement about the appropriateness of some diagnoses under *DSM-5* and some controversy concerning the influences of interested parties in the course of its creation (Francis, 2012; NHS Choices, 2013). The existence of dispute about the underlying reference volume within the expert population renders its usage in jurisdictions utilizing the

Frye standard subject to challenge. There is a substantial likelihood that the admission of testimony about a *DSM-5* diagnosis of a particular claimant will be preceded by a protracted "mini-trial" on the issue of the reliability of the science underlying the proposed testimony in such states, at least with respect to one of the diagnoses that are the subject of controversy.

With respect to testimony concerning the degree of impairment of function caused by a behavioral health concern, the same legal considerations apply to expert opinion, but there are sometimes other modes of approaching the issue. The law of evidence allows a non-expert to give one's opinion about one's own experience or about matters for which special expertise is not regarded as necessary, such as matters within the general knowledge of the average person. Thus, the person with a behavioral health concern generally can testify as to what s/he experience and how it affects her or him. To translate the experience of the plaintiff into a quantified measure of impairment of his or her functioning usually requires the assistance of a behavioral health expert.

The sixth edition of the AMA *Guides to the Evaluation of Permanent Impairment* incorporates a chapter on "Mental and Behavioral Disorders" (American Medical Association, 2008a, 2008b) that relied heavily on the *DSM-IV-TR* for its diagnostic underpinning. The chapter provides, unlike prior editions of the *Guides*, numerical ratings for some selected and well-documented major mental illnesses. Even where applicable, the majority of states have not adopted the sixth edition of the *Guides* for purposes of workers' compensation cases, although its use for tort cases may be more widespread. No other document with the credibility of the Guides that provides numerical impairment guidance is available. This deficit in objective impairment guidance leaves the determination of impairment of function due to behavioral health concerns largely unconstrained from the legal perspective, opening the door to vigorous litigation of the issue.

This litigation usually takes the form of "dueling experts." The plaintiff and defense arrange for opinion evidence to support higher or lower assessments of impairment. Both sides examine the plaintiff to assess the impairment claimed. The plaintiff is subjected to a process that has a tendency to entrench existing impairment and may create additional behavioral health concerns (see, Sect. 15.5, below).

The assessment of impairment in a legal context is usually limited to the assessment of current impairments of functioning for the purpose of determining and quantifying liability. Little or no analytical energy or emphasis is placed on the prospective restoration of functioning in this process, and the plaintiff may incorporate the message that his or her recovery of functionality is of little importance to the legal system.

A judge or a jury will be put into the role of making a determination concerning the relative weight to be given to the evidence presented in the case. In workers' compensation cases, juries are seldom utilized. In tort cases, the use of juries as the "trier of facts" is much more common. With respect to determination of the degree of impairment caused by a behavioral health concern, the trier of facts must make determinations concerning the basis of testimony and credibility of experts discussing a highly technical and specialized area of knowledge. The degree to which most judges can reasonably understand and distinguish credible testimony about behavioral health concerns can reasonably be questioned, given that most have not institutionally received training in the interpretation of such evidence. The expectation that a jury of people with wide variations in education and experience could make accurate determinations in this area is naïve.

15.4 Case Coordination and Coordination of Care

With regard to cases involving monetary compensation for a harm, people go to lawyers when they feel aggrieved as to their rights or feel that they are unable to comfortably perfect their rights without professional assistance. If the lawyer feels that it would assist in making a claim, he or she may attempt to steer the client to a health-care provider that, from prior history or reputation, is likely to support the claim (for an interesting study of the outcome of this behavior, see Victor, Barth, & Neumark, 2005). The defense bar also often has its stable of sympathetic health-care providers to whom the defense advocate will turn when a sympathetic opinion about the case is desired. The Model Rules of Professional Conduct (American Bar Association, 1993) for attorneys are silent on the issue of referrals to or from other professions, except for a general prohibition against receiving payment from another to represent a client without the client's informed consent (American Bar Association, 1993, Rule 1.8). These practices are reportedly widespread, but not meaningfully quantified.

Such referrals as do exist, in either direction, are generally for the development of a particular position in the case rather than for the purpose of advancing the care of the party. The greater the harm demonstrated to the judge or jury deciding the facts, the greater the compensation, and the greater the plaintiff's attorney's fee. The less harm shown, the more successful the defense and the greater credit to the defense attorney, resulting in a continuing stream of case referrals. Accordingly, the focus of referrals in a litigation context is the demonstration (or questioning) of disability and its quantification, rather than the restoration of functional ability.

Follow-up services provided by the advocate to the client after the end of the case are relatively rare, and focused attention on the restoration of client's functional ability is usually lacking. There is no economic incentive for such follow-up impacting either the plaintiff or defense bar, and services provided for such coordination are often uncompensated. Orders from the resolving adjudicatory body to continue jurisdiction over a case after its resolution, for the purpose of ensuring functional restoration of the claimant, are generally not permitted. In the legal system, once the decision is made in the case in front of them, the advocates and adjudicator move on to the next case. There is some reason to believe that this "abandonment" of the claimant after the development of a dependency on the advocate during the course of the claim exacerbates the harm suffered by the claimant. (See Chap. 16.)

In litigation to resolve the rights that have been alleged to be violated (particularly alleged workplace violations), it is more common for the advocate of the claimant to continue involvement, if only to be on the lookout for retaliation against the claimant by the employer, which may give rise to another cause of action. Moreover, in that context, it is more common for the remedy to involve restoration of some sort of relationship between the parties, rather than simple monetary award. The remedy that is fashioned may be monitored concerning its success and the good faith of the parties in implementing it.

Coordination of care between various health-care providers may or may not be a priority during litigation, depending on which party is being considered. The plaintiff's advocate has no economic motivation to expend time and effort on the coordination of care, other than that needed to ensure that a consistent message is presented to the judge or jury deciding the case. There is sometimes a motivation for the claimant's advocate to seek assistance in client control during the process, especially where behavioral health concerns make controlling the client's behavior problematic. The defense advocate has greater motivation in seeking coordination between health-care providers but usually for the purpose of limiting the overall expenditures for services, discovering inconsistencies between the representation made by the claimant to various health-care providers, or discovering inconsistencies with the statements or behavior exhibited by the claimant generally. Although individuals vary in their behavior, neither the plaintiff's or defense's advocate is institutionally concerned with the outcome of care, as they will have moved on to the next case before care issues are resolved. Accordingly, coordination of care is most often delegated to other professionals.

15.5 Medicalization of Claims

The legal system unintentionally encourages "medicalization" of a claim. Diagnosis, particularly diagnosis supported by some authoritative reference, tends to fulfill the *Frye* or *Daubert* criteria for admissibility of evidence concerning the behavioral concern that is connected with the plaintiff's claim. By giving it a name, the diagnosis demonstrates the general acceptability of the assessment of disability or adds weight to the independent assessment of the court, creating conditions that allow the admission of evidence of disability. Without such evidence, the cause of action or the limitations that give rise to an award of damages under the cause of action cannot be proven. Thus there is significant pressure created by the legal system to find a diagnosis for the plaintiff as part of the process of bringing a claim. These pressures impact the behavior of the attorneys as well as the attending behavioral health professionals. Even without improper economic motivation, the attorney seeks to win, and the strength of the case is improved by the appending of an established diagnosis to the symptoms.

Once the diagnosis is determined, individual variations among claimants for development of disability really come into play. Research has demonstrated that psychosocial factors are good predictors of the development of disability after injury (Bruns & Disorbio, 2009; Fayad et al., 2004; Jellema, van der Horst, & Vlaeyen, 2006; Main, Sullivan, & Watson, 2007; Van der Windt, Hay, Jellema, & Main, 2008). Many claimants recover fully and are not affected adversely by the dynamics of the legal system. For some, the outcome is much more difficult.

The claimant hears the diagnosis and sees it being built into the litigation strategy of the attorney. There is discussion of the claim for damages, and through questioning about the limitations experienced, the claimant quickly learns that the more disabled he or she is, the larger the claim for damages is likely to be. The attorney begins to refer to the plaintiff as a disabled person, and the perceptions of both shift to match the requirements of the task at hand – proving the disability. Claimants may hear and internalize the subtle messages imbedded in the language commonly used in the system and may start identifying with the role of the "injured worker," "accident victim," or "person whose rights have been violated." Surveillance and other documentation of daily activities becomes a factor, particularly in workers' compensation cases, and claimants understand that they may not do things that are inconsistent with their claim. Normal movement and activities of daily life are curtailed, either through reaction to the perceived expectations created in the litigation environment or through a natural guarding of an injured area from reinjury, and the physical effects of inactivity exacerbate the already existing symptoms of injury. The process of incorporating chronic limitations into daily life begins. As this process extends over time, the probability of the worker ever returning to one's pre-injury employment is significantly diminished (Bartley, 1994; Bellamy, 1997; Gerdtham & Johannesson, 2003; Guirguis, 1999; Harris, Multford, Solomon, van Gelder, & Young, 2005; Jin, Shah, & Svoboda, 1995; Johoda, 1983; Martikainen & Valkonen, 1998; Mathers & Schofield, 1998; McGill, 1968; McKee-Ryan, Kinicki, Song, & Wanberg, 2005; Nachemson, 1983; Organisation for Economic Co-operation and Development [OECD], 2009; Sander & Meyers, 1986; Stewart, 2001; Strang, 1985).

In the process of presenting the best possible case for a large award of damages, the natural tendency is for attorneys to project the worst possible case into the future, for the purpose of creating motivation for the award of maximized future damages. When an individual projects the worst-case scenario into the future, behavioral health experts are likely to refer to the phenomenon as "catastrophic thinking" and take therapeutic steps to assist the person in recasting one's thinking into more useful directions. When the same behavior takes place in the courtroom, litigators consider it good advocacy and seem unconcerned that the claimant may internalize the characterization, engage in his or her own catastrophic thinking about one's condition and prospects, and create behavioral conditions conducive to one's failure to restore full functioning (Barsky & Borus, 1996; Horwitz & Wakefield, 2007). Indeed, conversations with plaintiff attorneys about their clients are usually scattered with reference to lives that have been irretrievably shattered, with no hope of meaningful restoration and only a large award as solace. If the guide to this mysterious process has given up hope for the claimant's recovery, the claimant's opinion is likely to follow (Aurbach, 2013).

The legal process is one where the claimant is almost always subject to a loss of sense of control. Control is lost to the lawyers and judges running the process of dispute resolution, a health system that casts the patient in to the role of passive recipient and claims examiners who may control the means to obtain the basic needs of day-to-day living. This loss of control may combine with increasing focus on physical limitations, resulting in the litigant becoming increasingly identified with their cause of action and diagnosis. The claimant may change one's perceptions to fit one's new identity. When the new identity is entrenched, it is difficult for the worker to regain a sense of wholeness and independence. This is a systemic variant of "medicalization" of a claim, involving the larger actions of the entire medicolegal system in the process. The resulting encouragement of an identity as a disabled person, internalization of limitations consistent with that role, and change of perceptions so that experience in the world is interpreted to reinforce those limitations have been sometimes called "attorneyogenic disability." The legal system has shown no conscious awareness of the impact of this "medicalization" on the plaintiff's long-term well-being, although there is a tendency for the plaintiff's advocate to assert that the original diagnosis, once established, is a permanent condition. Unfortunately, the legal process itself may help fulfill this prophecy.

15.6 Professional Enabling

Lawyer audiences, and individual practitioners, inevitably assert that the behaviors described elsewhere in this chapter are certainly not the way they personally conduct business. Often they will protest that it is wrong to generalize with regard to the lawyers at all and certainly that it is unfair to characterize the entire profession as motivated solely or even primarily by personal gain.

The criticism is justified, to an extent. Legal education in the United States has been focused, during much of the last 50 years, on training students to "think like a lawyer." The term is often used as shorthand for the process of training someone to take any side of an argument, without regard for one's personal beliefs. While the socialization of students to disassociate from one's personal values has been widespread, there are certainly many individuals who make career choices that allow them to feel a personal sense of comfort with the positions that they take. These positions are often taken without regard to the remunerative nature of the representation. However, the attorney who avoids the trap of being influenced by pecuniary gain should not be secure in the belief that one's actions do not contribute to the disability of one's clients.

"Enabling" is a term applied, often in the context of alcoholism, or other issues involving familial dysfunction, to describe the behavior of protecting someone from the consequences of their actions. An alcoholic's enabler might make excuses to the alcoholic's work supervisor to keep him or her from getting fired, create explanations to friends and family, and deceive him- or herself into thinking that everything is normal or at least a reasonable response to abnormal stressors. The enabler does so in the belief that one is helping keep the family together and providing for stability and normalcy (Wegscheider-Cruse, 1989).

Professionals can also take the role of an enabler. When a lawyer acts as an enabler, he or she may act to save the client from the consequences of one's actions. The most obvious example of this behavior is the defense of criminal matters. If the aim of defense is to help the client "get off" with respect to the charges, then the professional role is to spare the client the consequences of one's actions. This enabling behavior often separates the client from the resources needed to address the underlying behavioral health issues. Indeed, the archetypical criminal defense lawyer only resorts to treating the underlying problem as a less onerous outcome to incarceration in cases where the guilt of the client can clearly be proven such that a plea bargain is advised under the circumstances. Similar kinds of services are performed in assisting the client deal with employment difficulties, marital and familial situations, economic obligations, and other aspects of everyday life.

Other types of professional enabling are subtler and more pervasive. The ads on television loudly proclaim that "you may be entitled to a cash award" or a similar phrasing. The message to clients is that they are owed something by the world, that is, that they should focus not on their own choices, options, and empowerment but rather on the notion that "fairness" demands that they receive something in compensation for what has been done to them by someone else. This focusing of the client on an outside agency as the source of one's problems, and one's ultimate salvation, protects the client from having to take psychological responsibility for one's circumstances. This enabling behavior allows the client to become "stuck" in the identity of a victim. It is not hard to conjure up examples of individuals who became controlled by their identity as a victim to the extent that they psychologically foreclosed the possibility of change in their circumstances. In this context it is not surprising that Dr. Christopher Brigham refers to attorneys as "the victim makers" (Brigham, 2015).

Interestingly, the author's personal experience speaking to audiences demonstrated that when offered the opportunity to write himself or herself a check for any amount of money in exchange for accepting a disabling injury or condition, virtually, no one indicates that one would find the exchange acceptable. The terms used by the legal system to refer to the payment at the end of the case are interesting in that context. The term "cash award" is often used – including the connotation of an award as recognition for some achievement. The term "settlement" is often used, implying that once the money is paid, the whole matter is settled, notwithstanding the fact that the client still has to live with the disability thereafter. Sometimes the reference is just to "cash" or "money." In all these cases, the concept that a payment is the appropriate mechanism for compensation has the tendency to objectify the client's condition and divorce the client from the consequence of choosing to be disabled rather than making the best of the life available to a person in one's present condition. This form of enabling distracts the client from one's power to make meaningful choices concerning the life one leads and saves the person from the emotional and psychological consequences of those choices. In this sense, the reduction of behavioral health disability to the product of an outside agency for which pecuniary compensation is the only appropriate redress has insidious consequences and may combine with or exacerbate the underlying behavioral health issues in ways that may be difficult to predict.

15.7 Symptom Magnification and Malingering

The issue of symptom magnification and malingering is one that varies substantially depending on the point of view of the parties. Not surprisingly, these terms are frequently used imprecisely, giving rise to confusion in discussion of the phenomena.

15.7.1 The Importance of Language

What we say about people with behavioral health concerns in the legal system has an impact on their future recovery and reintegration. The goal of the zero-sum game of litigation is to obtain the largest possible award or defeat the claim entirely. In this context, both sides utilize language that has a tendency to force the claimant into the position of defending and rendering habitual, the behavior that underlies the behavioral health claim.

In the process of making the best possible case for a large award, the claimant's advocate seeks the most inflammatory description available, because that will likely result in the largest award (and fee). The claimant hears that description and understands that his or her job is to ratify the description with his or her behavior and model the description credibly as a witness. See discussion of "medicalization of claims," in Sect. 15.5. The description of a behavioral health concern becomes a role that the claimant plays during the (often extended) pendency of the claim. Behaviors practiced over time become habitual. Thus the attachment of terminology to a set of symptoms in the context of litigation has consequences that tend to increase the possibility of needless, iatrogenic disability.

At the same time, the claims examiner and defense counsel question the credibility of the diagnosis, as part of the process of opposing each item of liability or damages. Attacking the diagnosis either requires the attorney to attack the qualifications or methods of the examining behavioral health practitioner or to attack the validity of the behavioral data on which it was based. This second form of attack looks, sounds, and feels to the claimant like an attack on one's personal credibility and integrity. In response, the claimant has a natural tendency (sometimes encouraged by plaintiff's counsel) to defend one's status and make one's behavior more obvious and pronounced so that it will not be questioned. This behavior, in turn, may occasion claims of symptom magnification or malingering from the defense. This overt attack on credibility results in further defense of the behavior that is being questioned (Lippel, 1999; Guthrie & Monterosso, 2009).

This might be seen as an inevitable result of the litigation process, present whenever less confrontational dispute resolution measures are not availing. The trouble is that language is misused frequently in litigation contexts and that this misuse exacerbates the long-term harm to the claimant (Talmage, 2007). One of the most egregious examples of this phenomenon is in the use of the terms "symptom magnification" and "malingering."

15.7.2 Symptom Magnification

"Symptom magnification" as used in legal context is a habitual focus on physical symptoms that exceeds "normal" expectations, but "normal" is in the eye of the beholder. Most people have had the experience of finding a cut or bruise and being unable to recall the circumstances of acquisition of the injury. Most people can recall instances when a minor incident caused completely focused attention on the immediate physical sensation and an overreaction to the objective harm incurred. "Normal" perception of symptoms falls within that rather broad range of experience. Symptom magnification occurs when the range of perceptions shifts toward the focused attention end of the spectrum. The person experiencing this shifted focus often experiences concurrent expectations of sensation and/or fear of sensation that reinforces the focused attention. Over time, focus upon one's sensations, and the emotional content associated with them, has a tendency, through normal processes of habit formation (the neuroscientists would refer to "brain plasticity" as the mechanism for this phenomenon), to become habitual and entrenched (Duffau, 2006; Kolb & Whishaw, 1998; Oakley & Halligan, 2009; Strang, 1985). Symptom magnification is established.

15.7.3 Malingering

"Malingering" is generally a more value-loaded concept in the law. The term is usually used to describe someone who emphasizes or extends his or her sensations or limitations in the expectation of secondary gain (Aronoff et al., 2007; Conroy & Kwartner, 2006; Mittenberg, Patton, Canyock, & Condit, 2002; Reid, 2000). *Secondary gain* is a neutral term that describes the seeking of external reward for behavior (Schultz & Gatchel, 2005). Secondary gains range from increased sympathy and attention from loved ones, through permission to avoid disagreeable tasks, to increased experience of disability in expectation of enhanced awards of damages. The seeking of *secondary gains* (at least at the lower levels of the continuum) is a natural behavior that is experienced by most of us in everyday life. The seeking of secondary gain can become destructive, however. The behavior can lead to avoidance of the activities and responsibilities of everyday life. When that happens, interference with normal activity and relationships can cause secondary physical or behavioral health harms.

Malingering is properly defined as the intentional display of behavior in the calculated attempt to obtain external benefits (secondary gain) that would not be otherwise forthcoming. Malingering is a species of fraud, involving an intentional misrepresentation of condition, known to be a misrepresentation when expressed, with the intent and for the purpose of obtaining a benefit to which the person would not otherwise be entitled.

15.7.4 Other Reward-Seeking Behaviors

There is another species of behavior that occurs quite frequently and is often mistaken for, or confused with, malingering. People learn to get what benefit they can out of conditions and circumstances with which they are presented. We say, "When life hands you lemons, make lemonade." All of us have learned that "feeling bad" sometimes gets us out of unpleasant activities. We may actually experience the stomach ache that gets us out of going over to dinner with relative who is a dreadful cook. When we are ill or hurt, we often get extra nurturance and attention. We do not stop and think of the causal connection but sometimes "make a fuss" and get a little extra warmth from those close to us. These behaviors are part of our everyday primary (internal) reward-seeking behavior (Schultz & Gatchel, 2005), established over time by classic operant conditioning. Most of the time, the mechanism operates without our conscious direction or decision. We might call this class of behavior "reward seeking" in the absence of an established term. But in the context of the law, there is a tendency to treat any reward-seeking behavior as evidence of malingering. Since both the focus of the behavior (*primary* vs. *secondary gain*) and the intention (unconscious vs. premeditated) distinguish "reward seeking" from "malingering," this is error. The mislabeling of reward-seeking behavior as malingering forces the reward seeker to defend and focus upon that behavior. The result is the entrenchment of the behavior and magnification of the perceived intensity. Thus the mislabeling of innocent normal behavior as malingering increases symptom magnification behavior and the probability of unnecessary disability.

15.7.5 Control of Symptom Magnification and Malingering by the Plaintiff's Advocates

As discussed above, it is unsurprising in the legal context that some claimants intentionally adopt behaviors or limitations that enhance the probability of success of their claim. Since in the legal system disability is rewarded and ability is not, these adopted behaviors are often inconsistent with activity that would assist the claimant in regaining function. Malingering and symptom magnification work contrary to the regaining of full function. Thus, control of those behaviors is a legitimate systemic concern.

The question of control of symptom magnification and malingering by the plaintiff's advocate is really a question of motivation. The greater the apparent disability of the plaintiff, the greater the award in fee-generating cases and the greater the emotional appeal of the case in causes of action that are intended to perfect or secure rights. In this paradigm, there is no institutional reason to suppress these behaviors.

As noted above, *symptom magnification* has a tendency to become an entrenched behavior. Such behaviors are more likely to be consistently displayed to treating healthcare providers and be employed to subjectively support a diagnosis. The existence of a diagnosis is highly useful in establishing the admissibility of evidence of harm, which is particularly important in cases where the harm is not visible or objectively verifiable to the judge or jury. Typically, a diagnosis is buttressed by the plaintiff's overt display of symptoms to the jury. Behavior on the witness stand is often coached, and the plaintiff's lawyer may speak to the claimant in terms that objectify and reinforce his or her sense of disability. In these ways, symptom magnification is often intentionally or unintentionally encouraged by the plaintiff's advocate.

An ethical attorney will not intentionally encourage malingering. Moreover, symptom magnification and malingering can make the attorney's job more difficult and less efficient by making the client more demanding or more logistically difficult to deal with. The legal system does not provide plaintiffs' attorneys with financial compensation, resources, or training for the purpose of assisting their clients with behavioral health concerns that bring them to the legal system or that are exacerbated by the inherent stressors in the system.

15.7.6 Control of Symptom Magnification and Malingering by Defense Advocates

When defense of cases is treated as a zero-sum game, there is a natural tendency to look for any possible "pry point" in which to get leverage to limit or avoid liability. In this context, questioning the objective existence of the symptoms claimed by the claimant is a popular approach to case defense. The defense directly, and through its experts, often question the veracity of the symptoms claimed. The claimant is put into a position of "defending" his or her symptoms from an adverse judgment. This requires the claimant to focus more attention upon those symptoms. This situation is exacerbated by accusations of symptom magnification or malingering, which bring the claimant's character and integrity into issue as well as one's behavioral symptoms. The claimant often feels that she or he is under personal attack. This dynamic forces the claimant to focus on the continuation and justification of one's symptoms, rather than upon symptom resolution and reintegration into normal life. Thus, defense against a behavioral health claim may extend or exacerbate it inadvertently.

15.8 Facilitating Return to Work and Stay at Work Behaviors

Attorneys involved in the process of litigation are not generally overly concerned about the process of returning the injured person to work (or keeping him or her at work in the first instance). The tendency is to focus upon the zero-sum game of litigation and move on to the next case as soon as the current case is resolved. The principle exception to this phenomenon arises when the claimant's work activity affects the damages that may result from the case. It is not uncommon to hear workers' compensation claimants complain that their attorney "won't let them" return to work, despite current economic hardship caused by the discrepancy between disability benefits and wages before the work stoppage. It is likewise common for such claimants to complain that the employer, defense doctors, or the defense counsel is trying to force the worker back to work prematurely. This dynamic arises primarily in those causes of action that seek monetary compensation as a remedy (Kilgour et al., 2015).

In civil and employment rights litigation, there is more opportunity built into the system for the parties to engage in pre-litigation attempts to mitigate or avoid the claim. In this context, it is possible for behavioral health issues to be raised in a more informal pre-litigation context and for them to be addressed as a problem to be solved rather than as an item of damages. If an attorney is employed prior to the initiation of a claim, the attorney may accept a private retainer, or a promise of future payment by the offending governmental entity or private employer, to represent the claimant in an effort to avoid litigation. In this role, the claimant's attorney seeks to encourage the cooperation of the employer and to resolve the issue prior to (threatened) litigation. In this context, return to work and specific accommodations in the workplace to facilitate staying at work are commonly negotiated. This procedural posture allows negotiation about work conditions and accommodation of behavioral health needs that is often unavailable once the party's positions are solidified by the pendency of litigation.

This kind of interaction carries its own psychosocial dynamic. The claimant may feel a sense of personal immunity from discipline and a sense of empowerment to make demands upon the employer for special treatment in the workplace, due to the backing of the attorney and the continuing threat of litigation. In the alternative, or at the same time, the worker may feel a sense of alienation due to one's unique status and the reaction of management and one's co-workers to his or her special status.

The employer in this situation may feel like he or she constantly has a "gun to the head" and may seek to find ways to make the claimant want to leave, may ignore the claimant, or may give in to every demand. The response may be similar to the response of an employer to being given a political appointee (in governmental service) or a relative of the boss (in private industry). Employers tend to mix recovery and personnel issues inappropriately. An injury becomes an excuse to get rid of a troublesome employee rather than facilitate their return to the workplace. The worker's time off for recovery may be seen by the employer as their vacation from the stress of supervising someone who is less than fully compliant or controllable, and early return to work may not be seen as a virtue in such cases. Contact with the employee, which is crucial to keeping them engaged in their identity as a worker, may be avoided. Even enlightened employers, who realize that prolonged absence from work increases the chances of permanent disability, can fall into inappropriate avoidance behaviors and inadvertently or intentionally encourage iatrogenic disability.

Excellent attorneys are aware of these dynamics and seek to heal the relationship between the employer and worker, before moving on to the next case. The healed relationship is more likely to be valued by both sides, resulting in more opportunity and willingness to return to work. The attorney may proceed by addressing the emotional components of the underlying experience of each through mediation, team building, and other conciliatory exercises. These efforts may emanate from either the plaintiff or defense advocate.

15.9 Appropriate Documentation of Objective Impairment and Limitations of Functioning

The process of determining what is reliable evidence of impairment and functioning is of great significance in the fashioning of an enlightened approach to behavioral health in the workplace. The responsibility for providing and coalescing such information falls on several parties in the system. The employer has the responsibility to provide accurate information concerning the functional demands of the job. The physical health-care provider has the responsibility for assessing the current physical condition of the worker and to obtain an accurate assessment of the duties of the job before making an assessment of duty limitations. The behavioral health professional has the duty of determining whether there are limitations based directly or derivatively on the injury. Optimally, the attorney advocates have the role of coordinating all these sources of information and bringing them together in a sensible manner. Regrettably, the dynamics of litigation (or even the threat of litigation) undermine these optimal roles by introducing outcomes that influence the behavior of the parties.

15.9.1 Distinguishing Between Objective and Subjective Evidence

In the context of claims of injury, the documentation of objective evidence of impairment and functional limitations begins substantially before the report of a behavioral health concern. It is important to have the actual job duties and performance standards documented and available for review. Often, when a health-care provider attempts to make a decision concerning the ability of a worker to return to work, they will interview the worker as to the nature and requirements of the job and seek no further information. The worker's view of the job is likely to be affected by his or her perceptions, the interpersonal relationships between the worker and his or her supervisor and co-workers, his or her perception of their current health status, and other psychosocial issues, such as symptom exaggeration. Provision of an existing objective description of essential job functions, working conditions and production demands, as well as other medical records, including mental health, to the examining health-care provider may create increased accuracy in the prognosis concerning return to work.

Similarly, prompt and thorough investigation and documentation by the employer concerning the circumstances of the injury can be important, although it is usually seen as being of greater significance in physical injuries than in behavioral health concerns. If it is well known how the behavioral health concern is reported to have occurred, there is a much better chance of distinguishing whether the concern is related to an event or if it was a preexisting concern. Investigation and documentation by the employer of the circumstances where the behavioral health concern arose may also help establish when harm was caused in a manner related to the workplace (workers' compensation) or by the actions of the defendant (other tort claims).

The objective assessment of impairment and limitations on functioning is dealt with elsewhere in this volume. It is important for the parties to be aware of the history of judicial acceptance with respect to scientific evidence in their jurisdiction. If the creation of objective evidence of impairment and limitations of function is based upon a methodology that has not been previously judicially tested, then much of the benefit associated creating the documentation may be lost. If the results of a novel testing protocol are not accepted by one party or the other, litigation under the applicable admissibility standard is likely to follow.

Attempts to reintegrate the person with a behavioral health concern into the workforce should also be carefully documented. The issue of good faith by the employer in accommodating the limitations of the worker in an employment context can give rise to its own cause of action for "retaliation" against the worker for the act of making a claim. Objective recording of the placement, efforts to make the worker successful, and actual performance of the worker are critical to avoiding inappropriate claims. Accurate recording of the actual performance of the worker in the placement will also give guidance to managers.

15.9.2 *Impact of Objective and Subjective Evidence*

When the parties focus upon subjective evidence of impairment and limitations, such as the worker's self-reporting of physical conditions or job duties, the possibility of greater variations in the outcome changes the litigation dynamics. If subjective evidence is introduced into the litigation process and treated as credible, then the possibility of a much larger award is created for the plaintiff. If the plaintiff relies on subjective evidence and is unsuccessful in establishing its credibility, then the defense has a better chance of defeating the claim outright or sharply limiting the liability exposure. Thus advocates for both sides have strong motivation to focus their attention on the subjective evidence, as its presence in the case creates a "risk-reward" calculus that makes their involvement in the case valuable. It is this "risk-reward calculus" that makes the adversarial process so difficult for injured workers and employers. The definition of "winning" has changed from rehabilitation and reintegration of the worker to maximizing or minimizing the extent of the award, and the possibility that the legal system will create disability that was avoidable becomes significant.

In contrast, when only objective evidence of behavioral health concerns (such as testing results verified for reliability and validity and diagnoses based upon clear causal evidence and objective criteria) is present in the case, there is little role for traditional litigation approaches. Based upon a rational analysis of the objective evidence, the "winner" of the case is usually easy to determine. If objective evidence determines that the plaintiff has a valid claim, then it can be paid appropriately and the energy and expense that would have been spent upon litigation can be devoted to return to work efforts and prevention of future harms. If objective evidence shows the claim to be invalid, then the probability of it being brought by the attorney relying on a contingent fee for compensation is diminished.

It would be naïve to think that the presence of objective evidence in a case will persuade parties to rely upon it exclusively. However, the presence of well-documented objective evidence of impairment and loss of function will inform the parties of what the likely outcome of the claim will be and the likely range of liability exposure and allow better choices concerning allocation of resources to be made. The addition of empirically based practice guidelines for the treatment of behavioral health concerns only increases the predictability of the outcome and reduces the costs associated with dispute resolution. When the outcome is predictable, there is less economic gain to be had by pursuing a dispute, and rational resolutions are encouraged.

15.10 Dispute Resolution Outcomes

When considering dispute resolution in the legal system, formal litigation is the model that most often comes to mind. This is true despite the fact that the overwhelming majority of cases are settled before the parties ever present their cases to a judge or jury. The reasons for this misperception probably arise from popular entertainments – settlement of cases does not make for good drama, in the way that a good confrontation in the courtroom does. The litigants are not unaffected by this dynamic. The desire for a "day in court" probably arises from the conditioned expectation that "justice" is the product of court proceedings. As noted previously, the law is not a justice engine, but rather a dispute resolution engine. It is not nearly as important to society that an individual dispute be resolved fairly as it is that the dispute be resolved finally, allowing society (if not the individuals) to pick up the pieces and move on in relative peace. Thus, the outcomes of dispute resolution after traditional litigation are not often stories of successful restoration of function and reintegration into the pre-harm lifestyle. The litigants are left in much the same (or worse) behavioral health circumstances as they were in before, except now the plaintiff may or may not be richer and the defendant (or his insurer) has spent money to defend the lawsuit and perhaps to pay damages.

If resolution of claims is the ultimate outcome, then approaches other than formal litigation can also achieve the desired results. The possibility exists to view disputes as an opportunity to fix problems, improve the system in which the problem occurred, and prevent future occurrences of harm. This role, in a legal context, has been called "counselor at law."

When a lawyer adopts the role of "counselor at law," the focus shifts from winning disputes to the prevention and solving of human problems in a legal context. The purpose of the counselor at law in a case is not to gain advantage for one side at the cost of the other but to find solutions that enhance the outcomes of both. The role of litigation advocate is not consistent with the role of counselor at law, and the roles tend to attract different personalities. However, some attorneys have developed the capability of switching between roles, as the needs of the situation dictate.

The advantages of the counselor's role to the plaintiff's interest in the ultimate outcome of the case are evident. In traditional litigation, dispute resolution is defined by one party winning and the other losing. The aftermath of this system is not conducive to the recovery of the parties, particularly in the context of behavioral health concerns. The complaining party has had to adopt the role of victim to pursue their claim. This attitude may become internalized and persistent. Especially in behavioral health claims, this may be the beginning of iatrogenic disability. The defendant has been placed into the role of denying the claim and questioning the veracity and character of the plaintiff. Mutual distrust after the system has finished with them is common. The distrust may create or exacerbate a behavioral concern. Each blames the intractability of the other for the need to expend the psychological energy and economic resources needed to reach a resolution. The threat that one side or the other will find a way to retaliate for an unfavorable outcome casts a pall on the continuing relationship. The claim is resolved, but the parties may not be able to resume their previous lives.

In a counselor's role, the outcome for the plaintiff is much better. Objective assessment of the case keeps expectations realistic in many cases. The stresses of litigation may be avoided altogether, or the litigation may be limited to a few unresolved issues, allowing the behavioral health client to avoid some of the rigors of the process. There is a recognition that an economic settlement will not really make the plaintiff whole, and the focus thus changes to what is needed to give the plaintiff an opportunity to regain as much of one's former life as is possible. The risk of an "all-or-nothing" outcome is reduced, as the approach allows the defendant to reallocate some of the resources originally devoted to defense of the claim to improvement of the situation that gave rise to it. The possibility of reintegration between the plaintiff and defendant is preserved, as the search for a mutually acceptable solution inherently engages both parties and is optimally designed to help them each achieve an improved situation. The parties tend to see each other in less extreme terms when neither wins at the expense of the other, and the possibility of a sense of peace that would allow the rebuilding of their relationship is created.

One difficulty for the adoption of the counselor's role by plaintiff attorneys is the lack of any formal mechanism for compensation of them in that role. Particularly in workers' compensation and tort claims work, the tradition of compensation by contingent fee is strong, and the tradition is reinforced by the relative inability of litigants who have already suffered harm to finance attorney intervention in their cases out of personal resources.

The defense side of the case also has much to gain from the counselor's approach. The defense is usually in reactive mode. When the defense lawyer is engaged in a case, the harm has usually occurred, and the possibility of avoiding it or mitigating it significantly has often been lost. Moreover, the defense is at the mercy of the cause of action chosen by the plaintiff and the theory, evidence, and experts the plaintiff chooses to pursue. The defense must respond to the plaintiff's case or face the possibility that it will be regarded as meritorious simply because it has not been confronted. This task is all the more difficult when the theory of recovery or the evidence of harm is unique or novel, as is more likely in behavioral health claims. A perfect defense to the cause of action that the plaintiff ought to have brought for the harm complained of may fail miserably if the plaintiff's case proceeds on a different theory. This reactive mode does not allow the defense advocate to help the parties avoid foreseeable harm or to mitigate the effects of harm before they are irretrievable. Prevention of a problem through early intervention is almost always more cost-effective than resolution of a problem in reactive mode, when the claim has been left to mature. Resources spent mitigating present, and preventing future, behavioral health claims are almost always more cost-effective than "rolling the dice" in court. However, the mechanisms are lacking for compensating attorneys who serve outside of an "in-house counsel" role for these kinds of services in workers' compensation and insurance defense environments.

15.11 Some Possibilities for an Improved Systemic Approach

The current legal system contains systemic features that tend to exacerbate, and in some instances create, behavioral health issues for the litigants who find themselves cast into the system for the purpose of resolving a dispute. There are two kinds of approaches to these challenges. One approach looks to the attorneys involved to change the way that they practice, while the other suggests peripheral changes to the structure of the legal system to assist needed changes in behavior.

15.11.1 Changes Lawyers Can Make

The role of counselor at law has been discussed above. The advantages to both sides in a behavioral health concern dispute run to increased possibility of recovery and reintegration and decreased risk of iatrogenic disability. The role is not often taught in law schools and is not always encouraged by clients, who have been conditioned to expect a more aggressive model of dispute resolution. Yet the benefits, particularly in behavioral health cases, are undeniable.

Barriers to this role include mechanisms for compensation, client education, inexperience and lack of training, and personal disinclination. Of these, compensation is the easiest to address. An alternative to normal contingent fee pricing structures should be offered to plaintiff seeking this kind of approach. For the plaintiff's side, a diminished fee percentage is already often used for settlements prior to litigation. A third tier of pricing or an hourly rate for exploring reconciliation before filing litigation could be established. Successful resolutions can contain a provision for payment of the fee of the counselor at law, and unsuccessful attempts at resolution will simply move on to the existing system.

The legal system is structurally designed to compensate with cash awards for harm that has been done. Even disregarding the emotional and psychological toll of injury, this system is inadequate to completely compensate the disabled person for the loss of one's productivity. Non-punitive awards virtually never replace the income that a person would have made had she/he kept working, and in workers' compensation cases, statutory limits on compensation are clearly not even designed to "make the victim whole." Clients need to be reeducated to understand that a cash award and permanent disability are almost always economically a worse financial outcome than return to productive life (Biddle, Boden, & Reville, 2001). In the absence of that kind of information, the client cannot truly make an informed choice about his or her litigation options; so the provision of this information has an ethical component as well (American Bar Association, 1993, Rule 1.2).

Lawyers need to become skillful in the basic recognition of existence of behavioral health concerns, the evaluation of the professional qualifications of behavioral health professionals, and the interpretation of the objective testing and other output of such evaluations. They need to become familiar and comfortable with the practice of the counselor's role and the use of the tools particular to that role. The tools of the counselor at law are often the tools of the counseling arts: listening, seeing the larger picture, finding commonly held values and goals, and helping people to find agreed solutions. In particular, true mediation, where a neutral facilitator assists the parties in an effort to voluntarily come to a mutually acceptable resolution, is a valued approach. Most importantly, counselors need to learn to look for solutions that allow both sides to "win" during the resolution process, instead of focusing on zero-sum outcomes.

Some law schools currently offer postgraduate programs in specialty areas of law, such as the law of taxation. A postgraduate specialization in the skills of a counselor at law would assist in the recognition of the role and perhaps lead to the kind of acceptance enjoyed in the British legal system for the separation between barristers and solicitors. Such a specialization would likely be embraced by law schools (whose faculty, after all, opted out of the traditional legal role) and over time would become an accepted part of the legal framework. The relatively recent flourishing of so-called "alternative dispute resolution" techniques is indicative of a readiness of the public to accept a less expensive and less confrontational method of solving our legal problems. Behavioral health concerns, especially where they are imbedded in traditional legal disputes, would particularly benefit from separation and separate processing in this more gentle and constructive paradigm.

Some attorneys will not accept this role. They choose, for whatever reasons, the adversarial nature of courtroom litigation. Such lawyers should look to the British model of barristers (who try cases before the court) and solicitors (who do nearly all other legal work) and associate lawyers who can take referrals of cases that can be settled while accepting referrals of cases where settlement was attempted unsuccessfully.

15.11.2 Disengagement of the Profit Motive from the Litigation Process

As seen earlier, the mechanism for the compensation of attorneys in the tort and workers' compensation system creates an incentive for attorneys to seek the largest possible awards for their clients, without regard to the unintentional adverse consequences to litigant behavioral health created in the process. When the incentive is to reduce the human problem to the largest possible monetary award, "medicalization" of the presenting condition, internalization of catastrophic thinking about the future, the creation of identity as a disabled person, and alteration of perceptions to reinforce that identity are outcomes affecting far too many litigants.

It is, perhaps, unrealistic to think that plaintiff's attorneys, who may earn millions from a single settlement, will willingly change their ways. Attorneys do, however, change their practice patterns in response to the demands of clients. As the public has become more aware of the nature and impact of litigation upon the individual and society as a whole, alternative dispute resolution has become more popular. A key issue in achieving these changes is the education of the public. Scholarly study of the economic impact of attorney involvement has been limited (Bernacki & Tao, 2008; Swedlow, 2003). As the public becomes aware of the real impact of litigation in our society and the practical alternatives such as alternative dispute resolution, their taste for the courtroom may be reduced. A few peripheral changes in the structure of the legal system could help reeducate the public and create an acceptable level of lawyer participation in changes that will help prevent "attorneyogenic" disability.

Defense counsel generally charges fees on an hourly basis. Attorney motivation to "churn" a case with excessive and time-consuming research, motions, discovery, and other activity is often suppressed by scrutiny from sophisticated clients. Nonetheless, systemic incentives are not designed to reward efficiency.

Attorney compensation on the basis of contingent fees for plaintiff's advocates and hourly fees for defense advocates is not the only possible model. We do not assume that doctors are unmotivated to do the best for their patients because they are paid on the basis of the work they complete. Certainly, the diagnosis of ailments of the human body and the restoration of heath is as challenging as legal practice, and the stakes are as high or higher. Some jurisdictions (notably Massachusetts and Western Australia) have adopted fees schedules for attorney work that compensates them by the task completed, rather than by the outcome or the hours consumed in workers' compensation cases. While studies of the impact of that fee structure continue to be conducted by groups such as the Workers' Compensation Research

Institute, indications are that claimant outcomes are not adversely affected and that overall systemic costs are reduced.

It might be argued that a fee schedule based upon work completed is a compensation system that is more available in workers' compensation than in tort, because in workers' compensation proof of fault is not part of the cause of action and therefore the risk of non-recovery is diminished. The contingent fee mechanism is also justified on the grounds that many injured people do not possess the resources to fund litigation except out of the recovery. It should be noted that the "American system" of attorney compensation, which presumes that the litigants will pay their own attorneys, is not universally followed even in the United States. Civil rights and employment cases (including those that enforce the rights of those with behavioral health concerns) and divorce cases are examples of decisions, as a matter of public policy, to allocate the cost of representation to the losing party. Reevaluation of the "American system" of attorney compensation should be undertaken in light of the unintentional harm to the litigants caused by the economic motivation the system imparts to the advocates.

Punitive damages also deserve a closer look. It might be advantageous to society to encourage an individual litigant to act as societal champion in an effort to create an economic deterrent to future wrongdoing. The resulting individual overcompensation of the successful claimant in such cases is hard to justify. When the defendant is a corporate entity with vast economic resources, the "punishment" must be large enough to get the corporation's attention to have the desired impact. But then a single litigant, who has already been compensated for one's actual damages, is the recipient of a massive redistribution of wealth unrelated to their personal harm. The plaintiff's lawyer, of course, gets a percentage of the award, which explains the popularity of the damage category. Arguably, it would be better to fashion the remedy requiring expenditures to undo the damage the defendant has done to others, or to make the punitive award a donation to a worthy cause, rather than to enrich one particular litigant and his or her attorney. Appropriate compensation for the work actually done could be paid to the attorney for seeking the punitive award, removing motivation based upon the expectation of a multimillion dollar fee.

15.11.3 Beyond Professional Enabling

Lawyers should be aware of the role that they play as professional enablers. It may not be possible to entirely avoid this role. Members of the general public do not generally engage lawyers unless there is a specific situation with which they need assistance. The resolution of the presenting situation is the reason the lawyer is involved in the first place. Yet a responsible lawyer must recognize that the client may not have his or her own best interests at heart. Sometimes "getting off" of charges will not lead to a life as a good citizen, or getting the largest settlement possible is not the solution that will lead to a life untainted by the continuing identity as a victim. Additional services, beyond those needed to resolve the presenting crisis, may provide the best hope for regaining a full and healthy life. A responsible attorney should look to the whole client and make referrals to other professionals and services. Just as doctors take the Hippocratic Oath, perhaps, it is time for attorneys to adopt the mind-set with regard to their clients to "first, do no harm."

15.12 Conclusion

The legal system causes unnecessary disability for many classes of claimants. Those suffering from behavioral health concerns are particularly vulnerable to the impact of structural and behavioral components in the system. Structural components include the win-lose nature of the dispute resolution system, the emphasis on reduction of all harms to a monetary award, and the mechanism for attorney compensation. Behavioral components include the effects of imprecision of language used in the process and the unintentional discouragement of recovery and reintegration that goes with making the claimant with a behavioral health issue defend the existence of the concern to obtain any recompense. These problems are deeply entrenched, but there are several examples of more enlightened dispute resolution approaches available as a guide.

What would the world look like under such a system? US litigation rates, estimated as of 2000 at 74.5 cases per 1000 population (Wollschlager, 1998), would likely fall, as more disputes are resolved prior to litigation. More persons with behavioral health concerns would resolve the issues that gave rise to their claims, resulting in fewer lives broken by the process of dispute resolution itself. Some attorneys would make less money, and others will flourish as they learn to help others solve their problems rather than merely resolving their disputes.

Behavioral concerns in the legal system are less often resolved by simple determination of rights and liabilities than by planning for the restoration of function and the healing of broken relationships. Flexibility in the way that we think about the law can open the possibility for roles and approaches that are more helpful in encouraging behavioral health.

References

American Bar Association. (1993). Model rules of professional conduct. Retrieved from http://www.abanet.org/cpr/mrpc/mrpc_toc.html.

American Medical Association. (2008a). *Guides to the impairment of permanent disability* (6th ed.). Chicago: American Medical Association.

American Medical Association. (2008b). *Guides to the evaluation of permanent impairment (Chapter 14)* (6th ed.pp. 347–382). Chicago: American Medical Association.

Annual Statistical Report on the Social Security Disability Insurance Program. (2015). Retrieved from http://www.ssa.gov/policy/docs/statcomps/ssi_asr/2007/index.html

Aronoff, G. M., Mandel, S., Genovese, E., et al. (2007). Evaluating malingering in contested injury or illness. *Pain Practice, 7*(2), 178–204.

Aurbach, R. (2013). Suppose hippocrates had been a lawyer: A conceptual model of harm to litigants, parts 1 and 2. *Psychological Injury and Law, 6*(3), 217–237.

Aurbach, R. (2015, January 7). Your biggest unmeasured cost, insurance thought leadership, *Insurance Thought Leadership.* http://insurancethoughtleadership.com/your-biggest-unmeasured-cost/

Barsky, A. J., & Borus, J. F. (1996). Somatization and medicalization in the era of managed care. *Journal of the American Medical Association, 274*, 1931–1934.

Bartley, M. (1994). Unemployment and ill health: Understanding the relationship. *Journal of Epidemiology and Community Health, 48*(4), 333–337.

Bellamy, R. (1997). Compensation neurosis: Financial reward for illness as nocebo. *Clinical Orthopaedics and Related Research, 336*, 94–106.

Bernacki, E., & Tao, X. (2008). The relationship between attorney involvement, claim duration and workers' compensation costs. *Journal of Occupational and Environmental Medicine, 50*(9), 1013–1018.

Biddle, J., Boden, L., & Reville, R. (2001). *Permanent partial disability from occupational injuries, earnings losses and replacement in three states*. Santa Monica, CA: Rand.

Brigham, C. (2015). *Living abled & health: Your guide to injury and illness recovery*. Honolulu, HI: Healthy Living Publications.

Bruns, D., & Disorbio, J. M. (2009). Assessment of biopsychosocial risk factors for medical treatment: A collaborative approach. *Journal of Clinical Psychology in Medical Settings, 16*, 127–147. https://doi.org/10.1007/s10990-009-91-48-9

Conroy, M. A., & Kwartner, P. P. (2006). Malingering. *Applied Psychology in Criminal Justice, 2*(3), 29–51.

Duffau, H. (2006). Brain plasticity: From pathophysiological mechanisms to therapeutic applications. *Journal of Clinical Neuroscience, 13*(9), 885–897.

Fayad, F., Lefevre-Colau, M. M., Poiraudeau, S., et al. (2004). Chronicity, recurrence, and return to work in low back pain: Common prognostic factors. *Annales de Réadaptation et de Médecine Physique, 47*(4), 179–189.

Francis, A. (2012). DSM 5 is guide not bible—Ignore its ten worst changes, *Psychology Today*. https://www.psychologytoday.com/blog/dsm5-in-distress/201212/dsm-5-is-guide-not-bible-ignore-its-ten-worst-changes

Gerdtham, U. G., & Johannesson, M. (2003). A note on the effect of unemployment on mortality. *Journal of Health Economics, 22*, 505–518.

Goldberg, J. (2013). *Case law update: ADA Amendments Act of 2008*. Washington, DC: U.S. Equal Employment Opportunity Commission. https://eeo.okstate.edu/sites/default/files/15-case%20law%20update.pdf

Guirguis, S. (1999). Unemployment and health: Physicians' role. *International Archives of Occupational and Environmental Health, 72*, S10–S13.

Guthrie, R., & Monterosso, S. (2009). Preventing further harm to the harmed – Towards a therapeutic approach to workers' compensation. *Journal of the International Association of Industrial Accident Boards and Commissions, 46*(1), 115–143.

Harding, T. (2004). Psychiatric disability and clinical decision making: The impact of judgment error and bias. *Clinical Psychology Review, 24*, 707–729.

Harris, I., Multford, J., Solomon, M., van Gelder, J. M., & Young, J. (2005). Association between compensation status and outcome after surgery. *JAMA, 293*(13), 1644–1652.

Horwitz, A. V., & Wakefield, J. C. (2007). *The loss of sadness: How psychiatry transformed normal sorrow into depressive disorder*. New York: Oxford University Press.

Jellema, P., van der Horst, H. E., Vlaeyen, J. W., et al. (2006). Predictors of outcome in patients with (sub)acute low back pain differ across treatment groups. *Spine, 31*(15), 1699–1705.

Jin, R. L., Shah, C. P., & Svoboda, T. J. (1995). The impact of unemployment on health: A review of the evidence. *Canadian Medical Association Journal, 153*(5), 529–540.

Johoda, M. (1983). *Employment and unemployment*. Cambridge: Cambridge University Press.

Kilgour, E., Kosny, A., McKenzie, D., & Collie, A. (2015). Interactions between injured workers and insurers in workers' compensation systems: A systematic review of qualitative research literature. *Journal of Occupational Rehabilitation, 25*(1), 160–181.

Kolb, B., & Whishaw, I. (1998). Brain plasticity and behavior. *Annual Review of Psychology, 49*, 43–64.

Lippel, K. (1999). Therapeutic and anti-therapeutic consequences of workers' compensation. *International Journal of Law and Psychiatry, 22*(5–6), 521–546.

Main, C. J., Sullivan, M. J., & Watson, P. J. (Eds.). (2007). *Pain management: Practical applications of the biopsychosocial perspective in clinical and occupational settings* (2nd ed.). Edinburgh, Scotland: Churchill Livingstone.

Martikainen, P. T., & Valkonen, T. (1998). The effects of differential unemployment rate increases of occupation groups on changes in mortality. *American Journal of Public Health, 88*, 1859–1861.

Mathers, C. D., & Schofield, D. J. (1998). The health consequences of unemployment: The evidence. *The Medical Journal of Australia, 168*, 178–182.

McGill, C. M. (1968). Industrial back problems: A control program. *Journal of Occupational Medicine, 10*, 174–178.

McKee-Ryan, F., Kinicki, A. J., Song, Z., & Wanberg, C. R. (2005). Psychological and physical well-being during unemployment: A meta-analytic study. *Journal of Applied Psychology, 90*(1), 53–76.

Melhorn, J. M., & Ackerman, W. E. (Eds.). (2008). *Guides to the evaluation of disease and injury causation*. Chicago: American Medical Association.

Mittenberg, W., Patton, C., Canyock, E., & Condit, D. (2002). Base rates of malingering and symptom exaggeration. *Journal of Clinical and Experimental Neuropsychology, 24*(8), 1094–1102.

Nachemson, A. (1983). Work for all – For those with LBP as well. *Clinical Orthopaedics and Related Research, 179*, 77–85.

NHS Choices. (2013, August 15) *News analysis: Controversial mental health guide DSM-5*. National Health Service, UK. http://www.nhs.uk/news/2013/08August/Pages/controversy-mental-health-diagnosis-and-treatment-dsm5.aspx

Oakley, D., & Halligan, P. (2009). Hypnotic suggestion and cognitive neuroscience. *Trends in Cognitive Sciences, 13*(6), 264–270.

Organisation for Economic Co-operation and Development – OECD (2009, May 14 – 15). Sickness, disability and work: Keeping on track in the economic downturn. Stockholm, Organisation for Economic Co-operation and Development.

Reid, W. H. (2000). Malingering. *Journal of Psychiatric Practice, 12*(2), 116–118.

Sander, R., & Meyers, J. (1986). The relationship of disability to compensation status in railroad workers. *Spine, 11*, 141–143.

Schultz, I. Z., & Gatchel, R. J. (Eds.). (2005). *Handbook of complex occupational disability claims*. New York: Springer.

Stewart, J. M. (2001). The impact of health status on the duration of unemployment spells and the implications for studies of the impact of unemployment on health status. *Journal of Health Economics, 20*, 781–796.

Strang, J. P. (1985). The chronic disability syndrome. In G. M. Aronoff (Ed.), *Evaluation and treatment of chronic pain* (pp. 247–258). Baltimore: Urban & Schwarzenberg.

Swedlow, A. (2003). *Attorney involvement in California workers' compensation, 1993–2000*. Oakland, CA: CWCI Research Notes.

Talmage, J. B. (2007). Failure to communicate: How terminology and forms confuse the work ability/disability evaluation process. *Journal of Insurance Medicine, 39*, 192–198.

van der Windt, D., Hay, E., Jellema, P., & Main, C. (2008). Psychosocial interventions for low back pain in primary care: Lessons learned from recent trials. *Spine, 33*(1), 81–89.

Victor, R., Barth, P., & Neumark, D. (2005). *The impact of provider choice on workers' compensation costs and outcomes*. Workers' Compensation Research Institute, WC05-14.
Warren, P. A. (2009). Behavioral health as a causation issue in workers' compensation and disability claims. *IAIABC Journal, 46*(2), 17–57.
Wegscheider-Cruse, S. (1989). *Another chance: Hope and health for the alcoholic family* (2nd ed.). Palo Alto, CA: Science and Behavior Books.
Wollschlager, C. (1998). Exploring global landscapes of litigation rates. Cited in Kritzer, H.(2001). Litigation. *International Encyclopedia of the Social and Behavioral Sciences, 13*, 8989–8995.

Chapter 16
A Neuroplastic Model of Secondary Contribution to Behavioral Health Disability: Theory and Implications

Robert M. Aurbach

16.1 Basic Neuroplasticity

Over the last two decades, there has been an explosion of understanding of the manner in which the brain functions. Sophisticated imaging techniques, physical mapping of connections between brain cells using microelectrodes, studies of the chemistry of the brain, and other research have all contributed to our understanding of how the organ functions.

One facet of that research looks at neuroplasticity, which is the ability of the brain to alter the structure of connections between brain cells in response to stimuli. Neuroscientists tell us that the physical structure of the brain changes throughout our lives. This phenomenon is pervasive – "Neuroplastic research has shown us that every sustained activity ever mapped – including physical activities, learning, thinking, and imagining – changes the brain as well as changing the mind" (Doidge, 2007).

Logic tells us that the brain must process together all of the inputs that it receives at any one moment. Thoughts, emotions, and physical sensations from inside the body and from the external world that are presented at the same time are connected through a network of the various neurons involved (Kolb & Whishaw, 1998). If the stimuli are presented together repeatedly, physical changes in the connections between neurons occur that allow processing across those connections to proceed faster and more automatically (Merzenich, Tallal, Peterson, Miller, & Jenkins, 1998). With time and repetition, the neural network becomes "facilitated" so that the stimulation of a part of the network stimulates all of its components (Butler & Moseley, 2003). Memories of events that were formed at closely spaced intervals are also stored in the same brain area in overlapping populations of neurons (Cai et al. 2016; Silva, 2017).

R. M. Aurbach (✉)
Uncommon Approach, Inc., Melbourne, VIC, Australia
e-mail: Rob@uncommonapproach.com

P. A. Warren (ed.), *Handbook of Behavioral Health Disability Management*,
https://doi.org/10.1007/978-3-319-89860-5_16

Many complex behaviors are learned in this way. We learn to speak without having to concentrate on pronunciation. If the network is damaged by stroke or brain injury, it may be possible to relearn the same skills through painstaking repetition that will build a new facilitated neural network (Overman & Carmichael, 2014). Complex physical skills like walking, playing sports or music, and driving are learned in this manner. We say "practice makes perfect" to encourage the repetition necessary to create the necessary changes in the brain to habituate a new skill. The accepted protocol for teaching a person to walk again after brain injury is to recapitulate the experience of an infant. Crawling, "cruising," and walking skills are practiced until the necessary facilitated networks are reformed (Cramer et al., 2011).

Similarly, there is evidence that complex mental behavior and even beliefs are learned through similar mechanisms. Practicing multiplication tables is a common method for developing efficiency in that simple mathematical function. While never attributed to this mechanism, the creation of irrational behavior patterns was described by B.F. Skinner in a context that is entirely consistent with the neuroplastic development of beliefs (Skinner, 1948).

Common experience again provides an instructive example: many people can recall an image, a song, or a smell that invokes emotions associated with another time and place. "Our song" doesn't cause feelings of first love to occur. Rather, the memories of the feelings that were associated with the song in the neural network formed at the time are stored in the same area of the brain, and the memory of feeling in love is triggered upon hearing it (Silva, 2017).

There are several important manifestations of this phenomenon. We say "someone pushed our buttons" when an inadvertent behavioral pattern occasions an emotional reaction that is unexpected under those circumstances. Chronic pain that is triggered when there is no physical cause evident for its manifestation has similarly been attributed to the existence of facilitated neural networks that contain the experience of acute pain (Butler & Moseley, 2003; Doidge, 2015).

But sufficient focus on the stimulus is necessary to create the connection. Many of us have discovered a wound or bruise without the ability to recall the incident that generated the injury. There can be little doubt that the affected body part sent a message to warn us of the injury at the time it occurred. When we are sufficiently focused on other things at the time, the message can sometimes be ignored (Cleary, 2011; Ellner & Aurbach, 2009).

The repetition necessary to create a facilitated neural network is not necessarily literal reoccurrence of all of the stimuli on multiple occasions. The necessary "practice" to facilitate connections occurs when we use internal resources as the source of the repetition. Elite athletes and sports psychologists have long understood that "visualization" improved performance. Mental repetition of a skill is nearly as effective as physical repetition in improving performance (Brouziyne & Molinaro, 2005; Isaac, 1992; Martin & Hall, 1995).

There is good reason to expect that this sort of "practice" is also effective in shaping behavior. Advertising that links images of children, small animals, or pleasurable events with a product is so prevalent precisely because the associations with the positive image carry over to the product and influence purchasing decisions.

An application of this model has led to significant practical improvements in the treatment of conditions previously thought to be untreatable. Individuals have regained function after stroke has killed brain tissue (Duffau, 2006) or regained functional "eyesight" after the optic nerve has been destroyed (Doidge, 2007). "Phantom pain" has been relieved, despite the lack of a limb to treat (Flor et al., 1995; Ramachandran and Ramachandran, 1996).

The research has been summarized in two simple rules. "Neurons that fire together wire together" (Doidge, 2007) describes the formation of facilitated neural networks. At the same time, the brain will recycle neural connections that are out of use. "Use it or lose it" is a common description of this phenomenon, familiar to anyone who has tried to use foreign language skills learned in school but unused for a number of years thereafter.

16.2 How Does This Relate to Behavioral Health?

Behavioral health concerns, including the efforts taken to treat symptoms and maintain function, are part of the experience that is processed together with the other thoughts, memories, emotions, and sensations experienced by the person with the concern. This means that the behavioral health concern and associated systemic responses can become part of a facilitated neural network involving unrelated stimuli that happen to be experienced at the same time.

The inclusion of a behavioral health concern in a facilitated neural network has at least two significant consequences. The behavioral health concern can act as a perceptual filter, creating a "confirmation bias" (Kahneman, 2012) that colors the interpretation of new stimuli, and with it the perceiver's evolving model of the world and one's place in it (Brigham, 2015; Hadler, 2008). Second, the inclusion of the mental health concern in the neural network means that there will be multiple stimuli that can trigger expression of the mental health concern that is not necessarily tied to the mental health concern by anything stronger than temporal association of the stimuli and the concern.

This would present a complex picture of interactions between the mental health concern and the person's functional ability or disability on its own. There are, however, significant additional factors in the environment that may join the evolving neural network, complicating the picture further.

16.3 Additional Factors Impacting Upon the Experience of Behavioral Health Concerns

If all of our thoughts, feelings, memories, emotions, and sensations have impact upon and are impacted by our behavioral health concerns, then it follows that additional "external" factors may impact on our experience. Collectively, we will refer to these external factors as "external messages." What follows is not intended as an exhaustive list nor as a representation of the experience of every person with behavioral health concerns. The important thing to remember is that each of them can becomes a point in the growing facilitated neural network that is capable of being stimulated and therefore stimulating all or most of the other features of the network.

16.3.1 Adverse Childhood Events (ACE)

Adverse childhood events (ACE) have been associated with a wide range of behavioral phenomena: recidivism among juvenile offenders (Wolff, Baglivio, & Piquero, 2015) child abuse (Felitti et al., 1998) development of alcoholism (Anda et al., 2002) and poor outcomes in recovery from illness or injury (Larkin, Felitti, & Anda, 2014). The mechanism facilitating the impact of such events is understandable in neuroplastic terms. The adverse childhood event may create a reaction, usually one of worthlessness, self-deprecation, and/or powerlessness. This reaction is far from universally experienced, and people experiencing adverse childhood events may or may not experience subsequent mental illness or behavioral dysfunction. But when the person experiencing the adverse childhood event internalizes the event as a negative self-judgment, the message may become part of the inner voice of the person, repeating as a background message sufficiently frequently to be incorporated into subsequently formed neural networks. The "message" likewise may act as a perceptual filter that colors incoming messages and creates the illusion of external validation of the belief. We often perceive what we anticipate (Kahneman, 2012), and the filtered message of low self-worth reinforces an experience of the world consistent with the expectation.

16.3.2 Stigma: Efforts to Overcome Stigma and Medicalization

Since Corrigan wrote about the adverse effects of stigmatization 15 years ago (Corrigan & Watson, 2002a, 2002b), it seems evident that organizations in many countries have attempted to counter the impact of stigmatization in mental health and get more people into treatment. Organizations such as the World Health Organization, beyondblue, and the Black Dog Institute in Australia, the Depression and Bipolar Support Alliance and National Mental Health Association in the United States, and Depression UK and the Depression Alliance in the United Kingdom spend considerable efforts on normalizing mental health concerns so that those experiencing them will seek qualified help. Yet the World Health Organization reports that the prevalence of people living with depression has increased 18% between 2005 and 2015 and that "Lack of support for people with mental disorders, coupled with a fear of stigma, prevent many from accessing the treatment they need to live healthy, productive lives" (World Health Organization (WHO), 2017). There is controversy about whether the increase in occurrences reported is a result of the destigmatization, more complete reporting of the existing phenomenon or other causes.

At the same time, efforts to destigmatize may have an unanticipated impact as well. The "normalization" of mental health concerns by well-meaning organizations has proceeded through the use of "sound bite"-sized messages such as "One in five Australian suffer from a mental illness" (Oneinfive, 2017) and the availability of unsupervised self-diagnosis tests (Mindspot, 2017). While well-meaning in intent, such messages allow people temporarily suffering from subclinical symptoms to self-diagnose and self-define as having a mental health concern. Once the person labels themselves as unwell, the label may become part of the inner dialogue that runs in the background of experience and can be joined into the neural networks that form while the label is actively accepted (Brigham, 2015). This is the essence of medicalization of a concern.

In this manner, attempts to destigmatize may have an unintended effect of creating "hypersensitivity" and self-labeling. A study of comorbidities to depression followed over a 15-year period in Australia showed that "psychological hypersensitivity" had become the most frequently diagnosed comorbidity to depression over the last 10 years, even though it was not even recognized at the beginning of the study (Tinker, 2014). It is unknown if similar results appear in other countries, but the study demonstrates a risk of increased comorbidity as a result of attempts to destigmatize, and the phenomenon is worthy of further study.

16.3.3 Interpersonal Reactions

While destigmatization has been considered largely from the perspective of getting a higher percentage of people the care that they need, it is clear that the efforts need to be addressed to nonclinical instances of stigmatization as well. When a mental health condition forms part of a facilitated neural network by temporal proximity, its expression may be triggered by seemingly unrelated events that are part of the network. To the unsophisticated observer, it looks like the expression of the mental health concern is "from left field" or a personal reaction to something the observer did or said. The phrase commonly used in such circumstances is that we have "pushed someone's buttons" or had our "buttons pushed" by someone else. What has happened is that a component of the facilitated neural network containing the response that is observed has been stimulated, triggering a behavioral expression that appears to be unrelated to, or exaggerated with respect to, the stimulus (Corrigan & Watson, 2002a, 2002b).

It is reasonably anticipatable that a percentage of such observers, including strangers, colleagues, employers, and even friends and non-treating professionals, will react to what is perceived as an aversive stimulus with withdrawal or revulsion. The experience of these social reactions (and their consequences with regard to employment) can become a part of a growing facilitated network of negative experience. The unexpected tends to cause reactions of fear or anxiety. Even in an environment where there is substantial public education concerning mental health concerns, observers may take the reaction "personally" or react from fear or discomfort before conscious compassion and understanding can assert itself (Rusch, Angermeyer, & Corrigan, 2009). A sort of "feedback loop" can form and provide "practice" to solidify the formation of neural networks that contain an expectation of future repetition of adverse reactions. The natural tendency to avoid aversive stimuli may tend to create isolation or a sense of exclusion and may be experienced as inhibiting the functions of everyday life (Corrigan & Watson, 2002a, 2002b).

16.3.4 Impact of Accessing Support Systems for Behavioral Health Disability

As noted above, much work has been done to allow access to mental health services without stigma. The inclusion of mental health concerns into the Americans with Disabilities Act Amendments of 2008 (see Chap. 15) also appears to be a helpful development.

At the same time, payment for treatment of mental health concerns is still a potential source of difficulty. Medical health insurance has traditionally contained limitations with respect to the mental health treatments that are covered. Co-payment requirements may be significant and exceed the assets of the person attempting to obtain treatment. But even before the limitations or co-payments are reached, the attitudes and actions of the claims manager with respect to the acceptance of such claims, the level of verification and documentation required, and the difficulty of dealing with an insurance system that is likely opaque to the claimant can present significant frustration, delay, and disincentive for treatment. Distrust is a common descriptor of the attitude of insurance claims managers for claims for payment for conditions that are difficult to see or objectively verify. Even where proof of the medicolegal "cause" of the condition is not a ground for rejecting coverage, the existence of the condition is a "fact" that will often be meant with skepticism by insurance examiners.

Even where the work of accessing treatment for the mental health system goes smoothly, efforts at destigmatization have reportedly resulted in increased waits for services in some markets (Warren, 2017). Delay in receiving treatment, especially when coupled with a perceived need for treatment, can be as frustrating as any barrier created by a claims manager.

16.3.5 Anger, Perceived Injustice, and Other Emotional Reactions

Strong emotional reactions to the combination of factors discussed above are reasonably anticipatable. Similar reactions have been noted with respect to the stressors in injury compensation systems (Sullivan et al., 2009; Sullivan, Yakobov, Scott, & Tait, 2014). Strong emotional reactions such as anger, perceived injustice, grief at what is perceived as lost, frustration, and catastrophic thinking can become part of the growing network of associated thoughts, emotions, memories, and sensations. This creates a situation where the emotional response is likely to be triggered by stimulation of other parts of the network in a manner that may not be anticipated by observers. The unexpected expression of the strong emotions can then invoke a response from observers, occasioning further emotional responses and locking them into the network in a self-reinforcing feedback loop.

The creation of self-reinforcing strong emotional responses to environment can be isolating, disempowering, and intensely frustrating. Depression, mood disorders, anxiety disorders, and similar mental health concerns can result (Corrigan, 2004). These mental health concerns are "secondary" to the original presenting mental health concern.

16.4 Secondary Contributions to Behavioral Health Disability

Medicalization, the unintended consequences of efforts at destigmatization, and the consequences of attempts to access systems of mental health treatment, can be seen as "secondary" behavioral health concerns in the sense that they are complications of the original presenting mental health concern. They are capable of exacerbating the experience of behavioral health concerns, contributing to the development of comorbid behavioral health conditions and making treatment more complex. They are iatrogenic, in the sense that they are occasioned by the interaction between the person experiencing the behavioral health concern and the global/systemic response to their condition. They engender new or additional harms to the person with a mental health condition in that they complicate treatment of the behavioral health concern itself and present additional points of contact with the facilitated neural network resulting in additional triggering of the expression of the behavioral health concern.

As with strong emotional responses, medicalization and unintended consequences of attempts to destigmatize exist in potential feedback loops. Medicalization may result in perceptual filters or confirmation biases that color the interpretation of "normal" experience of subclinical variation in daily experience and reinforce the existing network of associated thoughts, memories, emotions, and sensations. The reinforcement of the pattern and inclusion of the new way of thinking about the significance of symptoms means that the pattern, including the medicalised thinking, will be stimulated more often and by a wider range of phenomena. The person with the mental health concern may start offering their condition as an explanation, justification, or excuse for unrelated aspects of his or her life. The reactions of unsophisticated observers to that pattern of behavior will vary but may include rejection, avoidance, compassion, and attempts to assist. In each case, the reaction of observers will become part of the growing neural network, providing additional opportunities for stimulation of the components of the pattern. These subsequent reactions may be "explained" with reference to the mental health condition (albeit more likely through self-talk) and a feedback loop established.

The same pattern of self-reinforcing feedback can exist with respect to any difficulties experienced with respect to accessing economic support for treatment for the mental health condition. Claims managers in virtually any line of insurance commonly experience a small cohort of claimants that become "difficult" – meaning that they act in a highly demanding manner, engage in combative responses to any questioning of their demands, and view most encounters as a zero-sum game (my winning must be at the cost of you losing). These claimants are very resistant to shifting into a problem-solving approach. The model of neuroplastic experience of behavioral health concerns suggests that, whether correctly or not, some claimants "learn" that the claims manager working on their claim is the source or cause of blockage to access (through payment) to services that they perceive as needed. The interaction and the emotional reaction to frustrated treatment expectations become embedded in the network of associated experiences (facilitated neural network) that includes the behavioral health concern. The interaction itself becomes a trigger for a flare-up of the behavioral health concern, and the claims manager may react, engendering a feedback loop. Even where there is no insurance interaction, similar patterns can develop between persons with a behavioral health concern and virtually any helping professional.

A diagram of the potential interaction of the various factors discussed will demonstrate the significance of the addition of these factors (Fig. 16.1).

One feature of this model has particular significance with regard to functional limitations arising from behavioral health concerns, otherwise known as behavioral health disability. One of the key understandings of a facilitated neural network is its power to stimulate seemingly unrelated behavior that is associated with it in the network. Many of the functional limitations associated with mental health concerns arise from the reactions of others to unanticipated expressions of the mental health concern, secondary mental health concerns, and emotional reactions to the experience of having a mental health concern (Holzinger & Matschinger, 2010). The complexity of the network of associated experiences contributing to the expression of those attributes means that efforts to address the mental health concern may not fully alleviate the limitations on daily living that result from the entire pattern. This has implications for both clinical treatment and systemic responses to behavioral health disability.

16.5 Implications for Societal Response to Behavioral Health Concerns

The network of associated experiences is a societal concern because of the unnecessary additional harm that it creates. Harm is caused by creating additional trigger points for the expression of the mental health condition. This, in turn, creates additional opportunities for self-labeling and self-fulfilling prophecy, additional complexity of treatment, additional opportunities for adverse interactions with

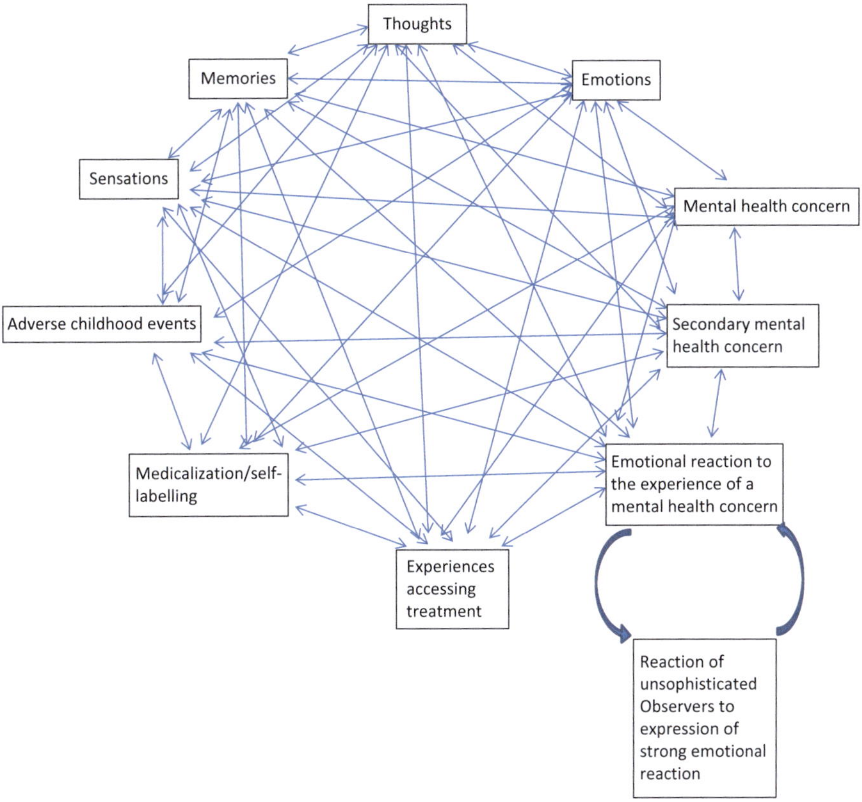

Fig. 16.1 Network of potential interactions contributing to mental health concerns

unsophisticated observers, and additional reinforcement of the tendency to allow beliefs to become a perceptual filter and/or create a confirmation bias. The quality of life experienced in this setting is likely to be compromised.

If adding trigger points is the problem, then there are at least two strategies for avoiding the result: avoidance of the problem creating the trigger or avoidance of the repetition of the trigger in connection with the rest of the associated experiences of the behavioral health concern. If there is insufficient repetition of the trigger, it does not become part of the facilitated neural network.

16.5.1 Implications for Clinical Treatment

Behavioral health disorders are associated with multiple risk factors and often have a significant developmental component. However the outcome of treatment is influenced by experiential factors and can be influenced by stress substance abuse trauma, the actions of others, and self-talk (Cramer et al., 2011). They tend to be chronic and/or episodic. The possibility of relapse is relatively high, with instances of relapse increasing the chance of further episodes (Patten, 2008).

This strongly suggests that, regardless of the source of behavioral health concerns, the treatment of them has to address the environmental concerns in which the person experiencing the behavioral health issue is functioning. Whatever treatment regimen is attempted will have to compete with already established patterns of association supportive of the behavioral health concern. The reactions of others, including social stigma and "change-back" behavior in social units (Wegscheider-Cruse, 1989), isolation, memories of triggering events and subsequent experiences, self-labeling and self-talk, and emotional reactions to the mental health concern and subsequent experiences still exist in a complex web of association together with the behavioral health concern. Triggering any point of contact triggers the entire facilitated network. For this reason, successful treatment may be frustrated unless disruption of the pattern is part of the treatment plan.

There appear to be at least two strategies that are available to accomplish this disruption of such a maladaptive pattern: therapies that are specifically designed to break established patterns of association, such as cognitive behavioral therapy (CBT), have demonstrated significant positive outcomes. It is also possible to strengthen the ability of an individual to quiet, redirect, or distract their self-talk, reducing repetition of a potential trigger to the point that it does not become incorporated in the neural network. Collectively, it is possible to characterize this latter strategy as the building of individual resilience.

Use of strategies that suppress symptoms does not attempt to change the environment in which the stimulation or development of the neural network occurred. Pharmacological approaches, while often effective in suppressing symptoms, do not impact the conditions that are present when the medication is not present. Thus reoccurrence of the symptoms of a wide range of behavioral health concerns is a concern associated with medication termination, and medication compliance is seen as a significant problem (Owiti & Bowers, 2010). Similarly, strategies that focus on the source of the behavioral concern, such as "talk therapy," may have limited impact on the underlying pattern of associations that has developed around the behavioral health concern, except to provide a "reason" for being unwell for uninformed self-labeling and medicalization. If the pattern still exists, stimulation of any of its parts will still stimulate the associated behavioral condition.

16.5.1.1 Pattern-Altering Therapies

Cognitive behavioral therapy (CBT) has been recognized as an effective treatment for a wide range of behavioral disorders (Beck, 2011; Butler, Chapman, Forman, & Beck, 2006; Coupland, 2009). It is based upon the "cognitive model" of psychological disturbances (Beck, 2011) that posits that "automatic thoughts" arise from combinations of beliefs and perceptions and can lead to maladaptive behavior (Beck, 2011). The "automatic" nature of these thoughts suggests that they arise from facilitated neural networks. Those networks associate thoughts from the inner of external environment with beliefs, sensations, thoughts, and emotions presented in temporal proximity until the presentation of one portion of the network stimulates all their network components. The associations do not require conscious recall and largely take place before our conscious control is asserted. Thus, there is a sense in which we can say that cognitive behavioral therapy works by replacing neural networks containing associations between environmental stimuli and specific maladaptive responses with patterns that do not include the unwanted behaviors.

Claims of success in alleviating behavioral health conditions have been made for other therapies such as eye movement desensitization and reprocessing (Shapiro, 2001), neuro-linguistic programming (NLP) (Andreas & Andreas, 1989), and hypnosis (Ellner & Aurbach, 2009). Since there is little controlled research demonstrating the efficacy of these approaches, they will not be addressed in detail. In each case, however, the therapy appears to be based upon techniques for making or breaking associations between specific thoughts or emotions and the triggers within the same facilitated neural network that occasions their expression.

16.5.1.2 Changing Self-Talk

Formation of facilitated neural networks requires repetition of the connection between the components of the network sufficiently often for the connections between neurons to change in characteristics. Oftentimes the repetition does not take place sufficiently frequently to accomplish this result, but a thought or emotion still becomes part of a facilitated neural network. A lawyer may say "You'll never be able to work again" only on one occasion, yet clients quite often end up internalizing the prediction and letting it become part of their identity. The principle mechanism for the necessary repetition of the message appears to be internal dialogue, or "self-talk." The ability to control or quiet self-talk or to modulate the nature of the message to be imbedded in the neural network may explain the difference between people subjected to adversity that succumb to it and those that thrive notwithstanding their circumstances. This is the essence of what we commonly call "individual reliance," and an approach for addressing the enhancement of resilience skills will be discussed below.

16.5.2 Systemic Responses

The model of a neuroplastic component of behavioral health disability demonstrates that addition of elements to a network of associated experiences can complicate the life of the affected person and make treatment more complex and challenging. Reduction of this unnecessary harm requires that avoidable additional elements of the pattern are not required by the circumstances of systemic interaction. It also requires avoidance of unnecessary repetition of unavoidable elements, thereby minimizing the opportunity for new elements to be incorporated into the pattern. Thus, the model provides guidance for development of systems that are less unintentionally harmful to those they attempt to assist.

16.5.2.1 Efforts to Address Stigmatization

It has been suggested that efforts at destigmatization of behavioral health concerns in North America have been increasingly successful, as evidenced by increasing difficulty in obtaining appointments with behavioral health professional in many areas (Warren, 2017). Waiting times for appointments are an important indicator of the comparison between the number of people seeking treatment and the resources available for delivering it, and a sudden change in the balance would appear to indicate that more people are seeking treatment than previously. The development of additional resources for treatment delivery is an important part of systemic response to behavioral health. Frustration and anger at delays and difficulty in accessing treatment is likely to impact both upon the willingness of people to come forward for treatment and the prevalence of secondary emotional responses to the system that is frustrating the desire to get what is viewed as necessary treatment.

But waiting times for treatment are probably not the entire story with regard to the impact of stigmatization on people with behavioral health issues. Destigmatization efforts may have been somewhat effective in increasing the number of people who will come forward for treatment. The reactions of others to a person with a mental health concern may not be similarly affected by attempts to normalize the idea of treatment. Classic cognitive dissonance reactions – I prefer not to "see" the person with a mental health concern because the thought that it could happen to me is too threatening – often mean that people with behavioral health conditions are "invisible," resulting in social isolation (Corrigan, 2004). As noted above, the unpredictability of the triggers to the expression of a mental health concern may cause a fear reaction in others, increasing isolation and the feeling of being adversely judged in the mind of the person with the behavioral health concern. Lifestyle impacts resulting from behavioral health concerns may cause avoidance by others and may become a self-fulfilling prophecy with negative impacts on housing availability and similar necessities (Thorincraft, 2006). These secondary impacts add to the facilitated neural network containing the behavioral health condition and set the stage for an increasingly multifaceted condition.

Public policy with regard to behavioral health could make efforts to address this sort of stigmatization by others. Efforts are being made to "mainstream" children with mental health concerns in classrooms with unaffected children. To the extent that proximity and familiarity reduce reactions to behavior outside the unaffected norm, the reduction of this form of stigmatization would be expected over time.

In the shorter term, efforts at educating the public could benefit from some of the more effective examples of popular media campaigns to normalize other conditions and raise money for research into cures. Cancer and AIDS were regarded with fear and distancing behavior relatively recently. A spate of popular movies depicting relationships between afflicted people and their friends, lovers, and carers have broken down some of the fear and discrimination for those segments of the population. Given the aggressive attempts to normalize mental health conditions and get people to seek treatment, this additional step would seem likely to be timely. High-profile telethons and other events designed to raise money for research combine entertainment and information and may provide a platform for compassionate education as well.

16.5.2.2 Legal Issues

Legal protections for people with behavioral health conditions can be strengthened. Access to housing is a critical step in breaking the feedback loop of rejection and isolation suffered by many. Similarly, access to gainful work is critical to beneficial outcomes (Thorincraft, 2006).

Additional clarification of existing laws or legislation of additional protections against discrimination in housing may be appropriate. The Fair Housing Act and Fair Housing Act Amendments (42 U.S.C. 3601–3619, 3631) leave the ascertainment of the right of rejection of a prospective tenant with a mental disability in the hands of the landlord. The Act asks the landlord to make objective determinations of the nature and severity of the risk of injury, likelihood of injury, and reasonableness of accommodations. Few landlords are qualified to make such objective determinations, and the protection against rejection based upon speculation or fear is largely illusory. First, the Act, as amended merely, creates a federal cause of action and does little to facilitate the assertion of rights by someone with a behavioral health concern. Second, the case law under the Fair housing Act is not particularly helpful, primarily pertaining to cases of failure to accommodate the needs of people with behavioral health disabilities (Kanter, 1994, 1998). Second, in housing markets where there are multiple applicants for a rental, the ability to prove the underlying discriminatory intent of a landlord is hampered by the ability of the landlord to argue that nondiscriminatory factors were the basis for the decision to reject the applicant.

As noted in Chap. 15, the Americans with Disabilities Act has been applied to discrimination by employers against people with mental health conditions in a few reported cases. Most of the reported cases that have recognized mental health concerns as discriminatory relate to depression. Incentives for the extension of ADA protections, such as access to attorney fee subsidies or guarantees or a pool of money to fund expert testimony in cases where legal aid is providing representation might help develop the case law further.

The Equality Act of 2010 in the United Kingdom may provide a useful comparison of approaches for ADA and the Fair Housing Act. If the Equity Act proves successful, it may be useful as a model of further revisions to legal protections for people with behavioral health concerns.

16.5.2.3 Systemic Responses to Issues of Access to Treatment

Treatment for behavioral health concerns may be provided on a private or public basis. In either event, there are forces at work that may create adverse impacts on the person needing treatment.

It has already been suggested that the interactions with claims managers in the role of gatekeepers for payment of claims associated with treatment can be difficult for both the claimant and the claims manager. The difficulty is that property/casualty lines of insurance are seen by that industry as a zero-sum game. Payment of a claim by the insurer means that the claimant gets a benefit at the expense of the insurer's profits. Nonpayment maximizes profits at the expense of denial or delay of the provision of services to the claimant. In such a system, it is not surprising that a culture of distrust of claimants pervades much of the claims management side of that industry.

The impact of distrust is to require proof that one is harmed to be eligible for treatment payments. In harms that are not immediately visible or objectively verifiable, such as behavioral health concerns, the requirements for repetitious recital of the circumstances in which the harm originated, multiple medical and psychiatric examinations (each accompanied by a retelling of the relevant medical history), and requirements for proof that the impacts of the condition are sufficiently bad to require the level of treatment proposed are common. In addition, it is common for insurers to delay payment of claims in hopes that the claimant will become frustrated and simply go away, resulting in a "win" for the insurer. Distrust generally begets distrust, and a percentage of claimants routinely become aggressive, belligerent, demanding, and focused upon the claims manager or the insurer as the source of their problems.

In the realm of behavioral health, these impacts are particularly egregious because of the comorbidities to the original condition that they may create. The balance between protection against false or inflated claims and the appropriate provision of funding for care requires that proof of condition is obtained in a way that minimizes the additional harm. At a minimum, the personnel assigned to such claims should have minimum qualifications ensuring that they understand the nature of the conditions and treatments that they are likely to encounter. Such personnel should also be specifically trained to be aware of and to take steps to minimize the repetition of narratives of the signs and symptoms, circumstances of the initiation of the harm, and other details that may contribute to self-labeling. The setting of realistic expectations both for overall outcomes and for step-by-step progression of the claim should be clearly communicated. Sharp practices intended to create pressure on claimants to get them to abandon their claim should be prohibited and the prohibitions enforced by insurers or regulators.

In the public realm, the problem is often somewhat different. The demand for resources often exceeds the supply, and access to treatment can be delayed or overly complicated by resource allocation forces. While the glib answer to this difficulty is the addition of resources to the problem, it seems unlikely that more resources will be made available until a crisis is perceived. It would be advisable for governments to plan the allocation of additional resources before the crisis becomes full blown, so that the regrettably common pattern of ineffective use of public funds "thrown at the problem" is not replicated. Unfortunately, that sort of planning is not often available in an environment where the existence of the problem is not given official recognition until a crisis perceived.

In this connection, the efforts of the National Health Service in the United Kingdom with regard to the mental health of its citizens are of interest. Improving Access to Psychological Therapies (IAPT) is a program that includes a variety of products, including 14 that are digitally accessed. Approximately 900,000 people access services through the program each year (NHS England, 2017). Of particular note is an online approach to the provision of CBT for mild to moderate depression and phobia and panic, which appears to be more effective as services provided by a human therapist at less cost (National Institute for Health and Clinical Excellence, 2008). These sorts of innovations may be replicable in North America, allowing for increased service provision without the cost or lead time inherent in increasing the available professional resources.

16.5.2.4 Systemic Issues Regarding the Setting of Expectations

Destigmatization efforts seem to share a common, if problematic, feature. In the course of raising public awareness of the prevalence of behavioral health concerns and urging people experiencing signs and symptoms to seek help, it would be helpful if the public awareness efforts could help set positive expectations regarding recovery. The vast majority of behavioral health concerns have a good prognosis if properly treated (Satcher, 1999). Unfortunately, there is little evidence that information about the success of proper treatment is widespread either among patients or even general practitioners.

The result is the likely promulgation of the unintended message that behavioral health concerns are of indefinite or permanent duration, creating a risk that the message that is incorporated into the developing neural network is that the condition is incurable. Obviously, such a message will have emotional components and is capable of creating confirmation bias or self-fulfilling prophesy. The ability of the system to set an expectation of recovery is likely to have positive impacts on individuals and the system as a whole.

One example of a behavioral health concern that has been somewhat successful in setting a positive expectation is the messaging that is provided to problem gamblers. Public advertisements provide examples of gamblers that were able to get help and improve their lives and the lives of the people around them. It is curious that advertisements raising awareness of other common behavioral health concerns, such as Major Depressive Disorder or an anxiety disorder, and PTSD, do not have the component of hope for a cure as a prominent part of the message.

Addressing the expectation of cure is a two pronged matter. Public education needs to expend the message to include a realistic positive prognosis where such is supported by the evidence. The more difficult part will likely be the education of medical professionals that are points of first contact with the person with a behavioral health concern. The casually delivered or well-intentioned unnecessarily poor prognosis from a family doctor can be repeated through self-talk sufficiently to become incorporated in the network of associated thoughts, memories, emotions, and sensations and become part of the reality of the listener. Other helping professions are also capable of inadvertently contributing to harm in this manner. Efforts to educate at the initial professional training will have a long lead time in having significant impact. Peer-to-peer efforts may be possible in the interim.

16.6 Building Individual Resilience

The primary approach of systemic suggestions for minimizing the unintended harm that has been discussed to this point has been minimization of the presentation of negative inputs into the neural network developing around the behavioral health concern. Each new "message" creates additional trigger points for stimulation of the entire network. There is an additional strategy for that potential to be effective.

The behavioral use of the term "resilience" traces back to studies in the 1980s about children from disadvantaged backgrounds (Masten, 2001). When researchers found that some children succeeded despite crushing social and economic disadvantages, the term was borrowed from materials science to describe the phenomenon. Since that time the research into this ability to "bounce back" after setback or adversity has been studied, and attempts have been made to offer advice through the use of correlation to observed resilient populations or through extension of personal anecdotal experience ("It worked for me, so it will look for you too"). Curiously, none of these attempts have sought to delve deeper into the operational mechanism of resilience.

As noted above, facilitated neural networks are created by repetition of thoughts, memories, emotions, and sensations in close temporal proximity. There is a phenomenon observable in common experience that requires an additional mechanism to explain. Sometimes a person will hear a message from the environment only one time (e.g., "Please don't sing – it's hurting my ears"), but the message will nonetheless become imbedded into a network of associated experience such that the content and associated emotions can be triggered by stimulation of other content in the network. The event is not literally repeated in temporal proximity with the other associated events. How does it get sufficient repetition to become part of a facilitated neural network?

Most of us have had the experience of ruminating on an event, repeating it over and over in your mind. Often it happens at night, when attempting to fall asleep and when there are few external distractions. The little girl who heard the message from her mother (who was suffering from a headache at the time) remembered that "she couldn't sing" whenever she wanted to sing along with music, friends, or school events. She "practiced" the inaccurate message that she had a terrible voice internally, through the way she talked to herself until it became her reality and an acquired inability to sing was born.

This sort of internal practice has been shown to be effective where other behaviors were being learned. Elite athletes have long known that mental practice (also known as visualization) helps improve performance (Warner & McNeill, 1988). In same way, repetition by internal practice is effective for facilitating connections between thoughts, memories, emotions, and sensations that make up the experience of living with a behavioral health concern. "Practice makes perfect" is applicable to thoughts and emotions just as much as it applies to physical skills.

If associations between thoughts, emotions, memories, and sensations are created by temporally proximate repetition and if an important source of such repetition is that which occurs through internal self-talk, then the ability to control one's self-talk is the ability to create or prevent the creation of networks of associated experiences. The intentional exercise of control over our self-talk requires discipline and energy and awareness of the challenge that we are trying to confront. The original observations concerning disadvantaged children suggest that such conscious control may not always be present. But if the habit of controlling "negative" self-talk is itself habitual, it will act to calm the negative messages whenever they are presented. To put it another way, if we can take control of our mental repetitio with adaptive habits of thought, we can prevent the repetition necessary to associate negative mental or physical events with other thoughts, memories, emotions, and sensations. If it doesn't become part of the network, then it does not take on special significance, and we are likely to be able to "bounce back" from the event. In short, the habituated ability to control self-talk allows us to take a measure of control over the extent that an internal or external event impacts us. This leads to a new operational definition of individual resilience: *Individual resilience is the habituated ability to quiet, change, or modulate negative self-talk about experience.*

All of the popular techniques for "teaching resilience" address this understanding in one way or another. Positive psychology techniques attempt to habituate a form of conscious optimism. They build skills in reframing challenges into opportunities and focusing attention on things that are going well in one's life. Mindfulness mediation works by quieting the mind and focusing on gratitude. These techniques are based in sound theory, but experience with them is mixed. Both suffer from rejection by some participants in training, and the effects of training tend to become less effective over time (Abbott, Klein, Hamilton, & Rosenthal, 2009; Bullen & Gardner, 2008; Horan 2016). A systemic review of resilience training literature found tentative evidence for the efficacy of resilience training in a workplace environment but cautioned that individualized training and content "would appear wise" (Robertson, Cooper, Sarkar, & Curran, 2015).

The problems with current "resilience training" stem from a failure of understanding of the operative mechanism. There is no single technique for quieting self-talk that fits across the broad range of personality types found in persons living in Western cultures. A quick look at our common experience demonstrates that different people with different thought processes and different habits of mind can all "bounce back" from adversity, even if they look very different from one another. The entrepreneur who has just lost a fortune but who isn't concerned because he or she can "always make more money" looks quite different from the Zen master, who regards all events on earth as a mere distraction from enlightenment. The single mom, working two jobs, studying at night, and making time to bake cupcakes for the school fair, looks quite different from the person who is comforted simply by finding a reasonable explanation for what has occurred. Each of them is demonstrating a high degree of resilience, yet they seem to have quite different skill sets in play quieting their respective inner voices. The second problem is that resilience skills must be learned as any other habituated skill – in association with other experiences that trigger its use. All our habituated skills associate a set of temporally related experiences, so that each of those experiences has the ability to "trigger" the utilization of the skill. When the pattern is not habituated in that way, the necessary effort to use the skill is much higher. Try to carry on a conversation with the native speaker of a language, using only phrase book knowledge of that language. The level of necessary effort and the overall effectiveness of the attempt are quite different than that experienced when speaking a language in which both participants are fluent. The key to learning to calm self-talk is to learn the skill under circumstances where its invocation becomes habituated to the situation in which the skill is needed.

16.6.1 A Heuristic Tool for Classifying Resilience Skills

To make sense of differing approaches to self-regulation of internal dialogue requires that some organizing principle be applied to observations of the world. Within Western cultures people seem to use resilience skills that can be placed into four categories, based upon the overall strategy. Within those categories, skill orientation can be either inwardly focused or outwardly focused, generating eight heuristically useful groupings. Other groupings are undoubtedly possible.

16.6.1.1 "Believer" Skills

Strong belief can calm or drown out negative messages from the world, allowing the possessor of that belief to continue on as if the negative message was not present (Aurbach, 2016). Entrepreneurs and politicians are classic examples of people that appear to have great faith in their own abilities. They often can shrug off external criticisms and continue in the face of adverse events. People with this preference may assess a wide range of life challenges as being well within their personal capabilities, with varying degrees of accuracy. These internally focused believer skills can quiet self-doubt or discount negative experience, allowing decisive action.

Believer skills can also be externally focused. Strong spiritual faith or strong belief in a cause or ideal can allow people to persevere in the face of nearly overwhelming opposition. The focus on an external belief does at least two things – it creates a confirmation bias, where we interpret events as confirming what we already thought would happen. If a person has a belief that a Higher Power will personally look after him, then external events will be interpreted as confirming that belief. He has no need to look for another explanation, so there is no inner doubt or conflict. Where the belief is in an external source of intervention or protection, it can provide strong reassurance in the face of doubt and anxiety. Betrayal of such a belief can be particularly devastating, as when a child suffers abuse or neglect negating the faith that parental figures will keep him or her safe from harm (Larkin et al., 2014; Uncommon Approach, 2016).

16.6.1.2 "Reframer" Skills

Evolutionary forces have placed value on learning from past experiences. Sometimes a negative message from the world can be placed into nonthreatening perspective by the act of understanding what has happened (Aurbach, 2016). For people relying on reframer skills, the ability to find an explanation or a lesson to be learned puts them comfortably back in control of the situation. Explanation allows the message to be viewed without being seen as personally intended or directed. The externally focused reframer may replay an unpleasant event for the purpose of finding a meaning. But once having found a "silver lining" to the cloud or a lesson from the event, the inner voice is quieted, and the memory can be safely filed away without a disruption of the reframer's sense of self or place in the world. The credo of an externally focused reframer is "Learn the lesson and leave the baggage." Cognitive behavioral therapy approaches to resilience training utilize this approach.

The internal manifestation of reframing is optimism. Stability is achieved by focusing on the best of people, gratitude for the things that are going well in one's life, or other affirming messages. When something unpleasant happens, the internal reframer holds onto the underlying principle and creates an explanation that explains the event as an aberration. The unusual can be discounted as not impacting the optimist's view of the world. If an optimist is disappointed by someone's behavior, he or she can quiet the concern by deciding that "people are still good even if that person is having a bad day." With the explanation in place, the belief system remains, and the optimist's sense of control over his or her life can remain intact without fundamental dislocation. The positive psychology approaches to teaching resilience incorporate these and similar techniques (Raftery, Murphy, O'Shea, Newell, & McGuire, 2013).

16.6.1.3 "Achiever" Skills

The achiever uses constant activity to remove the opportunity for negative messages to be considered (Aurbach, 2016). While engaged in activity, planning, or preparation, the achiever can push out concerns about success, consequences, and appropriateness. The externally focused achiever may "soldier on" filling their time with work, study, parental duties, activities, or a combination of them. The single mom, who works two jobs, takes care of her children, and studies in the evening, simply leaves no room or energy for rumination about anything but the tasks at hand. Achievers who are internally focused tend to set aside their concerns when engaged in activities that have been determined by primarily internal motivations. People "driven" to achieve their own goals, such as amateur athletes, musicians, sportsmen, and craftsmen, can ignore their concerns and regain a measure of their sense of control while engaged in their activity. In recognition of the power of this approach, people who have retired from working life are told to "get a hobby" to deal with their sense of lost purpose.

16.6.1.4 "Distancer" Skills

The distancer is able to avoid the negative messages of the inner voice by selectively focusing on something else (Aurbach, 2016). The quieting of the inner voice, relative to the object of focus, creates a "breathing space" allowing the restoration of a sense of control. By creating this "time-out," the distancer is able to get perspective and act going forward in a more considered manner.

A distancer focused on inner resources presents an outwardly calm image, although he or she may be expending significant effort in maintaining the state. Images of the Zen master or the yoga practitioner in the *savasana* pose come to mind. The practice of mindfulness meditation is a manifestation of internal distancer practice that is commonly promoted as benefiting resilience (Tang, Hölzel, & Posner, 2015). Internal visualization practices used by athletes and others also fit into this category, and they are shown to have to positively impact performance, suggesting that visualization is a form of neuroplastic repetition (Brouziyne & Molinaro, 2005; Isaac, 1992; Martin & Hall, 1995; Warner & McNeill, 1988). In this way, the practice of internal distancer techniques also serves to train new pathways and engrain new behaviors.

The external distancer uses outward focus to achieve the same sort of result. Computerized video games are designed to provide a focus for attention and are valued when they are "addictive" precisely because they allow the creation of space between the person and the messages that self-talk is attempting to deliver. Other forms of external distancing include many hobbies and activities such as golf, gardening, and fishing.

16.6.2 Assessing Different Styles

All of the different strategies outlined above are effective in allowing people to take more control over their self-talk and therefore more control over what messages get incorporated into the associated ideas, thoughts, emotions, and memories. But, different people demonstrate that their personality organization is more accepting of some strategies than others. Mindfulness meditation (Meiklejohn et al., 2012) and positive psychology (Suniya, Luthar, Lyman, & Crossman, 2014) approaches have been two commonly taught methods of achieving greater resilience. They both work, but only if they are "practiced" enough to become habituated as a response to a specific challenge or to challenges generally. If a person feels uncomfortable with the approach that they are taught, the probability is low that they will habituate the skill through sufficient practice.

The most common results of such training are outright rejection of the approach by some percentage of the population or poor retention of the results of the training by a substantial portion of the rest of the cohort (Horan, 2016). What has happened is that some of the participants simply will not engage in the recommended activity and some of the remainder may participate during the training period, but are not sufficiently comfortable with the skill to "practice" it for a sufficient time to make it habitual.

A more logical approach is to individualize the skills training offered and design the individual offering to be something comfortable enough to practice and internalize. This raises two questions: How do we help the individual to select an appropriate skill to develop, and how do we offer individualized training in a manner that facilitates habituation?

16.6.3 Resilience Style Preferences

A resilience skill preference profiling tool was constructed (Uncommon Approach, 2016), which takes a current snapshot of an individual's preferences among the various resilience skills. Forced choice among juxtaposed archetypical statements exemplifying different resilience styles was used to yield a picture of current skill preferences and the tendency toward inward or outward focus. A 22 question profiling tool was developed, and facial validity was established through feedback of 91 of 219 participants who also volunteered to rate accuracy of their profile. The instrument was rated as having acceptable or better accuracy of results by 96.7% of respondents. The preference profile can be administered in less than 5 min.

Analysis of the results of people taking the profiling tool appears to verify the hypothesis that different people have substantially different skill preferences. Figure 16.2 suggests that there is a wide variation among individual preferences, despite the nonrandomness of the sample. Participants volunteered for participation and were not otherwise screened.

Interestingly, mindfulness meditation, which has been the focus of significant training emphasis, falls within a skill set that is the first or equal first preference of approximately 3% of the test population.

The profile of existing skills preferences is just the starting place. For most of us, life will have taught us one or more skills fairly well. For people with behavioral health disability, existing skills appear to be inadequate or inappropriate for the presenting challenge. Development of a skill that is habituated for use when a current challenge presents itself allows greater ability to "bounce back" and retain function. Development of these backup resilience skills creates the "defense in depth" that we value when observing highly resilient people.

Interactions with multiple audiences in workshop settings and feedback solicited through the web-based testing site have yielded a long list of skills that people have self-identified as significant parts of their "resilience toolbox" (Uncommon Approach, 2016). Such a list can be broken down by skill category and inward or

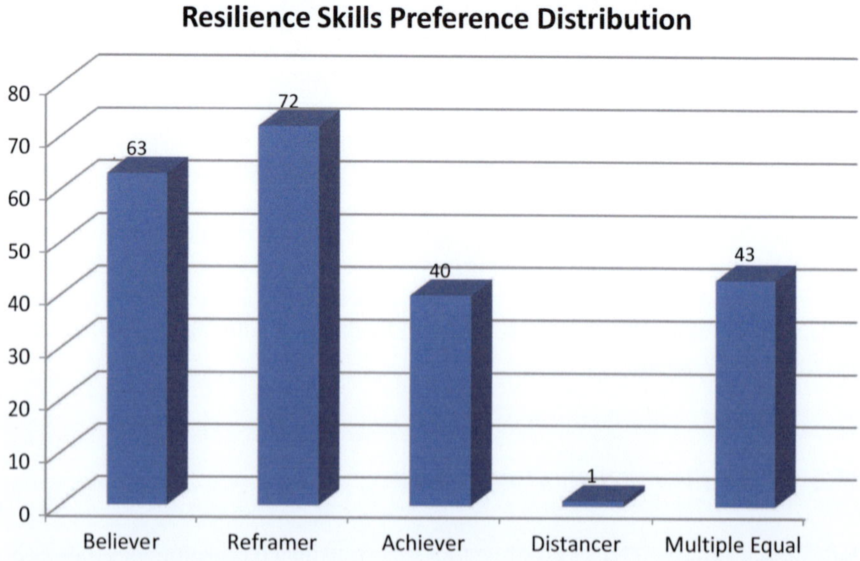

Fig. 16.2 Sample collected from 3 July 2016 through 29 January 2017, $n = 219$; five instances of "distancer" as an equal first choice

outward focus; it is possible for most individuals to find a skill that they do not currently rely upon but that fits sufficiently in their preference profile to be an acceptable subject for the kind of focus necessary to habituate the skill.

16.6.4 A Case Study

An individual moves to a "maritime" environment after living in a desert environment that featured an average of 325 days of sun a year. The long periods of cloudy, cool, breezy, and wet weather resulted in symptoms of seasonal affective disorder, with mood alterations, during the extended winter months. During one such period of low mood, the person serendipitously noticed a particularly beautiful landscape despite the day being dreary and wet. The person stopped and took a few minutes to appreciate it. With the beautiful image in mind, it was possible to stop focusing on the disagreeable aspects of the weather. Mood elevation and relief from the depressive symptoms occurred immediately after the experience and lasted the entire day. The individual decided to consciously pair the practice of looking for natural beauty in the environment to instances where he felt an adverse reaction to the weather. The pairing of the new skill with the stimulus was habituated by the end of the winter, and the individual learned that "stopping to smell the roses" was more than just a saying. The habit was sufficiently solidified by the end of the season that it was unconsciously applied from the beginning of the next winter season, resulting in lasting relief from the seasonal affective disorder symptoms. Moreover, the distancer skill that was habituated generalized to other situations where the person felt their other coping resources overwhelmed (Aurbach, 2016).

16.6.5 Habituation of the New Skill

The advent of "chatbot" technology has provided an opportunity to deliver training on the new skill to be acquired in an efficient manner. A smartphone application can be developed that provides programed interaction to encourage paired practice of the challenge and the new resilience skill that has been chosen. This technology has been demonstrated effective with regard to medication compliance for chronic conditions and exercise (Bickmore et al., 2013; Clevertar Digital Coaches Website, 2017), and it may provide an effective tool to allow people to build individual resilience and avoid some behavioral health disability.

16.7 Conclusion

The medical world has long recognized that iatrogenic harm sometimes occurs to patients in the care of the system. Physicians and medical administrators have taken steps to raise awareness of that harm and to eliminate its causes to the extent possible. This chapter argues from an extension of well-established neuroplasticity theory that the observed phenomenon of people with behavioral health disabilities experiencing increased symptoms or new harm is another instance of iatrogenic harm. It suggests clinical interventions, protocols for professionals working in the system, and policy formulation direction that can address this source of preventable harm.

References

Abbott, J., Klein, B., Hamilton, C., & Rosenthal, A. (2009). The impact of online resilience training for sales managers on wellbeing and work performance. *Electronic Journal of Applied Psychology: General Articles, 5*(1), 89–95.

Anda, R., Whitfield, C., Felitti, V., Chapman, D., Edwards, V., Dube, S., et al. (2002). Adverse childhood experiences, alcoholic parents, and later risk of alcoholism and depression. *Psychiatric Services, 53*(8), 1001–1009.

Andreas, C., & Andreas, S. (1989). *Heart of the mind*. Boulder, CO: Real People Press.

Aurbach, R. (2016). Recalibrating resilience. www.uncommonapproach.com/publications/RecalibratingResilience. (Also published through workcompcentral.com, https://www.workcompcentral.com/columns/show/id/b9b0011ccf70b88a11405ef0e7376ca4095ba4f8), both accessed on 29 Sept 2017

Beck, J. (2011). *Cognitive behavioral therapy: Basics and beyond* (2nd ed.). New York: The Guilford Press.

Bickmore, T., Silliman, R. A., Paasche-Orlow, M. K., Nelson, K., Cheng, D. M., Winter, M., et al. (2013). A randomized controlled trial of an automated exercise coach for older adults. *Journal of the American Geriatrics Society, 61*(10), 1676–1683.

Brigham, C. (2015). *Living abled and healthy: Your guide to injury& illness recovery*. Kailua, HI: Healthy Living Publishing LLC.

Brouziyne, M., & Molinaro, C. (2005). Mental imagery combined with physical practice of approach shots for golf beginners. *Perceptual and Motor Skills, 101*(1), 203–211.

Bullen, L., & Gardner, D. (2008). Resilience training in a restructuring organization. *Journal of Occupational Health and Safety, 24*(4), 309–319.

Butler, A., Chapman, J., Forman, E., & Beck, A. (2006). The empirical status of cognitive-behavioral therapy: A review of meta-analyses. *Clinical Psychology Review, 26*(1), 17–31.

Butler, D., & Moseley, L. (2003). *Explain pain*. Adelaide, SA: Noigroup Publications.

Cai, D., Aharoni, D., Shuman, T., Shobe, J., Biane, J., Song, W., et al. (2016). A shared neural ensemble links distinct contextual memories encoded close in time. *Nature, 353*, 115–118.

Cleary, D. (2011). *Targeting pain: A practitioner's guide to relief.* North Palm Beach, FL: Clearway Communications.

Clevertar Digital Coaches Website. (2017). http://www.clevertar.com/. Accessed 14 Sept 2017.

Corrigan, P. (2004). How stigma interferes with mental health care. *American Psychologist, 59*(7), 614–625.

Corrigan, P., & Watson, A. (2002a). Understanding the impact of stigma on people with mental illness. *World Psychiatry, 1*(1), 16–20.

Corrigan, P., & Watson, A. (2002b). The paradox of self-stigma and mental illness. *Clinical Psychology: Science and Practice, 9*(1), 35–53.

Coupland, M. (2009). CBT for pain management. *Journal of the International Association of Industrial Accident Boards and Commissions, 46*(2), 77–93.

Cramer, S., Sur, M., Dobkin, B. H., O'Brien, C., Sanger, T. D., Trojanowski, J. Q., et al. (2011). Harnessing neuroplasticity for clinical applications. *Brain, 134*, 1591–1609.

Doidge, N. (2007). *The brain that changes itself.* New York: Penguin Books.

Doidge, N. (2015). *The brain's remarkable way of healing: Remarkable discoveries and recoveries from the frontiers of neuroplasticity*. New York: Penguin Group New York.

Duffau, H. (2006). Brain plasticity: From pathophysiological mechanisms to therapeutic applications. *Journal of Clinical Neuroscience, 13*(9), 885–897.

Ellner, M., & Aurbach, R. (2009). Hypnosis in a disability setting. *Journal of the International Association of Industrial Accident Boards and Commissions, 46*(2), 57–77.

Felitti, V., Anda, R., Nordenberg, D., Williamson, D., Spitz, A., Edwards, V., et al. (1998). Relationship of childhood abuse and household dysfunction to many of the leading causes of death in adults: The adverse childhood experiences (ACE) study. *American Journal of Preventative Medicine, 14*(4), 245–258.

Flor, H., Elbert, T., Knecht, S., Weinbruch, C., Pantev, C., Birvaumers, N., et al. (1995). Phantom limb pain as a perceptual correlate of cortical reorganization following arm amputation. *Nature, 375*(6531), 482–484.

Hadler, N. (2008). *Worried sick*. Chapel Hill, NC: University of North Carolina Press.

Holzinger, A., & Matschinger, H. (2010). Emotional reactions to people with mental illness. *Epidemiologia e Psichiatria Sociale, 19*(1), 26–32.

Horan, C. (2016). Resilience training in the workplace: The role of trainee motivation, transfer climate and practice in prevention of psychological injuries, *Australian National University, open access thesis*. https://openresearch-repository.anu.edu.au/handle/1885/117264. Accessed on 14 Sept 2017.

Isaac, A. (1992). Mental practice- does it work in the field? *The Sport Psychologist, 6*, 192–198.

Kahneman, D. (2012). *Thinking fast and slow*. London, UK: Penguin Books.

Kanter, A. (1994). A home of one's own: The Fair Housing Amendments Act of 1988 and housing discrimination against people with mental disabilities. *American University Law Review, 43*, 925–994.

Kanter, A. (1998). Homeless but not helpless: Legal issues in the care of homeless people with mental illness. *Journal of Social Issues, 45*(3), 91–104.

Kolb, B., & Whishaw, I. (1998). Brain plasticity and behaviour. *Annual Review of Psychology, 49*, 43–64.
Larkin, H., Felitti, V., & Anda, R. (2014). Social work and adverse childhood experiences research: Implications for practice and health policy. *Social Work in Public Health, 29*(1), 1–16.
Martin, K. A., & Hall, C. R. (1995). Using mental imagery to enhance intrinsic motivation. *Journal of Sport and Exercise Psychology, 17*(1), 54–69.
Masten, A. S. (2001). Ordinary magic: Resilience processes in development. *American Psychologist, 56*, 227–238.
Meiklejohn, J., Phillips, C., Freedman, M. L., Griffin, M. L., Biegel, G., Roach, A., et al. (2012). Integrating mindfulness training into K-12 education: Fostering the resilience of teachers and students. *Mindfulness, 3*(4), 291–307.
Merzenich, M. M., Tallal, P., Peterson, B., Miller, S., & Jenkins, W. M. (1998). Some neurological principles relevant to the origins of – And the cortical plasticity-based remediation of – Developmental language impairments. In J. Grafman & Y. Christen (Eds.), *Neuronal plasticity: Building a bridge from the laboratory to the clinic* (pp. 169–187). Berlin: Springer-Verlag.
Mindspot. (2017). https://mindspot.org.au/our-services. Accessed 15 Sept 2017.
National Institute for Health and Clinical Excellence. (2008). *Technology appraisal 97 computerised cognitive behaviour therapy for depression and anxiety (review)*. London, UK: U.K. National Health Service.
NHS England. (2017). https://www.england.nhs.uk/mental-health/adults/iapt/. Accessed 15 Sept 2017.
One In Five. (2017). https://oneinfive.com.au/. Accessed 15 Sept 2017.
Overman, J., & Carmichael, S. (2014). Plasticity in the injured brain: More than molecules matter. *The Neuroscientist, 20*(1), 15–28.
Owiti, J., & Bowers, L. (2010). *A literature review: Refusal of psychotropic medication in acute inpatient psychiatric care*. London, UK: Institute of Psychiatry at the Maudsley, Section of Mental Health Nursing.
Patten, S. (2008). Sensitization: The sine qua non of depressive disorders? *Medical Hypotheses, 71*, 872–875.
Raftery, M., Murphy, A., O'Shea, E., Newell, J., & McGuire, B. (2013). Effectiveness of a cognitive behavioral therapy-based rehabilitation programme (Progressive Goal Attainment Program) for patients who are work-disabled due to back pain: Study protocol for a multicentre randomised controlled trial. *Trials, 14*, 290. https://doi.org/10.1186/1745-6215-14-290
Ramachandran, V. S., & Ramanchandran, D. (1996). Synaesthesia in phantom limbs induced with mirrors. *Proceedings of the Royal Society B: Biological Sciences, 263*(1369), 377–386.
Robertson, I., Cooper, C., Sarkar, M., & Curran, T. (2015). Resilience training in the workplace from 2003 to 2014: A systematic review. *Journal of Occupational and Organizational Psychology, 88*(3), 533–562. https://doi.org/10.1111/joop.12120
Rusch, N., Angermeyer, M., & Corrigan, P. (2009). Mental illness stigma: Concepts, consequences, and initiatives to reduce stigma. *European Psychiatry, 20*(8), 529–539.
Satcher, D. (1999). Mental health: A report of the surgeon general–executive summary. *Professional Psychology: Research and Practice, 31*(1), 5–13.
Shapiro, F. (2001). *Eye movement desensitization and reprocessing* (2nd ed.). New York: The Guilford Press.
Silva, A. (2017). Memory's intricate web. *Scientific American, 317*, 30–37.
Skinner, B. F. (1948). "Superstition" in the Pigeon. *Journal of Experimental Psychology, 38*, 168–272.
Sullivan, M., Davidson, N., Garfinkel, B., Siriapaipant, N., & Scott, W. (2009). Perceived injustice is associated with heightened pain behavior and disability in individuals with whiplash injuries. *Psychological Injury and Law, 2*(3–4), 238–247.
Sullivan, M. J. L., Yakobov, E., Scott, W., & Tait, R. (2014). Perceived injustice and adverse recovery outcomes. *Psychological Injury and Law, 7*, 325–334.
Suniya, S., Luthar, E., Lyman, L., & Crossman, E. (2014). Resilience and positive psychology. In M. Lewis & K. D. Rudolph (Eds.), *Handbook of developmental psychopathology* (pp. 125–140). New York: Springer.

Tang, Y., Hölzel, B., & Posner, M. (2015). The neuroscience of mindfulness meditation. *Nature Reviews Neuroscience, 19*, 213–225.
Thorincraft, G. (2006). *Shunned: Discrimination against people with mental illness*. Oxford: Oxford University Press.
Tinker, K. (2014). *Psychological injury and the role of emotional resilience*. Presentation to the Territory Insurance Organization Conference.
Uncommon Approach. (2016). www.uncommonapproach.com/resilience. Accessed on 29 Sept 2017.
Warner, L., & McNeill, E. (1988). Mental imagery and its potential for physical therapy. *Physical Therapy, 68*(4), 516–521.
Warren, P. (2017). Private email correspondence with the editor in preparation of this chapter.
Wegscheider-Cruse, S. (1989). *Another chance: Hope and health for the alcoholic family* (2nd ed.). Palo Alto, CA: Science and Behavior Books.
Wolff, K., Baglivio, M., & Piquero, R. (2015). The relationship between adverse childhood experiences and recidivism in a sample of juvenile offenders in community-based treatment. *International Journal of Offender Therapy and Comparative Criminology, 61*(11), 1210–1242.
World Health Organization. (2017). http://www.paho.org/hq/index.php?option=com_content&view=article&id=13294&Itemid=42050. Accessed 15 Sept 2017

Index

P. A. Warren (ed.), *Handbook of Behavioral Health Disability Management*,
https://doi.org/10.1007/978-3-319-89860-5

D

E

Q

R

MIX
Papier aus verantwortungsvollen Quellen
Paper from responsible sources
FSC® C105338

If you have any concerns about our products,
you can contact us on
ProductSafety@springernature.com

In case Publisher is established outside the EU,
the EU authorized representative is:
Springer Nature Customer Service Center GmbH
Europaplatz 3, 69115 Heidelberg, Germany

Printed by Libri Plureos GmbH
in Hamburg, Germany